Edited by

RAFAEL ANDRADE, M.D., F.A.A.D., F.A.C.P.

Professor and Chairman, Department of Dermatology, LaSalle Medical School,
La Salle University of Mexico; Consultant in Dermatology, and Chief, Section
of Dermatopathology, Departments of Dermatology and Pathology, General
Hospital of Mexico City. Formerly Associate Professor of Dermatology,
New York University School of Medicine, and Director, Laboratory of Skin Pathology,
Skin and Cancer Unit, New York University Medical Center.

STEPHEN L. GUMPORT, M.D., F.A.C.S.

Professor of Clinical Surgery, New York University School of Medicine; Co-Director
of the Tumor Service, Department of Surgery, New York University Medical Center;
Visiting Surgeon, Bellevue Hospital; Consultant, Manhattan Veterans Administration
Hospital; Attending Surgeon, University Hospital, New York.

GEORGE L. POPKIN, M.D.

Professor of Clinical Dermatology, New York University School of Medicine;
Attending in Dermatology, University Hospital, New York.

THOMAS D. REES, M.D., F.A.C.S.

Clinical Associate Professor of Surgery (Plastic Surgery), Institute of
Reconstructive Plastic Surgery, New York University School of Medicine;
Attending Surgeon, University Hospital and Doctors Hospital; Visiting
Surgeon, Bellevue Hospital; Consultant, U.S. Naval Hospital, St. Albans;
Surgeon Director, Manhattan Eye, Ear and Throat Hospital, New York.

Volume Two

CANCER
of the
SKIN

Biology-Diagnosis-Management

1976

W. B. SAUNDERS COMPANY

Philadelphia • London • Toronto

W. B. Saunders Company: West Washington Square
Philadelphia, PA   19105

1 St. Anne's Road
Eastbourne, East Sussex BN21 3UN, England

833 Oxford Street
Toronto, Ontario M8Z 5T9, Canada

Library of Congress Cataloging in Publication Data

Main entry under title:

Cancer of the skin.

Includes index.

CONTENTS: v. 1. Biology-diagnosis-management.

1. Skin—Cancer.   I. Andrade, Rafael. [DNLM: 1. Skin
   neoplasms. WR500 C215]

RC280.S5C36   616.9′94′77   73–91274

ISBN 0–7216–1245–8 (v. 1)

Cancer of the Skin

ISBN Vol 1: 0-7216-1245-8
ISBN Vol 2: 0-7216-1246-6

Print No.:   9   8   7   6   5   4   3   2   1

Contents

v

PART III   TOPOGRAPHIC CONSIDERATIONS

35

Basal Cell Epithelioma

George L. Popkin, M.D., and Charles P. DeFeo, Jr., M.D.

DEFINITION

Basal cell epithelioma (basal cell carcinoma, rodent ulcer, basalioma) is a malignant tumor arising from the epidermis (Lever, 1967) or its appendages (Sanderson, 1968). Usually found in hair-bearing skin (Lever, 1967), the tumor is characterized by slow growth and failure of the cells to mature, keratinize, and desquamate (Van Scott, 1971). It manifests a stromal dependency (Van Scott and Reinertson, 1961; Pinkus, 1965) and very rarely metastasizes. Its potential for localized destructiveness and its tendency to recur after therapy are well known.

ETIOLOGY

Among the predisposing causes, chronic actinic exposure seems to be of great importance — particularly in those individuals with fair skin and blue eyes who sunburn easily (Gellin, et al. 1965). Individuals with more darkly pigmented skin are subject to fewer basal cell epitheliomas (Urbach, et al. 1965; Sanderson, 1968). While there seems to be general agreement about the overall effect of sunlight, some investigators have noted discrepancies in this

regard. Urbach et al. (1965), using a special chemical dosimeter system and mannequin heads exposed to sunlight under varying conditions, determined the amount of radiation received by different portions of the head and neck. Comparing these areas with the prevalence and distribution of squamous and basal cell carcinomas in a series of selected hospital and clinic patients, he noted some discrepancies in the location of basal cell epitheliomas.

Squamous cell carcinoma occurred in skin areas most heavily exposed to ultraviolet light. However, about one-third of all the basal cell lesions were found on skin areas receiving less than 20 percent of the maximum possible dose of ultraviolet radiation. Geographic studies cited by Urbach further supported these mannequin chemical dosimeter observations. Brodkin et al. (1969) stated that areas showing dermal elastosis as a criterion for sunlight skin damage do not always correlate with sites of basal cell epitheliomas.

Ingestion of inorganic arsenic in Fowler's solution, insecticide residues, on food, or in drinking water may give rise to skin tumors, including the superficial type of basal cell epithelioma, after a long latent period.

Norins (1962) showed that ultraviolet ir-radiation can cause ionization and produc-tion of free radicals. He also noted that melanin is a free radical trap and that sulfhydryl conversion into disulfides takes up free radicals, thereby lessening the pool of free radicals, which in turn lessens the likelihood of skin damage.

Repeated solar insult produces injury first in subpapillary and later in papillary layers of the dermis, resulting in wide-spread collagen degeneration (Mackie and McGovern, 1958). They felt that damage to these layers caused impaired metabo-lism with a subsequent effect on overlying epidermis.

From the results of skin transplantation experiments, Orr (1961) showed that dermis damaged by chemical carcinogens is important as a determinant in skin grafts exchanged between normal and diseased skin. Dermis of chemically damaged skin covered with normal undamaged epi-dermis resulted in formation of skin tumors. Chemically damaged epidermis transplanted to "nondamaged" dermis did not result in formation of tumors if trans-plantation took place after chemical insult but prior to actual development of skin tumors.

Olson (1971) demonstrated dispersion of pigment throughout the epidermis in well-tanned Caucasian skin. Negro skin showed similar dispersion of melanosomes throughout the epidermis.

The skin of fair individuals who burn easily, freckle, but do not tan showed ir-regular dispersion of pigment with large melanosome complexes (Olson, 1971). Pa-tients with xeroderma pigmentosum showed deficient transfer of melanin from melanocyte dendrites to keratinocytes, re-sulting in poor protection from sunlight (Olson, 1971).

Utilizing fibroblasts cultured from actin-ically damaged skin of patients with xero-derma pigmentosum, Cleaver (1969) and Cleaver and Trosko (1970) demonstrated a failure in these fibroblasts to repair sun-light-damaged DNA strands. His work showed that the fibroblasts lack an endo-nuclease essential for this repair process. This important work may help to elucidate some of the mechanisms involved in car-cinogenesis.

CLINICAL PICTURE

Types of Basal Cell Epithelioma

A common story heard from male pa-tients is that several months prior to their clinic or office visit they nicked themselves with a razor while shaving. Since the origi-nal injury, the area has slowly enlarged and formed a persistent crust. This crusted basal cell epithelioma may reveal a telangiectatic, translucent portion or border when the crust has been removed. Such an erythematous lesion 4 to 7 mm. in size is quite common in private dermato-logic practice. The slowly growing, translu-cent papule with or without pigment, dis-playing a few telangiectatic vessels on its surface, is also a common type of basal cell epithelioma (Fig. 35–2). Both are found on the exposed surfaces of the face, neck (Freeman, and Knox 1967; Baferstedt, 1970), and ears. Rarely basal cell epithe-lioma lesions will be found on the legs and very rarely on the palms and soles.

The superficial type of basal cell epithe-lioma (Fig. 35–3) is usually found on the thorax. In its very early stage it is an ery-thematous, macular lesion with some

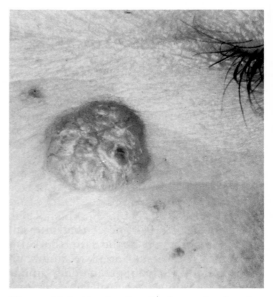

Figure 35–2 Basal cell epithelioma showing fine telangiectasia on surface.

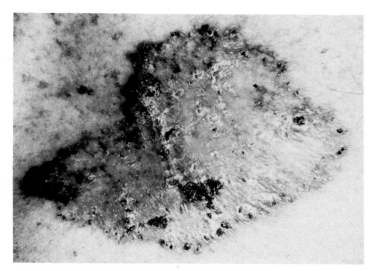

Figure 35–3 Superficial type of basal cell epithelioma.

scaling and may not show the threadlike, rolled edge of the more fully developed lesion. Moreover, it does not show as much scaling and tendency toward central clearing as the older and more well-developed carcinomas. The early lesion can be suspected only if the patient has had one or more superficial basal cell epitheliomas. Superficial basal cell epithelioma lesions tend to be multiple.

Older lesions have an eczematous or psoriasiform picture and frequently a violaceous hue that may be characteristic.

Another clinical type of basal cell epithelioma shows a centrally depressed area with an elevated translucent border. This type is usually seen on the face.

An unusual type of basal cell lesion is the slowly enlarging pore. The patient will note unequivocally that there has been a chicken pox–like pit on the face. Unlike an ordinary pit, it slowly increases in size. Sometimes the border will show telangiectasia.

The lesions of basal cell nevus syndrome (see Chapter 37) often may be mistaken for small, slightly pigmented, intradermal nevi. However, the multiplicity of lesions in association with the distinctive palmar pits, dentigerous cysts, broadened nasal root, increased interpupillary distance, and other stigmata place the patient into the basal cell nevus syndrome.

Odd locations for basal cell epithelioma lesions have been in vaccination scars (Weary, 1967) and in nevus pigmentosus (Sigal and Saunders, 1967, who also cite Pinkus, Meltzer, and Stegmaier with similar experience).

Lesions may arise in nevus syringocystadenomatosus papilliferus (Zugerman, 1961) and in trichoepithelioma (Lever, 1967). Hyman and Michaelides (1963), Lewis et al. (1965), and Goldberg (1968) reported basal cell epithelioma on the sole. An eccrine gland origin has been postulated for the lesions arising on the sole.

Another clinical variant one sees is the

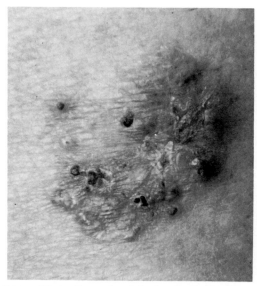

Figure 35–4 Crusted nodular basal cell epithelioma.

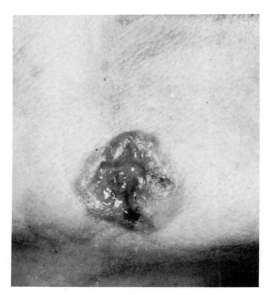

Figure 35–5 Ulceronodular basal cell epithelioma.

so-called "field fire" type of basal cell epithelioma. This shows central scaling and scarring peripheral spread with crusting at the margins (Fig. 35–4). This type is probably a clinical variant of the ulceronodular type (Fig. 35–5) and may become quite destructive.

Another uncommon clinical variant is the morphea type of basal cell epithelioma (Fig. 35–6). Often it presents as a firm, superficially telangiectatic, yellowish white or ivory plaque on the face. At times, the outlines are quite distinct, and at other times the lesion may blend with normal surrounding skin. Histologically, this lesion shows an intimate admixture of fibrous stroma and islets of basal cell epithelioma (Fig. 35–7). Botvinnick (1967) found in one series of 3000 basal cell epitheliomas an incidence of 0.6 percent for the morphea type of lesion.

Another distinct clinical type of basal cell epithelioma is the fibroepithelioma of Pinkus (1965) (Fig. 35–8). It resembles a pink, nonpigmented, seborrheic keratosis. This lesion is most frequently found on the skin of the lower portion of the back and also the abdomen. It may be found in multiples and is either sessile or slightly pedunculated.

Clinical Course

Most basal cell epitheliomas grow very slowly as far as patient and physician can observe. Van Scott (1964) noted that, despite numbers of basal cell epithelioma cells in active mitosis, the growth rate of the lesion is slow. Weinstein and Frost (1970) found a total germinative cycle of 217 hours for basal cell epithelioma. They suggested that a possible explanation for the clinically observed very slow rate of growth, despite the doubling time of nine days, may be that cell death occurs at nearly the same rate as cell division. Jackson (1965) mentioned a growth rate of

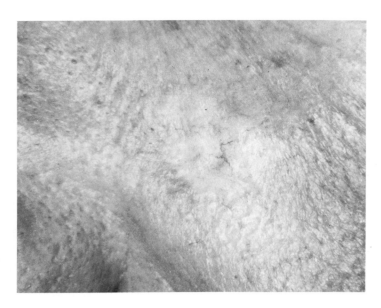

Figure 35–6 Morphea type of basal cell epithelioma. There is a lack of sharply defined margins at some portions of the border.

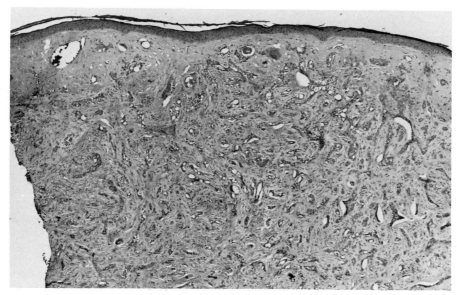

Figure 35–7   Histopathology of the morphea type of basal cell epithelioma, showing intimate admixture of islets and strands of basal cell epithelioma in a dense stroma.

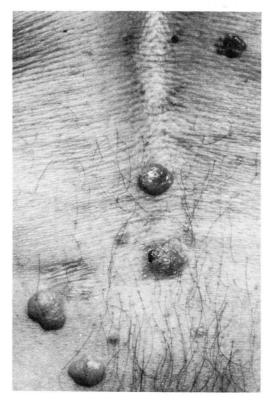

Figure 35–8   Fibroepithelioma of Pinkus. [Photograph used by permission of New York University School of Medicine (Skin and Cancer Unit).]

about 0.5 cm. per year. Certain basal cell epitheliomas pursue a true rodent ulcer course, i.e., slow destruction of the skin and the underlying structures.

Basal cell epitheliomas may invade along the nerve sheaths (Mohs, 1956). They may also invade along the walls of the orbit, eventually resulting in loss of the eye. Rarely, long-standing lesions may invade the tables of the skull and extend into the brain, resulting in death.

Basal cell epithelioma metastasizes very infrequently. Wernmuth and Fajardo (1970) were able to find 76 cases in the literature. Obviously these cases represent a minute fraction of the total number of cases of basal cell epitheliomas. Regional nodes and lungs were the commonest site of metastasis, but other organs were also involved. Metastasis appeared to be most common in white men between the third and sixth decades. Solitary metastasis was most common. Primary lesions were unusually large and ulcerated and had failed to respond to several modalities of therapy.

DIFFERENTIAL DIAGNOSIS

Common skin lesions that resemble basal cell epithelioma include papules of sebaceous hyperplasia (Fig. 35–9). The diagnosis of sebaceous hyperplasia is not difficult when multiple lesions are present. The typical lesion shows a central depression and has a rim which is yellowish, white, or skin-colored. These lesions are covered frequently with fine telangiectatic vessels. When only one lesion is present, there may be difficulty in clinical differentiation from basal cell epithelioma. A shave-type biopsy in questionable cases will quickly settle the problem. Lesions of sebaceous hyperplasia measure from a few mm. to 7 to 8 mm. in size.

Pigmented and nonpigmented intradermal nevi may give some difficulty in differential diagnosis. Usually nevi on the face are more firm on palpation and have been present for many years with little change in size or shape. Nevi previously damaged by shaving can be particularly difficult to differentiate from a small basal cell epithelioma. Often hairs will be seen growing in the nevus. Baden (1970) noted that palpation of basal cell epithelioma of the face yielded a sensation of central depression, as distinguished from other common benign facial tumors. However, one of the author's (CDF) clinical experiences did not support these findings.

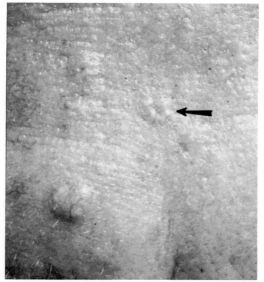

Figure 35–9 Sebaceous hyperplasia—some lesions showing typical central "pore." Lesion lower left might be mistaken for a basal cell epithelioma.

Solitary translucent molluscum contagiosum lesions on the face may resemble basal cell epithelioma. Often a light spraying with Freon, Freon–ethyl chloride combinations, or ethyl chloride alone will cause light surface frosting, accentuating the characteristic central plug or depression usually present in molluscum contagiosum. However, biopsy confirmation may be necessary in the final analysis to distinguish between these two lesions.

Basal cell epitheliomas with pigment may be confused with melanotic malignant melanoma. Usually the latter lesion shows a play of dark brown shades with less translucency than basal cell epithelioma. Sanderson (1968) noted that the margin of basal cell carcinoma usually displays telangiectasia, is rolled and multinodular, and has no pigmented halo. Bart (1971) found that patients with blue eyes are unlikely to have basal cell epithelioma with pigment. Therefore, a suspicious pigmented tumor in a blue-eyed patient should arouse the clinician's interest and suggest the possibility of melanoma.

Superficial basal cell epithelioma ordinarily offers no problem in diagnosis of the well-developed lesion. Pink to reddish purple, this lesion usually shows scaling with some tendency to central clearing and a border displaying a threadlike rolled margin under hand lens magnification. If such lesions occur in a psoriatic patient (usually with a history of inorganic arsenic ingestion 15 to 20 years earlier), diagnosis from a psoriatic patch may at times pose some difficulty and necessitate biopsy. Usually long-standing lesions of superficial basal cell epithelioma display slow peripheral growth and a tendency toward less central activity, and ordinarily are not as thickened as chronic psoriatic patches.

The more unusual pit variety of basal cell epithelioma superficially resembles a chicken pox scar. However, unlike a chicken pox scar, the patient notes that the pit is slowly and steadily increasing in size.

Morphea types of basal cell epithelioma usually occur on the face and have a white to yellowish color with overlying telangiectasia. The typical play of color seen in a single lesion of morphea is absent.

Jackson (1964) reports on ulcers of the

face resembling rodent ulcer. These non-epitheliomatous factitial lesions may arise following section of the fifth cranial nerve for trigeminal neuralgia. Patients pick, rub, or scratch the affected area to relieve paresthesia of the involved skin.

With a high index of suspicion on the part of clinicians, Lightstone et al. in one series (1965) reported errors in diagnosis. Twenty-five percent of the cases suspected of being basal cell carcinoma turned out to have other diagnoses.

Biopsy verification of the diagnosis of basal cell epithelioma is suggested for most cases prior to proceeding with treatment. With unequivocal histopathologic confirmation that the biopsied lesion is a basal cell epithelioma, the physician will proceed with more assurance in eradicating the lesion. Exceptions to this are when hundreds of small lesions occur, as in the case of basal cell nevus syndrome, or when many lesions typical of superficial basal cell epithelioma are found on the thorax. In such cases representative biopsies may be sufficient before proceeding to treatment.

Biopsy may be of several types. Not favored by pathologists but providing sufficient material for diagnosis is the use of curetted skin fragments. When curettage and electrodesiccation are contemplated for therapy within several weeks after biopsy, the scalpel "shave-type" biopsy parallel to the skin surface is preferred. This provides an adequate specimen for diagnosis but does not yield information concerning depth of involvement. When the actual curettage is performed, no punch or scalpel incisional biopsy defect is present for the curet to drop into. Such a "hole" may confuse the operator, leaving some doubt whether the defect is subcutis extension of the lesion or merely the defect caused by previous biopsy.

The scalpel incisional biopsy yields material sufficient for diagnosis and also gives some information about the depth of involvement. Punch biopsy will yield similar information. When this is performed by stretching the skin between index finger and thumb perpendicular to the natural wrinkle lines, an oval lesion is produced. This defect may be closed more readily with a few skin sutures than can the ordinary round hole resulting from a circular punch biopsy (Whyte, 1970).

In certain areas, such as the tip and ala of the nose, when the basal cell lesion is not elevated above the surface of the skin a scalpel incisional biopsy is preferred. The proposed fusiform biopsy site (3.5 to 4.5 mm. by 1 to 1.5 mm.) is marked with gentian violet and the area anesthetized. A miniature scalpel blade (such as the Beaver-type blade) is used to excise the specimen parallel to the wrinkle lines (Fig. 35–39). There is brisk bleeding, and the physician will be able to stop this quite simply with two or three nylon or dacron sutures (6–0 gauge). These sutures may be removed in three days to minimize suture marking, and sterilized tapes such as Steri-Strips, 1/8 inch in size, may be applied after an adhesive coating, such as Pre-Tac (Minnesota Mining Company) or compound tincture of benzoin, has been applied with a cotton applicator to each side of the wound. It is wise to remove surface skin oil with a cleanser prior to applying the adhesive coating. These strips may be left on for four more days. This thin type of incisional biopsy is practical though somewhat more time consuming. It is recommended for the tip and ala of the nose when a cosmetic type of biopsy is desired and methods of treatment other than sharp curettage and electrodesiccation are contemplated.

TREATMENT

In selecting the method most suited for the individual lesion in the patient under consideration, several factors should be given close attention. These include location of the lesion, histopathologic picture (i. e., extent of infiltration and presence or absence of fibrous stoma, as in morphea-type basal cell epithelioma), complexion of the patient, amount of actinic damage or solar elastosis present, age of patient, occupation of patient, general health and medical status, and finally, the personality of the patient. The last is not the least important. When a choice of therapy modality exists, as it frequently does in basal cell epithelioma, the psychologic considerations of the scar and its location must be considered. However, the primary concern is with eradication of the lesion. Cosmetic result, while important, is of secondary concern.

Ideally, the specialty of the physician should not enter into the choice of treatment in the particular case. In practice, this factor will be of some importance, depending upon whether the patient has access to a dermatologist, radiologist, or surgeon and upon whether the patient is close to a medical center where a multispecialty group is available.

Complicated, recurrent, or difficult therapeutic problems are best managed by consultation with a combined specialty skin tumor conference. Ideally, this consists of a dermatopathologist, dermatologist, radiotherapist, plastic surgeon, tumor surgeon, Mohs' chemosurgeon, and other specialists when the need arises.

Cure rates are high for the uncomplicated, small, basal cell epithelioma under 1 cm. in size. When treated by sharp curettage and electrodesiccation, excisional surgery, or x-ray therapy, the cure rate approaches 95 per cent (Popkin, 1968).

Unless specifically contraindicated, x-ray

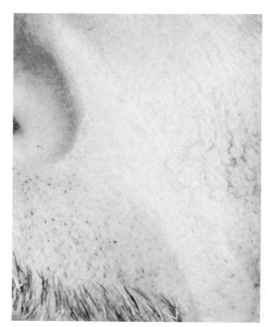

Figure 35–11   Seven years after excision of basal cell epithelioma.

therapy is preferred for treatment of uncomplicated and not deeply infiltrating basal cell epitheliomas of the canthus, eyelid margins (when the tumor is over a few mm. in size), lip vermilion–skin junction, and tip and ala of the nose. In these areas therapy by x-ray results in the smallest

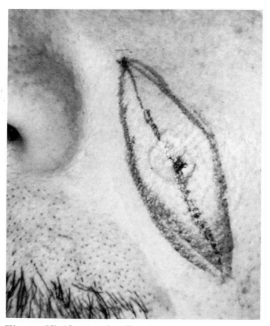

Figure 35–10   Basal cell epithelioma prior to excision.

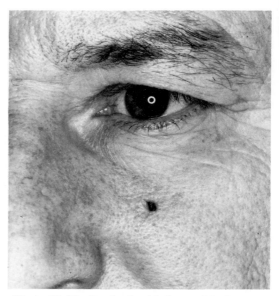

Figure 35–12   Basal cell epithelioma of the fibrosing type.

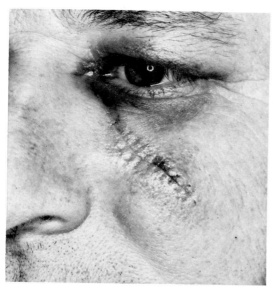

Figure 35–13   The same patient as in Figure 35–12, four days after excision of the basal cell epithelioma.

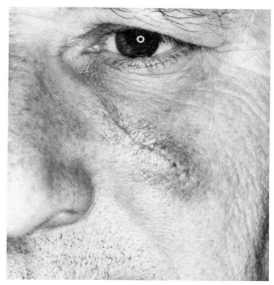

Figure 35–14   One week after excision.

possible anatomic or functional deficit. A drawback to x-ray therapy is the fact that over the years x-ray scars become telangiectatic and show atrophy. In general, surgically induced scars tend to improve in cosmetic appearance over the years.

In those small lesions in which the surgical excision may easily be placed so that the final scar will fall into normal wrinkle lines, a good cosmetic and functional end result can be achieved (Figs. 35–10 to 35–16). The method of surgical excision has much to recommend it. A total excisional biopsy specimen may be submitted for histopathologic verification of clear normal skin

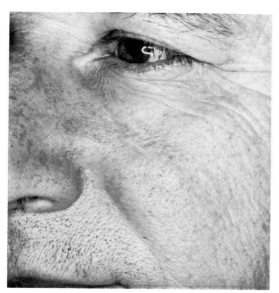

Figure 35–15   Eleven months after excision.

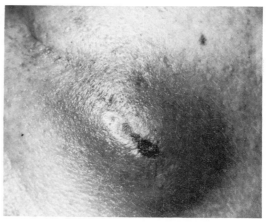

Figure 35–16   Hematoma of the face following excision of basal cell epithelioma.

margins in depth and around the lesion. Healing time is usually one week on the face, and as mentioned previously the resultant scar tends to improve with age. Disadvantages of this method are that it requires further training in surgical technique. It also requires a sterilized excision pack of instruments, sutures, and so forth. The actual operating time may be considerably longer than that of other acceptable dermatologic methods of therapy. Obviously, multiple lesions on the face and elsewhere may not readily lend themselves to excisional surgery techniques.

When complicated lesions are surgically excised and the use of skin flaps is contemplated for repair of the defect, it is wise to delay the definitive flap reconstruction, when possible, for 6 to 12 months. Temporary resurfacing with a split- or full-thickness graft is desirable so that, if tumor recurrences take place, they will not be masked by a thick flap.

The dermatologic method of sharp curettage and electrodesiccation (see Chapter 67) is a relatively simple, quick, bloodless, and nonfrightening approach to the treatment of small lesions of basal cell epithelioma. This technique depends upon the fact that the diseased epithelial tissue and its underlying fibroblastic mucopolysaccharide-rich stroma are soft in consistency.

By means of a skin curet, the diseased tissue and stroma may be scraped away readily under local infiltration anesthesia. For an additional safety margin, the electrodesiccating current or electrocautery is used to destroy a margin of normal tissue around and under the lesion (Figs. 35–17 to 35–29). These two processes of sharp

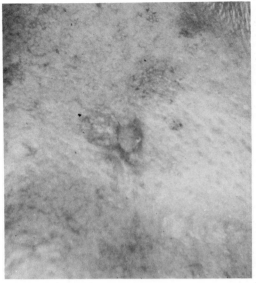

Figure 35–18 Basal cell epithelioma at junction of side of nose and face below eyelid prior to treatment by curettage and electrodesiccation.

curettage and electrodesiccation are repeated one or more times. The number of times curettage and electrodesiccation are repeated beyond two times and the amount of apparently normal tissue to be destroyed will vary with the extent and size of the lesion. The main advantage of this type of therapy is that the operator uses the curet to separate diseased from healthy tissue.

This method of treatment is well adapted to office or clinic management of the patient and his tumor. The wound that results from this method of treatment is slower to heal than an excisional surgical wound, taking two to three weeks or longer, depending upon the extent of the

Text continued on page 836

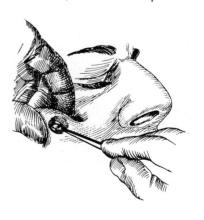

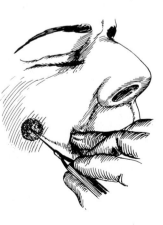

Figure 35–17 Curettage and electrodesiccation for treatment of basal cell epithelioma. (*From* Converse: Reconstructive Plastic Surgery. Ed. 2, Philadelphia, W. B. Saunders Company, 1977.

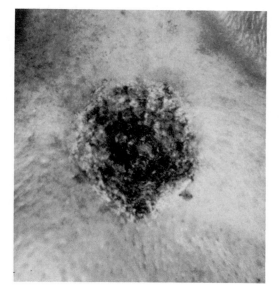

Figure 35-19 Immediately after completion of curettage and electrodesiccation, the procedures in this case having been repeated a total of three consecutive times.

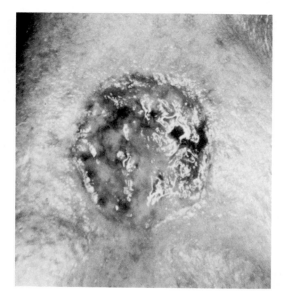

Figure 35-20 Appearance of treated site one week after curettage and electrodesiccation of basal cell epithelioma.

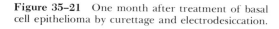

Figure 35-21 One month after treatment of basal cell epithelioma by curettage and electrodesiccation.

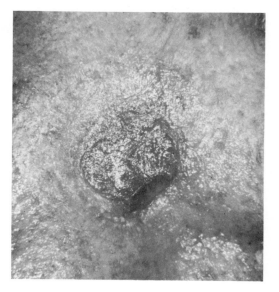

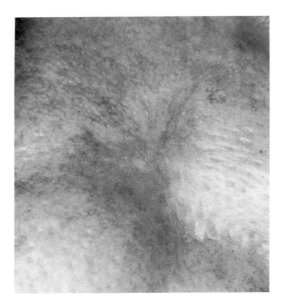

Figure 35–22 Healed end result one year after treatment of basal cell epithelioma by curettage and electrodesiccation.

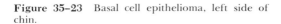

Figure 35–23 Basal cell epithelioma, left side of chin.

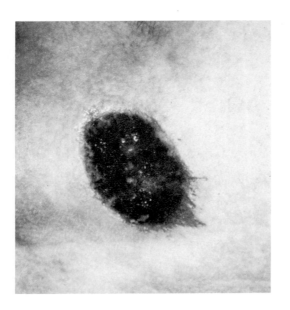

Figure 35–24 Immediately after treatment of basal cell epithelioma by curettage and electrodesiccation, showing full-thickness central defect and extent of treatment beyond borders of lesion.

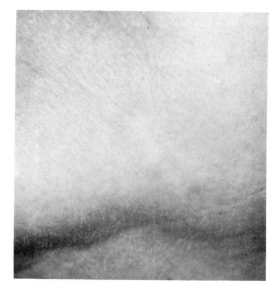

Figure 35-25   End result one year after treatment of basal cell epithelioma by curettage and electro-desiccation.

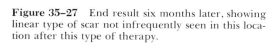

Figure 35-26   Immediately following treatment of basal cell epithelioma by curettage and electro-desiccation.

Figure 35-27   End result six months later, showing linear type of scar not infrequently seen in this location after this type of therapy.

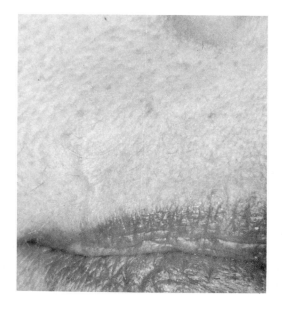

lesion. Simple aftercare with ordinary dressings, which the patient changes, is the rule following curettage and electrodesiccation.

Objections to this technique are the absence of a histopathologic specimen for verification of skin margins and a scar which, while often excellent, may at times show a sharp contrast with adjacent actinically damaged and discolored skin.

While superficial basal cell epithelioma is also readily treated by this technique, other methods yield a result which is superior in appearance to the hypertrophic or thickened scar which not infrequently results from the treatment of large lesions on the thorax.

Liquid nitrogen appears to offer an excellent alternative approach. Freezing the lesion gives good cosmetic results with occasional hypopigmentation but less overt scarring. The use of liquid nitrogen therapy for this type of basal cell epithelioma, as well as for ordinary types of basal cell epithelioma, is relatively new in comparison with other more well-established modalities. However, work by Torres (1971) (see Chapter 72), Zacarian (1969), and Wooldridge (1971) shows considerable promise.

Mohs' (1956) chemosurgery, a highly accurate, at times painful, painstaking

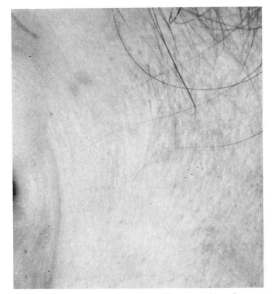

Figure 35–29 Scar five years later at site of treatment by curettage and electrodesiccation for basal cell epithelioma.

method of microscopically controlled excision of fixed tissue is recommended for difficult, recurrent, invasive, and destructive lesions (see Chapters 70 and 71).

Radiation therapy (see Chapters 68 and 69) of lesions in special locations as well as in certain age groups is well accepted. Large lesions of the face, neck, and ears, particu-

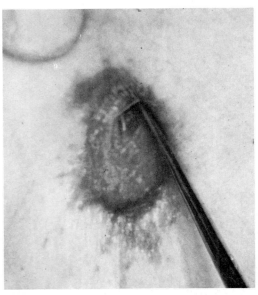

Figure 35–28 Use of curet to probe for and eradicate pockets of basal cell epithelioma tissue.

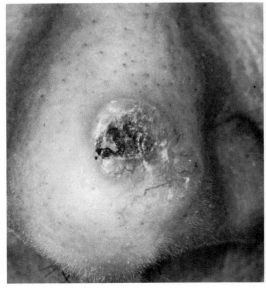

Figure 35–30 Basal cell epithelioma prior to x-ray therapy.

larly in older individuals, may be handled with little disability to the patient. Also, lesions involving the tip of the nose (Figs. 35–30 to 35–32), the ala, the vermilion margins of the lips, and the eyelid margins and canthi of the eyelids are suitable in selected cases for radiation therapy. While x-ray scars tend to worsen in appearance with the passage of time, this is of relatively less importance to patients in the older age group.

One of the techniques of x-ray therapy used at New York Skin and Cancer Unit, New York University, is described. The basal cell epithelioma lesion is shielded with lead of appropriate thickness to within 5 to 10 mm. of its clinically visible and palpable border. The 5-mm. shielding is used for simple uncomplicated lesions with clearly visible borders. Larger borders are used in lesions that may be recurrent from other methods of therapy or in those lesions in which the borders are difficult to define (such as the morphea type of basal cell epithelioma). Additional shielding is used to protect the eyes, thyroid, and gonadal areas. Appropriate cones are used to further reduce the amount of radiation scatter. When eyelid and canthal lesions are treated, special brass eyeshields or

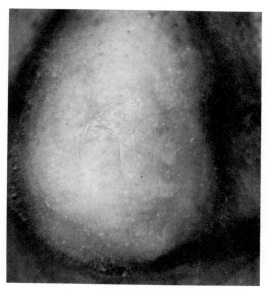

Figure 35–32 One month following x-ray treatment.

lead "tongue-type" eyeshields are inserted into the conjuctival sac and overshielded with lead shields of appropriate sizes.

Using a half value layer (HVL) of 0.8 to 1.0 mm. of aluminum, 65 to 100 kvp., 5 ma., and a target skin distance (TSD) of 15 to 20 cm., the lesion is given 680 R. per treatment three times a week for a total of 3400 R.

Using such a schedule in a series of 500 lesions treated at New York Skin and Cancer Unit, Bart and coworkers (1970) found cure rates of 92.7 per cent at 5 years and 88.9 per cent at 10 years.

Since chapters are devoted to treatment of skin by x-ray therapy, the reader is referred to those chapters for further information on technique and results.

Several topically applied chemicals have been used either alone or in combination to treat basal cell epithelioma. These include demecolcine (Jackson, 1959), 5-fluorouracil (Stoll, 1967), colchicine, thiocolchicine, methotrexate, chloroquine, podophyllin, and vitamin K_5 (Belisario, 1970). At the present time, the use of these preparations is still in the investigative stage. It is to be hoped that further experimental work will provide physicians with simple methods for eradicating basal cell epithelioma with suitable topical medications.

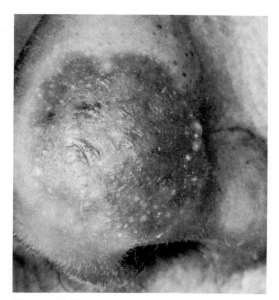

Figure 35–31 Acute radiodermatitis two weeks after last x-ray treatment for above lesion (4200 R. administered in 600-R. doses three times a week, 103 kvp, 5 ma., 0.9 mm. HVL Al, 15 cm. TSD).

Complications of Therapy

A complication of sharp curettage and electrodesiccation is low grade secondary pyoderma under the crust. When the patient returns for follow-up visits, the physician should look for the development of erythema and accumulation of purulent exudate. Pressing on the crust with an applicator stick may force out this purulent exudation. The crust should be removed and topical antibiotic therapy instituted. If granulation tissue is excessive under the crust, 10 per cent silver nitrate applied with a cotton applicator may be helpful.

Following curettage and electrodesiccation of lesions medial to the inner canthus of the eye, a permanent fold of tissue (Figs. 35–33 and 35–34) not infrequently results. Ordinarily, this does not disturb the patient but may be corrected by surgery if desired.

Hypertrophic scars are frequently seen when the lesion and treatment involve full thickness of the skin (Figs. 35–35 and 35–36). Such thickened scars usually subside spontaneously over a period of time. If not, they may be treated by intralesional infiltration with a few drops of diluted triamcinolone acetonide suspension (2.5 to 5 mg. per ml.) injected at monthly intervals.

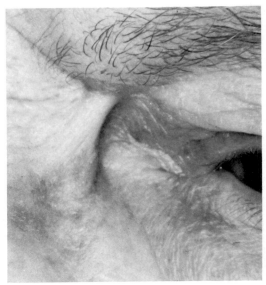

Figure 35–34 Skin fold following treatment of basal cell epithelioma by curettage and electrodesiccation.

Keloids may be a complication of treatment by sharp curettage and electrodesiccation or by surgical excision in certain locations, such as the deltoid portion of the arm, the chest, and the upper lip. Management of such keloids may prove satisfactory if treated early by intralesional injection of triamcinolone acetonide suspension (10 to 40 mg. per ml.), depending upon the size and bulk of the keloid. This treat-

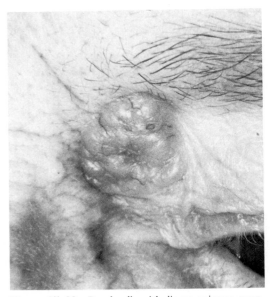

Figure 35–33 Basal cell epithelioma prior to treatment.

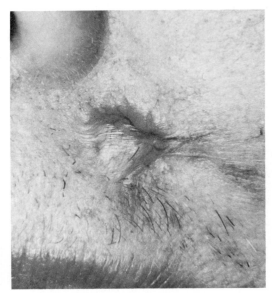

Figure 35–35 Hypertrophic scar after curettage and electrodesiccation of basal cell epithelioma.

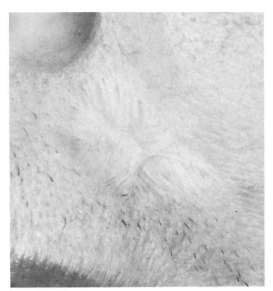

Figure 35-36   Hypertrophic scar two years later.

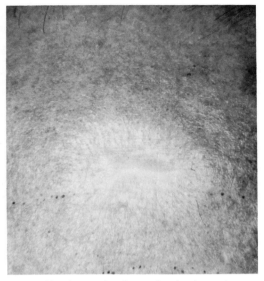

Figure 35-37   Forehead scar showing hypopigmentation following treatment by curettage and electrodesiccation for basal cell epithelioma.

ment may be pursued at monthly intervals, depending upon response.

Hypopigmented (Fig. 35-37) and on occasion hyperpigmented scars may result from x-ray therapy of skin cancers. Usually the hyperpigmentation tends to return to normal over a long period of time.

Suture marks on the face (Fig. 35-38) may be minimized by early removal of sutures and by using multiple, small-gauge, 5 and 6-0 synthetic sutures (nylon or dacron) carefully placed to distribute tension properly. Undermining of the wound edges and making the excision wound approximately 3 to 4:1 in length to width

ratio are both important aids. As mentioned previously, placement of excisions in or parallel to normal skin wrinkle lines further increases the likelihood of a good cosmetic end result (Figs. 35-10, 35-11, and 35-39).

Hematoma (Fig. 35-16), infection, and, later, wound disruption may be minimized by proper attention to technique. Gentle tissue handling by means of skin hooks and very fine forceps reduces crushing forces on the wound margins and minimizes devitalization of tissues.

By grasping the bleeding vessel with a fine, stainless steel, jewelers' forceps and

Figure 35-38 Complication of suture marks and cross-hatching following excision on forehead.

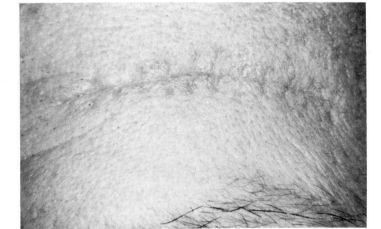

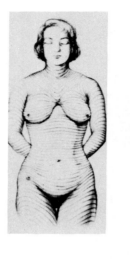
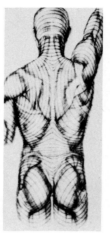
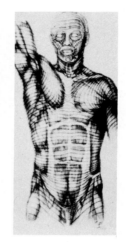
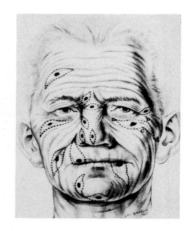
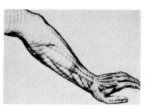
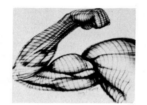
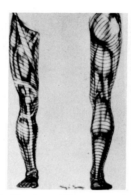

Figure 35–39 Wrinkle lines for elective placement of excision lines. (*From* Kraissl: Plastic and Reconstructive Surgery. Vol. 8. Copyright © 1951, The Williams and Wilkins Company, Baltimore.)

applying a bipolar coagulating current, proper hemostasis is obtained. This obviates burying foreign material, such as catgut, immediately under the skin. The absence of such foreign material greatly decreases the possibility of infection.

When drainage is indicated because of oozing, dead space, or the presence of infection, placement of a small (⅛-inch or ¼-inch) rubber dam type of drain is very helpful. A stab wound is made with a no. 11 type blade at the dependent portion of the wound, and the drain is inserted through this incision to the central and dependent portion of the wound. The drain is fixed by one suture to the skin. In closing the wound, care must be taken not to permit skin apposing sutures to pass through the drain, so that it can be removed two to three days later by severing the one suture fixing it to the stabe wound. This technique permits healing of the primary wound without disturbing the suture line.

Applying a pressure dressing with a moderate degree of firmness for two to three days postoperatively also helps to minimize the likelihood of hematoma. In vascular areas, such as the scalp, forehead, and neck, where hair interferes with placement of tape for this purpose, an elastic roller bandage placed over the dressing and around the head is very useful for one to two days after surgery. A particularly useful elasticized dressing for this purpose is Coban of Minnesota Mining Corporation. It does not adhere to the hair and is easily applied and removed.

RECURRENCES (Fig. 35–40)

Basal cell epithelioma is a skin tumor which has a distinct tendency to recur after therapy (Andrews, 1954; Lauritzen et al.,

1965). Lauritzen et al. (1965), citing Hayes to the effect that 83 per cent of recurrences were noted in the first two years after therapy, reviewed 2900 lesions treated over a 10-year period at the Ellis Fischel State Cancer Hospital in Missouri. They noted an accumulative low recurrence rate of 3.5 per cent in patients who had advanced skin cancers when first seen. Of the 101 recurrences, 79 were in surgical excision sites, and the remaining 22 were following radiotherapy. It is of interest that 50 per cent of the lesions recurred in the first two years in surgically excised cases reported with clear margins. The remainder of the recurrences took place over the next six years. In those specimens reported as inadequately excised, 70 per cent of the recurrences were noted within two years. The remaining 30 per cent were found in four to six years, in contrast to six years in the previously mentioned group. Following x-ray therapy, recurrences of 63 per cent were seen by one to two years, with the remainder occurring up to six years after therapy.

Patients with basal cell epithelioma remain at risk for recurrence (or new lesions or both) for long periods of time (i.e., eight years). Lauritzen et al. suggested that patients should be instructed to communicate with physicians regarding any suspicious activity in previously treated areas. Also, based on their study, it is reasonable to extend the follow-up period from five to eight years, even though the percentage yield after five years may be very small.

In an analysis of the treatment of recurrences of basal cell epithelioma, Menn et al. (1971) showed that retreatment by curettage and electrodesiccation, surgical excision, or x-ray resulted in cure rates of only 50 per cent. He suggested that the method of management for recurrences is Mohs' (1956) chemosurgery.

Table 35–1 shows a summary of reported cure rates after several modalities of therapy. It can be seen in general that cure rates of 95 per cent or better can be expected when treatment is performed by x-ray therapy, surgical excision, or sharp curettage and electrodesiccation in selected cases by experienced therapists.

When lower cure rates were reported, as in the case of Williamson and Jackson (1962), it was due to the lack of experience of the operator—in this case, most dermatology residents. Sweet (1963) did not perform curettage and electrocautery treatment two times (or more) at the time of the first treatment. When he retreated his recurrences by the same technique, he increased his cure rate from 88 per cent to 95.1 per cent. This suggests that, if he had performed curettage and electrocautery treatments two or more times, his overall cure rate may have been higher than 95 per cent.

Gooding et al. (1965), in a series of 1197 lesions surgically excised, showed that,

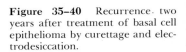

Figure 35–40 Recurrence two years after treatment of basal cell epithelioma by curettage and electrodesiccation.

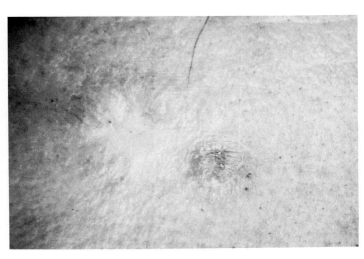

TABLE 35–1 BASAL CELL EPITHELIOMA: REPORTED CURE RATES

Author	Number of Lesions	Five-Year Cure Rate (%)	Method of Therapy, Comments
Knox et al. (1960)	56	96.67	curettage and electrodesiccation
Williams and Jackson (1962)	76	97.4	curettage and electrodesiccation
Sweet (1963)	593	88	curettage and electrodesiccation; single treatment; with retreatment, 95.1% cure rate
Freeman et al. (1964)			
105 patients	540	97	curettage and electrodesiccation; lesions < 2 cm.
12 patients		100	curettage and electrodesiccation; lesions > 2 cm.
68 patients	112	98	x-ray therapy; lesions < 2 cm.
11 patients		91	x-ray therapy; lesions > 2 cm.
25 patients	103	84	surgical excision; lesions < 2 cm.
8 patients		87	surgical excision; lesions > 2 cm.
Lauritzen et al. (1965)	2900	96.6 (10-year follow-up)	surgical excision
Gooding et al. (1965)	1197	98.1	surgical excision; 5.5 per cent reported showing marginal excision; only 34.8 per cent of these 5.5 per cent required retreatment; "corrected" cure rate, 98.1 per cent
Tromovitch (1965)	75	96	curettage and electrodesiccation
Mohs (1967)	4000 plus	99.1	microscopically controlled chemosurgical excision
Bart et al. (1970)	50	92.7 (88.9 at 10 year)	x-ray therapy

when the pathologist reported extension of the basal cell epithelioma to the margins of the excised tissue, only 34.8 per cent of those cases would recur clinically and require further treatment. They speculated that:

1. Marginal extension was due to an artifact during sectioning of tissue.

2. Trauma of surgery devitalized remaining basal cell epithelioma cells left in situ.

3. Marginal involvement did not extend beyond surgically excised specimen borders.

It can be seen that the method of Mohs' (1967) chemosurgery yields the best overall cure rates (see Chapters 70 and 71).

REFERENCES

Acker, D. W., and Helwig, E. B.: Rhinophyma with carcinoma. Arch. Dermatol., 95:250, 1967.

Anderson, N. P., and Anderson, H. E.: Development of basal cell epithelioma as a consequence of radiodermatitis. Arch. Dermatol. Syph. (Berl.), 63:586, 1951.

Andrews, G. C.: Diseases of the Skin. Philadelphia, W. B. Saunders Company 1954, p. 656.

Auerbach, H.: Geographic variation in incidence of skin cancer in the United States. Public Health Rep., 76:345, 1961.

Baden, H. P.: Palpation of basal cell epithelioma (letter to the Editor). J.A.M.A., 231:299, 1970.

Baferstedt, B.: Symposium on the treatment of skin cancer. Acta Derm. Venereol. (Stockh.), 50:475, 1970.

Bart, R. S.: Personal communication, 1971.

Bart, R. S., Kopf, A. W., and Petratos, M. A.: X-ray therapy of skin cancer, evaluation of a standardized method for treating basal cell epitheliomas. Sixth National Cancer Conference Proceedings. Philadelphia, J. B. Lippincott Company, 1970, pp. 559–569.

Belisario, J. C.: Topical cytotoxic therapy of cutaneous cancer and precancer. In Epstein, E. (Ed.): Skin Surgery. Springfield, Ill., Charles C Thomas, Publisher, 1970.

Blum, H. F.: Carcinogenesis by Ultraviolet Light. Princeton, N. J., Princeton University Press, 1959.

Botvinick, I., Mehregan, A. H., and Weissman, F.: Morphea-like basal cell epithelioma in a child. Arch. Dermatol., 95:67, 1967.

Brodkin, R., Kopf, A., and Andrade, R.: Basal cell epithelioma and elastosis: A comparison of distribution. In Urbach, F. (Ed.): Biologic Effects of Ultraviolet Radiation. New York, Pergamon Press, 1969.

Cleaver, J. E.: DNA, damage and repair in light sensitive human skin disease. J. Invest. Dermatol., 54:181, 1970.

Cleaver, J. E., and Trosko, J. E.: Xeroderma pigmentosum: A human disease defective in an initial stage of DNA repair. Proc. Natl. Acad. Sci. Cited in an editorial in J.A.M.A., 210:90, 1969.

Daniels, F., Jr.: Ultraviolet Carcinogenosis in Man. Natl. Cancer Inst. Monograph No. 10. Washington, D.C., U.S. Dept. of HEW, 1963, pp. 407–422.

Eastcott, D. F.: Epidemiology of Skin Cancer in New Zealand. Natl. Cancer Inst. Monograph No. 10. Washington, D.C., U.S. Dept. of HEW, 1963, pp. 141–151.

Freeman, R. G., and Knox, J. M.: Treatment of skin cancer. *In* Recent Results in Cancer Research. New York, Springer-Verlag, 1967, p. 38.

Freeman, R. G., Knox, J. M., and Heaton, C. L.: The treatment of skin cancer. Cancer, 17:535, 1964.

Gellin, G. A., Kopf, A. W., and Garfinkel, L.: Basal cell epithelioma, a controlled study of associated factors. Arch. Dermatol., 91:38, 1965.

Goldberg, L. C.: Plantar basal cell carcinoma. Cutis, 4:973, 1968.

Gooding, C. A., White, G., and Yatsuhashi, M.: Significance of marginal extension in excised basal cell carcinoma. New Engl. J. Med., 273:923, 1965.

Hyman, A. B., and Michaelides, P.: Basal cell epithelioma of the sole. Arch. Dermatol., 87:481, 1963.

Jackson, R.: The histological findings in normal skin and multiple superficial basal cell carcinoma treated with an ointment containing demecolcine. Dermatologica, 119:20, 1959.

Jackson, R.: Skin ulcerations simulating rodent ulcer following section of fifth cranial nerve for trigeminal neuralgia. Can. J. Surg., 7:319, 1964.

Jackson, R.: Observations on the natural course of skin cancer. Can. Med. Assoc. J., 92:564, 1965.

Jung, E. G., and Trachsel, B.: Molecular-biolozische untersuchunger Zur, Aisencarernozenese. Arch. Klin. Exp. Dermatol., 237:819, 1970.

Kligman, A. M.: Early destructive effect of sunlight in human skin. J.A.M.A., 210:2377, 1969.

Knox, J. M., Lyles, T. W., Shapiro, E. M., and Martin, R. D.: Curettage and electrodesiccation in the treatment of skin cancer. Arch. Dermatol., 82:197, 1960.

Knox, J. M., Rossman, R. E., and Freeman, R. A.: Environment and skin cancer. *In* Tumors of the Skin. Chicago, Year Book Medical Publishers, 1964.

Lauritzen, R. E., Johnson, R. E., and Spratt, J. S.: Pattern of recurrence in basal cell carcinoma. Surgery, 57:813, 1965.

Lever, W. F.: Histopathology of the Skin. Ed. 4. Philadelphia, J. B. Lippincott Company, 1967.

Lewis, H. M., Stensaas, C. O., and Okun, M. R.: Basal cell epithelioma of the sole. Arch. Dermatol., 91:623, 1965.

Lightstone, A. C., Kopf, A. W., and Garfunkel, L.: Diagnostic accuracy—A new approach to its evaluation. Arch. Dermatol., 91:497, 1965.

Litzow, T. J., and Engel, S.: Multiple basal cell epitheliomas arising in linear nevus. Am. J. Surg., 101:378, 1961.

MacDonald, E. J., and Bubendorf, E.: Some epidermiologic aspects of skin cancer. *In* Tumors of the

Skin. Chicago, Year Book Medical Publishers, 1964, pp. 23–65.

Mackie, B. S., and McGovern, V. J.: The mechanism of solar carcinogenesis. Arch. Dermatol., 78:218, 1958.

Meara, R. H.: Epithelioma after radiotherapy of the spine (correspondence with the Editor). Br. J. Dermatol., 80:620, 1968.

Menn, H., Robins, P., Kopf, A. W., and Bart, R. S.: The recurrent basal cell epithelioma. Arch. Dermatol., 103:628, 1971.

Mitchell, J. C., and Hardie, M.: Treatment of basal cell carcinoma by curettage and electrosurgery. J. Can. Med. Assoc., 93:349, 1965.

Mitchell, R. E.: Aspects of carcinogenesis in solar damaged skin. Aust. J. Dermatol., 11:14, 1970.

Miyaji, T.: Skin Cancers in Japan: A Nationwide 5 Year Survey, 1956–1960. Conference in Biology of Cutaneous Cancer. Natl. Cancer Inst. Monograph No. 10. Washington, D.C., Dept. of HEW, 1963, pp. 55–70.

Mohs, F. E.: Chemosurgery in Cancer, Gangrene and Infections. Springfield, Ill., Charles C Thomas, Publisher, 1956, p. 189.

Mohs, F. E.: Personal communication, 1967.

Norins, A. L.: Free radical formation in the skin following exposure to ultraviolet light. J. Invest. Dermatol., 39:445, 1962.

Olson, R. L.: Skin color, pigment distribution and skin cancer. Cutis, 8:225, 1971.

Orr, J. W.: Permutation of stromal tissues during carcinogenesis. Acta Un. Int. Cancr., 17:64, 1961.

Pantangco, E. E., Canlas, M., Basa, G., and Sin, R.: Observations on the Incidence, Biology and Pathology of Skin Cancer Among Filipinos. Conference in Biology of Cutaneous Cancer. Nat. Cancer Inst. Monograph No. 10. Washington, D.C., U.S. Dept. of HEW, 1963, pp. 109–119.

Pinkus, H.: Epithelial and fibroepithelial tumors. Arch. Dermatol., 91:24, 1965.

Popkin, G. L.: Curettage and electrodesiccation. N.Y. State J. Med., 68:866, 1968.

Rook, A.: Naevi and other developmental defects. *In* Rook, A., Wilkinson, D. S., and Ebling, F. J. A. (Eds.): Textbook of Dermatology. Oxford, Blackwell Scientific Publications, 1968.

Sanderson, K. V.: Tumors of the skin. *In* Rook, A., Wilkinson, D. S., and Ebling, F. J. A. (Eds.): Textbook of Dermatology. Oxford, Blackwell Scientific Publications, 1968, p. 1770.

Sarkany, I., Fountain, R. B., Evans, C. D., Morrison, R., and Szur, L.: Multiple basal cell epitheliomas following radiotherapy of the spine. Br. J. Dermatol., 80:90, 1968.

Schreiber, M. M., Shapiro, S. I., Berry, C. Z., Dahlim, R. F., and Freidman, R. D.: The incidence of skin cancer in southern Arizona (Tucson). Arch. Dermatol., 104:124, 1971.

Shu, Y.: Skin Cancer in Chinese in Taiwan. Conference in Biology of Cutaneous Cancer. Natl. Cancer Inst. Monograph No. 10. Washington, D.C., U.S. Dept. of HEW 1963, pp. 71–74.

Sigal, C., and Saunders, T. S.: Basal cell epithelioma and nevus pigmentosus. Arch. Dermatol., 96:520, 1967.

Stoll, H. L.: Effects of basal cell carcinoma of varying concentrations of locally administered 5-fluorouracil. J. Invest. Dermatol., 49:219, 1967.

Sulzberger, M. B., Baer, R. L., and Borota, A.: Do roentgen ray treatments as given by skin specialists produce cancers or other skin sequelae? Arch. Dermatol. Syph. (Berl.), 65:639, 1952.

Sutton, R. L.: Diseases of the Skin. Ed. 11, St. Louis, Mo., C. V. Mosby Company, 1956, p. 1073.

Sweet, R. D.: The treatment of basal cell carcinoma by curettage. Br. J. Dermatol., 75:137, 1963.

Ten Selden, R. E. J.: Skin Cancer in Australia. Conference in Biology of Cutaneous Cancer. Natl. Cancer Inst. Monograph No. 10. Washington, D.C., U. S. Dept. of HEW, 1963, pp. 153–166.

Torres, D.: Cryosurgery of premalignant and malignant skin lesions. Cutis, 8:123, 1971.

Traenkle, H. L.: X-ray induced skin cancer in man. *In* Tumors of the Skin. Chicago, Year Book Medical Publishers, 1964, pp. 67–74.

Tromovitch, T. A.: Skin cancer, treatment by curettage and desiccation. Calif. Med., 103:107, 1965.

Urbach, F., Davies, R. E., and Forbes, P. D.: Ultraviolet radiation and skin cancer in man. *In* Carcinogenesis, Advances in Biology of Skin. Vol. VII. Oxford, Pergamon Press, 1965, pp. 195–214.

Van Scott, E. J.: Definition of epidermal cancer. *In* The Epidermis. New York, Academic Press, 1964, p. 573.

Van Scott, E. J.: Basal cell carcinoma. *In* Fitzpatrick, J. B., Arndt, K. A., Clark, W. H., Eisen, A. Z., Van Scott, E. J., and Vaughan, J. A. (Eds.): Dermatology in General Medicine. New York, McGraw-Hill Book Company, 1971, p. 466.

Van Scott, E. J., and Reinertson, R. A.: Modulating influence of stromal environment on epithelial cell studies in human auto transplants. J. Invest. Dermatol., 36:109, 1961.

Weary, P.: Basal cell carcinoma arising at site of smallpox vaccination. Cutis, No. 10, 3:1114, 1967.

Weinstein, G. D., and Frost, P.: Cell proliferation in human basal cell carcinoma. Cancer Res., 30:724, 1970.

Wernmuth, B. M., and Fajardo, L. F.: Metastatic basal cell carcinoma. Arch. Pathol., 90:458, 1970.

Whyte, H. J., and Perry, H. O.: A simple method to minimize scarring following large punch biopsies. A.M.A. Arch. Dermatol., 81:520, 1960.

Wilgrim, G. F., Kidd, R. L., Krawczyk, W., and Cole, P. L.: Sunburn effect on keratinosomes. Arch. Dermatol., 101:505, 1970.

Williamson, G. S., and Jackson, R.: Treatment of basal cell carcinoma by electrodesiccation and curettage. Can. Med. Assoc. J., 80:855, 1962.

Wilson Jones, E., and Heyl, T.: Nevus sebaceous, A report of 140 cases with special regard to development of secondary malignant tumors. Br. J. Dermatol., 82:99, 1970.

Wooldridge, W. E.: Cryosurgery of Skin Cancer, One Man's Opinion, an oral presentation at the American Academy of Dermatology, 1971.

Zacarian, S. A.: Cryosurgery of Skin Cancer. Springfield, Ill., Charles C Thomas, Publisher, 1969.

Zugerman, I.: Basal cell epithelioma on nevus. Arch. Dermatol., 84:672, 1961.

36

Pathology of Basal Cell Epithelioma

André Kint, M.D.

The basal cell epithelioma is a tumor characterized histologically by the presence of a special cell that resembles those of the basal cell layer of the epidermis. Because of this analogy, the term "basal cell carcinoma" was introduced by Krompecher (1903).

Several forms can be distinguished clinically: epithelioma planum cicatrisans, nodular epithelioma, superficial basal cell epithelioma, rodent ulcer, morphea-like epithelioma, and vegetative epithelioma.

The presence of the same cell type in all the forms of basal cell epithelioma does not mean that the microscopic structure of the tumor is uniform. Differences in the histologic picture are due to variations in the general architecture, and to the differentiating and dedifferentiating capacities of the cells. The occurrence of these many variations causes most of the difficulty in interpreting the origin of a basal cell epithelioma.

HISTOLOGY OF BASAL CELL EPITHELIOMA

General Architecture

With Favre et al. (1936), Dupont and Piérard (1961), and Gottron and Nikolowsky (1960), we discern two principal tumor types: solid or massive, and reticular or adenoid. In the former, more or less compact cell masses with various forms and sizes are present in the dermis (Fig. 36–1); in the latter, the cells are arranged in intertwining strands, presenting a lacelike pattern (Fig. 36–2). Between the two types, many transitional forms can be found. In some tumors solid masses and reticular structures may be observed side by side.

Cell Types

In the tumor masses peripheral (or basal) and central cells are classically distin-

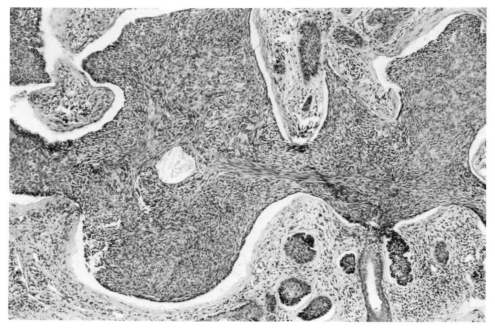

Figure 36–1   Solid or massive type of basal cell epithelioma. *H&E*, ×95.

guished. The peripheral cells are cylindrical, high, and narrow; they show a palisade arrangement and have little, poorly visible cytoplasm and an ovoid regular nucleus with a small nucleolus. The central cells are polyhedral, oval, round, or elongated and arranged irregularly (Fig. 36–3). The nucleus is regular and surrounded by a thin cytoplasmic rim. Intercellular bridges are seldom seen in routine sections; they can, however, always be found with iron-hematoxylin stains on thin sections.

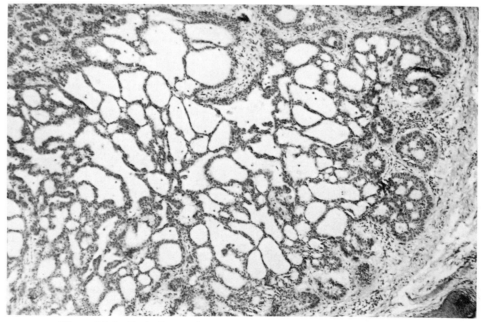

Figure 36–2   Reticular or adenoid type of basal cell epithelioma. *H&E*, ×95.

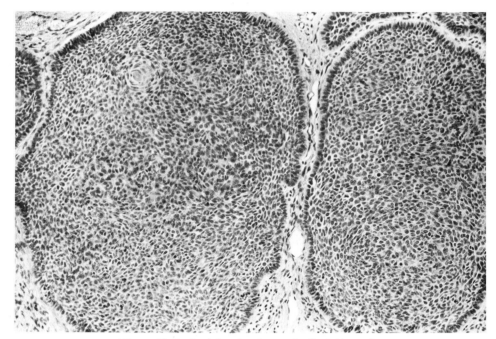

Figure 36–3   Peripheral and central cells. *H&E, ×175.*

In the center or on the margin of the tumor buds, a third cell type is sometimes found (Dupont and Piérard, 1961; Lever, 1948). It is a narrow, elongated cell, looking like a fibrocyte and having little cytoplasm and a dark, bar-shaped nucleus (Fig. 36–4).

Okun and Blumental (1964) and Rupec

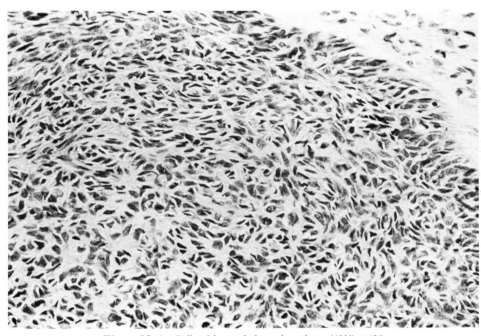

Figure 36–4   Cells with a rod-shaped nucleus. *H&E, ×430.*

and Vakilzadeh (1969) described giant cells with multiple nuclei; these cells are mostly grouped in some areas of the tumors. Their nuclei are closely packed and often atypical, have a variable chromatin content, and are surrounded by little cytoplasm.

Darier and Ferrand (1922) and Juon (1929) described a "metatypic epithelioma," in which they distinguished intermediary and mixed types. These tumors were called "basal squamous cell epithelioma" by Montgomery (1929). In the intermediary type the cells have features of basal cell and of squamous cell epithelioma cells and are considered to be intermediary between both cell types. With Welton et al. (1949), Lennox and Wells (1951), Smith and Swerdlow (1956), Dupont and Piérard (1961), and Lever (1967), we can hardly accept the existence of such a tumor type as a specific lesion. These tumors are more probably less specific basal or squamous cell epitheliomas, and careful examination of histologic sections will allow a distinction to be made between the two.

The mixed type consists of the presence, side by side, of a basal cell and a squamous cell epithelioma. This coexistence is frequently seen and cannot be questioned (Dupont and Piérard, 1961).

The Peritumoral Stroma

The stroma around the basal cell epithelioma consists of preexisting connective tissue bundles, newly formed fibrous strands, and more or less pronounced infiltrates of lymphocytes, histiocytes, and plasma cells; the number of mast cells is increased (Dupont and Piérard, 1961), and foreign body granulomas are sometimes found.

The appearance of the connective tissue bundles is, like that of the tumor itself, not consistent and can vary in the same patient from location to location. Generally, one finds around the tumor masses a loose network of fine undulating fibers, analogous to the connective tissue around hair follicles. In other cases compact fibrous strands or homogeneous mucoid or sometimes hyaline masses are found. This transformation toward a mucoid substance (cylindromatous degeneration) is rather frequent. It is often the result of the degeneration of connective tissue masses isolated by the progressing tumor, but it

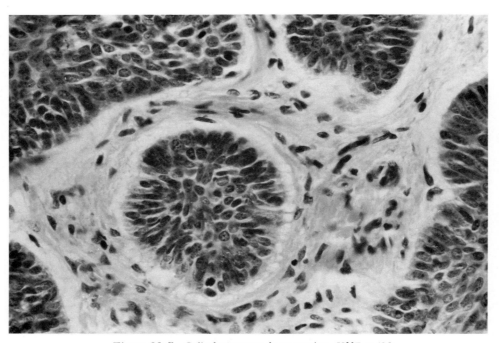

Figure 36–5   Cylindromatous degeneration. *H&E, ×430.*

can also be found around isolated tumor buds. These buds are then surrounded either by a relatively large band of mucoid tissue or, inversely, by only a narrow festooned rim, with each tip corresponding to the basis of a palisade cell (Fig. 36–5). Whether this peritumoral mucoid substance originates from primary connective tissue degeneration or from the tumor itself is not completely clear. Bazex et al. (1959 and 1961) favored the former opinion. It is difficult, however, to exclude an influence of the tumor cells on the connective tissue. Masson (1956) ascribed the phenomenon to a sweat gland differentiation of the tumoral cells; the secretion would be delivered in the direction of the connective tissue (*polaritée inversée*). Favre et al. (1936) and Woringer (1961) defended a similar opinion. However, objective proof of this interpretation is not given.

Pigmentation

Pigmentation is not rare and can occur in every type of the tumor. The pigment may be seen only microscopically or can be evident clinically. Differentiation from malignant melanoma can sometimes be difficult for the uninitiated; careful analysis of the clinical signs generally gives the solution. According to Touraine (1935), 75 percent of pigmented skin tumors are basal cell epitheliomas, and Becker (1930) found pigment histologically in 33 percent of his basal cell epitheliomas. Reviews on pigmented skin tumors were written by Bloch (1927), Becker (1930), Beck (1933), Eller and Anderson (1933), Touraine (1935), Gaté et al. (1937), and Puente-Duany (1950); readers are referred to these authors for more details.

The pigment in basal cell epithelioma is always melanin. Its localization is variable: it can be found in the epidermis and in the dermis as well as in the tumor itself. In the epidermis one can find an increase in the number of melanocytes located between the cells of the basal layer, or an accumulation of melanin in the basal cells. Frequently the pigment is concentrated in the upper dermis, between the epidermis and the tumor masses, and it is sometimes found in the peritumoral connective tis-

sue. In the tumor itself, melanin is mostly found in dendritic cells which are preferentially located at the periphery of the basalioma lobes; they are more frequent in superficial than in deeper structures. The shape and distribution of these starlike cells reminds one very much of the dendritic cells found between the bulbar cells of active hair follicles.

From time to time pigment-containing cells are found in the central parts of large epithelioma structures; when pseudocysts are formed through necrosis of these zones, the melanophages remain floating in the cavity for a certain period of time. The origin of these pigment-containing cells has been a matter of dispute for a long time: Masson (1956) thought that they penetrated from the epidermis into the tumor; Bloch (1927) and Pautrier and Diss (1929) considered them to be modified basal cells. In the connective tissue they could be macrophages (Pautrier and Diss, 1929). At this moment they are considered to be dendritic cells of neural origin, analogous to those found in the epidermis. These cells can easily be stained with the osmic acid–zinc iodide technique (Niebauer, 1957; Thies, 1962; Wiedmann, 1963; Niebauer and Sediko, 1965; Kint, 1966), which is specific for the demonstration of cells of neural origin.

DIFFERENTIATING AND REGRESSIVE CAPACITIES OF THE CELLS

Differentiating Capacities

Basal cell epitheliomas may include cells evolving toward keratinization, pilary formations, sweat glands, or sebaceous glands.

In evolving toward keratinization the cells become larger, diamond-shaped, and eosinophilic (Fig. 36–6), and they may contain a few keratohyalin granules.

Pilary formations are found in nearly every basal cell epithelioma and represent the most frequent type of differentiation in these tumors. Structures can be interpreted as pilary formations when they imitate the primary epithelial germ, the normal hair follicle or one of its cell types, or

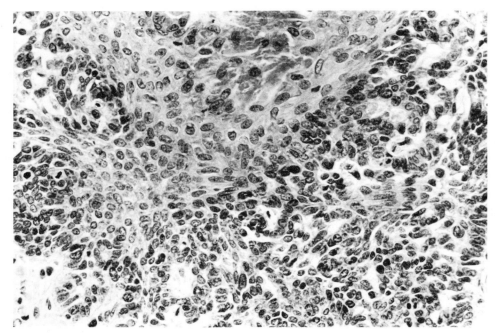

Figure 36–6   Evolution toward keratinization. *H&E, ×430.*

cellular aspects seen in the catagen follicle. They most often appear as bundles of spindle-shaped cells crossing the tumor buds in various directions and resembling the cells of the upper hair bulbus evolving toward the inner root sheath of the follicle (Fig. 36–7).

Concentrically arranged cell groups having one or more keratinized cells in their center can frequently be found (Fig. 36–8).

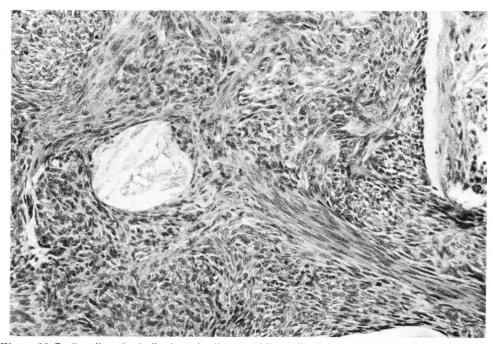

Figure 36–7   Bundles of spindle-shaped cells, resembling cells of the upper hair bulbus. *H&E, ×240.*

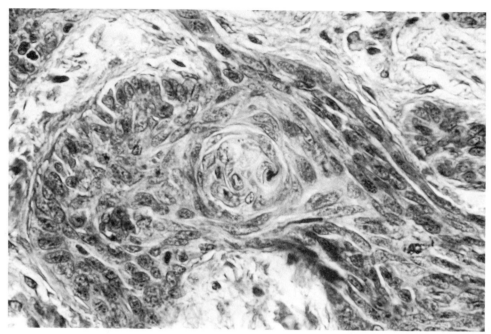

Figure 36-8   Concentrically arranged cell groups. *H&E*, ×520.

These structures are considered by Foot (1947) to be sweat gland formations; such structures, however, appear regularly in regressing hair follicles and never show any sign of sweat secretion (Kint, 1966).

Rudimentary follicles or structures imitating the shape of primary hair buds are regularly found at the periphery of the tumor buds (Fig. 36–9).

Differentiation toward sweat glands is characterized by the presence of intertwining cell strands with two or more cell layers, sometimes having a small lumen. In our experience sweat gland differentiation is rarely seen (Kint, 1966 and 1970), and our results confirm the data of Lennox and Wells (1951), who found only two sweat gland structures in 150 tumors. We seldom found apocrine gland formation and never saw eccrine glands; nevertheless, eccrine glands were found by Lapière and Piérard (1954) in morphea-like epithelioma, and Freeman and Winkelmann (1969) described two basal cell tumors with eccrine differentiation.

Foot (1947) described glandular differentiation in more than 30 percent of his cases. This high proportion can be explained by the fact that he considered concentrically arranged cell groups, often having a keratinized center, to be sweat gland formations. With Haythorn (1931), Warren et al. (1936), Hueck (1947), and Piérard and Dupont (1948), we consider these structures to be pilary formations.

Intratumoral fluid accumulation should not be interpreted as an evolution toward sweat glands; it results from cell degeneration or from liquefaction of connective tissue.

Differentiation toward sebaceous glands, whereby the cytoplasm becomes abundant, foamy, and clear, is very rare.

Regressive Changes

The most frequently found regressive change is stellar atrophy; it is due to degeneration and liquefaction of tumor cells. In this process some liquid is accumulated in the intercellular spaces, so that the tumor cells are no longer closely packed, but separated from each other, remaining connected only by narrow cytoplasmic threads. The cells themselves have only a thin cytoplasmic rim surrounding the oval nucleus (Fig. 36–10).

Pseudocysts are frequently observed in

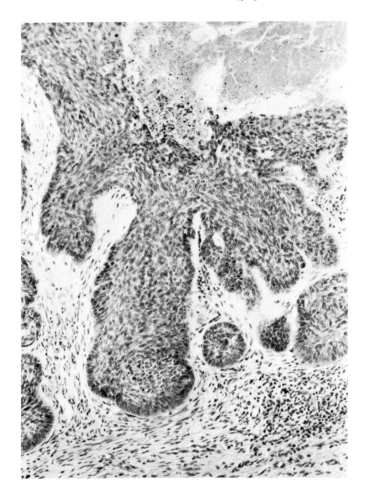

Figure 36–9 Structures imitating the shape of primary hair buds. *H&E, ×175.*

the tumor buds. They are formed in various ways:

1. By extension of stellar atrophy, resulting in the disappearance of the fine intercellular threads and in the formation of intercellular vacuoles or cysts (Fig. 36–11).

2. By massive cell necrosis, which is frequently seen in large tumor masses: the central cells first become more basophilic than ordinary basal cell epithelioma cells; afterwards the nuclei become pyknotic and the cells disappear (Fig. 36–12). Dubreuilh and Auché (1901) and Favre et al. (1936) thought that the process was due to deficient cellular nutrition; Beck (1933) ascribed it to aging.

3. By cylindromatous degeneration— that is, a destruction of the tumor stroma, which is changed into an amorphous and structureless material. The process can be seen around isolated tumor buds, but is generally found in those parts of the connective tissue that are enclosed by growing tumor buds. These pseudocysts are completely surrounded by tumor cells, and it may sometimes be difficult to distinguish them from pseudocysts resulting from another mechanism.

Hyaline degeneration is characterized by the accumulation of amorphous eosinophilic masses in one or more cells.

In the periphery of the tumor buds a special form of degeneration can be seen, consisting of an accumulation of liquid in the palisade cells (Fig. 36–13), which leads to necrosis of the nuclei and liquefaction of the peripheral cell layer (Fig. 36–14). Thus the tumor is separated from the peritumoral stroma, and large lacunae are formed, wherein necrotic cells and pyknotic nuclei can be found (Fig. 36–15). These lacunae are quite typical for basal cell

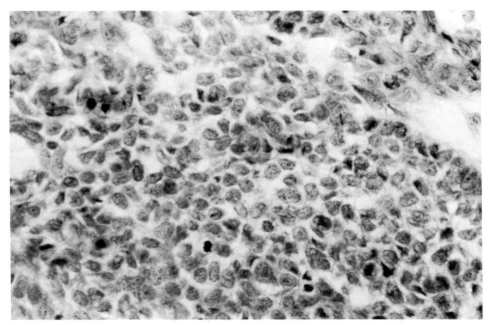

Figure 36–10 Stellar atrophy; the intercellular spaces are widened, and the cells are connected by narrow cytoplasmic threads. *H&E, ×430.*

epithelioma and have been attributed by most authors to fixation artifacts (Krompecher, 1903; Favre et al., 1936; Lund, 1957; Niebauer and Raab, 1962; Lever, 1967) and by Beck (1933) to decreased cohesion between the tumor and the surrounding connective tissue. According to Umiker and Director (1954), they result from an enzymatic depolymerization of the connective tissue. These peritumoral

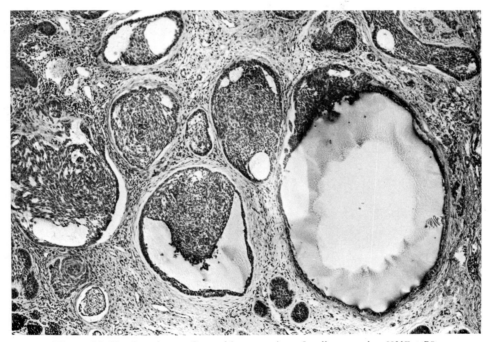

Figure 36–11 Pseudocysts formed by extension of stellar atrophy. *H&E, ×70.*

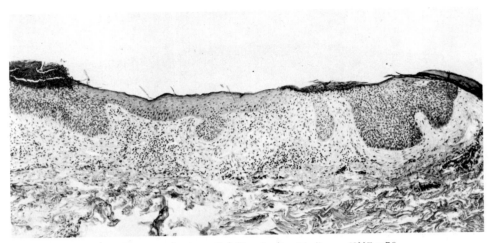

Figure 36–19   Superficial basal cell epithelioma. *H&E, ×70.*

massive necrosis of cells in the middle of some tumor buds; or from necrosis or liquefaction of connective tissue enclosed by the tumor.

The morphea-like epithelioma is rare and is composed of narrow basal cell strands of various shapes (Fig. 36–21); generally they have only one or two cell rows and are surrounded by an intense fibrosis.

The vegetative epithelioma has no specific histologic structure; it consists of neoplastic masses whose cells do not show any differentiation tendency.

The histology of the premalignant fibroepithelioma of Pinkus (Pinkus, 1953) is very characteristic. One finds long, thin, branching, and anastomosing strands, growing from the epidermis into the cutis (Fig. 36–22). They generally do not reach

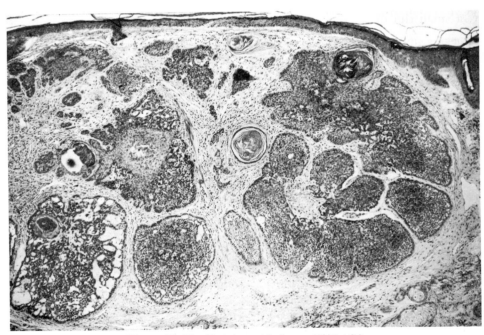

Figure 36–20   Nodular epithelioma. *H&E, ×70.*

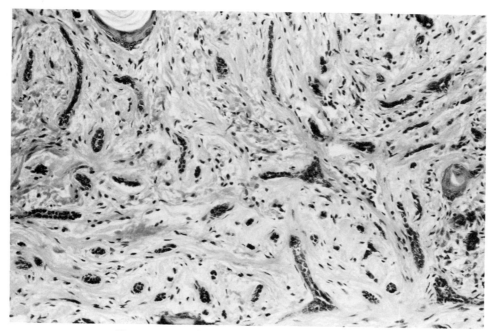

Figure 36-21 Morphea-like epithelioma. *H&E, ×175.*

beneath the level of the epidermis because a dense connective tissue reaction accompanies the tumor proliferation and pushes it upward. The peritumoral stroma is usually fibrous but may be loose or reticular. The tumor strands generally contain only two or three cell rows; from their sides, small cell groups grow into the stroma, resembling a bud on a branch.

Transition cases between the fibroepithelioma and the ordinary basal cell epithelioma have been described. For this reason Pinkus (1953), Degos and Hewitt (1955), Jaegher and Delacrétaz (1956), Dupont

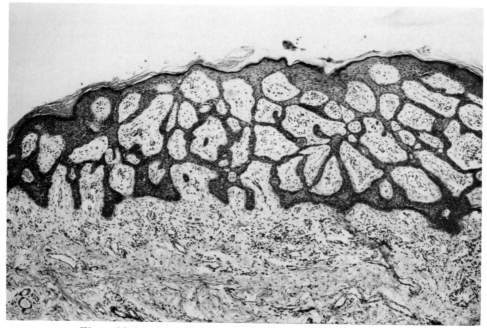

Figure 36-22 Premalignant fibroepithelioma of Pinkus. *H&E, ×70.*

and Piérard (1961), and Cramer (1960) think that it is a rare form of basal cell epithelioma.

HISTOCHEMISTRY OF BASAL CELL EPITHELIOMA

Carbohydrates

Glycogen. Glycogen has often been studied in basal cell epithelioma. Some authors did not find the substance in this tumor (Braun-Falco, 1954; Brett and Rathjens, 1953; Dutu and Longhin, 1960; Goltz et al., 1958 and 1959a and b; Niebauer and Raab, 1962; Steiner, 1955), while others described a large amount of glycogen (Beck, 1933; Dubreuilh and Auché, 1902; Fanger and Barker, 1957; Jessner and Biberstein, 1953; Wood et al., 1958).

In fact, the amount of glycogen is quite variable; some tumors contain a lot of glycogen, others show zones with and zones without glycogen, and in some tumors no glycogen can be found (Kint, 1966; Piérard and Kint, 1967). The localization is variable too: in some tumors glycogen is found in the palisade cells, and in others it is, on the contrary, localized in the center of the tumor buds. The distribution of glycogen is similar in the various forms of basal cell epithelioma.

Neutral Polysaccharides. Braun-Falco (1954 and 1961a), Steiner (1955), Goltz et al. (1959), and Sams et al. (1963) described PAS-positive and diastase-resistant substances, which are localized in the cells or resemble hyaline bodies. The basement membrane is homogeneous and distinct around massive tumor buds; it can be reticular in infiltrating tumors (Braun-Falco, 1954; Brett and Braun-Falco, 1955; Gottron, 1957; Ochoa et al., 1957).

Basal cell epitheliomas generally have but little neutral mucopolysaccharide content, which may be found in the tumor parenchyma as small intracytoplasmic granules, or in the horn pearls. A basal membrane is generally seen around the tumor; it is often discontinuous. This fact does not correspond to the invasive character of the lesion. When peritumoral lacunae are formed, the basal membrane generally adheres to the connective tissue.

Acid Mucopolysaccharides

METACHROMATIC SUBSTANCES. Metachromasia around basal cell epitheliomas was described by Fromme as early as 1906 and has been studied by numerous authors (Bunting, 1950; Braun-Falco, 1954 and 1957; Hieronymi, 1954; Lengyel and Vertes, 1956; Fanger and Barker, 1957; Steiner, 1957; Andrade, 1958; Pinkus, 1958; Swerdlow, 1958; Bazex et al., 1961; Christol-Jalby, 1959; Sams et al., 1963; Johnson and Helwig, 1963; Johnson et al., 1964).

Metachromatic substances are often found around the tumor and are frequently seen in the intercellular spaces of the tumoral buds. There is a relation between the histologic aspect of the tumor and the presence of the intratumoral metachromasia. It is most pronounced when the intracellular spaces are enlarged by accumulation of edema, and especially in cases with cylindromatous degeneration. In superficial basal cell epithelioma, in epithelioma planum cicatrisans, and in rodent ulcer, the intercellular substance is sometimes metachromatic, but generally not; in these tumors the reaction is principally seen around the tumor buds and is always less extensive than in nodular epithelioma.

Peritumoral metachromasia remains unchanged after treatment with hyaluronidase; the intratumoral metachromasia may, however, disappear with this enzyme. We infer from these facts that hyaluronic acid is not found around the tumor, but that it may be present in the intercellular spaces.

HALE- AND ALCIAN BLUE—POSITIVE MATERIAL. Such substances were described around and within the tumor buds by Moore et al. (1960), Sanderson (1962), and Sams et al. (1962 and 1963). Johnson and Helwig (1963), Godlewski (1964), Johnson et al. (1964), and Majewska et al. (1965) found the acid mucopolysaccharides around the tumor rather than within it.

The reactions are always intensely positive around the tumor and in the intercellular spaces, and the results with both techniques are thus more uniform than with toluidine blue. In contrast to the latter method, these techniques show no difference among the various histologic types of basal cell epithelioma.

The Nucleic Acids

Ribonucleic Acid. Lund (1957) found no or very little RNA in basal cell epitheliomas, and Pruniéras (1954) described less RNA in the tumor than in the surrounding epidermis. Grixoni and Ventura (1951), however, found an increased RNA content in the nucleoli and the cytoplasm of the cells. Moberger (1954) got the same dry weight of RNA in tumor cells as in normal epidermis; ultraviolet spectrophotometry showed an increased absorption in the tumor cells.

With the Unna-Brachet method and with gallocyanin, the RNA content of basal cell epithelioma cells always appears lower than that in the surrounding normal epidermis: the cytoplasm of the cells is in every case barely stained, and the nucleoli are small and intensively stained. The staining of the nucleoli does not, however, disappear completely after exposure to ribonuclease.

Deoxyribonucleic Acid. With histophotometry high DNA values have been described (Laquerrière et al., 1961). The DNA content of the nuclei varies according to the localization of the cells (Kint, 1963, 1964, and 1966). The palisade cells have higher DNA values than normal epidermal cells at a distance from the tumor, but the value is never tetraploid. In the center of the tumor, the DNA content decreases. Normal-looking epidermal cells situated above the tumor contain more DNA than epidermal cells distant from the tumor.

In basal cell epitheliomas of the solid and adenoid types, Ehlers (1966) found DNA values similar to those of normal somatic cells. In intermediate, or metatypic forms, the DNA values are much higher. In these tumors the author observed furthermore that the histone content increases in the same way as the DNA; this is not the case in solid tumors, where he found relatively more histone than DNA. That difference could be due to the presence of pyknotic nuclei in the solid tumor (Ehlers, 1968).

De Bersaques (1966), using a biochemical method, found 2½ times more DNA in basal cell epitheliomas than in normal epidermis. This difference could be due to technical reasons (measurement of separated nuclei in the histophotometry; determination of DNA per unit of dry weight in the biochemical method).

Distribution of –SH and S–S Groups

Steigleder (1957) described staining for –SH groups in the tumor similar to that in the normal epidermis. Foraker and Wingo (1956) found no alteration of the amount of –SH in these tumors. Steiner (1960) found spectrophotometrically a decrease of sulfhydryl-containing proteins. With amperometric titration, Ogura et al. (1961) found, on the contrary, an increased –SH content, suggesting a relation between the –SH content and the degree of differentiation of the tumor.

With Barnett and Seligman's method (1954) one generally finds a lower –SH content in basal cell epithelioma than in the basal cell layer of the normal epidermis above the tumor. The palisade cells may sometimes react more strongly than the central cells; however, the difference is so small that no importance can be given to it. The cells in the vicinity of the peritumoral lacunae are darker than normal palisade cells; that feature could be due to the liberation of –SH groups that are normally masked. There is no difference in the –SH content of the various forms of basal cell epithelioma.

The S–S groups, which can be demonstrated by the Barnett-Seligman method after exposure of the sections to thioglycolate, are seen only in the horny layer of normal epidermis. The basal cell tumor does not react, but we did find granules containing S–S in some cells of an epithelioma planum cicatrisans.

Enzymes

Enzyme histochemistry studies the distribution of enzymes in the tissues and gives an idea of the metabolism of the cells.

Hydrolytic Enzymes

ALKALINE PHOSPHATASE. Kopf (1957), and Nishiyama (1964) described zones reacting strongly and other zones without alkaline phosphatase in the peripheral cell layers of basal cell epithelioma. In contrast to these authors, Wood et al. (1958) did not find any difference between the tumor and the surrounding normal epidermis. In the peritumoral stroma, containing many capillaries, fibroblasts, and infiltrating cells, these authors often found a positive reaction. Wolff and Holubar (1965) did not observe any reactivity in the tumor, finding alkaline phosphatase only in the capillary walls and sometimes in the peritumoral tissue.

With Gomori's method (1952) no alkaline phosphatase can be found in basal cell epitheliomas; the peritumoral stroma is most often negative too. Around tumors with a strong connective tissue reaction, some activity is present. The capillaries always react strongly (Fig. 36–23). The method shows further that the number of vessels is variable around basal cell epitheliomas, some tumors being surrounded by a dense network of capillaries and others by only a few. There is no relation between the type of tumor and the number of vessels, or the intensity of the reaction for alkaline phosphatase.

ACID PHOSPHATASE. Acid phosphatase has been studied in basal cell epitheliomas

by Spier and Martin (1956), by Willinghagen (1960), and by Wolff and Holubar (1965), who described weak activity of this enzyme. Acid phosphatase activity can be demonstrated by several methods. The technique of Grogg and Pearse (1952), using sodium glycerophosphate as a substrate, shows that the epidermis above the tumor reacts more weakly than the one situated at a distance from the tumor. In the epithelioma itself, the reaction is always very weak and less than in the basal cell layer of the epidermis (Fig. 36–24). The tumor cells with keratinizing tendencies contain more acid phosphatase than the undifferentiated cells, and the keratinized grains are clearly positive. Acid phosphatase is absent from the peritumoral stroma and from the inflammatory infiltrate. There are no differences in these findings between the various types of basal cell epithelioma.

NONSPECIFIC ESTERASES. Steigleder and Löffler (1956) and Steigleder (1957) found little nonspecific esterase activity in basal cell epitheliomas; keratinizing cells react more strongly than undifferentiated tumor cells. Wells (1957) did not find an increase of the enzyme in the tumor. For demonstration of nonspecific esterases, the

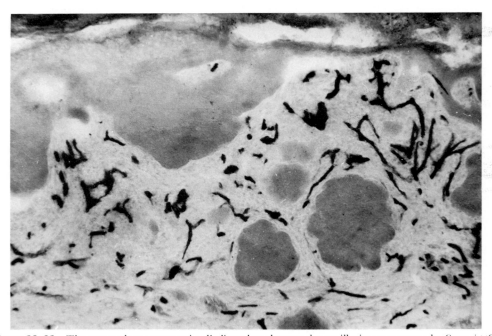

Figure 36–23   The tumor does not contain alkaline phosphatase; the capillaries react strongly. *Gomori,* ×95.

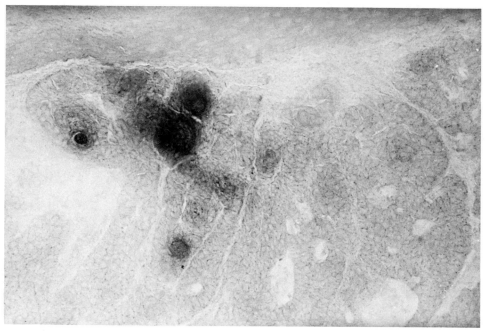

Figure 36–24. The tumor cells contain little acid phosphatase; around the horn pearls the reactivity increases. *Acid phosphatase, ×240.*

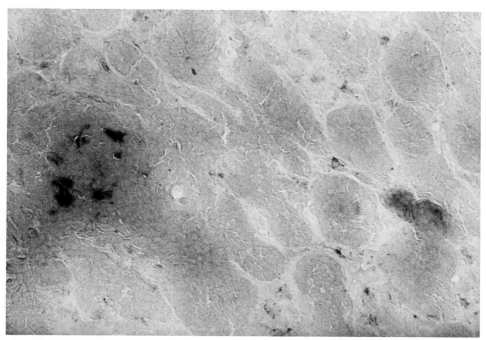

Figure 36–25 The tumor cells contain little esterases. The enzyme activity is stronger in some places than in others. *Esterases, ×240.*

method of Nachlas and Seligman adapted by Gomori, with α-naphthylacetate as a substrate (Gomori, 1952; Pearse, 1962), can be used. With that method basal cell epitheliomas generally appear to contain a weak, nonspecific, esterase activity; the activity is increased only around horn pearls (Fig. 36–25). There is, however, a positive reaction in the cells of the peritumoral infiltrate. All types of basal cell epitheliomas react in the same way.

OTHER HYDROLYTIC ENZYMES. Braun-Falco (1957) described a variable phosphorylase activity in the tumor buds and found no relation between the enzyme activity and the glycogen content of the tumor. Braun-Falco (1956) and Wolff and Holubar (1965) found a moderate diffuse reaction for β-glucuronidase in the tumor buds and an increased activity around keratinizing cells. The activities of nucleosidetriphosphatase and of 5-nucleotidase have also been studied by Wolff and Holubar (1965). The activity of the former enzyme appeared to be similar to that in normal epidermis; in some basal cell epitheliomas, however, the reaction was strongly positive in the palisade layer. The peritumoral stroma was often positive. The 5-nucleotidase was found in the peritumoral stroma, but not in the tumor itself.

Naphthylamidases. In a first paper Braun-Falco (1957b) described a moderate enzymatic activity in the tumor buds and considered the reaction negative in the vicinity of the tumor. The examination of new cases showed, however, a strongly positive reaction in the peritumoral connective tissue (Braun-Falco, 1957c). With the Burstone-Folk naphthylamide reaction, Steigleder and Kamei (1963) found only a weak proteolytic activity in the tumor cells; around the tumor buds the reaction was strongly positive. Wolff (1963) observed a moderate intratumoral activity with L-leucyl-β-naphthylamide as substrate; with L-leucyl-4-methoxy-β-naphthylamide, the reaction was positive only around the tumor. With biochemical methods, high naphthylamidase and di- and tripeptidase activities were found in tumor buds and in the surrounding stroma (De Bersaques, 1969).

With the substrate L-leucyl-β-naphthylamide (Nachlas et al., 1960; Pearse, 1962;

Wolff, 1963), there is in most cases a strongly positive reaction. In the tumor the reaction is not uniform: the peripheral cells generally contain more enzyme activity than the central ones (Piérard and Kint, 1966). The intensity of the reaction is, however, not constant; it changes not only from tumor to tumor but also from tumor bud to tumor bud (Fig. 36–26).

With the substrate L-leucyl-4-methoxy-β-naphthylamide, the basal cell epithelioma is always negative; in the peritumoral stroma the reaction is more positive than with the previous substrate (Fig. 36–27).

Enzymes of the Energy-Producing Metabolism

GLYCOLYSIS. The various enzymes of glycolysis have been studied in basal cell epitheliomas by Petzoldt and Braun-Falco (1968), who found that the intensity of the reactions is not uniform throughout the tumor and is generally less than in the surrounding epidermis. The adenoid forms react more intensely than the other types.

CITRIC ACID CYCLE

Succinic Dehydrogenase. Braun-Falco and Rathjens (1955), Foraker and Wingo (1956), and Serri (1958) all described increased enzymatic activity in the epidermis above and around the tumor; these authors found, moreover, a strongly positive reaction in the peripheral zones of the tumor buds. Braun-Falco and Rathjens drew attention to the fact that the intensity of the reaction may vary from one part of the tumor to another.

With the method of Nachlas et al. (1957), using nitroblue tetrazolium, the enzyme activity does not appear to be uniform in basal cell epithelioma (Wolff and Holubar, 1965; Kint, 1966; Piérard and Kint, 1966). It is generally less in the tumor buds than in the epidermis above the epithelioma. The reaction is stronger in the palisade cells than in the central ones; all the cells of the tumor, however, do not react in the same way; next to very intensely reacting buds, negative ones may be observed (Fig. 36–28).

ENZYMES OF THE RESPIRATORY CHAIN

NADPH-Tetrazolium Reductases. As Braun-Falco and Petzoldt described (1965), one finds only a weak activity with

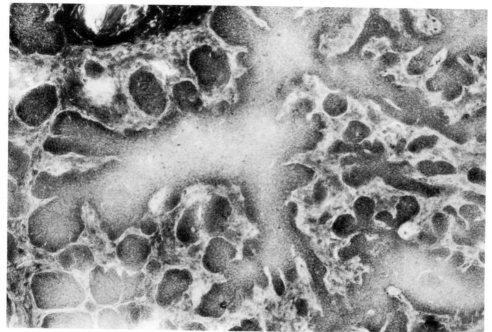

Figure 36–26   Tumor buds containing naphthylamidases. The peritumoral stroma is moderately positive. *Naphthylamide reaction with LNA, ×95.*

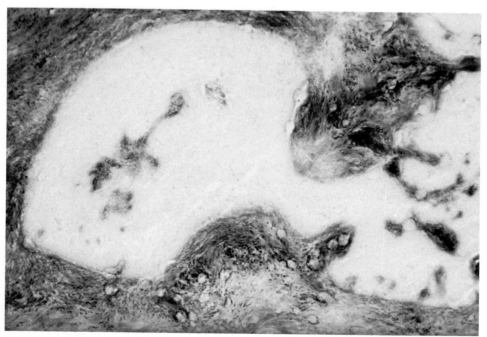

Figure 36–27   No naphthylamidase activity in the tumor buds. The peritumoral stroma is strongly positive. *Naphthylamide reaction with LMNA, ×95.*

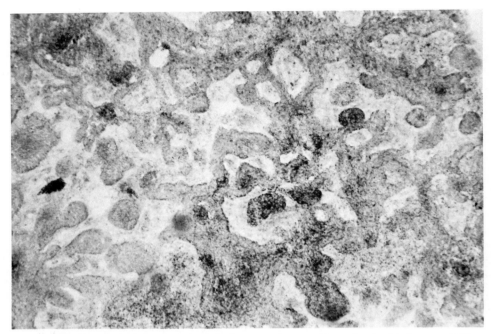

Figure 36–28   The activity of succinodehydrogenase is not uniform. *Succinodehydrogenase,* ×95.

the method of Nachlas et al. (1958a and 1958b). Around keratinizing centers the reaction is more positive, and sometimes a whole bud may react strongly. The enzyme is always located in the cytoplasm of the cells.

NADH-Tetrazolium Reductases. In contrast to the NADPH-tetrazolium reductases, there is a homogeneous positive reaction in basal cell epithelioma (Wolff and Holubar, 1965; Kint, 1966; Piérard and Kint, 1966).

Cytochromeoxidase. In three cases of basal cell epithelioma, Braun-Falco (1961) described an intense enzyme activity. Using the method of Burstone (1959, 1960, and 1961), one finds less enzyme activity in the tumor than in the basal cell layer of the surrounding epidermis (Fig. 36–29). Although the tumor buds react homogeneously in most of the cases, the enzyme activity may be stronger in some places than in others.

Ubiquinone. The distribution of ubiquinone is described by Petzoldt and Braun-Falco (1968), who found an uneven distribution of the substance in the tumor. The basal cell epithelioma of the adenoid type was more positive than the other types.

ELECTRON MICROSCOPY

Classic histologic ideas about the structure of the basal cell in epithelioma proved to be incomplete or incorrect in electron microscopy. The ultramicroscope has indeed revealed the presence of tonofilaments (Sirsat, 1956; Piérard and Kint, 1961 and 1962; Bonneau and Césarini, 1967) and desmosomes (Piérard and Kint, 1961 and 1962; Bonneau and Césarini, 1967), structures that had not been previously described in such tumors. Kobayasi (1970) found thickening and discontinuities of the dermal membrane, with disappearance of anchoring filaments, anchoring fibrils, and elastic fibril anchorings.

The tumor cell displays the same ultramicroscopic features as the undifferentiated ectodermal cell and can, up to a certain point, mimic the differentiations of the latter (formation of cells with malpighian characteristics, pilary evolution, keratin formation). According to Zelickson (1962), it would be analogous to that of the primary epithelial bud.

Lever and Hashimoto (1968) distinguished two cell types in basal cell epithelioma: clear cells, resembling those of

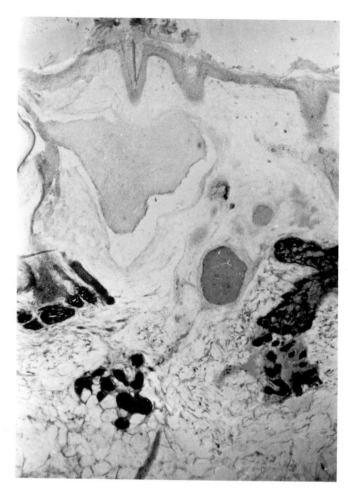

Figure 36–29 The epidermis above the tumor and the tumor react weakly. Sebum and sweat glands are strongly positive. *Cytochrome oxidase,×38.*

spinous cell carcinoma, and darker cells with the features of immature cells.

The presence of melanin pigment and melanocytes, already described by the histologists, has been confirmed by the electron microscope (Zelickson et al., 1961; Bonneau and Césarini, 1967; Zelickson, 1967). The melanin is located in dendrocytes and is not accepted by the tumor cells, which would not be able to phagocytize portions of the dendritic processes containing the melanin (Zelickson, 1967).

The following study comprises nine tumors: three superficial basal cell epitheliomas, three nodular epitheliomas, two tumors of the rodent ulcer type, and one morphea-like epithelioma.

The Basement Membrane

The appearance of the basement membrane is inconstant. It can be normal (an opaque band of 300 Å, separated from the plasma membrane by a structureless zone of 250 to 350 Å), but it is often thickened, not clearly delineated, or irregular (Fig. 36–30). Moreover, its continuity is frequently interrupted, and in several places tumor cells are directly in contact with the surrounding stroma (Fig. 36–31).

The Palisade Cells

The palisade cells are cubical; their lower cellular membrane is smooth, with occasional half-desmosomes, and their side walls are straight or slightly undulating. Few desmosomes are inserted in them, and they are separated from each other by narrow intercellular spaces. The nucleus is large, ovoid, and not very dense; nucleoli are mostly absent or poorly developed.

The ultrastructure of the cytoplasm is variable. In some cases, the nucleus is sur-

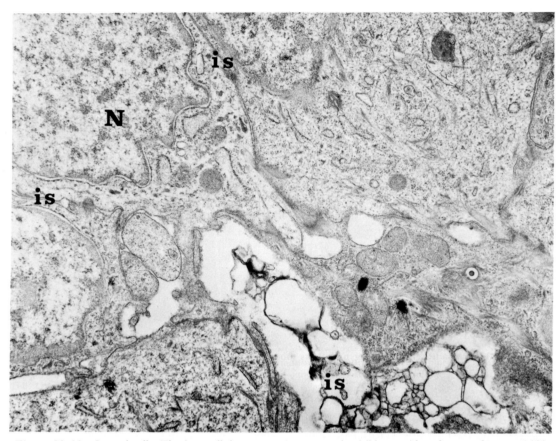

Figure 36–33   Central cells. The intercellular spaces (*is*) are poorly visible or widened. *N*, nucleus. ×24,000.

rectilinear filaments arranged lengthwise (Fig. 36–36). Oval, dark, and amorphous grains, with the aspect of trichohyalin, or melanin granules can be found. The presence of trichohyalin probably points to a differentiation toward components of the internal root sheath, while melanin would suggest evolution toward a cortical follicular cell.

Keratinization centers can be seen in isolated cells or in the middle of "onion skin" structures and can result from the two evolutionary types described above.

Regression Phenomena

The most frequent degenerative alteration is the phenomenon known by optical microscopy as "*stellar atrophy.*" It is mostly found in the nodular form. The most important transformation in that process is the alteration of the nuclear-cytoplasmic

ratio in favor of the nucleus; the latter fills the largest part of the cell and is encircled only by a narrow cytoplasmic border. The karyoplasm contains a nucleolus and small lumps of chromatin and is delimited by a double membrane. Mitochondria and tonofilaments are rare; the ribosomes are not numerous, and the endoplasmic reticulum is always absent. The intercellular spaces are widened owing to the deposition of a mucoid substance; the stellar aspect results from the fact that the cells remain attached by narrow cytoplasmic extrusions, at the center of which there remains a small desmosome (Fig. 36–37).

If the degeneration process goes on, the threadlike communications are ruptured, and lacunae appear within the tumor.

In so-called pseudocystic degeneration, the cytoplasm liquefies by an accumulation of intracellular edema. Round lacunae of various sizes, bound by an osmiophilic

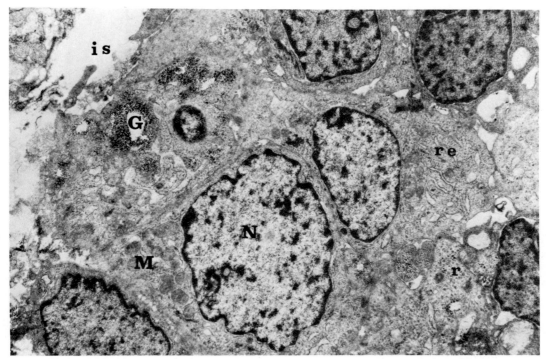

Figure 36–34 Cells situated in the center of a tumor bud. *G*, glycogen; *is*, intercellular space; *M*, mitochondria; *N*, nucleus; *r*, ribosomes; *re*, rough-surfaced endoplasmic reticulum. ×*13,250.*

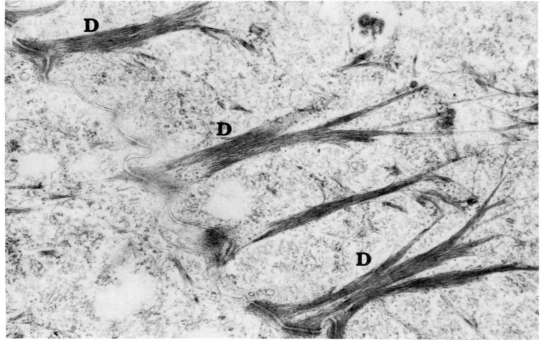

Figure 36–35 Evolution toward a malpighian cell. The desmosomes (*D*) are numerous. ×*31,500.*

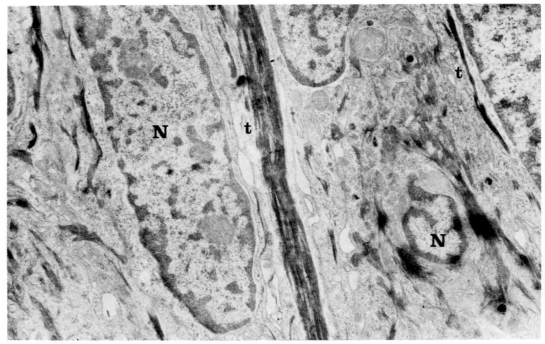

Figure 36–36 Evolution toward pilary formations. The cells become fusiform, and the cytoplasm contains numerous rectilinear filaments (*t*) arranged lengthwise. *N*, nucleus. ×21,500.

membrane, appear in the cell, whose volume increases and whose stretched plasma membrane ruptures, resulting in complete lysis of the cell content (Fig. 36–38). A special form of degeneration is seen at the level of the palisade cells: vacuoles accumulate in the infranuclear part of the peripheral cells and are accompanied by a lysis of the organelles. When they increase in volume, they separate the lower cellular membrane from the rest of the cytoplasm and are thus the starting point of the peritumoral lacunae that are so frequently seen in the optical microscope (Fig. 36–39).

Melanin

Melanin grains are generally found in the dendrites of the melanocytes, which penetrate into the intercellular spaces. They can also be seen in the cytoplasm of the tumor cells, where they float or are contained in small, round vesicles demarcated by a smooth membrane (Fig. 36–40). These are probably dendritic extrusions, included in the neoplastic cell.

The Surrounding Stroma

The surrounding stroma consists of a variable number of collagen fibers, between which histiocytes, fibroblasts, lymphocytes, and plasma cells are found. It is not rare to find neoformation of collagen fibers, as evidenced by the appearance of longitudinal fibrils in the fibroblasts and even the presence in some cells of fibrils with an apparent cross-striation. We will not insist here on this phenomenon, which we saw only at a glimpse and which requires further observation.

HISTOGENESIS

By analogy with normal basal cells, Krompecher (1903) thought that basal cell epitheliomas derived from the basal layer of the epidermis as well as from that of the appendages, whose cells would not be able to develop into mature forms. This assumption led to the term "basocellular." However, he understood the possibility that some cells of a basal cell epithelioma could differentiate toward structures re-

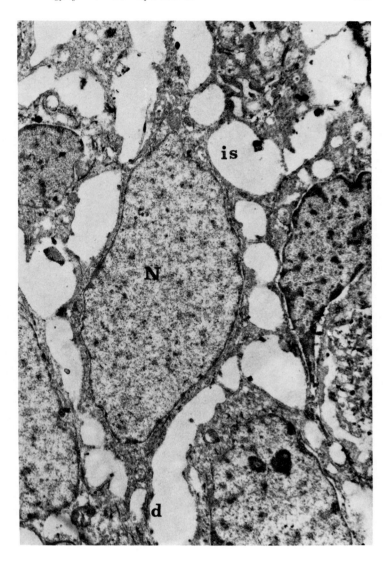

Figure 36–37 Stellar atrophy. The cells contain a large nucleus (*N*) and a thin, cytoplasmic rim. The intercellular spaces (*is*) are widened. Small desmosomes (*d*) are seen in the middle of the cytoplasmic extrusions. ×*14,250*.

sembling those of the appendages, and thought, therefore, that the tumor cells were pluripotential (Krompecher, 1919). Numerous histologists did not subscribe to that view and considered the skin appendages as possible tumor origins (Adamson, 1914 and 1917; Darier, 1922; Favre et al., 1936; Foot, 1947; Haythorn, 1931; Hernaman-Johnson, 1926; Mallory, 1910 and 1914; Smith and Swerdlow, 1956; Swerdlow, 1958; Wallace and Halpert, 1950; Welton et al., 1949).

According to Feyrter (1939), the basal cell epithelioma is not derived from ordinary basal cells but from special cells located in the basal layer and in the germina-

tive layer of the epidermis. This theory is only speculative and not based upon objective data.

Lever (1948) considered the tumor to be a hamartoma originating from the embryonic hair germ. The existence of embryonic germs in the adult skin cannot be proved, and such a germ can be imagined as a primary hair germ or even an undifferentiated ectodermal cell (Pinkus, 1959). Because the hair germ derives from the epidermal basal layer in embryonic skin, such a cell has to be located in the basal cell layer of the adult epidermis or perhaps in the regenerative zone of the hair complex. Moreover, it supposedly remains un-

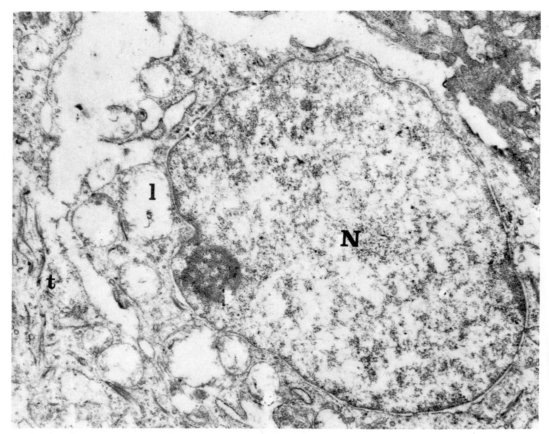

Figure 36–38   Pseudocystic degeneration. Lacunae (*l*) of various sizes appear in the cells, resulting in a lysis of the cell content. *N*, nucleus; *t*, tonofilaments. ×*12,500.*

changed for years and is not able to form keratinized epidermis.

Lever's argument that basal cell epithelioma appears only in zones with hair follicles is not consistent with the fact that these tumors have also been observed on the palms (Johnson, 1960; Kint, 1966), the soles (Pascher, 1953; Pascher and Sims, 1954; Zugerman, 1957), and the vulva (Siegler and Greene, 1951; Ward, 1956; Nel, 1957; Marcus, 1960; Schueller, 1965; Beans and Becker, 1968). Since basal cell epitheliomas cannot be produced experimentally and would never metastasize, Lever thinks that they are not truly malignant. However, basal cell epitheliomas have been produced experimentally in rats with methylcholanthrene (Zackheim et al., 1959; Zackheim, 1962 and 1963). Metastases have been described in about 80 cases (Pinkus, 1966–67). For these reasons we

cannot subscribe to the view that the tumor is a hamartoma.

In that connection we can mention that, in man, several factors can favor the formation of a basal cell epithelioma, such as light (Pinkus, 1953; Mackie and McGovern, 1958; Howell, 1960; Richter, 1960) and x-rays (Anderson and Anderson, 1951; Stein and Webster, 1958; Maron, 1963). Basal cell epitheliomas have been observed in burn scars (Treves and Pack, 1930; Lawrence, 1952; Gaughan et al., 1969), in smallpox vaccination scars (Goncalves, 1966; Zelickson, 1968), and in a keratoacanthoma scar (Burge and Winkelmann, 1969).

Pinkus (1953, 1959, and 1963) has pointed out the differentiating and dedifferentiating capacities of the epidermal and appendage cells and has thus extended the notion of pluripotentiality, pre-

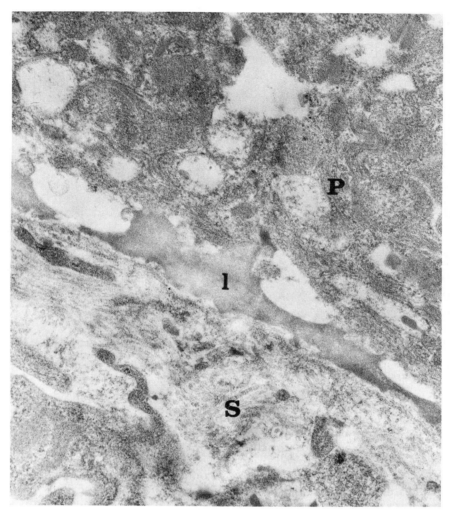

Figure 36–39 In the lower part of a palisade cell *(P)* a lacuna *(l)* is formed. *S*, peritumoral stroma. ×*36,000.*

viously introduced by Krompecher (1903). According to this principle, not only could the ectodermal cell differentiate in several directions, but also every differentiated cell could return again to the primitive cell and, if necessary, develop into other structures. According to Pinkus, the basal tumor cell is derived from a dedifferentiated cell and still has many potentialities, and the difference between it and a normal developing cell would be due to the surrounding stroma. Pinkus thinks that basal cell epithelioma is an aggressive tumor, which can originate anywhere from the ectoderm and which is accompanied by a more or less organized stroma.

This hypothesis, which has been ac-

cepted by many authors (Achten, 1959; Dupont and Piérard, 1961; Woringer, 1961; McMullan, 1962; Niebauer and Raab, 1962; Zackheim, 1963), does not take into account the different physiologic changes which occur in the skin and particularly in the hair follicle. Hair follicles are inconstant structures and undergo cyclic changes (F. Pinkus, 1927; Kligman, 1959). After a period of active growth (anagen phase), a regression of the infra-seboglandular part occurs (catagen phase); it is followed by a resting period (telogen phase). During the catagen period the cells of the prekeratogenous zone dedifferentiate and form a column of undifferentiated epithelial cells (Braun-Falco and

Congr. Dermatol. Syphiligr. Langue Française, Alger, 1959. Paris, Masson, 1961.

Beans, S., and Becker, F. T.: Basal cell carcinoma of the vulva. Arch. Dermatol., 98:284, 1968.

Beck, S. C.: Epitheliome. *In* Jadassohn, J.: Handbuch der Haut- und Geschlechtskrankheiten. Bd. XII/3. Berlin, Springer-Verlag, 1933.

Becker, S. W.: Cutaneous melanoma. Arch. Dermatol. Syph. (Chicago), 21:818, 1930.

Bloch, B.: Ueber benigne, nicht naevoide Melano-epitheliome der Haut nebst Bemerkungen über das Wesen und die Genese der Dendritenzellen. Arch. Dermatol. Syph. (Berl.), 153:20, 1927.

Bonneau, H., and Césarini, J. P.: Contribution des épithéliomas baso-cellulaires pigmentés de la peau à l'étude de la mélanogénèse en microscopie électronique. Bull. Soc. Fr. Dermatol., 74:587, 1967.

Braun-Falco, O.: Histochemische und morphologische Studien an normaler und patologisch veränderter Haut. Arch. Dermatol. Syph. (Berl.), 198:111, 1954.

Braun-Falco, O.: Histochemische Untersuchungen über das Verhalten der β-Glucuronidase—Aktivität bei Psoriasis, Basaliom und spinocellulärem Carcinom. Arch. Klin. Exp. Dermatol., 203:68, 1956.

Braun-Falco, O.: Zur Histotopographie der Phosphorylase bei Basaliom und Psoriasis. Arch. Klin. Exp. Dermatol., 204:175, 1957.

Braun-Falco, O.: Ueber die Histotopographie der Aminopeptidase bei Hauttumoren. Klin. Wochenschr., 35:50, 1957b.

Braun-Falco, O.: Beitrag zum Verhalten der Grundsubstanz bei malignen epithelialen Hauttumoren. Derm. Wochenschr., 135:417, 1957c.

Braun-Falco, O.: Die Histochemie der Haut. *In* Gottron, A., and Schoenfeld, W.: Dermatologie und Venerologie. Bd. I. Stuttgart, Thieme, 1961a.

Braun-Falco, O.: Zur Histotopographie der Cytochromoxydase in normaler und pathologisch veränderter Haut sowie in Hauttumoren. Arch. Klin. Exp. Dermatol., 214:176, 1961b.

Braun-Falco, O.: Histochemische Morphologie der abnormalen Verhornung. Proc. XIIth Int. Congr. Dermatol., Washington, 1962. Amsterdam, Excerpta Medica, 1963.

Braun-Falco, O., and Kint, A.: Zur Dynamik der Katagenphase bei der Albinoratte. Arch. Klin. Exp. Dermatol., 223:1, 1965.

Braun-Falco, O., and Petzoldt, D.: Über die Histotopie von NADH- und NADPH-Tetrazoliumreduktase in menschlicher Haut. II. Pathologisch veränderte Haut und Hauttumoren. Arch. Klin. Exp. Dermatol., 221:410, 1965.

Braun-Falco, O., and Rathjens, B.: Histochemische Untersuchungen über die Lokalisation und Grösse der Bernsteinsäuredehydrogenase-Aktivität bei M. Paget, Basaliom und spinozellulärem Carcinom. Arch. Dermatol. Syph. (Berl.), 199:152, 1955.

Braun-Falco, O., and Thianprasit, M.: L'istologia e l'istochimica del follicolo pilifero nell' alopecia areata. Minerva Dermatol., 38: 252, 1963.

Brett, R., and Braun-Falco, O.: Beitrag zur Differenzierung von Tumoren. Arch. Klin. Exp. Dermatol., 200:515, 1955.

Brett, R., and Rathjens, B.: Zur Differenzierung von Basaliomen, metatypischen Epitheliomen und spinozellulären Carcinomen. Derm. Wochenschr., 128:1195, 1953.

Bunting, H.: The distribution of acid mucopolysaccharides in mammalian tissues as revealed by histochemical methods. Ann. N.Y. Acad. Sci., 52:977, 1950.

Burge, K. M., Winkelmann, R. K.: Keratoacanthoma. Association with basal and squamous cell carcinoma. Arch. Dermatol., 100:306, 1969.

Burstone, M. S.: New histochemical techniques for the demonstration of tissue oxidase (cytochrome oxidase). J. Histochem. Cytochem., 7:112, 1959.

Burstone, M. S.: Histochemical demonstration of cytochrome oxidase with new amine reagents. J. Histochem. Cytochem., 8:63, 1960.

Burstone, M. S.: Modifications of histochemical techniques for the demonstration of cytochrome oxidase. J. Histochem. Cytochem., 9:59, 1961.

Christol-Jalby, B.: La métachromasie dans les épithéliomas basocellulaires. Thèse Toulouse, Imp. Saubiron, 1959.

Darier, J.: Des épithéliomes primitifs de la peau. Br. J. Dermatol., 34:145, 1922.

Darier, J.: *In* Précis de Dermatologie. Paris, Masson, 1923.

Darier, J., and Ferrand, M.: L'épithélioma pavimenteux mixte et intermédiaire. Ann. Dermatol., Série 6, 3:385, 1922.

de Bersaques, J.: Deoxyribonucleic acid in epidermis. J. Invest. Dermatol., 46:40, 1966.

de Bersaques, J.: Leucine aminopeptidase and naphthylamidases in human epidermis. II. Biochemical and histochemical data in psoriasis and basal cell tumors. Arch. Klin. Exp. Dermatol., 234:52, 1969.

Dubreuilh, W., and Auché, B.: De l'ulcus rodens. Clinique et anatomie pathologique. Ann. Dermatol. Syphiligr. (Paris), Série 4, 2:705, 1901.

Dubreuilh, W., and Auché, B.: Diagnostic clinique et histologique de l'ulcus rodens. Ann. Dermatol. Syphiligr. (Paris), Série 4, 3:318, 1902.

Dupont, A., and Piérard, J.: Etude histologique des épithéliomas cutanés basocellulaires et spinocellulaires. *In* Epithéliomas Cutanés. C. R. Xe Congr. Dermatol. et Syphiligr. Langue Française, Alger 1959. Paris, Masson, 1961.

Dutu, R., and Longhin, C.: Histochemical carbohydrate variations in malignant tumors of the skin. Derm. Venereol, 4:97, 1959; Roem. Ref. Z. Haut. Geschlechtskr, 105:91, 1960.

Ehlers, G.: Cytophotometrische Untersuchungen an Basalzellepitheliomen im ultravioletten und sichtbaren Licht. Arch. Klin. Exp. Dermatol., 224:329, 1966.

Ehlers, G.: Vergleichende quantitativ-cytochemische Untersuchungen über den Desoxyribonucleinsäure-und Nucleohiston-Gehalt von Basalzellepitheliomen. Arch. Klin. Exp. Dermatol., 232:102, 1968.

Eller, J. J., and Anderson, N. P.: Basal cell epitheliomas with excessive pigment formation. Arch. Dermatol. Syph. (Chicago), 27:277, 1933.

Falin, L. I.: Glycogen in the epithelium of mucous membranes and skin and its significance. Acta Anat., 46:244, 1961.

Fanger, H., and Barker, B. E.: Histochemical studies of some keratotic and proliferating skin tumours. Arch. Pathol., 64:143, 1957.

Favre, M., Josserand, A., and Martin, J. F.: Tumeurs malignes cutanées. Nouv. Prat. Dermatol., 6:693, 1936.

Feyrter, F.: Über diffuse endokrine epitheliale Organe. Leipzig, Barth, 1938; Ref. Z. Haut. Geschlechtskr., 61:104, 1939.

Foot, N. C.: Adnexal carcinoma of the skin. Am. J. Pathol., 23:1, 1947.

Foraker, A. G., and Wingo, W. J.: Protein-bound sulfhydryl and disulfide groups and succinic dehydrogenase activity in basal cell carcinoma of the skin. Exp. Med., 14:122, 1956.

Freeman, R. G., and Winkelmann, R. K.: Basal cell tumor with eccrine differentiation (eccrine epithelioma). Arch. Dermatol., 100:234, 1969.

Fromme, cited by Andrade, R.: Dermatol. Wochenschr., 173:120, 1958.

Gaté, J., Massia, G., and Delbos, J.: Les épithéliomas basocellulaires pigmentés (contribution à leur étude anatomo-pathologique). Ann. Dermatol. Syphiligr., Série 7, 8:337, 1937.

Gaughan, L. J., Bergeron, J. R., and Mullins, J. F.: Giant basal cell epithelioma developing in acute burn site. Arch. Dermatol., 99:594, 1969.

Godlewski, H. G.: Intracellular carbohydrates in epidermal tumors. IIe Int. Congr. Histochem. Cytochem. Frankfurt, Springer-Verlag, 1964, p. 117.

Goltz, R. W., Fusaro, R. M., and Jarvis, J.: Observations on glycogen in epithelial tumors. J. Invest. Dermatol., 31:331, 1958.

Goltz, R. W., Fusaro, R. M., Blazejowsky, R., and Jarvis, J.: Pathways of carbohydrate metabolism in normal and neoplastic cutaneous ectoderm. A histochemical study. J. Invest. Dermatol., 33:337, 1959a.

Goltz, R. W., Fusaro, R. M., and Jarvis, J.: The carbohydrates in basal cell epitheliomas. A histochemical study. J. Invest. Dermatol., 32:629, 1959b.

Gomori, G.: Microscopic Histochemistry. Chicago, The University of Chicago Press, 1952a.

Gomori, G.: The histochemistry of esterases. Int. Rev. Cytol., 1:323, 1952b.

Goncalves, J. C. A.: Malignant change in smallpox vaccination scars. Arch. Dermatol., 93:229, 1966.

Gottron, H. A.: Karzinomentwicklungen in der Haut. Dtsch. Med. Wochenschr. 82:761–764; 777–778, 1957a.

Gottron, H. A.: Karzinomentwicklungen in der Haut. Dtsch. Med. Wochenschr. 82:802–807; 815–816, 1957b.

Gottron, H. A.: Basaliomprobleme. Dermatol. Wochenschr., 150:220, 1964.

Gottron, H. A., and Nikolowski, W.: Karzinom der Haut. *In* Gottron, H. A., and Schoenfeld, W.: Dermatologie und Venerologie. Bd. IV. Stuttgart, Thieme, 1960, pp. 295–406.

Grogg, E., and Pearse, A. G. E.: A critical study of the histochemical techniques for acid phosphatase, with a description of an azo-dye method. J. Pathol. Bacteriol., 64:627, 1952.

Grixoni, F., and Ventura, B.: Gli acidi nucleinici nelle neoplasie cutanee dermatosi neoplasiformi. G. Ital. Dermatol. Syph., 92:296, 1951.

Haythorn, S. R.: Studies on the histogenesis of the so-called "basal-cell carcinoma." Am. J. Cancer Suppl., 15: 1969, 1931.

Hernaman-Johnson, F.: The treatment of rodent ulcer (basal cell epithelioma), with especial reference to recurrence. Lancet, 1:389, 1926.

Herzberg, J.: Das Stroma als wichtiges, gestaltendes Prinzip in der Klinik und Histologie der Basaliome. Z. Haut. Geschlechtskr., 16:340, 1954.

Hieronimi, G.: Über Vorkommen und Verteilung saurer Mucopolysaccharide in Geschwülsten. Frankfurt. Z. Pathol., 65:409, 1954.

Howell, J. B.: The sunlight factor in aging and skin cancer. Arch. Dermatol. 82:865, 1960.

Hueck, W.: Zur Morphologie der epithelialen Tumoren insbesondere der Basaliome. Virchows Arch. Pathol. Anat., 314:137, 1947.

Jessner, M., and Biberstein, H.: A sweat gland tumor. Dermatologica, 107:97, 1953.

Johnson, D. E.: Basal-cell epithelioma of the palm. Arch. Dermatol., 82:253, 1960.

Johnson, W. C., and Helwig, E. B.: Histochemistry of the acid mucopolysaccharides of skin in normal and in certain pathologic conditions. Am. J. Clin. Pathol., 40:123, 1963.

Johnson, W. C., Graham, J. H., and Helwig, E. B.: Histochemistry of the acid mucopolysaccharides in cutaneous calcification. J. Invest. Dermatol., 42:215, 1964.

Juon, M.: Ueber die "metatypischen" Formen der Hautepitheliome. Arch. Dermatol. Syph. (Berl.), 157:81, 1929.

Kabat, E. A., and Furth, J.: A histochemical study of the distribution of alkaline phosphatase in various normal and neoplastic tissues. Am. J. Pathol., 17:303, 1941.

Kint, A.: Histophotometric investigation of the nuclear DNA-content in normal epidermis, seborrheic keratosis, keratosis senilis, squamous-cell carcinoma and basal-cell carcinoma. J. Invest. Dermatol., 40:95, 1963.

Kint, A.: Contribution à l'étude des acides nucléiques au cours de la différentiation épidermique normale et pathologique. Arch. Belg. Dermatol., 20:243, 1964.

Kint, A.: Histogenetische Studie van het Basocellulair Epithelioma. Brussels, Arscia, 1966.

Kint, A.: Histogenetic study of the basal cell epithelioma. *In* Current Problems in Dermatology. Vol. 3. Basel, S. Karger, 1970, pp. 82–123.

Kligman, A. M.: The human hair cycle. J. Invest. Dermatol., 33:307, 1959.

Kobayasi, T.: Dermo-epidermal junction in basal cell carcinoma. Acta Derm. Venereol. (Stockh.), 50: 401, 1970.

Kopf, A. W.: The distribution of alkaline phosphatase in normal and pathologic human skin. Arch. Dermatol., 75:1, 1957.

Krompecher, E.: Der Basalzellenkrebs. Jena, G. Fischer, 1903.

Lapière, S., and Piérard, J.: Contribution à l'étude clinique et histologique de l'épithélioma morphéiforme. Ann. Dermatol. Syphiligr., (Paris), 81:365, 1954.

Laquerrière, R., Laumonier, R., and Stewart, W. M.: Essai d'étude histophotométrique des tumeurs cutanées. C. R. Xe Congr. Dermatol. Langue Fr., Alger. Paris, Masson, 1961, pp. 111–122.

Lawrence, E. A.: Carcinoma arising in the scars of

thermal burns. Surg. Gynecol. Obstet., 95:579, 1952.

Lengyel, J., and Vertes, B.: Hyaluronsäure – Untersuchungen an lokalen Myxödemen und im Stroma der Hautkrebse. Dermatologica, 113:219, 1956.

Lennox, B., and Wells, A. L.: Differentiation in the rodent ulcer group of tumours. Br. J. Cancer, 5:195, 1951.

Lever, W. F.: Pathogenesis of benign tumours of cutaneous appendages and of basal cell epithelioma. Arch. Dermatol., 57:679–708; 709–734, 1948.

Lever, W. F.: Histopathology of the Skin. Ed. 4. Philadelphia, J. B. Lippincott Co., 1967.

Lever, W. F., and Hashimoto, K.: Electron microscopic and histochemical findings in basal cell epithelioma and squamous cell carcinoma. Verh. XIII. Int. Congr. Dermatol., München, 1967. Berlin, Springer-Verlag, 1968.

Lund, H. Z.: Tumors of the Skin. Washington, D. C., Armed Forces Institute of Pathology, 1957.

Mackie, B. S., and McGovern, V. J.: The mechanism of solar carcinogenesis. Arch. Dermatol., 78:218, 1958.

Majewska, H., Majewski, C., Radzicki, J., and Leja, Z.: Acid mucopolysaccharides in the ground substance of connective tissue in cancer of the skin. Cancer, 18:388, 1965.

Mallory, F. B.: Recent progress in the microscopic anatomy and differentiation of cancer. J. Am. Med. Assoc., 55:1513, 1910.

Mallory, F. B.: The Principles of Pathologic Histology. Philadelphia, W. B. Saunders Company, 1914.

Marcus, S. L.: Basal cell and basal-squamous cell carcinomas of the vulva. Am. J. Obstet. Gynecol., 79:461, 1960.

Maron, H.: Basaliom bei Kindern. Dermatol. Wochenschr., 147:545, 1963.

Masson, P.: Tumeurs Humaines, Histologie, Diagnostic et Techniques. Paris, Maloine, 1956, pp. 328–341.

McMullan, F. H.: Basal cell tumors. Proc. 12e Int. Congr. Dermatol., 2:1595, 1962.

Moberger, G.: Malignant transformation of squamous epithelium. Acta Radiol., Suppl. 112, 1954, pp. 7–108.

Montgomery, H.: Superficial epitheliomatosis. Arch. Dermatol. Syph. (Chicago), 20:339, 1929.

Moore, R. D., Stevenson, J., and Schönberg, M. D.: The response of connective tissue associated with tumors of the skin. Am. J. Clin. Pathol., 34:125, 1960.

Nachlas, M. M., Tsou, K. C., De Souza, E., Cheng, C., and Seligman, A. M.: Cytochemical demonstration of succinic dehydrogenase by the use of a new *p*-nitro-phenyl substituted ditetrazole. J. Histochem. Cytochem., 5:420, 1957.

Nachlas, M. M., Walker, D. G., and Seligman, A. M.: A histochemical method for the demonstration of diphosphopyridine nucleotide diaphorase. J. Biophys. Biochem. Cytol., 4:29, 1958a.

Nachlas, M. M., Walker, D. G., and Seligman, A. M.: The histochemical localization of triphosphopyridine nucleotide diaphorase. J. Biophys. Biochem. Cytol., 4:467, 1958b.

Nachlas, M. M., Monis, B., Rosenblatt, D. H., and Seligman, A. M.: Improvement of the histochemical localization of leucine aminopeptidase with a new substrate L-leucyl-4-methoxy-β-naphthylamide J. Biophys. Biochem. Cytol., 7:261, 1960.

Nel, R. W.: Basal cell carcinoma of the vulva. S. Afr. Med. J., 31:381, 1957.

Niebauer, G.: Der Pigmentstoffwechsel als neurohormonales Problem. Arch. Klin. Exp. Dermatol., 206:770, 1957.

Niebauer, G., and Raab, W.: Ueber das Basaliom der Haut. Wien. Klin. Wochenschr., 74:476, 1962.

Niebauer, G., and Sediko, N.: Ueber die Dendritenzellen der Epidermis. Eine Studie über die Langerhans-Zellen in der normalen und ekzematösen Haut des Meerschweinchens. Arch. Klin. Exp. Dermatol., 222:23, 1965.

Nishiyama, S.: Capillardarstellung durch die alkalische Phosphatase-Färbung bei verschiedenen Dermatosen. VI. Epitheliale Tumoren. Hautarzt, 15:175, 1964.

Ochoa, P. C., Schmidt, O. D., and Swerdlow, M.: The dermal-epidermal junction. A preliminary study with periodic-acid–schiff stain. Arch. Dermatol. Syph. (Chicago), 75:70, 1957.

Ogura, R., Knox, J., and Griffin, C.: Quantitative studies of epidermal SH. J. Invest. Dermatol., 36:29, 1961.

Okun, M. R., and Blumental, G.: Basal cell epithelioma with giant cells and nuclear atypicality. Arch. Dermatol., 89:598, 1964.

Pascher, F.: Basal-cell epithelioma of the sole. Arch. Dermatol., 67:108, 1953.

Pascher, F., and Sims, C.: Basal cell epitheliomas of the sole. Arch. Dermatol., 69:475, 1954.

Pautrier, L. M., and Diss: Epithélioma baso-cellulaire pigmentaire du cuir chevelu. Bull. Soc. Fr. Dermatol. Syphiligr., 36:498, 1929.

Pearse, A. G. E.: Histochemistry. Theoretical and Applied. London, Churchill, 1962.

Petzoldt, D., and Braun-Falco, O.: Enzyme des energieliefernden Stoffwechsels in Basaliomen. Hautarzt, 19:509, 1968.

Piérard, J.: De l'épithéliome pagétoïde aux carcinoides d'Arning. Arch. Belg. Dermatol. 4:147, 1948.

Piérard, J., and Dupont, A.: Nodular epithelioma. Br. J. Dermatol., 60:50, 1948.

Piérard, J., and Kint, A.: A propos de l'histologie des épithéliomas basocellulaires. Note préliminaire. Arch. Belg. Dermatol., 17:297, 1961.

Piérard, J., and Kint, A.: Constatations récentes au sujet de la structure de l'épithélioma basocellulaire. Ann. Dermatol. Syphiligr. (Paris), 89:121, 1962.

Piérard, J., and Kint, A.: Etude histochimique de quelques enzymes dans l'épithélioma basocellulaire. Arch. Belg. Dermatol., 22:109, 1966.

Piérard, J., and Kint, A.: Distribution des hydrates de carbone dans l'épithélioma basocellulaire. Bull. Soc. Fr. Dermatol. Syphiligr., 74:735, 1967.

Piérard, J., de Bersaques, J., and Kint, A.: L'élastose sénile. *In* Maladies du tissu élastique cutané. C. R. XIIe Congrés Dermatol. Syph. Langue Française, Paris, 1965. Paris, Masson, 1968.

Pinkus, F.: Die normale Anatomie der Haut. *In* Jadassohn, J.: Handbuch der Haut- und Geschlechtskrankheiten. Bd. I/1. Berlin, Springer-Verlag, 1927, pp. 1–378.

Pinkus, H.: Premalignant fibroepithelial tumours of the skin. Arch. Dermatol., 67:598, 1953.

Pinkus, H.: Keratosis senilis. A biologic concept of its pathogenesis and diagnosis based on the study of normal epidermis and 1,730 seborrheic and senile keratoses. Am. J. Clin. Pathol., 29:193, 1958.

Pinkus, H.: Zur Entwicklung des Haarfollikels beim Menschen, insbesondere des Infundibulums und des bindegewebigen Anteils. Hautarzt, 10:164, 1959a.

Pinkus, H.: Clinical, histologic and differential considerations. *In* Rothman, S.: The Human Integument. Washington, D.C., American Association for the Advancement of Science, 1959b.

Pinkus, H.: Skin cancer and basic research in dermatology. J. Invest. Dermatol., 33:171, 1959c.

Pinkus, H.: Histogenesis of skin cancer. Proc. XIIth Int. Congr. Dermatology, Washington, 1962. New York, Excerpta Medica, 1963.

Pinkus, H.: Zur Begriffsbestimmung der Naevi, Organnaevi und naevoiden Tumoren. Hautarzt, 16:184, 1965a.

Pinkus, H.: Epithelial and fibroepithelial tumors. Arch. Dermatol., 91:24, 1965b.

Pinkus, H.: The border line between cancer and noncancer. Yearbook of Dermatology. Chicago, Year Book Medical Publishers, 1966–67, pp. 5–34.

Pruniéras, M.: Essai d'application du test de Brachet en histopathologie cutanée. Bull. Soc. Fr. Dermatol. Syphiligr. 64:117, 1954.

Puente-Duany, N.: Pigmented basal cell epitheliomas. Arch. Cuba. Cancer., 7:287, 1948. Ref.: Br. J. Dermatol., 62:341, 1950.

Richter, R.: Das Hautkarzinom in seinen Formen und seinen Beziehungen zu ethnologischen und klimatologischen Faktoren. Dermatol. Wochenschr., 142:1025, 1960.

Rothberg, S., and van Scott, E. J.: Absence of normal epidermal protein in basal cell tumour. J. Invest. Dermatol., 42:141, 1964.

Rupec, M., and Vakilzadeh, F.: Über das Vorkommen von mehrkernigen Riesenzellen in Basaliomen. Arch. Klin. Exp. Dermatol., 235:198, 1969.

Sams, W. M., Smith, J. G., and Davidson, E. A.: The connective tissue histochemistry of normal and some pathological skin. J. Histochem. Cytochem., 10:710, 1962.

Sams, W. M., Smith, J. G., and Finlayson, G. R.: The histochemistry of the basal cell epithelioma. J. Invest. Dermatol., 41:457, 1963.

Sanderson, K. V.: Interaction between epithelial and mesodermal elements in anthramine-induced tumours of the rat. Nature (Lond.), 194:95, 1962.

Schueller, E. F.: Basal cell carcinoma of the vulva. Am. J. Obstet. Gynecol., 93:199, 1965.

Serri, F.: The distribution of glycogen and succinic-dehydrogenase in certain skin diseases. Trans. St. John's Hosp. Dermatol. Soc., 40:57, 1958.

Siegler, A. M., and Greene, H. J.: Basal cell carcinoma of the vulva: A report of five cases and review of the literature. Am. J. Obstet. Gynecol., 62:1219, 1951.

Sirsat, S. M.: Electron microscopic studies of fine structure of basal cell carcinoma. Proc. 1st Reg. Conf. in Asia and Oceania, Tokyo, 1956, pp. 227–233.

Smith, O. D., and Swerdlow, M. A.: Histogenesis of basal-cell epithelioma. Arch. Dermatol., 74:286, 1956.

Spier, H. W., and Martin, K.: Histochemische Untersuchungen über die Phosphomonoesterasen der gesunden Haut mit Hinweis auf Befunde bei Hauterkrankungen. Arch. Klin. Exp. Dermatol., 202:120, 1956.

Steigleder, G. K.: Die Histochemie der Epidermis und ihrer Anhangsgebilde. Arch. Klin. Exp. Dermatol., 206:276, 1957.

Steigleder, G. K., and Kamei, Y.: Die Beziehung zwischen Tumoren der Haut und umgebendem Bindegewebe (proteolytische Aktivität im Parenchym und Stroma von Hauttumoren und ihre Beziehung zur Gewebsmetachromasie). Arch. Klin. Exp. Dermatol., 217:457, 1963.

Steigleder, G. K., and Löffler, H.: Zum histochemischen Nachweis unspezifischer Esterasen und Lipasen. Arch. Klin. Exp. Dermatol., 203:41, 1956.

Stein, H. L., and Webster, G. V.: Basal cell carcinoma in children. Am. J. Surg., 96:445, 1958.

Steiner, K.: A histochemical study of epidermal glycogen in skin diseases. J. Invest. Dermatol., 24:599, 1955.

Steiner, K.: Mucoid substances and cutaneous connective tissue in dermatoses. J. Invest. Dermatol., 28:387, 1957.

Steiner, K.: Sulfur levels in normal and pathologic epidermis. J. Invest. Dermatol., 34:189, 1960.

Swerdlow, M.: Histogenesis of basal-cell carcinoma. Arch. Dermatol., 78:563, 1958.

Thiery, M.: Bijdrage tot de Kennis van het Experimentele Cervico-Vaginale Carcinoma. Brussels, Arscia, 1962.

Thies, W.: Über die Brauchbarkeit einer modifizierten Osmiumjodidmethode zur Darstellung des Nervensystems der Haut. Hautarzt, 13:12, 1962.

Touraine, A.: Les épithéliomas pigmentés de la peau. Ann. Dermatol. Syphiligr. (Paris), Série 7, 6:785 1935.

Treves, N., and Pack, G. T.: The development of cancer in burn scars. Surg. Gynecol. Obstet., 51:749, 1930.

Umiker, W., and Director, W.: Fibrosing basal cell epithelioma. Arch. Dermatol. 69:486, 1954.

Wallace, S. A., and Halpert, B.: Trichoma: tumour of hair anlage. Arch. Pathol., 50:199, 1950.

Ward, J.: Five cases of basal cell carcinoma of the vulva. J. Obstet. Gynaecol. Br. Emp., 63:697, 1956.

Warren, S., Gates, O., and Butterfield, P. W.: The value of histologic differentiation of basal cell carcinomas. New Engl. J. Med., 215:1060, 1936.

Wells, G. C.: Esterases in cutaneous granulomata. Br. J. Dermatol., 69:415, 1957.

Welton, D. G., Elliot, J. A., and Kimmerstiel, P.: Epithelioma: clinical and histologic data on 1,925 lesions. Arch. Dermatol., 60:277, 1949.

Wiedmann, A.: Ueber das neurohormonale System der Haut. Hautarzt, 14:60, 1963.

Willinghagen, R. G. J.: Histochemisch onderzoek van de activiteit van alkalische en zure fosfatase in normaal en in pathologisch veranderd menselijk weefsel. Dissert., Leiden, 1960.

Wolff, K.: Zur Orthotopie der histochemisch erfassbaren Aminopeptidasenaktivität der menschlichen Haut. Arch. Klin. Exp. Dermatol., 217:534, 1963.

Wolff, K., and Holubar, K.: Zur Histochemie des Basalioms. Arch. Klin. Exp. Dermatol., 223:483, 1965.

Wood, G. M., Pranich, K., and Beerman, H.: Investigation of possible apocrine gland component in basal-cell epithelioma. J. Invest. Dermatol., 30: 273, 1958.

Woringer, F.: Classification et histogenèse des épithéliomas cutanés. Xe Congr. Dermatol. Langue Fr., Alger, 1959. Paris, Masson, 1961.

Zackheim, H. S.: The origin of experimental basal cell epithelioma in the rat. J. Invest. Dermatol., 38:57, 1962.

Zackheim, H. S.: Origin of human basal cell epithelioma. J. Invest. Dermatol., 40:281, 1963.

Zackheim, H. S., Simpson, W. L., and Langs, L.: Basal cell epitheliomas and other skin tumors produced in rats and mice by anthramine and methylcholanthrene. J. Invest. Dermatol. 33:385, 1959.

Zelickson, A. S.: An electron microscope study of the basal cell epithelioma. J. Invest. Dermatol., 39: 183, 1962.

Zelickson, A. S.: The pigmented basal cell epithelioma. Arch. Dermatol., 96:524, 1967.

Zelickson, A. S.: Basal cell epithelioma at site and following smallpox vaccination. Arch. Dermatol., 98:35, 1968.

Zelickson, A. S., Goltz, R. W., and Hartmann, J. F.: A histologic and electron microscopic study of a pigmented basal cell epithelioma. J. Invest. Dermatol., 36:299, 1961.

Zugerman, I.: Basal-cell epithelioma of the sole. Arch. Dermatol., 76:247, 1957.

37

The Nevoid Basal Cell Carcinoma Syndrome

J. B. Howell, M.D., and
David E. Anderson, Ph.D.

DEFINITION

The nevoid basal cell carcinoma syndrome is a genetic entity characterized by five major components: multiple basal cell carcinomas with an early age at onset; epithelium-lined jaw cysts with unique multiple mural cysts in the connective tissue stroma; diagnostic pits of the hands or feet or both; a variety of anomalies of the skull, ribs, and spine; and ectopic calcification. Other less frequent signs include multiple milia; cysts of the skin, ovaries, and mesentery; a hypophosphaturic response to parathyroid hormone with or without brachymetacarpalism; medulloblastoma; and various ocular anomalies (Clendenning et al., 1964; Howell et al., 1964; Maddox et al., 1964).

The occurrence of multiple basal cell carcinomas in association with various anomalies was first recognized and established as the basal cell nevus syndrome by Howell and Caro (1959). Although Binkley and Johnson (1951) had previously described the essential components of the syndrome, they had interpreted the tumors as epithelioma adenoides cysticum, an interpretation repeated by Gross (1953) and confirmed by Lund (1957). Howell and Caro, however, recognized that the behavior of the tumors was not consistent with the benign behavior of Brooke/Fordyce tumors, which fail to transform into multiple basal cell carcinomas and are not typically associated with developmental defects, although the microscopic features of the two types of tumors are sometimes strikingly similar. They retained Nomland's (1932) terminology of basal cell nevus until further investigation might clarify the nomenclature. They further emphasized the sinister character of the tumors in the young adult. The report by Gorlin and Goltz (1960) a year later served to confirm the concept of the basal cell nevus syndrome.

Since 1959, close to 300 cases have been reported in the literature, indicating not only increased awareness and recognition of the syndrome by a variety of medical specialists throughout the world but also a much more frequently occurring entity than was initially suspected. Although the entity is comprised of many varied components, the basal cell nevi or nevoid basal cell carcinomas, as they are now called, constitute the most obvious and serious component. The tumors have further interest since they represent a prototype of an inherited form of basal cell carcinoma.

GENETIC FEATURES

The syndrome, regardless of the degree of expression, has been repeatedly demonstrated to have a genetic basis and to follow an autosomal dominant mode of inheritance (Anderson et al., 1967). Penetrance of the gene is high and of the order of 97 percent; thus, virtually all individuals carrying the gene manifest the syndrome in one form or another. A hint of linkage between the gene locus for the syndrome and the Rh blood group was recently detected, raising the intriguing possibility that both genes are in close proximity on the same chromosome (Anderson, 1968). This finding is still in need of confirmation.

The syndrome gene is apparently influenced by other genetic or extraneous environmental factors or both, since expression of the syndrome varies more among than within families. Some families may be characterized by extreme multiplicity and early onset of cutaneous tumors and a low frequency of skeletal anomalies, while others may show a low degree of cutaneous involvement but a high degree of skeletal involvement, and so on. Some of this variability in expression is undoubtedly the consequence of age differences, because cutaneous lesions, ectopic calcification, and some other components increase at differing rates with increasing age. Skeletal anomalies, however, are congenital and thus show no age association, but yet they vary more in frequency and type among families than within families. This indicates that the variability among families is not entirely the consequence of age differences but also involves other genetic or environmental factors or both.

Although the syndrome has a genetic basis, not all patients will always have a positive family history of the syndrome. In fact, in a series of 47 index patients known to have the syndrome by cutaneous, microscopic, and radiologic examinations, family studies indicated that two-thirds of the patients had positive family histories of the syndrome, while the remaining one-third were sporadic occurrences, possibly representing new mutations or phenocopies (Anderson, 1970). A negative family history in a patient does not, however, necessarily argue against a genetic basis. Such a patient could still transmit the syndrome gene to approximately 50 percent of his or her subsequent children, as expected with dominant inheritance.

It should also be emphasized that a positive family history of multiple basal cell carcinoma may occur in the absence of other features of the syndrome. Among 20 other index patients with multiple basal cell carcinomas but with no other clinical or radiographic signs of the syndrome, over one-half had positive family histories of basal cell carcinoma, but not of the syndrome per se (Anderson, 1970). Whether these familial occurrences of basal cell carcinoma refer to a different entity caused by a different gene(s), to a different allele(s) at the syndrome locus, to minimal expression of the syndrome gene, or to other unrecognized causes is yet to be determined.

No constant abnormality in chromosome number or structure has been observed in patients with the syndrome. One report describes an abnormally long arm of one of the number 1 chromosomes in one patient with the syndrome, but the same chromosome abnormality was observed in relatives not having the syndrome (Yunis and Gorlin, 1963). Another report describes marker chromosomes in two cases of the syndrome (Mills and Foulkes, 1967); however, marker chromosomes have been observed in phenotypically normal individuals. An unpublished study of seven syndrome patients indicated no evidence of marker chromosomes or changes in chromosome number or structure (Anderson, 1970).

AGE AT ONSET

The various components comprising the syndrome are expressed at different ages (Anderson et al., 1967). Since some of the components are present at birth, the syndrome per se is congenital. The skeletal component is the most frequent anomaly present at birth. The skin tumors, although they may be present at birth, generally develop later during the first or second decades or possibly during the third decade, but rarely later. Their average age at onset varies for different families. In one well-documented family the average was 7 years (Anderson et al., 1963), and in another it was 14 years (Anderson and Cook, 1966). The cysts of the jaws in these same families occurred at an average age of 13 years. The onset of ectopic calcification, which is more difficult to document, is probably after the skin tumors or jaw cysts but usually before detection of the pitting defect of the hands and feet.

Of the various components, only the skin cancers and the jaw cysts typically cause signs and symptoms. They are thus the two components through which the syndrome is most frequently first encountered and detected (Maddox et al., 1964).

NEVOID BASAL CELL CARCINOMAS

Distribution

The face and neck area is a common site for tumor development in some patients, while the trunk is favored in others; in still others, the distribution is more generalized. The tumors may be few in number but usually they are numerous, occasionally numbering well into the hundreds. Multiplicity of tumors with early onset and unrelenting development of new tumors throughout life are the primary characteristics of the disease (Howell and Caro, 1959; Howell et al., 1964; Binkley and Johnson, 1951; Anderson and Cook, 1966; Clarkson and Wilson, 1959).

Tumors in the mid-facial area, i.e., the periorbital region, eyelids, nose, malar region, and upper lip, pose a serious threat to the tissues in these areas. Rapidly growing and deeply infiltrating tumors in the eyelids may lead to loss of one or both eyes, and tumors in the ala nasi may lead to loss of portions of the nose (Fig. 37–1). The tumors may also lead to loss of life from uncontrolled progressive disease (Taylor et al., 1968). The attending physician must

be alert to the seriousness of these tumors and the importance of early detection and tumor removal to avoid possible serious consequences of the disease.

The tumors may also develop, but less frequently, on the abdomen, limbs, and scalp, or occasionally, on the genitalia, nasal vestibule, helix, concha, external auditory meatus, or the hand and/or foot.

A previously unrecognized facet concerning tumor distribution is the heavy concentration of tumors in the neck region of children who have the syndrome and develop medulloblastoma. A collar of tumors, as shown in Figure 37–2, which is a composite drawing of previously reported cases, could serve to identify children at risk to medulloblastoma.

Natural History

Nevoid basal cell carcinomas behave as benign, nonaggressive tumors before puberty. To our knowledge, no examples of ulceration, infiltration, or destructive behavior have been observed during the first decade of life. The tumors grow slowly, vary in size from 0.5 to 2 or 5 mm., and remain relatively quiescent. The tumors in this age period, as a rule, do not require treatment except perhaps for cosmetic reasons. During adolescence and the early twenties, individual tumors may begin to enlarge and ulcerate. These tumors and/or those involving strategic sites around the eyes and nose should be treated at this time, preferably by curettage and electrodesiccation. The seriousness of the tumors in adult years must be recognized, because the trend is for accelerated growth and continued development of crops of new tumors at varying frequencies and different grades of severity throughout life. In later decades there appears to be little or no decrease in the number of new tumors and no decline in the destructive behavior of the tumors. Spontaneous regression has not been observed, except on grafted skin, as reported by Clarkson and Wilson (1959) and Blackwell and McComb (1969). From our experience and study of the literature, the eyelids, periorbital region, nose, and central facial area are particularly vulnerable to rapid growth

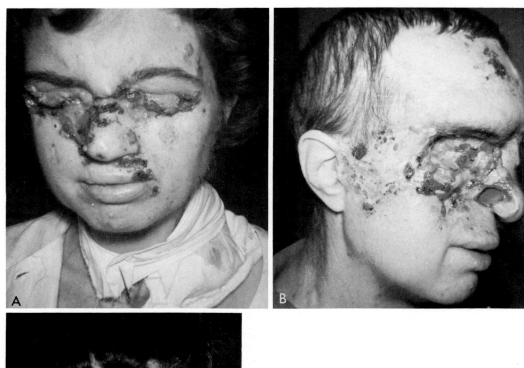

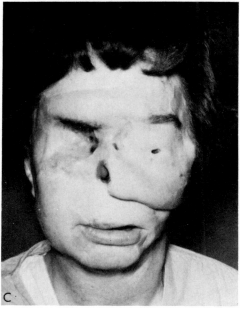

Figure 37–1   Multiple nevoid basal cell carcinomas infiltrating upper lip, nose, and eyelid areas, necessitating radical surgical treatment.

and deep infiltration of one or more tumors (Burgoon et al., 1968). The superficial flat lesion, if untreated, may slowly penetrate deeply into the soft tissues and, indeed, into the boney structures of the skull with disastrous consequence (Taylor et al., 1968; Clarkson and Wilson, 1959).

The aggressiveness of the nevoid tumors in some patients is no more than would be expected in patients with multiple basal cell carcinomas resulting from other causes. But too frequently, the nevoid tumors are more aggressive than those induced by arsenic, ionizing radiation, or ultraviolet light. Nevoid tumors, however, are less aggressive and have a better prognosis than most multiple basal cell carcinomas occurring in xeroderma pigmentosum, although they may approach the severity and destructiveness of that disease

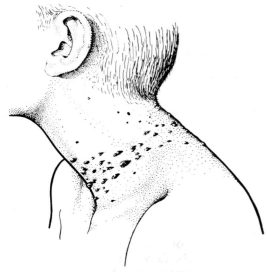

Figure 37–2 Composite drawing of collar distribution of multiple nevoid basal cell carcinomas seen in children also developing medulloblastoma.

in later decades. If the severity of multiple basal cell carcinomas is greatest in xeroderma pigmentosum, then next in severity, in our judgment, are the nevoid basal cell carcinomas, followed by those induced by ionizing radiation, arsenic, and, lastly, those resulting from prolonged ultraviolet light exposure, as in farmer's skin.

Clinical Types

All the clinical types of basal cell carcinomas have been observed in syndrome patients with the exception of the rare, morphea-like lesion. The tumors may be papular, pedunculated, pigmented, nodular, erythematous, or ulcerated, with several varieties occurring in the same patient. The flat lesions are predominant on the trunk, while the papular and nodular varieites are common in the facial area (Howell et al., 1964).

Microscopically, the nevoid tumors assume a wide spectrum of appearances, resembling benign adnexal tumors in some cases or frank basal cell carcinomas in others. There are no reported histopathologic, histochemical, or electron microscopic features that clearly differentiate the nevoid from the ordinary type of basal cell carcinoma.

A striking feature of the tumors, especially in children, is the wide discrepancy between their harmless, benign, clinical appearance and their histologic appearance. Incipient, nonaggressive tumors in children may resemble milia, molluscum contagiosum, or cystic lesions, but histopathologically they are, from initial onset, basal cell carcinomas.

Differential Diagnosis

Differentiation of nevoid basal cell carcinomas from a lengthy list of clinically similar tumors is simplified by histopathologic examination. Other distinguishing features include early age of onset, tendency to develop from multiple or multicentric foci, site of involvement, genetic etiology, and the occurrence of associated lesions in other tissue systems. Multiple benign cystic epithelioma, or the Brooke/Fordyce tumor, however, has several overlapping cutaneous, histopathologic, and genetic features and differentiation between these two diseases may sometimes be difficult. This commonality may explain why Brooke/Fordyce tumors were formerly confused with nevoid basal cell carcinomas (Graham et al., 1965).

Although an individual tumor in a patient with benign cystic epithelioma may transform into a basal cell carcinoma, multiple tumors do not undergo transformation in these patients, while in the syndrome, the cancers are typically multiple and aggressive. Graham et al. (1965) demonstrated the presence of bone in some of the cutaneous tumors in approximately one-third of their syndrome patients—a nondiagnostic feature, but one that was absent in the Brooke/Fordyce tumor. They also observed an abundance of sulfated acid mucopolysaccharides in nevoid basal cell carcinoma with the adenoid pattern, while most of the acidic substance in the Brooke/Fordyce tumor was hyaluronic acid. The blood vessels in Brooke/Fordyce tumors were also sparse and more organized, while a prominent proliferation of the capillary endothelial tissues characterized the syndrome tumors.

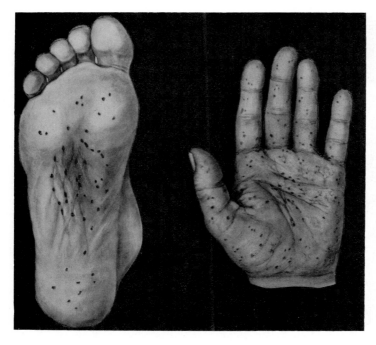

Figure 37–5 Composite drawing of pits of hand and foot. *(From* Howell and Mehregan: Arch. Dermatol., 102:587, 1970. Copyright 1970, American Medical Association.

years, while tumors have continued to develop on nongrafted areas of the skin (Figs. 37–3 and 37–4).

Dermabrasion and 5-fluorouracil are not recommended treatment modalities for nevoid basal cell carcinomas.

PITS OF THE HANDS AND FEET

In addition to the nevoid basal cell carcinomas, pits of the hands and feet are another and perhaps pathognomonic hallmark of the syndrome (Figs. 37–5 and 37–6). They are permanent and specific and, when present, permit a definite diagnosis of the disorder by visual inspection alone. They differ in numerous ways from porokeratosis of Mantoux (Howell and Mehregan, 1970).

They are found only on the hands and feet and are observed in approximately two-thirds of syndrome patients (Dodd et al., 1970). The pits are shallow, nonpalpable depressions, approximately 1 to 3 mm. in depth and diameter. Occasionally they may also occur as large depressions 5 to 10 mm. in diameter.

The pits, which usually are individual but may be grouped or confluent, are irregular and multiform in shape. They may follow the palmar or plantar creases or appear between the creases. The color at the base is flesh-colored, pink, or red. They give the impression of a depression caused by gouging of soft skin by a dull instrument, but they result from a partial or

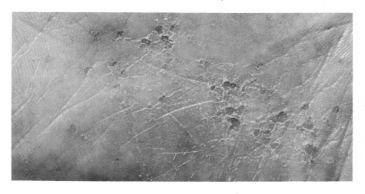

Figure 37–6 Pits of foot.

complete absence of the stratum corneum (Zackheim et al., 1966).

Because of the asymptomatic nature of the pits, the patients are usually unaware of them, and consequently their age at onset is not easily determined. We know of no reports of pits being present at birth or infancy, although they have been observed in children younger than 10 years of age (Anderson, 1970; Braverman, Personal communication). They seemingly become manifest in the majority of cases during or after the second decade of life.

Primary basal cell carcinoma of the hand or foot is a rarity, even in the syndrome. Ward (1960) has an illustration of a basal cell cancer of the foot, and Taylor (1970) observed one on the palm, which recurred two years after surgical excision of a basal cell cancer in a syndrome patient. Holubar et al. (1970) and Howell and Mehregan (1970) recorded the interesting microscopic finding of basal cell epithelioma of palmar pits.

Histopathologically, the palmo-plantar pits show distinctive changes (Howell and Mehregan, 1970). Each pit is characterized by a 2- to 3-mm. punched-out area, showing an absence of a compact keratin layer

(Zackheim et al., 1966). The epidermis at the floor of the pit is somewhat thinner than surrounding areas and shows irregularity in the size and shape of rete ridges and their corresponding papillae. The rete ridges are made up mainly of immature small basaloid cells. There is no sharp line of demarcation between the abnormal epithelium at the base of the pit and the surrounding epidermis. In some areas crowding of basaloid cells extends beyond the limit of the pit and may involve two or three rete ridges in the surrounding area. Maturation of the epidermal cells proceeds only within the suprapapillary plate. In this area, the large and polygonal prickle cells are not formed, and instead the small basaloid cells transform directly into flattened granular cells. At the surface of the epidermis, the keratin layer is very thin and appears noncoherent and flaky. The granular layer is much thinner than normal and absent in some areas. Dermal changes include papillary telangiectasia and engorgement of the dilated capillaries with erythrocytes. Other dermal changes include a mild perivascular lymphocytic infiltrate, relative increase in the number of mast cells, presence of scattered macro-

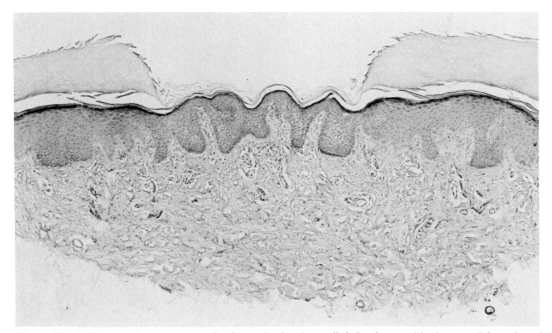

Figure 37–7 Microscopic appearance of palmar pit, showing well-defined area with absence of dense keratin layer and irregularity of epidermal rete ridges. *H & E,* ×75. (*From* Howell and Mehregan: Arch. Dermatol., 102:593, 1970. Copyright 1970, American Medical Association.)

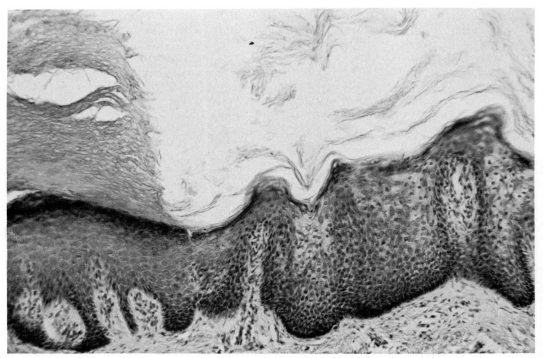

Figure 37–8 Border of pit from palm, demonstrating rete ridges populated by small basaloid cells. Note vacuolation of epidermal cells. Stratum granulosum consists of one or two layers of cells. Keratin layer is thin and flaky. *H & E, × 180.*

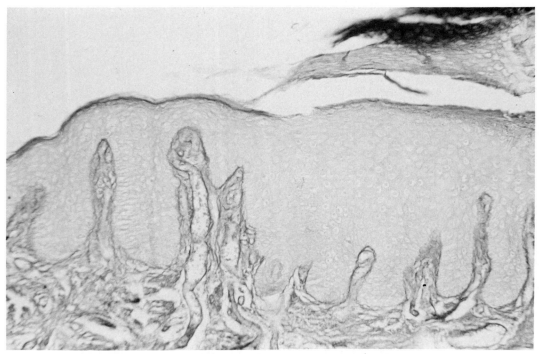

Figure 37–9 Border of pit from palm depicting telangiectatic capillaries within a dermal papilla. *Alcian blue–PAS, ×225.* (*From* Howell and Mehregan: Arch. Dermatol., 102:595, 1970. Copyright 1970, American Medical Association.)

phages containing melanin pigment, and disorganization or loss of the superficial network of elastic fibers (Figs. 37–7 to 37–9).

OTHER CUTANEOUS LESIONS

Multiple epithelium-lined cysts of the skin and milia of the face, both characterized by an early age at onset, are two other frequently observed stigmata of the syndrome. The milia are generally asymptomatic and only of cosmetic concern. They are too nonspecific to be of diagnostic importance. The cysts have a generalized distribution but often occur on the fingers, hands, or feet, where they may interfere with normal function. Some cysts have an open or enlarged pore with a comedone in the orifice. On the sole, the pore may be filled with keratin, and it resembles plantar hyperkeratosis (Howell and Mehregan, 1970). Infection of a cyst is not uncommon, particularly in those cysts subject to trauma or pressure on the hands and feet. Carcinoma developing from a cyst is a possibility but is apparently rare.

SKELETAL ANOMALIES

Skeletal anomalies are one of the most frequent and earliest manifestations of the syndrome. The majority are congenital. Although the anomalies in themselves are not individually specific, their highly frequent occurrence in combination is highly specific, and diagnosis of the syndrome can usually be made by radiologic findings alone, particularly in children who are still too young to manifest skin lesions. The frequencies of the various skeletal anomalies which follow are from a recent report (Dodd et al., 1970) that summarizes the radiologic findings in 90 patients examined in connection with a genetic study of the syndrome.

Skull

Complete or partial bridging of the sella turcica is a frequent congenital defect of the skull; it is observed in 75 percent of patients, compared with only 8 percent of controls. Ectopic calcification of intracranial structures is also highly frequent (81 percent) as are jaw cysts (78 percent). Hypertelorism, sometimes also denoted by the terms broad nasal root and dystopia canthorum, is another characteristic of this as well as other syndromes (Gorlin and Goltz, 1960). Discriminant function analysis has recently indicated that all width dimensions of the skull, and not only the ocular distances, are significantly increased in patients compared with their unaffected siblings (Anderson, 1970). Frontal and parietal bossing, large or asymmetrical calvaria, prognathism, hyperostosis frontalis interna, mottling of the calvaria, and platybasia are other reported defects of the skull (Pollard and New, 1964; Gorlin et al., 1965; Kennedy and Abbot, 1968; Bopp et al., 1969; Kedem et al., 1970).

Spine and Rib Cage

Anomalies of these structures generally involve the upper thoracic and cervical areas. The principle spine anomalies, observed in about 66 percent of patients, include spina bifida, scoliosis, hemivertebrae, and incompletely segmented vertebrae. Rib anomalies occur in 55 percent of patients and are composed of flared, bifid, fused, flattened, broad, hypoplastic, or cervical ribs. Sprengel's deformity of the scapula with or without dysplastic clavicles is observed in about 5 percent of cases. Pectus excavatum and other defects of the sternum are being reported with increasing frequency and may represent another skeletal anomaly (Nally, 1966; Ferrier and Hinrichs, 1967; Stevanovic, 1967; Lile et al., 1968; Sawyer and Braverman, 1969; Kedem et al., 1970).

Extremities

Subcortical cystic changes of the phalanges and occasional cysts of the long bones are observed in 46 percent of patients. Shortening of the fourth metacarpal, a defect emphasized by Clendenning et al. (1964), has a frequency of 28 percent, which contrasts with one of 9 percent in controls. Polydactyly and syndactyly also occur in a significant proportion of cases (Anderson et al., 1967). Other possibly associated anomalies of the extremities include hallux valgus and malleus (Block and Clendenning, 1963; Schønning and Visfeldt, 1964; Davidson and Key, 1964; Becker et al., 1967; Rubino et al., 1968), pes planus (Ferrier and Hinrichs, 1967), and excavatia equinovara and genu valgum (Stevanovic, 1967). Shortened distal phalanges of the thumbs, a bizarre rotation deformity of the thumbs, and small proximal phalanges of the large toes have also been noted in some few patients (Davidson, 1962; Anderson et al., 1967; Lile et al., 1968).

Interestingly, several syndrome patients have arachnodactyly or excessive height or both and have an increased arm span relative to height, or have actually been reported as examples of Marfan's syndrome (Calnan, 1953; Boyer and Martin, 1958; Jones et al., 1965; Kumar and Berenson, 1966; Nally, 1966; Stevanovic, 1967; Smith, 1968; Kopp et al., 1969). However, subluxation of the lenses or dissecting aneurysm of the ascending aorta, two integral features of Marfan's syndrome, have not been present in these patients. The gigantism reported in a syndrome patient by Kopp et al. (1969) was hereditary, but it was transmitted independently of the syndrome.

Hyperextensibility of the joints, hyperelasticity of the skin, and inguinal hernia are other connective tissue findings described in syndrome patients (Shroff, 1964; Gorlin et al., 1965; Nichols and Solomon, 1965; Becker et al., 1967; Clendenning et al., 1963; Graham et al., 1968; Ziprkowski et al., 1967; Grinspan et al., 1969), but whether these changes occur at higher frequencies than they do in the general population still remains to be determined.

JAW ANOMALIES

Cysts of the jaws are one of the most frequent and consistent characteristics of the syndrome. They vary in size, number, and onset and develop in the mandible or maxilla or both, including the maxillary sinuses, in many but apparently not all syndrome patients (Anderson et al., 1963; Van Erp, 1968; Rater et al., 1968). The cysts may occur unilaterally or bilaterally, either as a unilocular or multilocular lesion. Their proximity to one or more teeth may lead to malposed teeth. Cysts have been detected in patients as young as 5 years of age; they also develop as late as the fifth decade. However, the age at first detection averages 13 years (Anderson and Cook, 1966). The presenting complaint often includes pain, tenderness, swelling of the jaw, and/or a draining fistula (Howell et al., 1967). The trend is for continued development of new and recurring cysts at increasing frequencies until about age 30, when the rate of development tends to decrease (Anderson et al., 1967).

The jaw cysts are best treated by surgery; radiation is not indicated. Treatment should be directed toward either complete enucleation or removal of a portion of the cyst and its contents. Removal of the roof of a cyst is sometimes advocated, thus eliminating the cyst but retaining and facilitating the eruption of an involved tooth (Howell et al., 1967).

Histologically, the cysts are lined by a variable number of layers of flattened, stratified, keratinizing, squamous epithelium, surrounded by a thickened fibrous capsule. These cysts are indistinguishable from other odontogenic cysts, except when microcysts or daughter cysts are demonstrable in the connective tissue stroma. Foci of calcification have been observed in the cyst walls (Anderson and Cook, 1966), but whether or not this is a distinguishing feature of the cysts occurring in the syndrome requires further study.

Evidence is now beginning to accumulate that these cysts may have an increased propensity for tumor formation. Ameloblastoma developing from a cyst wall was reported by Clendenning et al. (1964) and Maddox et al. (1964), but the possibility of proliferation of odontogenic rests of Malassez is not excluded in these cases, according to Gorlin et al. (1963). One patient with a full complement of cutaneous and skeletal lesions, including an untreated cyst in the left maxillary antrum, developed a squamous cell carcinoma in that antrum three years after detection of the cyst

(Dodd et al., 1970). Another patient developed a calcifying maxillary myxoma (Walike and Karas, 1969), and another a spindle cell carcinoma (Shapiro, 1970). Reed (1968) and Tamoney (1969) recently described two patients with fibrosarcoma of the jaw. This neoplasm in the patient reported by Binkley and Johnson (1951) is speculated to have resulted from radiation therapy, and the diagnosis in the case of Howell and Caro (1959) is questioned. The latter patient is still living at age 72.

Other oral anomalies possibly associated with the syndrome include a high arched palate (Hermans et al., 1960; Gorlin et al., 1965; Jones et al., 1965; Graham et al., 1968; Van Erp, 1968; Worth and Wollin, 1968; Kopp et al., 1969), cleft lip or cleft palate or both (Anderson et al., 1963; Summerly and Hale, 1965; Shroff and Smith, 1966; Becker et al., 1967), lip pits (Shroff, 1964; Gorlin et al., 1965), and prognathism (Gorlin et al., 1965).

ECTOPIC CALCIFICATION

Ectopic intracranial calcification is a highly distinctive feature of the syndrome. It occurs most frequently in the falx cerebri, tentorium cerebelli, and petroclinoid ligaments. Calcification in one or more of these structures is observed in 70 percent of patients younger than 10 years of age and in 93 percent of patients 40 years of age or older, frequencies markedly in excess of the 6 percent reported for the general population (Dodd et al., 1970). In the falx cerebri, the calcification is distinctly lamellar in appearance, unlike the buttonlike or elliptical configuration noted in the general population. Ectopic calcification may also occur in basal cell lesions (Graham et al., 1965), subcutaneous tissues (Murphy, 1969), the lining of the jaw cysts (Anderson and Cook, 1966), mesenteric cysts, ovarian or uterine cysts or fibromas (Clendenning et al., 1963; Becker et al., 1967), and the sacrotuberous ligament (Anderson et al., 1963). This calcification is not known to be associated with any signs or symptoms, although Caron (1965) considered extreme calcification of the falx, cerebral cortex, and dura to be causally related to micturation difficulties in a 24 year old patient.

Calcification of soft tissues, shortening of the fourth metacarpals, and absence of significant phosphorus diuresis after intravenous injection of parathyroid hormone led Block and Clendenning (1963) and Clendenning et al. (1963) to propose that the syndrome may be a variant of pseudohypoparathyroidism. Approximately 30 patients have now undergone metabolic studies, about one-half of whom have manifested a normal response to parathyroid extract and the other half a refractive response (Berlin, 1966; Jones et al., 1965; Berke, 1970; Gorlin et al., 1965; Nichols and Solomon, 1965; Becker et al., 1967; Lile et al., 1968; Murphy, 1969; Dodd et al., 1970). Patients with a refractive response may be tall or short, may or may not have a shortened fourth metacarpal, and usually have normal levels of serum calcium and phosphorus before and after injection of parathyroid extract. Witkop (1968) considered syndrome patients to be refractive to the effects of the hormone at both kidney and bone sites, similar to the case in pseudohypoparathyroidism.

NEUROLOGIC ABNORMALITIES

Ectopic intracranial calcification is the most frequent neurologic abnormality, occurring in 81 percent of patients, as indicated in the preceding section. A variety of ophthalmologic problems are also encountered, including exotropia and strabismus (Anderson et al., 1967; Shear and Wilton, 1968), coloboma (Anderson and Cook, 1966; Gorlin et al., 1963) cataracts (Clendenning et al., 1964; Shapiro, 1970), congenital corneal opacities (Meerkotter and Shear, 1964; Shroff and Smith, 1966; Kahn and Gordon, 1967), micro-ophthalmia (Graham et al., 1968), and dysgenesis neuroblastica gliomatose (Hermans et al., 1960). Other lesions involving the eye or eyelids include basal cell carcinomas and chalazia. Probably an incidental occurrence is the malignant melanoma of the iris described by Kedem et al. (1970).

Medulloblastoma, although an infrequent brain tumor, is observed in a significant number of syndrome patients. In fact, of 90 patients included in one study, all of whom were examined or medically documented, 4 developed this tumor (Dodd et al., 1970). The literature includes 8 cases (including the above 4) in which this tumor occurred in association with the syndrome (see summary in Neblett et al., 1970). Other brain tumors described in children with the syndrome include cerebellar astrocytoma (Cawson and Kerr, 1964; Moynahan, 1964; Kahn and Gordon, 1967), meningioma (Telle, 1965), and meningioma and craniopharyngioma (Tamoney, 1969). Kennedy and Abbot (1968) described the syndrome in a mother and daughter of a family in which another daughter died of a "brain stem tumor." Hydrocephalus, which was primary and not secondary to a brain tumor, has been documented by Gorlin et al. (1963), Kumar and Berenson (1966), and Neblett et al. (1970). Cysts of either the choroid plexus, cerebral hemisphere, or diencephalon were noted by Kahn and Gordon (1967) and Taylor et al. (1968). Seizures are rare in syndrome patients but have been reported by Gorlin et al. (1965) and Mills and Foulkes (1967).

Although often reported, no special attempt has been made to determine if emotional and intellectual disturbances in patients with the syndrome differ in type and frequency from those observed in the general population. Graham et al. (1968) indicated that 17 percent of previously reported patients were mentally retarded. This is obviously a gross overestimate, since the majority of the patients had not been subjected to appropriate psychologic and psychiatric evaluation. Only one mentally retarded child (IQ = 63) was observed in a series of 56 examined patients (Anderson et al., 1963 and 1967). Another patient in this series was reported as mentally dull on the basis of clinical examination, but subsequent psychometric evaluation revealed a WAIS full-scale IQ score of 115. Emotional disturbances have been recorded by several workers (see review by Gorlin et al., 1965). A special study would be required to determine whether these are part of the syndrome, the consequence of cosmetic disfigurement, or a combination of both factors.

Agenesis of the corpus callosum has been noted in only one patient (Binkley and Johnson, 1951). Frontal atrophy was observed at autopsy in a patient reported by Taylor et al. (1968), and findings suggesting cortical atrophy were described by Caron (1965).

OTHER MALIGNANT TUMORS

The types of tumors occurring in patients with the syndrome other than those already discussed include adenocarcinoma of the colon, breast tumor or cancer, cutaneous melanoma, thyroid tumor, and rhabdomyosarcoma, all of which are likely incidental occurrences. However, uterine and particularly ovarian tumors seemingly occur at a high frequency (Clendenning et al., 1963; Gorlin et al., 1963; Pollard and New, 1964; Gorlin et al., 1965; Zackheim et al., 1966; Becker et al., 1967; Mills and Foulkes, 1967; Lile et al., 1968; Rater et al., 1968; Van Erp, 1968; Holubar et al., 1970), an occurrence which takes on significance in view of adenocarcinoma of the ovary in two syndrome patients reported by Dodd et al. (1970), and the fact that the patients are apparently not prone to other tumors.

MISCELLANEOUS

Two interesting associations have recently been reported: Katz et al. (1968) described a large family in which some members had ulcerative colitis or regional enteritis in association with or independent of the syndrome. The concurrence of these two genetic diseases is probably incidental and unique to this family. The association has not been observed in other family studies. Another unique association was reported by Swift and Horowitz (1969). They recorded a family with Charcot-Marie-Tooth disease in which several affected members also exhibited lamellar calcification of the falx cerebri and multiple recurrent jaw cysts. It is not yet known whether this association is fortuitous and represents the segregation of two gene loci or is the consequence of the pleiotropic effects of a single gene. This association has not been reported in other families.

REFERENCES

Anderson, D. E.: Linkage analysis of the nevoid basal cell carcinoma syndrome. Ann. Hum. Genet., 32:113, 1968.

Anderson, D. E.: Unpublished data, 1970.

Anderson, D. E., and Cook, W. A.: Jaw cysts and the basal cell nevus syndrome. J. Oral Surg., 24:15, 1966.

Anderson, D. E., McClendon, J. L., and Howell, J. B.: Genetics and skin tumors, with special reference to basal cell nevi. *In* Tumors of the Skin. Chicago, Year Book Medical Publishers.

Anderson, D. E., Taylor, W. B., Falls, H. F., and Davidson, R. T.: The nevoid basal cell carcinoma syndrome. Am. J. Hum. Genet., 19:12, 1967.

Becker, M. H., Kopf, A. W., and Lande, A.: Basal cell nevus syndrome: Its roentgenologic significance. Review of the literature and report of four cases. Am. J. Roentgenol. Radium Ther. Nucl. Med., 99:817, 1967.

Berke, M.: Basal cell nevus syndrome. Arch. Dermatol., 101:125, 1970.

Berlin, N. I.: Basal cell nevus syndrome. Combined clinical staff conference at the National Institutes of Health. Ann. Intern. Med., 64:403, 1966.

Binkley, G. W., and Johnson, H. H., Jr.: Epithelioma adenoides cysticum: Basal cell nevi, agenesis of the corpus callosum and dental cysts. A clinical autopsy study. Arch. Dermatol. Syph. (Berl.), 63:73, 1951.

Blackwell, J. B., and McComb, H.: The long-term results of autologous transportation of basal cell carcinoma in skin grafts. Cancer, 23:101, 1969.

Block, J. B., and Clendenning, W. E.: Parathyroid hormone hyporesponsiveness in patients with basal cell nevi and bone defects. New Engl. J. Med., 268:1157, 1963.

Bopp, C., Bakos, L., and Ebling, H.: Sindrome nevo baso celular. Rev. Amrigs, 12:39, 1969.

Boyer, B. E., and Martin, M. M.: Marfan's syndrome. Report of a case manifesting a giant bone cyst of the mandible and multiple (110) basal cell carcinomata. Plast. Reconstr. Surg., 22:257, 1958.

Burgoon, C. F., Jr., Gordon, M., and Lefing, W. M.: Multiple basal cell carcinomas (nevoid basal cell carcinoma syndrome). Arch. Dermatol., 97:349, 1968.

Calnan, C. D.: Two cases of multiple naevoid basal cell epitheliomata? Porokeratosis of Mantoux. Br. J. Dermatol., 65:219, 1953.

Caron, G. A.: Basal cell naevi with a neurological syndrome. Proc. R. Soc. Med., 58:621, 1965.

Cawson, R. A., and Kerr, G. A.: The syndrome of jaw cysts, basal cell tumours and skeletal anomalies. Proc. R. Soc. Med., 57:799, 1964.

Clarkson, P., and Wilson, H.: Two cases of basal cell congenital naevus. Proc. R. Soc. Med., 53:295, 1959.

Clendenning, W. E., Herdt, J. R., and Block, J. B.: Ovarian fibromas and mesenteric cysts: Their association with hereditary basal cell cancer of the skin. Am. J. Obstet. Gynecol., 87:1008, 1963.

Clendenning, W. E., Block, J. B., and Radde, I. C.: Basal cell nevus syndrome. Arch. Dermatol., 90:38, 1964.

Davidson, F.: Multiple naevoid basal cell carcinomata and associated congenital abnormalities. Br. J. Dermatol., 74:439, 1962.

Davidson, F., and Key, J. J.: Multiple naevoid basal cell carcinomata and associated congenital abnormalities. Proc. R. Soc. Med., 57:891, 1964.

Dodd, G. D., Jing, B. S., and Anderson, D. E.: Nevoid basal cell carcinoma syndrome. Unpublished observations.

Ferrier, P. E., and Hinrichs, W. L.: Basal cell carcinoma syndrome. Am. J. Dis. Child., 113:538, 1967.

Gorlin, R. J., and Goltz, R. W.: Multiple nevoid basal cell epithelioma, jaw cysts and bifid rib: A syndrome. New Engl. J. Med., 262:908, 1960.

Gorlin, R. J., Yunis, J. J., and Tuna, N.: Multiple nevoid basal cell carcinoma, odontogenic keratocysts and skeletal anomalies: A syndrome. Acta Derm. Venereol. (Stockh.), 43:39, 1963.

Gorlin, R. J., Vickers, R. A., Kelln, E., and Williamson, J. J.: The multiple basal cell nevi syndrome: An analysis of a syndrome consisting of multiple nevoid basal cell carcinoma, jaw cysts, skeletal anomalies, medulloblastoma, and hyporesponsiveness to parathormone. Cancer, 18:89, 1965.

Graham, J. H., Mason, J. K., Gray, H. R., and Helwig, E.: Differentiation of nevoid basal cell carcinoma from epithelioma adenoides cysticum. J. Invest. Dermatol., 44:197, 1965.

Graham, J. K., McJimsey, B. A., and Hardin, J. C., Jr.: Nevoid basal cell carcinoma syndrome. Arch. Otolaryngol., 87:72, 1968.

Grinspan, D., Abulafia, J., and Pomposiello, I. M.: Sindrome del nevo basocelular. Dermatol. Ibero Lat. Am., 10:255, 1969.

Gross, P. P.: Epithelioma adenoides cysticum with follicular cysts of maxilla and mandible: Report of case. J. Oral Surg., 11:160, 1953.

Hermans, E. H., Grosfeld, J. C. M., and Valk, L. E. M.: Eine funfte Phakomatoses; Naevus epitheliomatodes multiplex. Hautarzt, 11:160, 1960.

Holubar, K., Matras, H., and Smalik, A. V.: Multiple palmar basal cell epitheliomas in basal cell nevus syndrome. Arch. Dermatol., 101:679, 1970.

Howell, J. B., and Caro, M. R.: The basal cell nevus. Its relationship to multiple cutaneous cancers and associated anomalies of development. Arch. Dermatol., 79:67, 1959.

Howell, J. B., and Mehregan, A. H.: Pursuit of the pits of the nevoid basal cell carcinoma syndrome. Arch. Dermatol., 102:586, 1970.

Howell, J. B., Anderson, D. E., and McClendon, J. L.: The basal cell nevus syndrome. J.A.M.A., 190:274, 1964.

Howell, J. B., Byrd, L., McClendon, J. L., and Anderson, D. E.: Identification and treatment of jaw cysts in the nevoid basal cell carcinoma syndrome. J. Oral Surg., 25:129, 1967.

Jones, J. E., Desper, P. C., Welton, W. A., and Flink, E. B.: The nevoid basal cell carcinoma syndrome. Arch. Intern. Med., 115:723, 1965.

Kahn, L. B., and Gordon, W.: The basal cell naevus syndrome: Report of a case. S. Afr. Med. J., 41:832, 1967.

Katz, J., Savin, R., and Spiro, H. M.: The basal cell nevus syndrome and inflammatory disease of the bowel. Am. J. Med., 44:483, 1968.

Kedem, A., Even-Paz, Z., and Freund, M.: Basal cell nevus syndrome associated with malignant melanoma of the iris. Dermatologia, 140:99, 1970.

Kennedy, J. W., and Abbott, P. L.: Nevoid basal cell carcinoma syndrome. Oral Surg., 26:406, 1968.

Kopp, W. K., Klatell, J., and Blake, M.: Basal cell nevus syndrome with other abnormalities. Report of a case. Oral. Surg., 27:9, 1969.

Kumar, V., and Berenson, G. S.: The Marfan syndrome: Report of an interesting case with unusual anatomic findings. J. Louisiana Med. Soc., 118:511, 1966.

Lile, H. A., Rogers, J. F., and Gerald, B.: The basal cell nevus syndrome. Am. J. Roentgenol., Radium Ther. Nucl. Med., 103:214, 1968.

Lund, H. Z.: Tumors of the skin. *In* Atlas of Tumor Pathology. Section 1, Fascicle 2. Washington, D.C., Armed Forces. Institute of Pathology, 1957.

Maddox, W. D., Winkelmann, R. K., Harrison, E. G., Devine, K. D., and Gibilisco, J. A.: Multiple nevoid basal cell epitheliomas, jaw cysts, and skeletal defects: A clinical syndrome. J.A.M.A., 188:106, 1964.

Meerkotter, V. A., and Shear, M.: Multiple primordial cysts associated with bifid rib and ocular defects. Oral Surg., 18:498, 1964.

Mills, J., and Foulkes, J.: Gorlin's syndrome: A radiological and cytogenetic study of nine cases. Br. J. Radiol., 40:366, 1967.

Moynahan, E. J.: Basal cell naevus syndrome. Trans. St. John's Hosp. Dermatol. Soc. (London), 50:187, 1964.

Murphy, K. J.: Subcutaneous calcification in the naevoid basal cell carcinoma syndrome: Response to parathyroid hormone and relationship to pseudohypoparathyroidism. Clin. Radiol., 20:187, 1969.

Nally, F. F.: The Marfan syndrome: Report of two cases. Oral. Surg., 22:715, 1966.

Neblett, C. R., Waltz, T. A., and Anderson, D. E.: Neurological involvement in the nevoid basal cell carcinoma syndrome. J. Neurosurg., 35:577, 1971.

Nichols, L., and Soloman, L. M.: Basal cell nevi syndrome. Arch. Dermatol., 91:188, 1965.

Nomland, R.: Multiple basal cell epitheliomas originating from congenital pigmented basal-cell nevi. Arch. Dermatol. Syph. (Berl.), 25:1002, 1932.

Pollard, J. J., and New, P. F. J.: Hereditary cutaneomandibular polyoncosis. A syndrome of myriad basal cell nevi of the skin, mandibular cysts, and inconstant skeletal anomalies. Radiology, 82:840, 1964.

Rater, C., Selke, A. C., and Van Epps, E. F.: Basal cell nevus syndrome. Am. J. Roentgenol., 103:589, 1968.

Reed, J. C.: Nevoid basal cell carcinoma syndrome with associated fibrosarcoma of the maxilla. Arch. Dermatol., 97:304, 1968.

Rubino, V. H., Sammartino, C. A., and Johnson, E. S.: Basal cell nevus syndrome: Report of case. J. Oral Surg., 26:665, 1968.

Sawyer, C. S., and Braverman, I. M.: Basal cell nevus syndrome with inflammatory disease of the bowel. Arch. Dermatol., 99:131, 1969.

Schønning, L., and Visfeldt, J.: The syndrome of jaw cysts–basal cell carcinomas–skeletal anomalies: Clinical study with chromosomal analyses of a family. Acta Derm. Venereol. (Stockh.), 44:437, 1964.

Shapiro, M. J.: Basal cell nevus syndrome: A case report with associated carcinoma of the maxilla. Laryngoscope, 80:777, 1970.

Shear, M., and Wilton, E.: Cytogenetic studies of the basal cell carcinoma syndrome. J. Dent. Assoc. S. Afr., 23:99, 1968.

Shroff, F. R.: Multiple cysts of the jaw, basal cell carcinomas and bifid ribs — An unusual syndrome. New Zealand Dent. J., 60:115, 1964.

Shroff, F. R., and Smith, J. L.: Multiple cysts of the jaw, basal cell carcinomas and bifid ribs. New Zealand Dent. J., 62:37, 1966.

Smith, N. H. H.: Multiple dentigerous cysts associated with arachnodactyly and other skeletal defects. Report of a case. Oral Surg., 25:99, 1968.

Stevanovic, D. V.: Nevoid basal cell carcinoma syndrome. Arch. Dermatol., 96:696, 1967.

Summerly, R., and Hale, A. J.: Basal cell naevus syndrome. Trans. St. John's Hosp. Dermatol. Soc., New Series, 51:77, 1965.

Swift, M. R., and Horowitz, S. L.: Familial jaw cysts in Charcot-Marie-Tooth disease. J. Med. Genet., 6:193, 1969.

Tamoney, H. J.: Basal cell nevoid syndrome. Am. Surgeon, 35:297, 1969.

Taylor, W. B., and Wilkins, J. W.: The nevoid basal cell carcinoma syndrome of palm. Arch. Dermatol., 102:654, 1970.

Taylor, W. B., Anderson, D. E., Howell, J. B., and Thurston, C. S.: The nevoid basal cell carcinoma syndrome: Autopsy findings. Arch. Dermatol., 98:612, 1968.

Telle, B.: Multiple basaliome bei einem jungen Mann. Dermatol. Wochenschr., 151:1425, 1965.

Van Erp, I. F. R.: Naevus epitheliomatodes multiplex. Dermatologica, 136:257, 1968.

Walike, J. W., and Karas, R. P.: Nevoid basal cell carcinoma syndrome. Laryngoscope, 79:478, 1969.

Ward, W. H.: Naevoid basal celled carcinoma associated with a dyskeratosis of the palms and soles. A new entity. Australian J. Dermatol., 5:204, 1960.

Witkop, C. J., Jr.: Gardner's syndrome and other osteognathodermal disorders with defects in parathyroid functions. J. Oral Surg., 26:639, 1968.

Worth, H. M., and Wollin, D. G.: The basal cell naevi and jaw cysts syndrome. Clin. Radiol., 19:416, 1968.

Yunis, J. J., and Gorlin, R. J.: Chromosomal study in patients with cysts of the jaw, multiple nevoid basal cell carcinomata and bifid rib syndrome. Chromosoma, 14:146, 1963.

Zackheim, H. S., Howell, J. B., and Loud, A. V.: Nevoid basal cell carcinoma syndrome. Arch. Dermatol., 93:317, 1966.

Ziprkowski, L., Krakowski, A., and Schewach-Millet, M.: Hereditary epidermis tumors. Proc. Tel Hashomer Hosp., 6:70, 1967.

38

Squamous Cell Carcinoma of the Scalp, Face, and Neck

Harold H. Sage, M.D., and
Phillip R. Casson, M.D.

The incidence, etiology, and clinical course of squamous (epidermoid) carcinoma of the skin of the head and neck area have been well documented by several writers. There is a considerable body of precise knowledge concerning the development of squamous carcinoma, including precancerous states such as keratosis and hyperplasia. The precise point and time of cancer formation are not easily identified. Nevertheless, a relatively slow growth rate and ready accessibility for observation, palpation, and biopsy generally permit early diagnosis. This results in a high rate of cure in the early stages with several forms of treatment being used, including surgery, radiation, desiccation and curettage, and chemosurgery (Mohs, 1956).

As a group, squamous carcinomas of the skin of the head and neck can be categorized in the degree-of-malignancy range between basal cell carcinoma and malignant melanoma. Comparison with basal cell carcinoma reveals the growth rate of squamous carcinoma to be faster and the local invasiveness to be more wide-spread and less well defined. Unlike basal cell carcinoma, squamous carcinoma eventually metastasizes through lymphatics to lymph nodes in a significant percentage of persistent or recurrent cases. This results in a higher mortality.

Comparison with malignant melanoma reveals significant differences in spread of the cancer in the early as well as advanced metastatic stages. Lymphatic metastases are more frequent and occur at an earlier stage in malignant melanoma. Hematogenous spread is rare in squamous carcinoma of the skin, even in the most advanced metastatic stages. Malignant melanoma spreads through the blood frequently and sometimes in early stages. Such blood-borne distant metastasis is rarely curable.

Individual differences in behavior among the various subgroups of squamous carcinoma and at different stages are important. Failure to note such differences may result in poor end results in regard to cure, function, and cosmetic appearance. Overgeneralization is responsible for both

899

change. Genetic and other factors, including immunologic status, are important here as well as in all other states associated with carcinogenesis.

X-radiation has been administered in the head and neck area for treatment of malignant lesions as well as benign lesions, such as acne, hirsutism, and hemangiomas. Occasionally such radiation has been responsible for the production of squamous carcinoma, often as late as 10 to 30 years after the therapeutic use of the radiation. In some instances radiation has also induced basal cell carcinoma of the skin.

The relationship of x-radiation exposure to later occurrence of squamous carcinoma must be considered in terms of dosage and quality of radiation, including kilovoltage, filtration, shielding of surrounding areas, and the use of single or divided doses, as well as individual differences in the patient, including age and texture of the skin. Sulzberger et al. (1952) has reported that x-ray dosages of 1000 roentgens or less of superficial x-rays (60 to 100 kv.; half value layer of 0.5 to 1 mm. of aluminum) in fractional, small doses such as are used in the treatment of benign dermatoses did not produce significant skin sequelae. Dosages of between 1000 and 2630 roentgens resulted in chronic skin changes, which were relatively mild, in 1.5 percent of patients. No radiation-induced carcinomas were observed.

When larger doses of x-radiation were used, as in treatment of skin cancer, later follow-up has shown significant chronic roentgen sequelae in the radiated skin. Radiation changes, including atrophy and telangiectasia, may be demonstrated within a year following such exposure to x-radiation or as much as 30 years later (Pack and Davis, 1965). Carcinoma of the skin may be produced.

The process whereby x-radiation results in cancer is of interest. X-radiation above the level of the "erythema dose" can induce a chronic tissue process which is self-perpetuating and in many instances progressive. Atrophy and telangiectasia followed by hyperplasia are evident in the later stages of development of x-radiation dermatosis. This may progress to carcinoma when the skin is subject to the usual external exposures under average "wear-and-tear" conditions. No additional x-radiation or other unusual event is necessary. The previously radiated tissues have lost their ability to produce a complete and normal healing response to ordinary physical and chemical insults. Chronic ulceration may occur. Further hyperplastic response which may be accompanied by loss of immunologic resistance will occasionally result in carcinoma.

A somewhat similar situation exists with regard to the production of squamous carcinoma in burn scars. Here again, a single event is capable of inducing a chronic process. Cancer may develop in a burn scar within a matter of several months, generally in an ulcer which has progressed without healing. On the other hand, it may occur many years later in a wound which has healed initially with a residual scar which subsequently breaks down. Treves and Pack (1930) indicated the onset of carcinoma in the acute wound group was at 0.3 years, whereas in the chronic group the average age of the scars was 32.5 years prior to carcinoma formation. The acute burns resulting in carcinoma were more frequent in older people with atrophic and keratotic skin. The sequence of histologic changes occurring in burn scar carcinogenesis have been described by Arons et al. (1965) as acanthosis, basal cell hyperplasia, pseudoepitheliomatous hyperplasia, basal cell atypia, and finally squamous carcinoma.

A single trauma, such as occurs with a surgical incision or a clean wound, is rarely associated with the later production of skin cancer. Local wound healing is generally complete. Such a scar does not break down under average "wear-and-tear" conditions. There is no evidence of loss of immunologic resistance.

The effect of ultraviolet light and other sunlight on skin is documented in other sections of this book. Blum (1948) indicated that the carcinogenic wavelengths of sunlight are between 2900 Å and 3200 Å. The precancerous and cancerous changes in skin resulting from ultraviolet irradiation may be defined in clinical as well as histologic terms: atrophy, telangiectasia, chronic ulceration, and hyperplasia. One may, however, assume that biochemical changes have also occurred. For instance, possible to implant squamous cell carcinoma cells in the postexcision field if the instruments used for excision are also used for the closure of the wound.

Because of the proximity of vital structures, the principle of wide local excision, with normal surrounding margins of 1 to 2 cm. beyond gross disease, which is applicable in squamous carcinomas in other regions of the body, is often not feasible in squamous carcinomas of the face and scalp, even in the early stages.

For the small, previously untreated, superficial lesion, stage 0 and stage I, simple elliptical excision with a 1 to 2 cm. margin around the lesion and direct closure by lateral undermining is sufficient, taking care to place the incisions so that they lie parallel to the lines of minimal skin tension and naturally occurring skin creases of the face (Fig. 38–5). For the more extensive lesions of the face, for example, those over 2 cm. in diameter, direct closure after excision with a satisfactory margin of 1 to 2 cm. is often impossible, and a plastic closure becomes necessary.

The facial disfigurement must not interfere with adequate excision, and the physician should rely on reconstructive techniques to restore the appearance of the patient to a reasonable facsimile of normal. The possibility of injury to underlying but uninvaded structures must also be considered, particularly the branches of the seventh nerve, and when not in the field of cancer invasion, these branches should be identified and preserved. If it is necessary to sacrifice a main branch of the nerve because of possible invasion by carcinoma, consideration should be given to an immediate nerve graft.

Techniques used for repair of defects of the skin which are too large for direct closure are (1) split-thickness skin grafts; (2) full-thickness skin grafts; (3) local flaps from skin adjoining the defect; (4) transposition flaps from the forehead, neck, or shoulder; and (5) tube pedicle tissue brought from a distance.

The Split-Thickness Skin Graft

The split-thickness skin graft has little place in the permanent reconstruction of the face because of its well-known tendency to contract and the poor color match obtained from the use of donor sites on the thighs, buttocks, or abdomen. It may be used as a temporary covering when the surgeon is not optimistic about the chances of cure and so wishes to use the simplest method and still avoid the possibility of covering persistent disease with a flap; permanent reconstruction may be completed one or two years later if the local disease is controlled.

The Full-Thickness Skin Graft

A full-thickness skin graft taken from the retroauricular area or the supraclavicular fossa may be used to cover excisional defects on the face as large as 5 to 8 cm. in diameter. A delayed application technique (Stell and Brown, 1970) is advisable in the more extensive cancers; this also allows a detailed examination of the specimen by the pathologist for completeness of excision. The full-thickness graft provides a simple and cosmetically acceptable closure for the majority of defects encountered after excision of skin carcinomas 2 to 4 cm. in diameter where no underlying bone is exposed.

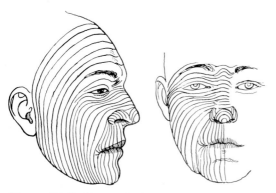

Figure 38–5 Lines of minimal skin tension and naturally occurring skin creases. (*From* Converse: Reconstructive Plastic Surgery. Philadelphia, W. B. Saunders Company, 1964.)

Flaps From the Adjoining Tissues

The skin and subcutaneous tissues immediately adjoining a defect created by the excision of carcinoma may be used for advancement, rotation, or transposition flaps (see Chapter 65) and are often employed in conjunction with a skin graft, which is used to cover the secondary defect.

In advanced carcinomas of the skin of the face when a radical neck dissection must be performed, the skin of the neck is available for reconstruction of the facial defect, the customary radical neck dissection incision being modified to provide a cervical flap. The shoulder and the anterior chest wall may be used to reconstruct defects of the lower and middle portions of the face, using part of the flap as a carrying pedicle to transport skin to the defect to be reconstructed. After three to four weeks this is divided and returned to its original position. Of special interest is the use of the forehead in total reconstruction of the nose (Converse, 1964); the tissue may also be used for reconstruction of the cheek or upper lip, leaving a bridge of normal skin with its blood supply between the base of the forehead flap and the defect to be reconstructed.

Tube Pedicles From a Distance

Tube pedicles may be constructed on the arm, neck, chest, or abdomen which may be transferred directly to the defect to be repaired, as when a cervical tube is used to repair a defect of the face, or indirectly by moving first one end of the pedicle and then the other toward the defect, when the arm may be employed as a carrier. This technique, which requires multiple stages over a considerable period of time, is therefore unsatisfactory for immediate reconstruction or early reconstruction and is used only when local tissues are unsuitable or unavailable.

Contraindications to the Use of Flaps

While the use of flaps may be indicated where bone is exposed, and while it offers other advantages in function and appearance, it presents the marked disadvantage of providing a covering of skin and subcutaneous tissue through which it may be difficult to detect persistent or recurrent cancer. In patients in whom the prognosis is poor, it may be advisable to obtain a skin closure by the use of a split-thickness skin graft with final reconstruction to be completed after an interval of one or two years free of disease. This applies particularly to patients with a history of several recurrences following surgery, chemosurgery, desiccation and curettage, or radiation therapy.

SPECIFIC PROBLEMS ASSOCIATED WITH SQUAMOUS CELL CARCINOMA OF DIFFERENT SITES

Neck

Squamous carcinoma of the skin of the neck under 2 cm. in size can usually be treated by a wide local excision, without the need for skin graft. Lesions 4 cm. or larger may require skin grafting or a flap to repair the defect. In the neck, invasion of superficial fascia, platysma muscle, and the deep fascia generally occurs in a predictable and readily definable sequence. Such invaded tissues can be excised without functional or cosmetic impairment and should therefore be included in the dissection, even when invasion is unproven. Underlying muscle and areolar and deeper tissues can also be excised, achieving 1 to 2 cm. of normal tissue margin in depth.

Eyelids

Squamous cell carcinoma may affect the upper or the lower eyelid. If surgical excision is used, immediate reconstruction is necessary to prevent ulceration of the cornea and perhaps loss of the eye. In the older age group in which squamous cell carcinoma occurs most commonly, there is often sufficient laxity of tissues so that up to one-third of either lid may be removed by the use of a simple excision and direct closure obtained, with little resulting deformity.

Extensive reconstructive procedures of

the lower eyelid may be accomplished by using either laterally placed rotational flaps or, if necessary, a mucosal graft obtained from the nose if there is insufficient conjunctiva remaining. Reconstruction of the upper lid is a much more difficult problem because of its protective function and the need for mobility. If extensive loss is present, the lower lid may be used to reconstruct the upper lid, replacing the lower lid with tissues lying lateral to it (Mustarde, 1966).

Lip

Squamous cell carcinoma of the skin may invade the upper or lower lip or both, requiring excision of the full thickness of the lip. If direct closure is not possible, as when more than one-third of the lip has been removed, a triangular, full-thickness flap on a narrow pedicle containing the labial artery may be rotated from the unaffected lip into the defect. This pedicle is divided at 10 to 14 days, permitting the patient to once again open the mouth. Total removal of upper or lower lip may be adequately reconstructed with local flaps. This is preferable to tissues brought in from a distance, such as a forehead flap which does not contain muscle. A combination of two techniques may be used, bringing tissues from the cheeks, laterally, to be sutured to an Abbe type of flap in the midline of the upper or lower lip (Fig. 38-6).

Squamous carcinoma which has invaded the lip is aggressive locally and also metastasizes to lymph nodes more frequently than carcinoma confined to the skin. Careful evaluation of neck lymph nodes must be made and consideration given to prophylactic as well as therapeutic neck dissection.

Tumors of the Scalp or Forehead Invading Bone

When squamous cell carcinoma of the skin of the scalp or forehead is clinically fixed to the skull, even in the absence of radiographic evidence of destruction, it should be assumed that there is invasion of bone. Full-thickness resection of the calvaria in the involved area should generally be performed (Fig. 38-7). A more limited excision, even including removal of the outer table of the skull, is frequently followed by recurrence. If the lesion overlies either the sagittal or lateral sinus, caution must be exercised in removing the bone to prevent exsanguination. The neurosurgeon should be part of the operative

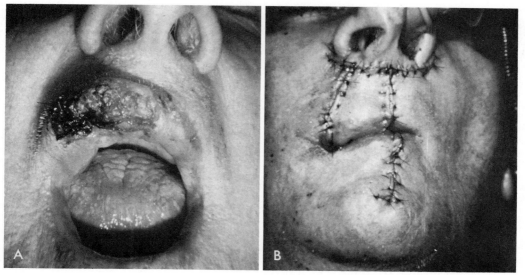

Figure 38-6 *A,* An extensive carcinoma of the upper lip treated by wide excision. *B,* Reconstruction of the upper lip by a combination of an Abbe flap from the lower lip and bilateral advancement flaps. (See also Color Plate II-C.)

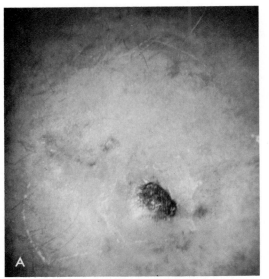

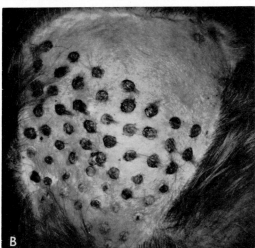

Figure 38–7 *A,* Recurrent squamous carcinoma of the scalp, previously excised and irradiated, in a 44 year old Haitian male. Radiographs revealed invasion of the cortex of the skull. This was treated by wide excision, including full-thickness skin grafts of the skull with replacement of the defect by an acrylic prosthesis. A rotation scalp flap was used to cover the defect.

B, The donor site, which was covered with a split-thickness graft, was later implanted with hair transplants.

(See also Color Plate II-D.)

team. Dural invasion, which is determined at the time of resection, requires excision of dura. When underlying brain is involved, salvage is unlikely.

Two alternatives are available for imme-diate reconstruction of skull. If any doubt exists as to the adequacy of cancer exci-sion, a split-thickness skin graft should be used. The graft will take well over dura or brain. The patient seems to be undistur-bed by the pulsating brain directly beneath the skin graft, and further reconstruction with a rotation flap of scalp or a pedicle flap may be undertaken at a later date. Im-mediate reconstruction may also be ob-tained by moving a large scalp rotation flap into position to cover exposed bone and dura. Bone loss may be replaced ei-ther by split rib graft or by the use of a sili-cone rubber plate, or Vitallium mesh tai-lored to fit the defect. The open area resulting from the flap rotation is closed by the use of a split-thickness skin graft.

Tumors Invading the Maxilla and Orbit

In instances of neglect or recurrence of cancer, deep invasion of the maxillary, frontal, and ethmoid sinuses may occur by direct extension. This is determined by radiographic examination, biopsies, and operative exposure. Maxillectomy with ex-cision of all involved sinuses and palate should be performed. The ultimate deci-sion as to the exenteration of the orbit may require operative exposure to determine whether there is direct extension of tumor into the floor of the orbit and into the eye itself. Preservation of the palate is not as critical a problem, since a prosthesis is readily available.

Parotidectomy

This may be required because of direct invasion through the capsule of the gland, or to allow adequate excision of parotid lymph nodes. The decision as to whether or not the facial nerve should be preserved depends on the extent of the individual cancer.

Auditory Canal

Squamous carcinoma of the skin may in-vade the external auditory canal or arise in the canal itself. In the invasive stage, recurrence is common following any treatment method which does not include the underlying cartilage. Surgical excision of the cartilage should be performed with closure utilizing the available local tissue or a split-thickness skin graft.

Deep invasion of the middle or internal ear requires excision of the temporal bone along with the overlying tissues.

REFERENCES

Allen, A. C.: Persistent "insect bites" (dermal eosinophilic granulomas) simulating lymphoblastomas, histiocytoses, and squamous cell carcinomas. Am. J. Pathol., 24:367, 1948.

Arons, M. S., Rodin, A. E., Lynch, J. B., Lewis, S. R., and Blocker, T. G.: Scar tissue carcinoma: II. An experimental study with special reference to burn scar carcinoma. Surg. Forum, 16:488, 1965.

Bennett, J. E., Moore, T. S., Vellios, F., and Hugo, N. E.: Surgical treatment of skin cancer of the nose. Am. J. Surg., 117:382, 1969.

Binder, S. C., and Catlin, D.: Epidermoid carcinoma of the skin of the nose. Am. J. Surg., 116:506, 1968.

Blum, H. F.: Review: Sunlight as causal factor in cancer of the skin in man. J. Natl. Cancer Inst., 9:247, 1948.

Carpenter, C., Derbes, V. J., and Jolly, H. W.: Carcinoma of the skin—A guidepost to internal malignancy? J.A.M.A., 186:621, 1963.

Conley, J.: Management of malignant tumors of the scalp. Ann. N.Y. Acad. Sci., 114:976, 1964.

Conley, J.: Cancer of the skin of the nose. Arch. Otolaryngol., 84:55, 1966.

Converse, J.: Reconstructive Plastic Surgery. Philadelphia, W. B. Saunders Company, 1964.

Freeman, R. G., Knox, J., and Heaton, C. L.: The treatment of skin cancer. Cancer, 17:535, 1964.

Glass, R. L., Spratt, J. S., and Perez-Mesa, C.: The fate of inadequately excised epidermoid carcinoma of the skin. Surg. Gynecol. Obstet., 122:245, 1966.

Jackson, R.: Observations on the natural course of skin cancer. Can. Med. Assoc. J., 92:564, 1965.

Lund, H. Z.: How often does squamous cell carcinoma of the skin metastasize? Arch. Dermatol., 92:635, 1965.

Modlin, J. J.: Cancer of the skin. Miss. Med., 51:364, 1954.

Mohs, F.: The chemosurgical method for the microscopically controlled excision of cancer of the skin. N.Y. State J. Med., 56:3486, 1956.

Mustardé, J. C.: Repair and Reconstruction in the Orbital Region. Baltimore, The Williams and Wilkins Company, 1966, p. 117.

Pack, G. T., and Davis, J.: Radiation cancer of the skin. Radiology, 84:436, 1965.

Pack, G. T., and Wuester, W. O.: The development of cancer in acrodermatitis chronica atrophicans. J.A.M.A., 118:879, 1942.

Ratzer, E. R., and Strong, E. W.: Squamous cell carcinoma of the scalp. Am. J. Surg., 114:570, 1967.

Reed, W. B., Landing, B., Sugarman, G., Cleaver, J. E., and Melnyk, J.: Xeroderma pigmentosum: Clinical and laboratory investigation of its basic defect. J.A.M.A., 207:2073, 1969.

Ridenhour, C. E., and Spratt, J. S.: Epidermoid carcinoma of the skin involving the parotid gland. Am. J. Surg., 112:504, 1966.

Roth, D., and Sage, H. H.: Defective photochemical repair in epithelium predisposed to field cancerization. Cancer, 24:511, 1969.

Sage, H. H.: Palpable cervical lymph nodes. J.A.M.A., 168:496, 1958.

Schewe, E. J., and Pappalardo, C.: Cancer of the external ear. Am. J. Surg., 104:753, 1962.

Sedlin, E. D., and Fleming, J. L.: Epidermoid carcinoma arising in chronic osteomyelitic foci. J. Bone Joint Surg. (Am.), 45-A:827, 1963.

Stell, P. M., and Brown, G. A.: Delibrate delayed primary skin grafting. Br. J. Surg., 57:702, 1970.

Sulzberger, M., Baer, R. L., and Borota, A.: Do roentgen-ray treatments as given by skin specialists produce cancers or other sequelae? A.M.A. Arch. Dermatol. Syph., 65:639, 1952.

Treves, N., and Pack, G. T.: The development of cancer in burn scars. Surg. Gynecol. Obstet., 51:749, 1930.

Warren, S., and Hoerr, S. O.: A study of pathologically verified epidermoid carcinoma of the skin. Surg. Gynecol. Obstet., 69:726, 1939.

39

Squamous Cell Carcinoma of the Body and Extremities

W. Robson N. Grier, M.D.

Squamous cell carcinoma, also called epidermoid carcinoma, prickle cell carcinoma, spinocellular carcinoma, spinalioma, Bowen's carcinoma, cornified epithelioma, and pavement epithelioma, is a malignant tumor arising from the epidermis or its appendages whose cells show some degree of maturation toward keratin formation (Rook, 1968).

CLASSIFICATION

Among the resolutions and recommendations of the International Conference on the Biology of Cutaneous Cancer, 1962, was the following:

It is suggested that, insofar as possible, diagnosis of cutaneous tumors conform to classification by histopathologic type, anatomic site and known environmental or genetic predisposing factors:

   a. Histopathologic Types
     1) Squamous cell carcinomas (of skin exclusive of mucosa of lip, penis, scrotum, vulva)
       i. Squamous cell carcinoma

       ii. Squamous cell carcinoma arising in burns, ulcers, scars
       iii. Senile keratosis with squamous cell carcinoma
       iv. Squamous cell carcinoma arising in other precancerous dermatoses
     2) Keratoacanthoma . . .
   b. All Lesions Should Be Accurately Identified as to Anatomic Site With as Great Specificity as Possible

The use of general anatomic sites such as "face" and "lower extremity" are not satisfactory, for they are likely to conceal differences in distribution that are significant. Distinction between the skin and mucous membranes of the lips, vulva, penis, scrotum and anus should always be made.

   c. Known Predisposing Exposures and Genetic Predispositions
     1) Environment
       i. Radiation
         a. Actinic
         b. Ionizing
       ii. Chemical
         a. Occupational
         b. Therapeutic
         c. Others, as specified
       iii. Social (custom and habit)
       iv. Burns, scars, and ulcers

2) Predisposing genetic disorder
  i. Albinism
  ii. Xeroderma pigmentosum
  iii. Basal cell hamartomas (basal cell naevi)

The above classification is designed to cover all histopathologic types of skin cancer. We are concerned in this chapter only with the squamous cell carcinoma; however, all the predispositions apply except basal cell hamartomas.

According to Bendl and Graham (1970), it is important to classify squamous carcinoma into solar (senile) keratosis with squamous cell carcinoma, adenoid squamous cell carcinoma, and de novo squamous cell carcinoma. The incidence of metastases was 0, 2, and 17 percent respectively. In addition, they would use the classification as mentioned above, e.g., x-ray keratosis with squamous carcinoma.

HISTORY

In the first century Celsus, a Roman physician, noted cancer developing in a burn scar. In 1775, Sir Percival Pott described squamous cancer of the scrotum due to soot in chimney sweeps. The cause of cancer of another site was not discovered for more than 100 years; it was not until 1879 that lung cancers in Schneeberg miners were shown to be caused by ionizing radiation (Stewart, 1963). In 1822, arsenic was recognized as a cause of skin cancer. In 1828, Jean Nicolas Marjolin gave an excellent account of burn scar cancer, and subsequently this entry became known as Marjolin's ulcer.

In 1835, Hawkins described the first case of squamous carcinoma arising in a sinus of chronic osteomyelitis. In 1875, Volkman reported scrotal cancer in paraffin workers, and in 1876 Bell added coal tar and shale oil to the list of skin carcinogens. In England, epitheliomas due to occupational hazards became so common that in 1920 they became a notifiable disease.

In 1900 the kangri burn cancer was described by E. F. Neve, and subsequently similar cancers were reported from Japan (kairo cancer) and northwest China (kang cancer).

Prior to the recognition of keratoacanthoma (also called self-healing squamous carcinoma), the statistics on squamous carcinoma would contain these cases. Therefore, the incidence of metastases would be lower and the results of treatment better. In an excellent review of the subject, Baer and Kopf (1963) credit a 1954 report by Levy, Cohn, Shaffer, and Beerman with giving impetus to the general recognition of keratoacanthoma. However, most statistics prior to 1960 are suspect. The incidence is one keratoacanthoma to three squamous carcinomas (Champion and Rook, 1962). Baer and Kopf reviewed series in which the ratio varied from 1 to 50 to almost 2 to 1, with an average of 1 to 4.

EPIDEMIOLOGY AND INCIDENCE

Since many of the etiologic factors involved in squamous carcinoma are known, the incidence of the disease is quite predictable, although it varies widely from one region to another and among races in the same area. The two main factors are the amount of sunlight and the susceptibility of the skin. It is very common in fair-skinned people living in sunny climates such as Queensland, Australia, and Texas, where skin cancer constitutes 50 percent and 33 percent, respectively, of all cancers (Belisario, 1959). In such areas of high insolation, the vast majority of skin cancer will be on the head and neck, and the basal cell epithelioma will be the predominant skin cancer. However, because the hands and forearms of farmers and other outdoor workers are exposed, there will be a moderate number of epitheliomas on the upper extremity, and these are mainly squamous cancers. The distribution of squamous carcinoma of the skin in a series from Texas (Freeman and Knox, 1967) was: head and neck, 81 percent; upper extremity, 16 percent (hands, 11 percent; arms, 5 percent); trunk, 1.5 percent; lower extremity, 1.3 percent.

Contrast the above distribution with the reports from New Guinea (Atkinson et al., 1963) and Uganda (Davies, 1968), where the people have dark skins; squamous carcinoma is much commoner than basal cell epithelioma, and the main etiologies are tropical ulcers, old burns, and traumatic scars. The squamous cancers in the report from New Guinea were distributed as follows: head and neck, 7 percent; upper extremity, 3 percent; trunk, 11 percent; lower extremity, 79 percent. The Uganda distribution was: head and neck, 13 percent; upper extremity, 5 percent; trunk, 2 percent; and lower extremity, 80 percent.

In Thailand (Transurat, 1963), where sunlight, chronic ulceration, and scars are all important in etiology, the distribution of squamous skin cancer is: head and neck, 50 percent; upper extremity, 10 percent; trunk, 18 percent; and lower extremity, 22 percent.

Most series report fewer women than men with squamous carcinoma of the skin. In the report from M. D. Anderson Hospital, Texas (Macdonald and Bubendorf, 1964), women formed 20 percent of the patients; in Minnesota the corresponding figure was 25.5 percent (Lynch et al., 1970); in the California Tumor Registry, 33 percent (Epstein et al., 1968); in Uganda, 37 percent; in Japan, 41 percent (Miyaji, 1963); in East Germany, 44 percent (Yung and Kolzsch, 1968). It appears that men have more exposure to the common carcinogens. They work outdoors more than women and receive more solar radiation. In those countries in which the squamous cancers are secondary to traumatic scars, burns, and tropical ulcers, these precancerous lesions are commoner in men.

There is one area, however, where women may develop more squamous cancer than men—the leg. Obviously because of women's dress, they receive more exposure from the sun on their legs. In a report from Sweden, Swanbeck and Hillstrom (1969) described 122 ulcerating squamous cancers on the lower extremity; 72 of these were in women and 50 in men. More specifically, of 89 on the legs, 53 were in women and 36 in men; moreover, if the cancers developing on specific lesions, such as scars and chronic fistulas, were eliminated, the figures showed 40 women and 15 men. Finally, considering the lesions on the lateral aspect of the lower third of the leg where you would expect the most sun exposure, 12 occurred in women and only 2 in men.

Haenszel (1963) has described the incidence of skin cancer in the United States by reviewing the figures from the ten-city and Iowa morbidity studies and the Upstate New York Cancer Registry. Table 39–1 is reprinted from this article and

TABLE 39–1 AGE-ADJUSTED* SKIN CANCER INCIDENCE PER 100,000 POPULATION BY SEX, HISTOLOGIC TYPE, SITE, AND REGION: EIGHT UNITED STATES CITIES** (1947)

Type and Site	Four Northern Cities		Four Southern Cities		Ratio: North/South	
	Male	Female	Male	Female	Male	Female
All skin cancers†	33.4	25.4	143.3	88.0	0.23	0.29
Melanoma‡	1.5	1.6	3.2	5.6	0.47	0.29
Face, head, neck, and upper extremities	0.5	0.7	1.3	2.6	0.38	0.27
Trunk and lower extremities	0.9	0.9	1.2	2.4	0.75	0.38
Basal and basosquamous cell carcinoma‡	15.7	12.4	61.2	40.6	0.26	0.31
Face, head, and neck	14.3	11.3	55.1	35.6	0.26	0.32
Upper extremities	0.1	0.1	2.3	1.2	0.04	0.08
Trunk	0.9	0.8	2.4	2.2	} 0.42	} 0.31
Lower extremities	0.2	0.1	0.2	0.7		
Squamous cell carcinoma‡	8.9	5.3	32.3	14.3	0.28	0.37
Face, head, and neck	5.9	3.5	22.2	9.6	0.27	0.36
Upper extremities	1.5	0.5	8.0	3.0	0.19	0.17
Trunk	0.8	0.8	1.3	0.9	} 0.70	} 0.75
Lower extremities	0.6	0.4	0.7	0.7		

From Haenszel: Variations in skin cancer incidence within the United States. National Cancer Institute Monograph, 10:238, 1963.
*Age-adjusted to total population of continental United States, 1950.
**Whites only.
†Includes newly diagnosed cases of all types and sites, with or without microscopic confirmation.
‡Includes other and unspecified sites.

shows the marked influence of sunlight and the general site and sex distribution of skin cancer. In the United States, squamous cancer is slightly more common than basal cell carcinoma outside of the head and neck. This is mainly due to squamous cancer of the upper extremity in men, which is about three times as common as basal cell epithelioma. On the lower extremity, the incidence of squamous cancer is about 1½ times that of basal cell carcinoma, while on the trunk, basal cell is twice as common as squamous cell cancer. There are approximately twice as many squamous cancers on the trunk as on the lower extremity, and twice as many on the upper extremity as on the trunk.

The incidence of squamous carcinoma occurring in chronic stasis (venous, varicose) ulcers of the leg must be very low. Halliday (1968) reports 1 case in 20 years from a clinic which sees 30 to 50 new patients with venous ulcers each year. The incidence of a squamous carcinoma developing in chronic osteomyelitis is about 0.5 percent (Sedlin and Fleming, 1963).

ETIOLOGY AND PATHOGENESIS

Squamous carcinoma arises on the body and extremities much less commonly than on the head and neck because the latter get more exposure to the sun. However, sunlight is still the major carcinogen accounting for the high incidence on the back of the hand and forearm of outdoor workers. Special habits may account for unusual distribution. Australian fishermen get squamous carcinoma on their legs, which are exposed to the sun while they are in their boats. In a careful survey of the incidence, site, and type of skin cancer in Minnesota, Lynch et al. (1970) found that both basal cell carcinoma and squamous carcinoma were commoner on the lower extremities of women than of men. For all other sites, these skin cancers were commoner in men than in women. Swanbeck and Hillstrom (1969) reported that the incidence of squamous carcinoma of the lower extremities in the southern half of Sweden was 1.74 times that in the northern half. Solar radiation will account for most squamous car-

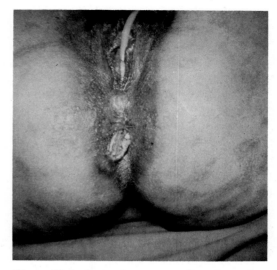

Figure 39-1 Perianal squamous cell carcinoma in a 31 year old female with Fanconi's anemia (see text). (See also Color Plate II-E.)

cinomas in a fair-skinned population living in a sunny climate. It is of little importance in other races and, of course, does not affect the unexposed skin of the body. Patients with xeroderma pigmentosum and albinism, without regard to racial origin, are extremely prone to develop solar-induced skin cancers (see Chapters 6 and 23).

There may be other genetic predispositions to squamous carcinoma of the skin. We have excised a squamous carcinoma from the perianal skin of a 31 year old woman with Fanconi's anemia (Figs. 39-1 and 39-2). This case (J.M.) has been reported by Swift and Hirschhorn (1966). Also, the case of her sister who has Fanconi's anemia and a perianal carcinoma was reported (Swift, 1971). Dyskeratosis congenita is another familial syndrome. It shares many of the features of Fanconi's anemia, including the propensity to develop squamous carcinoma of the mucocutaneous junctions as well as other malignancies (Selmanowitz et al., 1971).

Arsenical skin cancer is mainly on the body and extremities and is apparently unrelated to sunlight. Shu Yeh et al. (1968) has studied a group of cases in an area of Taiwan where the artesian wells supplying the drinking water have a high arsenic content. He found 72 percent of the le-

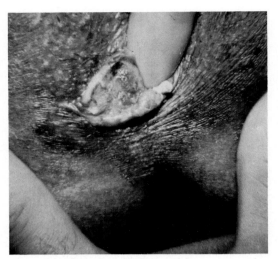

Figure 39–2   Close-up view of Figure 39–1 with a finger in the anus. This was a 2 × 2.5 cm. firm, nodular, squamous carcinoma.
(See also Color Plate II-F.)

sions on the trunk and 22 percent on the extremities, with 74 percent on unexposed skin. Ninety-nine percent were multiple. Of the 238 lesions examined by biopsy, 58 percent were intraepidermal carcinoma—mostly Bowen's disease, 19 percent squamous cancer, 15 percent basal cell epitheliomas, and 7 percent combined form. The 46 squamous carcinomas were distributed as follows: head and neck, 3; trunk, 17; hand, 10; lower extremity, 17 (7 of these on the foot).

Chemically induced skin cancer is usually squamous carcinoma, and most of the exposure is occupational and is a direct action of the chemical on the skin. The principal chemical carcinogens are soot, paraffin, tar, shale oil, spindle oil, mineral oil, anthracene, and asphalt. A chronic dermatitis may or may not precede the cancer and, if present, is quite similar to chronic solar or radiation dermatitis. According to Hueper (1963), workers handling coal tar and mineral oil develop cancers mainly on the hands, forearm, face, and neck; workers with pitch dust develop cancers of the legs and feet; mule-skinners, paraffin pressers, and chimney sweeps develop cancers of the scrotum or vulva and sometimes the groin. The incidence of these chemically induced cancers continues to increase with increased dura-

tion of exposure. Of the patients with skin cancer, the average exposure is 20 years.

Scar tissue carcinoma is a common type of squamous carcinoma of the body and extremities (Arons et al., 1965). In most series, and especially among dark-skinned people, scars will be the commonest predisposing condition. The best known of these is Marjolin's ulcer, the burn scar which was not grafted and which healed after months of treatment (Fig. 39–3). Probably of a similar etiology are the squamous carcinomas developing in chronic leg ulcers; acne conglobata (Dillon and Spjut, 1963); hidradenitis suppurativa (Humphrey et al., 1969); the sinuses of osteomyelitis (Figs. 39–4 and 39–5); other chronic sinuses and fistulas, such as empyemic, urethral, and pilonidal ones; old scars on amputation stumps; and vaccination scars. In the last category, unlike the other scar tissue malignancies, squamous carcinoma does not predominate. In a collected series of 24 cases, Marmelzat (1968) found 13 basal cell carcinomas, 6 melanomas, and 5 squamous carcinomas. One of the squamous carcinomas developed five weeks after vaccination, but the

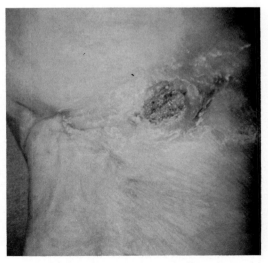

Figure 39–3   Two-cm. squamous cell carcinoma in old burn scar (Marjolin's ulcer); lateral aspect of knee.

This 57 year old white female suffered hot water burns to both legs at age 6. Healing occurred without grafting after one year. In the past 19 years she has developed four separate squamous carcinomas in the burn scars.
(See also Color Plate III-A.)

others had latent periods of 33, 40, 44, and 45 years.

A rare but interesting group of six cases of squamous carcinoma developing in skin tubes used as substitutes for the esophagus has been reported (Nakayama et al., 1971). Two of these cancers were related to chronic fistulas, but the other four developed in intact antethoracic skin tubes. The latent intervals were 21, 23, 24, 25, 30, and 34 years.

The kangri burn cancer was best described in 1923 by E. F. Neve, a surgeon at the Kashmir Mission Hospital. The kangri is an earthenware bowl 5 to 6 inches in diameter, surrounded by basket work, heated by burning wood and charcoal, and worn under a single loose garment against the skin of the abdomen or inner thighs. Many elderly Kashmiris who have used the kangri for years show a chronic heat dermatitis with many burn scars. There is pigmentation with dry horny skin. Squamous cancer develops as an infiltration under the horny surface with ulceration later. Since 1881, of the 2491 operations for epithelioma, approximately 2000 (84 percent) were for kangri cancer (Neve, 1923).

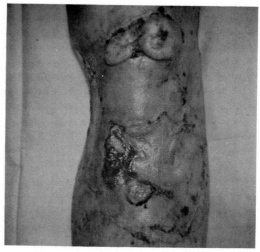

Figure 39–5 Same patient as Figure 39–4 five weeks postoperatively. Note large recurrence at upper margin of graft and smaller recurrence near lower margin. An above-knee amputation successfully controlled the local disease, but six months later a groin dissection was necessary for squamous carcinoma involving 5 of 16 nodes. The patient died six months later at home.
(See also Color Plate III-C.)

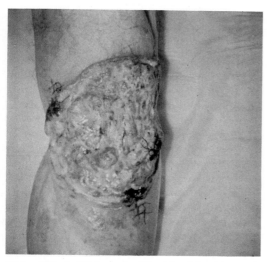

Figure 39–4 White male, 63, with a 10 × 12 cm. ulcerating squamous carcinoma just below the left knee. Severe bilateral compound fractures received in an automobile accident at age 5 resulted in much scarring. At age 27, a right above-knee amputation was done for osteomyelitis. Because a left above-knee amputation would confine him to a wheelchair, wide excision including the underlying cortex of the tibia was done.
(See also Color Plate III-B.)

Rather similar cancers have been reported from Japan resulting from the use of a kairo—a tin box filled with burning charcoal and worn against the skin of the abdomen (Treves and Pack, 1930). Cross (1967) of Dublin, Ireland, has seen 162 cases in five years of squamous carcinoma of the middle third of the lower leg in elderly Irish women. All these patients came from rural areas and gave a history of working close to turf (peat) fires most of their lives.

Squamous cancer of the skin has developed in association with many chronic skin diseases, especially those with much scarring and those chronic granulomas with pseudoepitheliomatous hyperplasia. In many of these, the treatment may have been more of a factor in the development of the squamous cell carcinoma than the disease. A recent report of squamous cell carcinoma in psoriasis vulgaris (Lagerholm and Skog, 1968) describes three cases and reviews the previously reported cases—about 50. Most of the 50 cases had been treated with arsenic, and many had received treatment with other carcinogenic modalities—tar or mineral oil ointments and radiation. The incidence is obviously very low, and four possible relationships between the two diseases are considered: (1) it is coincidence; (2) treatment causes the squamous carcinoma; (3) the squamous carcinoma develops with psoriasis around it—the Koebner phenomenon; and (4) squamous carcinoma develops secondary to psoriasis.

Squamous carcinoma has developed in association with granuloma inguinale (Davis, 1970), lichen planus (Kronenberg et al., 1971), lupus vulgaris, leprosy, syphilis, discoid lupus erythematosus, poikiloderma congenitale, dystrophic epidermolysis bullosa (Wechsler et al., 1970), and chronic fungal infections of the skin, such as chromoblastomycosis (Caplan, 1968). In cases with extensive pseudoepitheliomatous hyperplasia and in the absence of metastases, the diagnosis of carcinoma is always in some doubt.

Carcinoma develops in areas of radiation dermatitis, and in most cases on the body and extremities the histology will be squamous cell, while in the head and neck it will be basal cell. In a consecutive series of 105 basal cell or squamous skin cancers admitted to the hospital, there were 20 which developed in an area of radiodermatitis (Totten et al., 1957). This is a high incidence compared with other reports, and in the future, with better control of radiation exposure, radiation dermatitis should be rare. The fingers of doctors and dentists were a common site for radiation-induced squamous carcinoma.

Gerwig and Winer (1968) described three patients who developed radiodermatitis because of radioactive gold rings. One of these cases had a deeply invasive squamous carcinoma of the finger requiring amputation.

Several squamous carcinomas have been reported in association with nevus sebaceus (Jones and Heyl, 1970). However, only one of these metastasized; most tumors secondary to nevus sebaceus are benign. Rarely a skin cancer develops secondary to porokeratosis of Mibelli—always after prolonged presence of foci and always squamous cancer (Oberste-Lehn, 1968). Cutaneous horns may have a squamous carcinoma at the base. It is not clear whether the horn develops on top of the cancer, or whether the horn comes first

and the cancer develops at the base. Likewise, giant condylomata may develop a secondary squamous carcinoma. While squamous carcinoma has been reported in association with sebaceous (epidermoid) cyst and seborrheic keratosis, these benign lesions are so common and secondary carcinoma so rare that the association must be coincidental.

Recently a great deal of evidence has been accumulated that immunologic factors are important in the development and progression of human malignancies. The evidence suggests that lack of immunity allows a cancer to grow and metastasize. This may explain the different behavior of apparently similar squamous cancers in different patients.

Squamous carcinoma develops in the scars of patients with polydysplastic epidermolysis bullosa. This disease has its onset at birth or shortly thereafter and is characterized by bullous formation, erosion, and delayed healing with tissue paper–like scarring. Wechsler et al. (1970) described three cases with well-differentiated squamous carcinoma of the skin—all with lymph node metastases. One of the patients, as well as 1 of 12 previously reported cases, accepted an allograft, which implies altered immunologic competence. This may account for the very poor prognosis of squamous carcinoma in polydysplastic epidermolysis bullosa.

Another case of squamous carcinoma of the skin occurring in a patient with a congenital immune defect has been reported (Stritzler et al., 1971). This patient, a 33 year old man, had congenital dislocation of the hips, kyphoscoliosis, and a huge number of skin lesions resembling seborrheic keratoses, Bowen's disease, and verruca vulgaris.

There is probably an increased risk of development and spread of cancer in patients on immunosuppressive drugs. Harris (1971) reported the case of a 32 year old man treated for psoriasis with methotrexate and steroids who developed squamous carcinoma of the skin of the right leg with lymph node and lung metastases.

To discover impaired immunologic reactivity, Eilber and Morton (1970) tested cancer patients for their ability to develop delayed cutaneous hypersensitivity to 2,4-dinitrochlorobenzene (DNCB). Of those who failed to react, 93 percent (27 of 29) were inoperable or developed early recurrence, whereas 92 percent (50 of 54) of patients who reacted to DNCB were free of disease for six months. These 83 patients had a wide variety of malignancies, but 41 of them had squamous carcinoma (head and neck, 21; cervix, 14; skin, 6). This test may be valuable in predicting the rare occurrence of metastasis from squamous cancer of the skin.

CLINICAL DESCRIPTION

The patient with squamous cancer of the skin usually gives a history describing one of the various etiologies mentioned above. Typically he is a man who has worked outdoors most of his life; he is about 60 years of age, and he has had actinic changes in the skin for years. These consist of loss of elastic tissue, irregular pigmentation, telangiectasia, and keratoses. Many early squamous cancers are asymptomatic, but commonly the patient complains of enlargement of a skin lesion, bleeding with trauma, failure to heal, pruritus, or pain.

Clinically a squamous carcinoma is suspected when an area of induration is noted. This may be in what was previously a solar keratosis, and there is often accompanying hyperemia. The lesion may be a plaque with or without a crust, but most squamous cancers ulcerate early. The better differentiated tumors may retain a papillary or verrucous surface with little ulceration or discharge. The typical ulcerated cancer is a firm tumor in the skin and raised several millimeters above it, having an indurated edge and an eroded center with a purulent exudate.

Those cancers arising in arsenical keratoses and Bowen's disease may be flat and without ulceration, but there is always induration and usually hyperemia.

Patients with chronic diseases, such as stasis ulcers and hidradenitis suppurativa, usually have a 20-year history or more of the original disease with a short (several-month) history of the squamous carcinoma. However, it may be hard to differentiate a stasis ulcer with secondary carcinoma from an ulcerating squamous carcinoma on the ankle.

Anaplastic squamous carcinoma is a rare lesion, arising from apparently normal skin, growing and metastasizing rapidly. It appears first as a firm, slightly inflamed nodule and may be mistaken for a sebaceous cyst. However, it grows through the skin, ulcerates, and may kill the patient in a few months.

Epithelioma cuniculatum is a very well-differentiated squamous carcinoma reported on the sole of the foot (Aird et al., 1954). There is a bulbous mass with a squashy consistency which, when pressed, exudes greasy, rancid material from multiple sinuses on the surface "like toothpaste from a tube." The tumor extends through the foot and appears on the dorsum, so that amputation is necessary for cure.

A few cases of giant condylomata have become well-differentiated squamous carcinoma, and clinically this should be suspected if a condyloma develops induration or ulceration. Subungual squamous cancer may be missed because it presents as a nail deformity, paronychia, chronic fissure, or pyogenic granuloma. The thumb and index finger are most frequently involved, and only about 15 percent of cases occur on the toes.

Squamous cancer developing in a burn scar occurs at an average of 32.5 years after the burn (Treves and Pack, 1930). Commonly it is a flat, indurated, ulcerated lesion, and rarely an exophytic papillary growth. Squamous carcinoma may arise deep in an osteomyelitis sinus and not be evident until the pink, opaque, rounded edge of cancer grows out to the surface. It is well described by Sedlin and Fleming (1963), who reviewed 90 cases reported in the literature since 1940 and added 12 cases from the Detroit-Windsor area. The lower extremity accounted for 85 percent of the cases, with 50 percent in the tibia. The patient is usually a middle-aged man (ranging from 24 to 76 years) who has had osteomyelitis an average of 30.5 years. The cancer starts in the epithelial-lined sinus tract; usually there is a recent history of pain and increased discharge and fetor, and a growth appears at the opening of the sinus. The lymph nodes are often enlarged, usually due to inflammation, but often there are metastases (22 of 102 in this series).

INCIDENCE OF METASTASES

Lymph node metastases from squamous carcinoma of the skin have been reported with an incidence varying from 0.1 percent to more than 50 percent. Low rates are reported by dermatologists who usually treat small early lesions, by surveys which include office-treated cases, and by surveys which include all sites. High rates are found in the older articles because of late diagnosis, in reports from specialized institutions where advanced cases are treated, and especially in studies in which only certain sites are considered.

The lowest incidence of metastases was reported by Lund (1965). In 12 years of office practice as a dermatopathologist in Greensboro, North Carolina, he estimated he examined 3700 squamous cell tumors and that 780 of these were invasive cancers. Only four metastasized, for an incidence of 0.1 percent of the total group, or 0.5 percent of the invasive cancer group. In addition, he made a search and collected reports of 12 cases with metastases: 5 were of actinic origin and were all on the head and neck; 7 were not of actinic origin and were on the body and extremities.

Epstein et al. (1968) reviewed the squamous skin cancers in the California Tumor Registry (all hospital cases), and of 6900 cases, only 142 (2 percent) had distant metastases at the time of admission. In the 142 patients, there were 174 metastatic sites as follows: regional nodes, 115; subcutaneous tissue, 17; bone, 14; lung, 7; other, 12; and generalized, 9. At five years 25 percent were still alive, and only 57 percent died of skin cancer.

Kopf and Andrade (1967) reported, "In a consecutive series of 132 cutaneous squamous cell carcinomas . . . 4 patients had metastases before their first visit to our clinic and 2 developed metastases subsequently."

At the Roswell Park Hospital between January 1, 1946, and December 31, 1950, there were 413 patients with 601 squamous cancers of the skin. Metastases were found on admission in 20 patients and

during the follow-up in another 15 patients—a total incidence of 8.5 percent. The rate was slightly higher in men, but there was no difference between the various sites (Katz et al., 1957). Modlin (1954), reviewing the overall experience with squamous cancer of the skin at the Ellis Fischel State Cancer Hospital, found node metastases in 52 of 444 (11 percent) of those cases followed at least five years. Of the 52 metastasizing cancers, 42 were larger than 2 cm., and 30 were recurrent.

Mohs (1956) treated 100 squamous carcinomas of the skin of the body and extremities with chemosurgery. Recurrent cancers accounted for 40 percent. Eleven cases metastasized.

Abrao and Bastos (1967) reported 104 cases of squamous cancers of the upper extremity, 8 of which (7.6 percent) had axillary lymph node metastases. In the lower extremity, 6 of 52 cases (11.5 percent) had inguinal metastases.

In a series of 511 patients with squamous cancers of the extremities treated at the Mayo Clinic from 1908 to 1946, 43 (8.4 percent) had node metastases on admission, and 46 of 379 (12.1 percent) patients who were traced developed metastases later (Browne et al., 1953). Blood-borne metastases went to the lung, vertebrae, and bony pelvis.

In 1941, Taylor, Nathanson, and Shaw, going back over the records as far as 1915, reported the squamous cancers of the extremities at three Boston hospitals. Of 335 patients, 66 (19 percent) developed node metastases. A breakdown by site revealed metastases in 3 of 33 on the finger (9 percent), 30 of 205 on the hand (15 percent), 7 of 27 on the arm (26 percent), 10 of 24 on the foot (41 percent), and 16 of 46 on the leg (36 percent). There were 18 cases with epitrochlear node involvement and 1 case with popliteal node involvement.

Swanbeck and Hillstrom (1969) reported 22 cases of exophytic squamous cancer of the lower extremities, of which 3 had metastases to nodes only, and 3 had metastases to nodes and other organs. Of 122 ulcerating squamous cancers, 15 had node metastases, and 5 had metastases to nodes and other organs.

The commonest cause of squamous cancer of the skin in New Guinea is tropical ulcer, and of these cases, 20 percent had node metastases (Atkinson et al., 1963).

Reporting the experience at the Ellis Fischel State Cancer Hospital with epidermoid skin cancer of the lower extremity, Glass et al. (1964) found that 10 of 26 patients developed inguinal node metastases (3 on admission and 7 within one year). Of 13 cases with antecedent lesions, only 2 metastasized despite an average size of 12 cm. Of 13 cases without antecedent lesions (de novo cancers), 8 metastasized.

Of 72 squamous cancers of the fingers, hand, and forearm, 10 metastasized to axillary nodes and 1 to the epitrochlear nodes (Johnson and Ackerman, 1950). There were no metastases from those cancers which had not invaded the dermis below the level of the sweat glands.

Of 53 cases of chronic scar tissue carcinoma, 18 (34 percent) developed metastases (Arons et al., 1965). However, 7 of the 23 burn cancers were on the head and neck, and none of these metastasized. Therefore, of the 46 squamous cancers on the body and extremities, the incidence of metastases was 39 percent.

PATHOLOGY

The gross pathology of squamous carcinoma of the skin is what the clinician sees, although he may not be able to appreciate the depth of penetration exactly. The large lesion often keratinizing may show yellowish gray areas on cross-section. They are often heavily infected. Deep fixations, such as a lesion on the dorsum of the hand attached to the underlying tendons, may be due to either inflammatory or neoplastic tissue, and it is impossible to tell grossly which one (Ackerman and del Regato, 1970). The tumor may grow mainly outward, producing a burgeoning exophytic growth; it may develop inward, infiltrating and ulcerating the underlying tissue; or it may spread in the skin itself, involving only the epidermis and papillary layer. At times it may involve a large surface area of skin with little invasion in depth.

The local spread of skin cancer has been accurately studied by Mohs during chemosurgical treatment, which is a microscopically controlled excision (Mohs, 1952). He has described spread beyond the obvious clinical extent of the tumor in eight categories:

1. Dermis; commoner in basal cell cancer than in squamous cell cancer.

2. Fascial planes; muscle is rarely invaded, but the carcinoma may spread along the fascia on the surface of a muscle.

3. Periosteum; Mohs describes a squamous cancer that spread along the cranial bones for 10 cm.

4. Perichondrium; rarely spreads more than 5 to 6 mm.

5. Embryonic fusion planes; mainly applies to facial cancers.

6. Nerve sheath; this spread was found in 20 of 807 squamous cancers (2.5 percent). Most of these were on the face, and many were recurrent and far-advanced lesions.

7. Lymphatic vessels; by embolic spread in the local skin plexus. Only five cases.

8. Blood vessels; either along the walls (seen in seven squamous cancers) or in the lumen (seen in one squamous cancer).

Despite the above possibilities, it is usually easy to completely excise a small primary squamous cancer if a 5-mm. margin of normal tissue is included on all sides. In difficult cases frozen sections may be helpful during surgery, and every case should be checked microscopically for adequacy of excision both laterally and in depth.

For the clinician certain other points in the pathology may be helpful in managing the case. Most squamous cancers of the skin are well differentiated; however, if the histology is poorly differentiated, anaplastic, or spindle cell, the prognosis is grave. The depth of infiltration is important. In studying squamous carcinoma of the hand, Johnson and Ackerman (1950) found no metastases from lesions that had not invaded deeper than the level of the sweat glands. If the epidermis adjacent to the invasive squamous carcinoma shows changes of a solar keratosis, the lesion is less aggressive, according to the report of Bendl and Graham (1970). However, the adenoid squamous carcinoma (adenoacanthoma) which probably develops in a solar keratosis with acantholysis may be a more serious lesion. Of 155 patients with 213 lesions described by Johnson and Helwig (1966), 3 developed metastases and 2 others died of direct extension. The most serious squamous carcinoma is the one with no associated changes of solar keratosis, termed squamous carcinoma de novo by Bendl and Graham. Of 98 lesions reported by Johnson and Helwig (1966), 17 metastasized.

DIFFERENTIAL DIAGNOSIS

Clinically, squamous carcinoma may have no characteristic feature, especially if it is diagnosed early as most skin cancers are today. Bendl and Graham (1970) described two groups of squamous carcinoma. The first group of 156 were those cancers derived from solar keratoses, and the common initial clinical diagnoses were: basal cell carcinoma, 48; solar keratosis, 45; squamous carcinoma, 19; solar keratosis with squamous carcinoma, 14; keratoacanthoma, 11; seborrheic keratosis, 8. The second group of 92 were those squamous cancers with no microscopic changes of an associated solar keratosis, and the common initial clinical diagnoses were: basal cell carcinoma, 34; squamous carcinoma, 19; keratoacanthoma, 11; solar keratosis, 8. While the diagnostic accuracy appears low, the conditions diagnosed are closely related, and most require the same treatment. These were mainly small lesions; the median size was 1 cm. in the first group, and 1.2 cm. in the second.

A report in 1941 (Torrey and Levin) correlated the clinical and histologic diagnoses of 4213 skin lesions, 2806 of which were confirmed as being epitheliomas by biopsy. The clinical diagnosis of epithelioma was confirmed histologically in 90 percent, and the more specific clinical diagnosis of squamous carcinoma was confirmed in 75 percent. Of the 1403 histologically diagnosed squamous cancers, 953 (68 percent) were correctly diagnosed as such clinically. There were 317 incorrect positive clinical diagnoses of squamous carcinoma. Lightstone et al. (1965) calculated the diagnostic accuracy, taking into account both the incorrect positive clinical diagnoses and the incorrect negative clini-

cal diagnoses. According to their method, the figures here would be:

$$\frac{953}{953 + 450 + 317} \times .100 = 55.4 \text{ percent}$$
$$\text{(diagnostic accuracy)}$$

Basal cell epithelioma accounted for more than half the incorrect diagnoses. However, about 46 percent of these squamous cancers were on the oral mucosa, lower lip, or upper extremity where the confusion with basal cell carcinoma hardly exists. The diagnostic accuracy in the other sites would probably be under 50 percent. It is well to remember that in 1941, keratoacanthoma was not being separated from squamous carcinoma. And indeed keratoacanthoma has a characteristic clinical picture, while squamous carcinoma does not. From the same article the diagnostic accuracy for basal cell epithelioma would be 66 percent.

Applying the same calculations to another review (Freeman and Knox, 1963), the diagnostic accuracy for squamous carcinoma is 41 percent and for basal cell carcinoma, 70.5 percent.

If there is any suspicion, a biopsy should be done. For example, a chronic paronychia does not heal with standard therapy, a chronic osteomyelitis sinus develops unusual pain. It is well to remember that squamous cancers can become infected, so that the demonstration of some organism does not rule out the diagnosis. Likewise, squamous cancer can be secondary to a chronic infection or scarring type of dermatitis. It is important, in a lesion where two diseases coexist, to take the biopsy from the squamous carcinoma—the hard, indurated, opaque tissue. Inflammatory tissue and pseudoepitheliomatous hyperplasia do not have as much induration.

A squamous cancer, especially that developing in Bowen's disease, may look like psoriasis. Such a lesion may not be deeply infiltrating and may have no ulceration and yet have already metastasized to the regional nodes. A primary syphilitic chancre, especially in an unusual location, can mimic squamous cancer.

With the added information of the biopsy, the differential diagnosis narrows down to keratoacanthoma, pseudoepitheliomatous hyperplasia, metastatic squamous carcinoma, and, in the anaplastic tumor, melanoma and various metastatic malignancies. Keratoacanthomas usually grow much faster with a rounded, protruding, partially skin-covered contour and a central keratin plug. They often occur on normal skin and may be multiple and recurrent, but the only sure differentiation from squamous carcinoma is their "self-healing" feature. The diagnosis is made by a correlation of the clinical and pathologic evidence. For the latter to be of value, the whole lesion must be removed, or at least a deep biopsy through the center and edge of the lesion should be performed. If the clinical and pathologic evidence is not quite typical for keratoacanthoma, the lesion should be treated as a squamous carcinoma — provided the treatment is not mutilating. Fortunately, on the body and extremities such a lesion can usually be adequately excised without causing disability. The exception would be a lesion requiring amputation of a digit, especially the thumb. The spontaneous healing of such a large keratoacanthoma would cause some permanent destruction of tissue and scarring, but the loss of tissue would be less than that of a cancer operation. From a scientific viewpoint, it is more instructive to await spontaneous resolution. Once the lesion is removed, even when the pathologist diagnoses squamous carcinoma, the question always remains whether it might have regressed if left another few weeks.

Pseudoepitheliomatous hyperplasia associated with chronic granulomas may mimic squamous carcinoma. Foreign body granulomas may be caused by hairs, certain oils, and silica. Pseudoepitheliomatous hyperplasia occurs also in chronic ulcers, insect bites, molluscum contagiosum, granuloma inguinale, tuberculosis cutis, syphilis, bromoderma, ioderma, atebrin dermatitis, and deep mycoses (sporotrichosis, blastomycosis, chromoblastomycosis, coccidioidomycosis). Even in the presence of a confirmed chronic granuloma, there may be a secondary squamous carcinoma developing. The common tropical ulcer of the leg in Africa is an example.

Metastatic squamous carcinoma in the skin rarely presents a difficult diagnostic problem. However, Camiel (1969) described metastases from squamous carcinoma of the lung to the palm, sole, nail bed, nose, face, and scalp. These tumors were the presenting complaint of the patients, and some ulcerated and grossly looked like primary squamous cancer of the skin. In contrast to the primary lesions, the usual metastatic cancer involving the skin (1) arises at a deeper level — dermis or subcutaneous tissue; (2) ulcerates late; (3) does not involve skin showing premalignant changes (e.g., actinic or radiation dermatitis); (4) histologically does not arise from adjacent epithelium; and (5) is associated with a known primary cancer elsewhere. If the skin cancer is metastatic, there would be no metastases in the regional nodes, in keeping with the general rule that metastases do not metastasize (Sugarbaker et al., 1971). Anaplastic squamous carcinoma may be hard to differentiate from melanoma, metastatic tumors, reticulum cell sarcoma, and so forth.

Squamous carcinoma should be seriously considered in the differential diagnosis of skin tumors of the foot. In a study of such lesions at the Christie Street Hospital, London, Levene (1958) found 68 squamous cancers, 31 of which were on the sole. The other common malignancy was melanoma, a total of 67 being found with 32 of these on the sole. However, the melanomas were mainly in the region of the arch, while the squamous cancers tended to be on the metatarsal region and heel.

TREATMENT

Squamous carcinoma of the skin other than that of the head and neck is usually treated by surgery. Although the tumor is radiosensitive, there are more complications with radiation to the body and extremities, apparently due to poor blood supply. Topical chemotherapy may be useful in treating actinically damaged skin with multiple solar keratoses and some very early squamous cancers (see Chapter 73). Likewise, a dermatologist may elect to treat relatively superficial squamous cell carcinomas by curettage and electrodesiccation (see Chapter 67). Cryosurgery is a new technique of destroying cancer and may have a place in the treatment of small squamous cancers (see Chapter 72). Chemosurgery, the microscopically controlled excision of cancer developed by Mohs, has a definite place, especially in the treatment of squamous cancers on the fingers and hands (see Chapters 70 and 71).

Surgery performed on the body and extremities does not involve many of the difficulties encountered when it is performed on the face. There is less chance of proximity to a vital structure and, therefore, less hesitation in taking an adequate border of grossly normal tissue. The skin is on a more even plane, and the extent of the tumor both laterally and in depth may be easier to judge. There is usually enough laxity to permit a primary closure, and if not there is seldom any hesitation in using a split-thickness skin graft, because the cosmetic result is not as important as it is on the face. In many cases, these cancers on the extremities arise in precancerous lesions, such as sinuses, chronic ulcers, and burn scars, and these lesions should be excised along with the cancer. Finally, the pathologic specimen is intact, and the pathologist can give a more informed opinion than with any other method of treatment.

As a general rule, a skin lesion that may be a squamous carcinoma should be examined by biopsy prior to definitive excision. This should be done prior to any extensive procedure such as an amputation. Usually an incision biopsy is performed. While the biopsy should obtain adequate tissue, it should not extend, especially in depth, to the level at which the definitive cancer operation will be done.

If a lesion is less than 1 cm. and is not clinically aggressive, the diagnosis usually falls between solar keratosis and solar keratosis with squamous carcinoma. An excision biopsy with 2 to 3 mm. of normal tissue laterally and in depth may be done. When the pathologist reports invasion into the dermis (squamous cell carcinoma) in one small area, usually in the center of the solar keratosis, there is no need to do a wider excision. However, if a nodular squamous cell carcinoma is similarly removed, even though it is a similarly small lesion (i.e., less than 1 cm.), the 2- to 3-mm. margin should not be considered adequate. Such lesions should be excised with a minimum of 5 mm. of normal tissue all around, therefore, in the case cited above, the biopsy scar should be completely excised. The aim of the second operation should be to stay out of the previous wound; therefore, the excision should be on a deeper plane. This will usually include all the subcutaneous tissue and the fascia.

For a larger lesion diagnosis is confirmed by incision biopsy. An adequate excision is generally stated to be 5 to 10 mm. of normal surrounding tissue. Actually, the essence of a good operation is the clinical recognition of the extent of the tumor. If local anesthesia is to be used, it should not be injected until later. Very careful inspection and palpation from different angles and with a good light are necessary. The line of excision is carefully marked on the skin with dye and again the tumor is evaluated. Usually one part of the line is changed either farther away or closer. Despite its mobility, a large lesion should be removed with the fascia over the muscles.

From a tumor surgery viewpoint, the wound should now be closed with a split-thickness skin graft. This makes discovery of a recurrence very easy. Even a primary closure means the sliding of two flaps of skin together, and recurrences may take place in depth and be concealed (Baer and Kopf, 1965). However, primary closure is the usual procedure on the body and extremities, because there is excess skin in many areas (see Chapter 66).

If the pathologist reports that a squamous cancer has been inadequately excised, there is a 50 percent recurrence rate and a 25 percent mortality, according to Glass et al. (1966). Immediate re-excision is advised. In this series all 17 recurrences occurred within two years, and 13 of these occurred within six months of the initial excision. If the wound had originally been grafted, it may be adequate to excise only that margin where the pathologist found cancer at the surgical line of incision. If a primary closure had been done, it is usually necessary to re-excise the whole scar with particular attention to the area of probable residual cancer.

Burn scar cancers may be prevented by grafting third degree burns, keeping scars supple with lanolin or other creams, and releasing contractures at flexures. If there is any thickening or ulceration in an old burn scar, excise it. It may be cicatrix, pseudoepitheliomatous hyperplasia, or squamous carcinoma—in any case, it should be removed.

The incidence of squamous carcinoma in chronic leg ulcers is probably very low, but the ulcers which come to surgical excision are the most advanced ulcers which have not responded to other therapy. The usual excision of these ulcers including the underlying fascia is wide enough so that even if cancer is found in the specimen it is not necessary to reoperate (Arons et al., 1965). If the pathologist indicates that the cancer excision has not been complete, an amputation (usually above the knee) will probably be necessary.

The squamous cancer developing in the epithelial-lined tract associated with chronic osteomyelitis almost always involves the bone. The treatment is amputation to include all the involved bone. In one case of osteomyelitis of the calcaneus, the cancer did not involve the bone and was cured by a wide local excision (Sedlin and Fleming, 1963).

Spread of squamous cancer via the local skin lymphatics forming satellite nodules is rare (Roth et al., 1967). In such a case, a very wide local excision would be indicated. Infiltration involving the bone of an extremity requires amputation of that bone. It is rare to have involvement of the muscle in an extremity (Mohs and Lathrop, 1952) without bone involvement also. Regional lymph nodes may become involved owing to embolic spread of squamous cancer (for routes of spread, see Chapter 44). Because the incidence of lymph node metastases is low, prophylactic dissections are not done. However, it is important to do a dissection if the nodes are clinically positive, because approximately 33 percent of these patients will be cured. Ordinarily nodes are not examined by biopsy; if the nodes are clinically involved, a complete axillary or inguinal node dissection is done. If the epitrochlear nodes are involved, an axillary dissection is also done. It is well to remember that clinical examination of the nodes is more accurate in the groin than in the axilla. Involved axillary nodes are more likely to escape detection.

PROGNOSIS

The prognosis for most patients with squamous carcinoma of the skin is good. The usual small (less than 2 cm.) lesion, developing in an actinic keratosis and without obvious gross clinical morphology of invasive cancer, has the best prognosis. Even when larger, these actinic cancers seem to have a better prognosis. The squamous cancers developing in areas of radiation dermatitis also have a low incidence of metastases. The squamous cancers developing in scar tissue have an intermediate prognosis, and those developing from normal skin (squamous carcinoma de novo) have a very poor prognosis. Perhaps because of the different etiologies, squamous cancer of the skin of the head and neck has a better prognosis than that elsewhere, and the upper limb lesions have a better prognosis than those on the lower limbs.

Despite a high incidence, skin cancer (excluding melanoma) is not a common cause of death. In California there are approximately 6000 new skin cancers each year and 40 to 50 deaths from skin cancer (Dunn et al., 1965). Three-fourths of these deaths are due to squamous carcinoma.

In 1968, Hansen and Jensen reported a long-term follow-up of 1198 skin cancers treated primarily by radiation from 1937 to 1955. Of 46 deaths due to skin cancer, 43 were in the group of 450 squamous cancers, for a mortality rate of 9.5 percent.

Freeman and Knox (1967) reported only 10 recurrences after treatment of 368 squamous cancers followed five years—a cure rate of 97.3 percent. This report came from Texas, where there is a high incidence of solar-induced skin cancer; only 19 percent of lesions occurred on the body and extremities, and early diagnosis and treatment were the rule (only 13 percent of these lesions were larger than 2 cm).

Contrast these figures with the results of treatment of 26 invasive squamous cancers of the lower limb reported by Glass et al. (1964). Group I cases comprised 13 cancers with no recognized antecedent lesion. These averaged 4.9 cm. in diameter;

8 metastasized, and only 6 patients (47 percent) were alive at the time of the report. The 13 Group II cases developing on scars had a somewhat better prognosis despite their large size—on the average, 12.2 cm. Only 2 of these metastasized, and 10 patients survived (77 percent). This report came from the Ellis Fischel State Cancer Hospital, where advanced cases are referred. Only 1 of the 26 cancers was less than 2 cm.; probably none developed in actinic keratoses, and the 13 Group I cases were de novo cancers by all criteria.

Mohs (1956) reported a series of 100 patients with squamous cancers of the body and extremities with at least a six-year follow-up. Forty percent of the cancers were recurrent, and 11 percent metastasized. Of 81 determinate cases, 79 (97.5 percent) were locally controlled by chemosurgery. However, 9 unsuccessful results were due to uncontrolled metastases; therefore, the five-year cure rate was 70 of 81 (86.4 percent). In the same 1956 report, Mohs cited a five-year cure rate in squamous cancer of the skin of all sites of 84.8 percent, whereas he has more recently reported a five-year cure rate of 93.2 percent in 1562 determinate cases (Mohs, 1970).

Shu Yeh (1968) reported 46 arsenical epidermoid skin cancers in 35 patients. Over a five-year period, 12 patients died. Five of the deaths were due to metastases from the skin cancer. Of 46 patients with chronic scar tissue cancers of the body and extremities reported by Arons et al. (1965), 18 (39 percent) developed metastases, and 14 (30 percent) died. Of 71 patients with chronic osteomyelitis with squamous carcinoma followed 18 months or longer, 22 (31 percent) developed metastases, and 18 (25 percent) died (Sedlin and Fleming, 1963).

In a report from Brazil (Abrao and Bastos, 1967), the five-year survival rate for 82 patients with squamous cancers of the upper extremity was 88 percent, and for 42 patients with squamous cancers of the lower extremity 83 percent. In a series from Boston (Taylor et al., 1941), the mortality for 265 patients with squamous cancers of the upper extremity was 15.5 percent, and for 70 patients with cancers of the lower extremity 38.5 percent. Of the

68 deaths, 66 percent occurred in the first year and 93 percent in the first two years. Of 48 patients with squamous cancers of the upper extremity followed at least three years, Johnson and Ackerman (1950) reported 41 (85 percent) cured.

REFERENCES

Abrao, A., and Bastos, J. A. V.: Skin carcinoma of the extremities. Rev. Brasil. Cirurg., 54:124, 1967.

Ackerman, L. V., and del Regato, J. A.: Cancer: Diagnosis, Treatment and Prognosis. Ed. 4. St. Louis, Mo., C. V. Mosby Company, 1970.

Aird, I., Johnson, H. D., Lennox, B., and Stansfeld, A. G.: Epithelioma cuniculatum. Br. J. Surg., 42:245, 1954.

Arons, M. S., Lynch, J. B., Lewis, S. R., and Blocker, T. G.: Scar tissue carcinoma (review). Ann. Surg., 161:170, 1965.

Atkinson, L., Farago, C., Forbes, B. R. V., and Ten Seldam, R. E. J.: Skin cancer in New Guinea native people. Natl. Cancer Inst. Monograph, 10:167, 1963.

Baer, R. L., and Kopf, A. W.: Keratoacanthoma. In Year Book of Dermatology, 1962–1963. Chicago, Year Book Medical Publishers, 1963, pp. 7–42.

Baer, R. L., and Kopf, A. W.: Complications of therapy of basal cell epitheliomas. In Year Book of Dermatology, 1964–1965. Chicago, Year Book Medical Publishers, 1965, pp. 7–26.

Belisario, J. C.: Cancer of the Skin. London, Butterworth, 1959.

Bendl, B. J., and Graham, J. H.: New concepts on the origin of squamous cell carcinoma—a clinicopathologic and histochemical study. Proc. Natl. Cancer Conf., 6:471, 1970.

Browne, H. J., Coventry, M. B., and McDonald, J. R.: Squamous carcinoma of the extremities. Proc. Staff Meet. Mayo Clin., 28:590, 1953.

Camiel, M. R., Aron, B. S., Alexander, L. I., Benninghoff, D. L., and Minkowitz, S.: Metastases to palm, sole, nailbed, nose, face, and scalp from unsuspected carcinoma of the lung. Cancer, 23:214, 1969.

Cancer from mineral oil (editorial). Br. Med. J., 4:443, 1969.

Caplan, R. M.: Epidermoid carcinoma arising in extensive chromoblastomycosis. Arch. Dermatol., 97:38, 1968.

Champion, R. H., and Rook, A.: Keratoacanthoma. In Proceedings of the XII International Congress of Dermatology, 1962, p. 288.

Conway, H., Hugo, N. E., and Tulenko, J. F.: Surgery of Tumors of the Skin. Ed. 2. Springfield, Ill., Charles C Thomas, Publishers, 1966.

Cross, F.: On a turf (peat) fire cancer—Malignant change superimposed on erythema ab igne. Proc. R. Soc. Med., 60:1307, 1967.

Davies, J. N. P., Meyer, R., and Thurston, P.: Cancer of the integumentary tissues in Uganda Africans—The basis for prevention. J. Natl. Cancer Inst., 41:31, 1968.

Davis, C. M.: Granuloma inguinale – A clinical, histological and ultrastructural study. J.A.M.A., 211:632, 1970.

Dillon, J. S., and Spjut, H. J.: Epidermoid carcinoma occurring in acne conglobata. Ann. Surg., 159:451, 1963.

Dunn, J. E., Jr., Levin, E. A., Linden, G., and Harzfeld, L.: Skin cancer as cause of death. Calif. Med., 102:361, 1965.

Eilber, F. R., and Morton, D. L.: Impaired immunologic reactivity and recurrence following cancer surgery. Cancer, 25:362, 1970.

Epstein, E., Epstein, N. N., Brag, K., and Linden, G.: Metastases from squamous cell carcinoma of the skin. Arch. Dermatol., 97:245, 1968.

Freeman, R. G., and Knox, J. M.: Clinical accuracy in diagnosis of skin tumors. Geriatrics, 18:546, 1963.

Freeman, R. G., and Knox, J. M.: Recent Results in Cancer Research – Treatment of Skin Cancer. New York, Springer-Verlag, 1967.

Freeman, R. G., and Knox, J. M.: Recent experience with skin cancer. Arch. Dermatol., 101:403, 1970.

Gellin, G. A., and Possick, P. A.: Occupational cancer of the skin. Cutis, 5:543, 1969.

Gerwig, T., and Winer, M. N.: Radioactive jewelry as a cause of cutaneous tumor. J.A.M.A., 205:595, 1968.

Glass, R. L., Spratt, J. S., Jr., and Perez-Mesa, C.: Epidermoid carcinoma of the lower extremities. Arch. Surg., 89:955, 1964.

Glass, R. L., Spratt, J. S., Jr., and Perez-Mesa, C.: The fate of inadequately excised epidermoid carcinoma of the skin. Surg. Gynecol. Obstet., 122:245, 1966.

Haenszel, W.: Variations in skin cancer incidence within the United States. Natl. Cancer Inst. Monograph, 10:255, 1963.

Halliday, J. P.: Squamous carcinoma in a venous ulcer. Med. J. Aust., 1:449, 1968.

Hansen, P. B., and Jensen, M. S.: Late results following radiotherapy of skin cancer. Acta Radiol. (Stockh.), 7:307, 1968.

Harris, C. C.: Malignancy during methotrexate and steroid therapy for psoriasis. Arch. Dermatol., 103:501, 1971.

Hueper, W. C.: Chemically induced skin cancer in man. Natl. Cancer Inst. Monograph, 10:389, 1963.

Humphrey, L. J., Playforth, H., and Leavell, U. W.: Squamous cell carcinoma arising in hidradenitis suppurativum. Arch. Dermatol., 100:59, 1969.

International Conference on the Biology of Cutaneous Cancer, 1962. Natl. Cancer Inst. Monograph, 10:657, 1963.

Johnson, R. E., and Ackerman, L. V.: Epidermoid carcinoma of the hand. Cancer, 3:657, 1950.

Johnson, W. C., and Helwig, E. B.: Adenoid squamous cell carcinoma (adenoacanthoma). Cancer, 19:1639, 1966.

Jones, E. W., and Heyl, T.: Naevus sebaceus. Br. J. Dermatol., 82:99, 1970.

Katz, A. D., Urback, F., and Lilienfeld, A. M.: The frequency and risk of metastases in squamous cell carcinoma of the skin. Cancer, 10:1162, 1957.

Kopf, A. W., and Andrade, R.: Year Book of Dermatology, 1966–1967. Chicago, Year Book Medical Publishers, 1967, p. 229.

Kronenberg, K., Fretzin, D., and Potter, B.: Malignant degeneration of lichen planus. Arch. Dermatol., 104:304, 1971.

Lagerholm, B., and Skog, E.: Squamous cell carcinoma in psoriasis vulgaris. Acta Derm. Venereol. (Stockh.), 48:128, 1968.

Levene, M.: Distribution of skin tumours of the sole of the foot. Br. Med. J., 1:1519, 1958.

Lightstone, A. C., Kopf, A. W., and Garfinkel, L.: Diagnostic accuracy – A new approach to its evaluation. Arch. Dermatol., 91:497, 1965.

Lund, H. Z.: How often does squamous cell carcinoma of the skin metastasize? Arch. Dermatol., 92:635, 1965.

Lynch, F. W., Seidman, H., and Hammond, E. C.: Incidence of cutaneous cancer in Minnesota. Cancer, 25:83, 1970.

MacDonald, E. J., and Bubendorf, E.: Some Epidemiological Aspects of Skin Cancer. Tumors of the Skin. Seventh Clinical Conference on Cancer, M. D. Anderson Hospital. Chicago, Year Book Medical Publishers, 1964.

Marmelzat, W. L.: Malignant tumors in smallpox vaccination scars. Arch. Dermatol., 97:400, 1968.

Miyaji, T.: Skin cancers in Japan: A nationwide five year survey, 1956–1960. Natl. Cancer. Inst. Monograph, 10:55, 1963.

Modlin, J. J.: Cancer of the skin. Missouri Med., 51:364, 1954.

Mohanty, S., Federowicz, T. E., and Ueharra, H.: Metastatic lesions of the fingers. Surgery, 64:411, 1968.

Mohs, F. E.: Chemosurgery in Cancer, Gangrene, and Infections. Springfield, Ill., Charles C Thomas, Publisher, 1956.

Mohs, F. E.: Chemosurgery for the microscopically controlled excision of skin cancer. Proc. Natl. Cancer Conf., 6:517, 1970.

Mohs, F. E., and Lathrop, T. A.: Modes of spread of cancer of the skin. Arch. Dermatol. Syph. (Berlin), 66:427, 1952.

Nakayama, K., Yazawa, C., Sakakibara, N., Suzuki, H., Yano, M., and Ide, H.: A Report on three cases with carcinoma developing after antethoracic reconstructive surgery of the esophagus (by skin graft). Surgery, 69:800, 1971.

Nelson, L. W., and Hamilton, C. F.: Primary carcinoma of the nail bed. Arch. Dermatol., 101:63, 1970.

Neve, E. F.: Kangri burn cancer. Br. Med. J., 2:1255, 1923.

Oberste-Lehn, H., and Moll, B.: Porokeratosis Mibelli and prickle cell carcinoma. Hautarzt, 19:399, 1968.

Oettlé, A. G.: Skin cancer in Africa. Natl. Cancer Inst. Monograph, 10:197, 1963.

Oluwasanmi, J. A., Williams, A. O., and Alli, A. F.: Superficial cancer in Nigeria. Br. J. Cancer, 23:714, 1969.

Rook, A. J.: *In* Rook, A., Wilkinson, D. S., and Elibing, F. J. G. (Eds.): Textbook of Dermatology. Oxford, Blackwell Scientific Publications, 1968.

Roth, W. G., Klippenstein, H., and Weber, G.: Skin metastases in squamous cell carcinoma of the skin. Arch. Klin. Exp. Dermatol., 230:126, 1967.

Schreiber, M. M., Shapiro, S. I., Berry, C. Z., Dahlen, R. F., and Friedman, R. P.: The incidence of skin cancer in southern Arizona (Tucson). Arch. Dermatol., 104:124, 1971.

Schwartz, L., Tulidan, L., and Birmingham, D. J.: Occupational diseases of the skin. Ed. 3. Philadelphia, Lea and Febiger, 1957, p. 732.

Sedlin, E. D., and Fleming, J. L.: Epidermoid carcinoma arising in chronic osteomyelitis foci. J. Bone Joint Surg., 45A:827, 1963.

Selmanowitz, V. J., Van Voolen, G. A., and Steier, W.: Fanconi's anemia and dyskeratosis congenita. J.A.M.A., 216:2015, 1971.

Shapiro, L., and Baraf, C. S.: Subungual epidermoid carcinoma and keratoacanthoma. Cancer, 25:141, 1970.

Shu Yeh, How, S. W., and Lin, C. S.: Arsenical cancer of the skin. Cancer, 21:312, 1968.

Skipworth, G. B., and Flandermeyer, K. L.: Incidence of skin cancer. Arch. Dermatol., 102:561, 1970.

Stewart, H. L.: Foreword to the first conference on the biology of cutaneous cancer. Natl. Cancer Inst. Monograph, 10:IX, 1963.

Stritzler, C., Sawitsky, A., and Stritzler, R.: Bittner's syndrome. Arch. Dermatol., 103:548–549, 1971.

Sugarbaker, E. V., Cohen, A. M., and Ketcham, A. S.: Do metastases metastasize? Ann. Surg., 174:161, 1971.

Swanbeck, G., and Hillstrom, L.: Analysis of etiological factors of squamous cell skin cancer of different locations. Acta Derm. Venereol. (Stockh.), 49:427, 1969.

Swift, M.: Fanconi's anemia in the genetics of neoplasia. Nature (Lond.), 230:370, April, 1971.

Swift, M. R., and Hirschhorn, K.: Fanconi's anemia: Inherited susceptibility to chromosome breakage in various tissues. Ann. Intern. Med., 65:496, 1966.

Swift, M., Zimmerman, D., and McDonough, E. R.: Squamous cell carcinoma in Fanconi's anemia. J.A.M.A., 216:325, April, 1971.

Taylor, G. W., Nathanson, I. T., and Shaw, D. T.: Epidermoid carcinoma of the extremities with reference to lymph gland involvement. Ann. Surg., 113:268, 1941.

Ten Seldam, R. E. J.: Skin cancer in Australia. Natl. Cancer Inst. Monograph, 10:153, 1963.

Torrey, F. A., and Levin, E. A.: Comparison of clinical and pathologic diagnoses of malignant conditions of the skin. Arch. Dermatol. Syph. (Chicago), 43:532, 1941.

Totten, R. S., Antypas, P. G., Dupertius, S. M., Gaisford, J. C., and White, W. L.: Pre-existing roentgen-ray dermatitis in patients with skin cancer. Cancer, 10:1024, 1957.

Transurat, P.: Regional incidence and pathology of skin cancer in Thailand. Natl. Cancer Inst. Monograph, 10:71, 1963.

Treves, N., and Pack, G. T.: The development of cancer in burn scars. Surg. Gynecol. Obstet., 51:749, 1930.

Wechsler, H. L., Krugh, F. J., Domonkos, A. N., Scheen, S. R., and Davidson, C. L.: Polydysplastic epidermolysis bullosa and development of epidermal neoplasms. Arch. Dermatol., 102:374, 1970.

Woolridge, W. E., and Freirchs, J. B.: Multiple adenoid squamous cell carcinoma. Arch. Dermatol., 104:202, 1971.

Yung, H. D., and Kolzsch, J.: Epidemiology of precancerous and malignant skin tumors. Hautarzt, 19:151, 1968.

40

The Pathology of Squamous Cell Carcinoma of the Skin

Siria Poucell, M.D., and Jorge Albores-Saavedra, M.D.

Squamous cell carcinoma of the skin is a neoplasm which originates in the epidermis but which is rarely confined to it (Fig. 40–1) (for intraepithelial carcinoma of Bowen's disease, see Chapter 27). More often, however, squamous cell carcinoma invades the dermis, from which it may spread to the adjacent tissues. It may be encountered at any site in the skin and occasionally arises from certain keratinous cysts.

Almost always it occurs in previously damaged skin, such as in chronic ulcers, radiodermatitis, burn scars, and fistulas (Bowers and Young, 1960; Sedlin and Fleming, 1963; Giblin et al., 1965), as well as in relation to other premalignant lesions (Graham, and Helwig, 1966). Of these, the most important ones are arsenical and solar keratosis (Helwig and Graham, 1964) and the genetically conditioned disease, xeroderma pigmentosum (Keeler, 1963). Helwig and Graham (1964) found invasive squamous cell carcinoma in 12 percent of cases of solar keratosis, in 14 percent of cases of erythroplasia of Queyrat, in 5 percent of cases of Bowen's disease, and in 8 to 9 percent of cases of the intraepidermal epitheliomas of

Jadassohn. Occasionally squamous cell carcinoma of the skin appears as the result of chronic exposure to chemical carcinogens, such as arsenic (Montgomery, 1941), soot, tar, creosote, fuel oil, pitch, and anthracene oil.

Squamous cell carcinoma of the skin occurs most frequently in white people who have been chronically exposed to sunlight (Urbach et al., 1966). The low incidence of this tumor among Negroes (Hazen and Freeman, 1950) is explained by their greater amount of cutaneous melanin, which plays an important protective role against ultraviolet light rays. This has been proved both epidemiologically and experimentally.

In some countries, such as Australia (Belisario, 1959), this tumor represents approximately 50 percent of all malignant tumors, and in Texas (Phillips, 1941) it constitutes 33 percent.

Squamous cell carcinoma is more frequent in males. Clinically it appears as a superficial, erythematous nodule, which in its early stages is small and firm. As it increases in size, it develops ulceration in its central portion. Then its borders become wider and indurated. The ulcerated part is

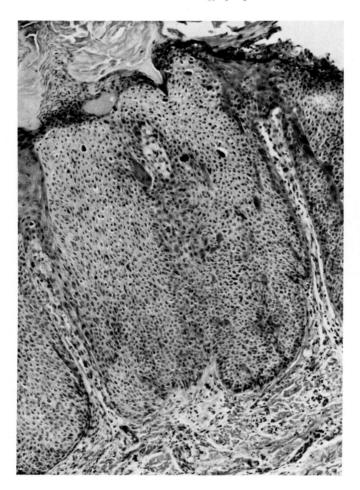

Figure 40-1 Bowen's disease. The epidermis is thickened and shows hyperkeratosis. Atypical cells are present at all levels. There are vacuolated cells, mainly in the upper layers. Multinucleated giant cells and mitotic figures may also be seen.

often crusted over. Some other tumors exhibit a verrucous or fungating appearance. Verrucous carcinoma is of a lower grade of malignancy than the ulcerated forms. However, the clinical course of squamous cell carcinoma is quite variable, and it is not possible to predict its clinical behavior on clinical grounds only. When the tumor originates from solar keratosis, it is less aggressive than when it is associated with Bowen's disease, Queyrat's erythroplasia, xeroderma pigmentosum, radiodermatitis, chronic ulcers, and fistulas.

Ulcerating squamous cell carcinoma of the lip, vulva, penis, and anus, which are covered by modified skin, grows more rapidly and is more prone to metastasize.

The incidence of metastasis of squamous cell carcinoma of the skin in general is very low, but it has been reported to range from 0 to 50 percent, according to different authors (Lund, 1965). There is a direct relationship between the depth of invasion and the ability to produce metastasis. The tumors that invade beyond the sweat glands more frequently give rise to metastases, and these tumors are usually more anaplastic.

HISTOPATHOLOGY

The tumor is made up of prickle cells, among which one sees variable degrees of differentiation. They are usually arranged in cords or sheets which invade the dermis. At least in some places it is possible to identify dyskeratosis and horn pearls (Fig. 40-2). Mitotic activity is quite variable, but in general the anaplastic tumors show more

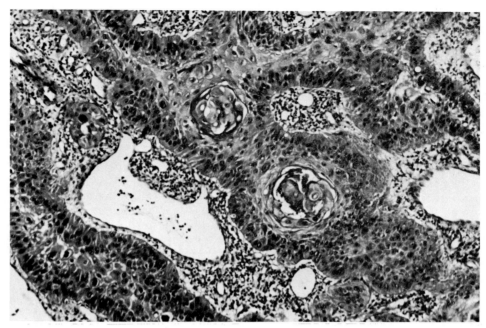

Figure 40-2   Anastomosing cords of neoplastic prickle cells. Two horn pearls are present. The stroma contains dilated blood vessels as well as a lymphocytic inflammatory infiltrate.

mitotic figures than do the well-differen-tiated ones (Fig. 40–3). Broders' (1932) system of classification is based on the proportion of well-differentiated and un-differentiated neoplastic cells. According to this system, there are four grades of squamous cell carcinoma. This system of grading is still utilized by some pathol-

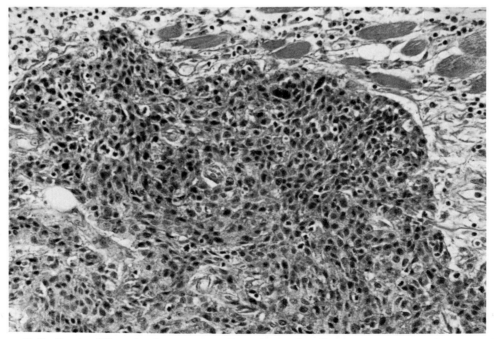

Figure 40-3   Poorly differentiated squamous cell carcinoma invading muscle. Nuclear pleomorphism is evident.

ogists. Many others, however, prefer to speak in terms of poorly, moderately, and well-differentiated tumors. In the well-differentiated squamous cell carcinoma, there usually is a chronic inflammatory infiltrate surrounding the tumor.

Recently De Moragas et al. (1970a) studied epidermal tumors for production of intercellular substance present in the normal epidermis. They found that individual cell keratinization was related to intercellular substance. In anaplastic squamous cell carcinoma, only the few cells that undergo keratinization show intercellular substance.

The same authors (De Moragas et al., 1970b) carried out immunofluorescence studies of basement membrane in epithelial skin tumors and found that the well-differentiated squamous cell carcinoma exhibited a clearly defined basement membrane, whereas in poorly differentiated or anaplastic tumors it was absent.

There are three special microscopic types of squamous cell carcinoma of the skin: spindle cell squamous carcinoma, adenosquamous (pseudoglandular or adenoid) carcinoma, and verrucous carcinoma. The former is often confused with a sarcoma or a pseudosarcomatous lesion. The opposite is also true. For example,

Hudson and Winkelman (1972) reported 10 cases of atypical fibroxanthomas which were originally diagnosed as the spindle cell variant of squamous cell carcinoma.

The adenoid or pseudoglandular squamous cell carcinoma is characterized by the formation of glandlike or tubular structures caused by acantholysis of the central portion of the cords (Figs. 40–4 and 40–5). At the present time, the pathogenesis of this phenomenon remains unknown. One of the proposed theories is that it is produced by an enzymatic defect. Adenoid or pseudoglandular squamous cell carcinoma appears more frequently in older individuals than do the usual types; this type appears mainly in the head and neck region or in exposed areas of the skin. Frequently it is multiple and is found in association with senile keratosis with or without acantholysis. In Johnson and Helwig's (1966) review of 155 patients, only three developed regional lymph node metastases, and one had lung metastases. Verrucous carcinoma occurs more frequently in the penis and vulva, and clinically it is often confused with condyloma acuminatum (Kraus and Pérez-Meza, 1966). Microscopically it is an extremely well-differentiated papillary squamous tumor. The frondlike papillary structures are com-

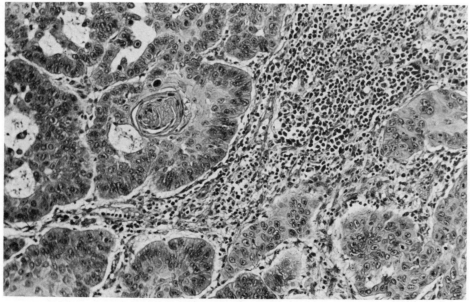

Figure 40–4 Pseudoglandular squamous carcinoma. A few glandlike structures are seen in the left upper corner.

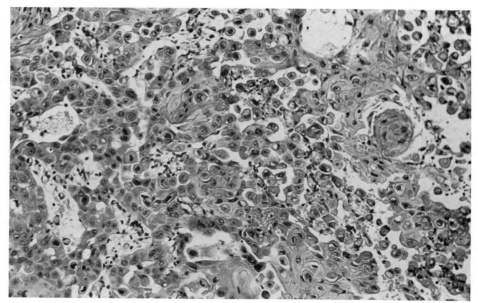

Figure 40–5 Extensive acantholysis in a pseudoglandular squamous cell carcinoma.

posed of cells with very little nuclear atypism. It seldom gives rise to metastasis.

HISTOCHEMISTRY

With histochemical techniques it has been shown that the mucin present in the adenoid or pseudoglandular squamous cell carcinoma gives reactions similar to that of the pilar portion of the epidermis. This substance has been identified as hyaluronic acid.

DIFFERENTIAL DIAGNOSIS

Although the diagnosis of squamous cell carcinoma of the skin is quite simple, the disease should be distinguished from senile keratosis, keratoacanthoma, and pseudocarcinomatous hyperplasia. In senile keratosis the qualitative changes are essentially the same as those already noted. The important difference between this entity and Bowen's disease is that it does not affect the whole thickness of the epidermis, and, with squamous cell carcinoma, that the basement membrane is completely intact.

Keratoacanthoma usually is of short duration and has a characteristic nodular ap-

pearance. When the lesion exhibits all the microscopic features of keratoacanthoma (see Chapter 32, Histopathology of Keratoacanthoma), the diagnosis should present no problem, even though cell pleomorphism and mitosis may be present. However, the microscopic diagnosis should always be correlated with the clinical data. If doubt remains, the best way to manage this lesion is to treat it as a squamous cell carcinoma.

In the lesions that produce pseudocarcinomatous hyperplasia, one sees epidermal prolongations of well-differentiated cells that occasionally show individual keratinization and horn pearls. However, the dermis contains an inflammatory infiltrate which is part of the main disease responsible for the epithelial changes. Some basal cell carcinomas show extensive squamous metaplasia, and for this reason they are sometimes confused with squamous cell carcinoma.

REFERENCES

Belisario, J. C.: Cancer of the Skin. London, Butterworth, 1959.

Bowers, R. F., and Young, J. M.: Carcinoma arising in scars, osteomyelitis and fistulae. Arch. Surg., 80:564, 1960.

Broders, A. C.: Practical points on the microscopic grading of carcinoma. N.Y. J. Med., 32:667, 1932.

De Moragas, J. M., Winkelmann, R. K., and Jordan, R. E.: Immunofluorescence of epithelial skin tumors I. Cancer, 25:1399, 1970a.

De Moragas, J. M., Winkelmann, R. K., and Jordan, R. E.: Immunofluorescence of epithelial skin tumors II. Cancer, 29:1404, 1970b.

Giblin, T., Pickrell, K., Pitts, W., and Armstrong, D.: Malignant degeneration in burn scars: Marjolin's ulcer. Ann. Surg., 162:291, 1965.

Graham, J. H., and Helwig, E. B.: Cutaneous premalignant lesions. *In* Montagna, W., et al. (Eds.): Advances in Biology of Skin. Vol. 7, Carcinogenesis. New York, Pergamon Press, 1966, pp. 277–327.

Hazen, H. H., and Freeman, C. W.: Skin cancer in the American Negro. Arch. Dermatol. Syph., 62:622, 1950.

Helwig, E. B., and Graham, J. H.: Pathology of precancerous dermatoses. *In* Tumors of the Skin. Chicago, Year Book Medical Publishers, 1964, pp. 131–148.

Hudson, A. W., and Winkelmann, R. K.: Atypical fibroxanthoma of the skin: Reappraisal of 19 cases in which the original diagnosis was spindle-cell squamous carcinoma. Cancer, 29:413, 1972.

Johnson, W. C., and Helwig, E. B.: Adenoid squamous cell carcinoma (adenoacanthoma). A clinico-pathologic study of 155 patients. Cancer, 19:1639, 1966.

Keeler, C. E.: Albinism, xeroderma pigmentosum and skin cancer. Natl. Cancer Inst. Monogr., 10: 349, 1963.

Kraus, F. T., and Pérez-Mesa, C.: Verrucous carcinoma; clinical and pathologic study of 105 cases involving oral cavity, larynx and genitalia. Cancer, 19:26, 1966.

Lund, H. Z.: How often does squamous cell carcinoma of the skin metastasize? Arch. Dermatol., 92:635, 1965.

MacDonald, E. J., and Bubendorf, E.: Some epidemiologic aspects of skin cancer. *In* Tumors of the Skin. Chicago, Year Book Medical Publishers, 1964, p. 23.

Montgomery, H. M.: Epithelioma attributable to arsenic. J. Invest. Dermatol., 4:365, 1941.

Phillips, C.: The relationship between skin cancer and occupation in Texas. Texas J. Med., 36:613, 1941.

Sedlin, E. D., and Fleming, J. L.: Epidermoid carcinoma arising in chronic osteomyelitic foci. J. Bone Joint Surg. (Am.), 45:827, 1963.

Urbach, F., et al.: Ultraviolet radiation and skin cancer in man. *In* Montagna, W., et al. (Eds.): Advances in Biology of Skin. Vol. 7, Carcinogenesis. New York, Pergamon Press, 1967.

41

Malignant Ulcers Following Trauma

Richard J. Coburn, D.M.D., M.D.

Carcinomatous degeneration of traumatic scars, although rare, has fascinated surgeons and oncologists since the observations of Marjolin and Hawkins in the nineteenth century. This evolution from tissue injury to tumorigenesis spawned and sustained the traumatic, irritative theories of carcinogenesis. A circumscribed model in which the source of trauma can be defined, the onset of neoplasia observed, and the chronology related has only one imperfection: the number of scars developing carcinoma is infinitesimal. Nevertheless, full-thickness wounds allowed to heal by second intention in areas prone to repeated trauma are Marjolin's ulcer candidates.

The literature records two varieties of Marjolin's ulcers: lesions which develop within one year of injury, and latent tumors which appear 20 to 60 years after the initial trauma. The former is an uncommon variant of an uncommon lesion and merits limited discussion. The latter is the more characteristic form of the disease.

The incidence of Marjolin's ulcer, the eponym originally applied to burn scar neoplasia but now loosely applied to carcinomas originating in scar tissue, is thought to be decreasing. Unlike most tumors, the underlying if not the precipitating cause is known, and prophylaxis can be applied by improved treatment of acute burns and early resurfacing of thermal and other skin defects. Despite the potential for eradication through prevention, the disease persists, and the remainder of this chapter will consider the clinicopathologic manifestations and treatment of traumatic scar neoplasia.

HISTORY

Although Celsus mentions tumors arising in scar tissue, the credit for describing scar neoplasia belongs to surgeons of the mid-nineteenth century. Jean-Nicolas Marjolin, a Paris surgeon, described in an 1828 French publication a tumor arising in a traumatic scar: "the surface of the ulcer was formed by a tissue composed of a large number of irregular firm nodules which was in all respects similar to skin cancer." Five years later, on December 10, 1833, Caesar Hawkins, an English surgeon, delivered a paper before the Medico-Chirurgical Society of London, recounting his observations on tumor growth in scar tissue. His first case was a soldier who had been repeatedly flogged 11 years prior to admission: "in the cicatrix several warts sprung up which coalesced to form a tumor." Were medical history more democratic, we might well ascribe Hawkins' ulcer to traumatic scar neoplasia and reserve Marjolin for burn scar tumors; alas, the literature acknowledges Hawkins but repeatedly attributes scar-related tumors to the more celebrated surgeon, Marjolin. Dupuytren in 1839 also observed tumor formation in an acid burn, but it was not until 1860 that Heurteux first described a thermal scar which became malignant.

Following these original descriptions, the second half of the nineteenth century produced a lengthy list of case reports citing additional forms of trauma in the genesis of carcinomatous ulcers. In 1970, Margolis noted 123 reports of Marjolin's ulcer in the literature. Treves and Pack in 1930 published the still classic reference on Marjolin's ulcer based on their 12-year experience at Memorial Hospital, New York. A more recent addition is the report by Arons and colleagues (1965).

Two unique examples of burn scar ulcers are the kangri and kairo cancers. The former is seen in India where the kangri, a bowl containing hot charcoal, is worn against the body for warmth (Neve, 1923). Tumors arise at points of contact. The kairo burn tumors are caused by a similar Japanese box applied to the abdomen for warmth. Both lesions are endemic to their cultural origins, and like the other causes of Marjolin's ulcer, they are slowly disappearing with changing customs.

INCIDENCE

Incidence figures for tumors arising in scar tissue range from a low of 0.1 percent in a general hospital population to a high of 2.59 percent in a cancer referral center. The actual number, somewhere between the extremes, is only an estimate, as most units diagnosing less than one case per year do not reach the literature. The relevant numbers are derived from patients seeking treatment of tumors in whom a history of previous scarring is elucidated; statistical data on the opposite spectrum, the percentage of scars which eventually form tumors, is unavailable.

The most well-researched report, that of Treves and Pack (1930), represents 2465 patients who were treated at Memorial Hospital, New York, for epidermoid or basal cell carcinoma. The authors found 21 squamous and 7 basal cell malignancies arising in scar tissue among this tumor-bearing population.

Conway et al. (1966), citing a 31-year period at the New York Hospital, observed only two cases of Marjolin's ulcer in a group of 1367 skin carcinomas. In a similar population of 644, Macomber et al. (1959) found a 2.3 percent incidence of tumors arising in preexisting scars; Schrek (1941) found an incidence of 2.8 percent; Murray and Cannon (1960), reviewing 41 patients under 30 years of age with basal cell tumors, noted six or 15 percent with a previous history of scarring or trauma. In a selected series of 265 patients with squamous cell lesions only, Broders (1921) noted a 24.5 percent incidence of previous thermal trauma.

Despite the variation in finite percentages, two observations regarding the occurrence of Marjolin's ulcer are significant. First, the entity is decreasing in regions where scar management is improving or tribal habits are being abandoned; second, as the number of cases wanes, the index of suspicion must increase if missed or late diagnoses are to be avoided.

The age and sex ratios are linked to the causes of injury and the latent period required for neoplasia to develop. Males, although less prone to burns and other scar-producing injuries, have three times the incidence of Marjolin's ulcer. Horton et al. (1958) stated that any race is susceptible, but no predisposition has been defined. Except for the rare acute carcinomatous ulcer, scar degeneration appears two to three decades following the injury, pushing the mean age into the fifties in most large series. The geographic incidence, except for the kangri and kairo tumors, is related to the level of concern for scar care.

ETIOLOGY

The postulated disease entities and physical agents which could be associated with carcinomatous ulcers are legion. It is reasonable to assume that any irritative process that persists for a significant portion of the patient's lifetime could result in neoplastic differentiation. There are interesting exceptions, however, the most common being the typical stasis ulcer complicating venous disease of the lower extremity. This indolent lesion constantly subject to trauma rarely degenerates into a malignant process (Halliday, 1968). On the other hand, certain chronic sores have an inordinately high potential for malignant change, an example being the cutaneous lesions of discoid lupus erythematosus (Mladick et al., 1968). However, this may be related to the various forms of local therapy (such as x-rays) rather than to the primary disease process.

Thermal, chemical, electrical, and cold burns produce the vast numbers of Marjolin's ulcers, and within this group the most noxious agent is the thermal burn. Although the literature quotes several exceptions, the influence of chronic irritation and delayed healing subsequent to the burn is essential in the evolution of a Marjolin's ulcer. Frostbite-related malignant ulcers are infrequent, only ten cases being described (DiPirro and Conway, 1966).

A partial list of diseases and insults known to be associated with scar neoplasia is recorded in Table 41–1. Following burns, fistulous tracts, chronic osteomyelitis, and amputation stump ulcers comprise a far less common second group. The third group is composed of pathologic entities following which a small number of patients have been observed to develop neoplasia; syphilis, lupus vulgaris, hidradenitis suppurativa, and smallpox vaccinations (Goncalves, 1966; Marmelzat, 1968) are examples.

Various theories have been proposed to explain, first, why a given scar incites neoplastic degeneration, and second, the propensity of such ulcers to develop following burns. Treves and Pack (1930) evoked the concept of a localized nutritional deficiency, leading to a weakened epithelial cover which ultimately produces a tumor, but they added the hypothesis that the burn scar releases a tissue toxin which acts as a superimposed carcinogen. In support of this Kennaway and Hieger (1930) demonstrated that human skin, when heated, yields a carcinogen for mouse skin. Hueper and Conway (1964) also felt that the tumor resulted from the reaction of carcinogenic material generated during thermal injury. MacKenzie and Rous (1941) postulated that latent or dormant neoplastic cells reside in the burn epithelium until some as yet unknown stimulus triggers neoplasia. Wolbach (1925) felt that the sustained attempt to repair resulted in an altered cornium and accounted for the malignant change. Castillo and Goldsmith (1968), adopting a more modern theory, believed that a depressed immunologic state is produced by the surrounding scar tissue which permits neoplastic development.

Nearly every article on Marjolin's ulcer in the first half of this century attempted to formulate or justify a theory of carcinogenesis. Recent papers pay homage to these irritative theories, the latent period, and the predilection for burn scars, but the seed which alters a benign reparative process into an undisciplined tissue destruction likely rests at the foundation of what is a cancer.

TABLE 41–1 TRAUMA AND DISEASES ASSOCIATED WITH SCAR NEOPLASIA

Most common	Burns, heat and electrical Fistulous tracts
Rare	Burns, cold and chemicals Stasis ulcers Osteomyelitic sinus Amputation stumps Lacerations
Isolated case reports	Syphilis Lupus vulgaris Smallpox vaccinations Hidradenitis suppurativa Vesicovaginal fistula Pilonidal sinus Lymphogranuloma inguinale

PATHOLOGY

The burn scar tumor with few exceptions is a carcinoma; the ratio of squamous cell to basal cells is approximately 3 to 1 but varies with the etiologic agent. Shallow lesions produce less virulent forms of the

TABLE 41–2

Authors	Patients	Acute	Chronic	Male	Female	Average Age (years)	Basal Cell	Squamous Cell
Arons et al., 1965	25	3	22	20	5	58.5	2	23
Bowers and Young, 1960	9	0	9	9	0	52	0	9
Byrd et al., 1961	66	13	53	48	18	50		
Cornil et al., 1937	15	1	14	9	6	40–50	4	11
Glover and Kiehn, 1949	7	0	7	5	2	49.1	0	7
Horton et al., 1958	7	2	5	3	4	43.5	2	3
Johnson, 1926	3	0	3	0	3	49	1	2
Josserand et al., 1957	16	4	12	12	4	53.2	0	16
Kayabali and Duman, 1970	24	0	24	17	7	46.3	0	24
Lawrence, 1952	10	0	10	8	2	50.5	1	9
Macomber and Traube, 1951	3	0	3	3	0	37	0	3
Ruffo and Gandolfo, 1934	25			12	13	40.9		
Schlosser et al., 1956	3	0	3	1	2	38	0	3
Touraine and Bour, 1938	200	71	128	183	51		36	123
Treves and Pack, 1930	28	6	22			53.5	7	21

disease. The tumor arises from the wound margin or from epithelial remnants trapped in the scar. Adjacent nonscarred tissue may be invaded, but initially the tumor is confined to the cicatrix. Lawrence (1952) observed several very early cases and found progressive thickening of the surrounding epithelium extending into the ulcer.

The gross lesion is typically found on an extremity and is single, despite the Treves and Pack (1930) report, in which two patients had multiple tumors in extensive scars, and Stone's and Montiel's patient (1970) with eight synchronous basal cells in a radiated burn scar. Clinically the more common squamous cell growth presents as an irregular, shallow, ulcerated defect; an exophytic variety is seen infrequently. The basal cell tumor resembles a typical rodent ulcer and is found primarily on the head and neck.

Microscopically, the carcinoma arises in the overlying scar epithelium and exhibits a distinct margin with the cellular characteristics of a low grade, well-differentiated malignancy; there are few mitoses and lit-tle tendency for invasion. Keratin pearls are described, as is an inflammatory component. The basal cell tumors are of two varieties, the commoner being nodular-ulcerative, the other a superficial multicentric lesion (Margolis, 1970). Sarcomas have been associated with scars in only isolated case reports (Horton et al., 1958).

Metastasis from scar-associated tumors occurs via the lymphatics in about one-third of patients. The slow growth and fibrotic barrier offered by the scar retards early spread, but with extension of the local lesion the incidence of spread rises sharply. Visceral metastases are uncommon. Treves and Pack (1930) noted only one in their series, a pulmonary nodule spreading from an extremity lesion. De-Bell and Stevenson (1936), in a review of 60 patients with squamous cell epitheliomas of the extremities, six of which were related to trauma, had only nine cases with microscopically positive regional nodes. Three of the nine, however, were from the trauma group, leading to the conclusion that, despite the fibrous barrier, the Marjolin's ulcer is more aggressive than its sister,

TABLE 41–2 *(Continued)*

Etiology	Treatment	Survival	Latent Period (years)	Meta- stasis	Miscellaneous
burns	surgery	5 of 22 died	36.5	8	31 cases related to sinuses and osteomylitis
burns, trauma	surgery	Short follow-up	4	0	1 case of adenocarcinoma in fistula
burns, laceration	surgery, x-ray	4 of 29 treated died			Cancer found in 36 lacerations
burns	Radium, x-ray, surgery		20–30	0	
burns, osteomyelitis	surgery	2 died	36.3	3	
burns	surgery		24		2 sarcomas
burns	surgery	66% 1 yr.	44	1	Prolonged wound healing
burns	surgery, x-ray, coagulation	7 of 12 died	30.8	1	Large percentage of fatal cases
burns	x-ray, surgery		40.8	33%	Good results with x-ray
	surgery				
burns	surgery, x-ray	50% 5 yrs.	36.1	4	
burns	surgery		24	0	1 cancer following good burn coverage
burns	surgery		27	1	
thermal, chemical	surgery, coagulation				Large number with cancer following injury
burns	surgery, radium	54% 3 yrs.	32.5	5	

the non–scar-related squamous cell cancer. Corroborating this conclusion, Taylor et al. (1941) noted a 30 percent incidence of metastasis in burn scar neoplasia and only 17 percent in a population of 335 skin carcinomas. They observed no metastasis in 11 patients with malignant ulcers secondary to chronic osteomyelitis.

The latent period prior to the clinical detection of neoplastic activity has two spectra. The acute lesion presenting within a year of injury is more often a basal cell carcinoma, but Gardner (1959) reported two patients with squamous cell carcinoma developing four and six weeks after trauma.

With the chronic ulcer, the latent period may last for many years (Table 41–2). Arons et al. (1965), in a report on 22 well-scrutinized patients, noted a median time interval of 36.5 years from scarring to neoplasia. Lawrence (1952) compiled statistics to document that the younger the patient at injury, the longer the latent period, i.e., those burned from age 0 to 4 years were found to have a 39.3 year delay, 30 and over a 19.8 year delay. He concluded that the aged skin is more conditioned to develop malignant degeneration if an irritative stimulant is applied.

CLINICAL FEATURES

The diagnosis of Marjolin's ulcer should be entertained from a history of injury followed by prolonged healing. Coupling this relationship between indolent repair and scar carcinogenesis helps establish a diagnosis in the early, treatable stage. Unfortunately the latent interval between injury and tumor formation is an inconstant clue; characteristically the cancer arises two to three decades following trauma, but acute lesions apparently associated with the injury can occur. Most observers have called attention to the inverse relationship between the age and the onset of carcinoma; the younger the patient when injured, the longer the latent period. Burn injuries have the highest frequency, but any unstable or chronically traumatized scar has the potential for malignant degeneration. Epidemiologically it would be convenient if the chronic ulcer which becomes malignant were brought to the knowing physician's attention immediately. The early Marjolin's ulcer, however, is not unlike the crusting, indolent sore that has healed and broken down on numerous occasions over the preceding years. There is no reliable warning for the patient or physician that malignant degeneration is occurring; thus there is a need for a high index of suspicion. Pain is an occasional clue; a chronic ulcer which gradually develops a dull ache or gnawing pain should be suspect.

On physical examination the tumor presents two characteristic forms; the more common is a shallow, flat, or depressed ulcer with well-defined margins. The surface is often irregular with grayish firm nodules of tumor tissue usually involving the margins (Browne, 1941). The lesion is normally mobile unless extension to the deeper tissues has occurred. The regional lymph nodes may be invaded in long-standing cases and are palpable. The second form is an exophytic proliferative tumor with papillary granulations. These lesions are less common and less aggressive and are rarely fixed to the underlying tissue.

Infection may be superimposed on either lesion, temporarily masking the true pathology and also causing lymphadenopathy. When present, infection produces a foul-smelling, wet, exudative sore which, unlike the tumor, may motivate the patient to seek treatment.

The lesion may be located anywhere; however, in contrast to non–scar-oriented skin cancer, Marjolin's ulcers have a predilection for the extremities. In the Lawrence series (1952), 60 percent involved the upper or lower extremities. Basal cell ulcers follow the pattern of the nonscarred sister lesion and characteristically involve the head and neck, but exceptions are recorded (Gaughan et al., 1969). Treves and Pack (1930) observed that 38 percent of their scar-based tumors involved the lower extremity, 22 percent the upper, 30 percent the head and neck, and 10 percent the trunk.

Once the diagnosis is entertained, a biopsy is mandatory. Any lesion thought to be a Marjolin's ulcer requires prompt excision and resurfacing, if only to prevent later degeneration, yet the width and depth should be more extensive if the presence of tumor is confirmed; hence the value of definitive biopsy. Since the earliest changes are difficult to appreciate in scarred, chronically inflamed tissue, a four quadrant biopsy is the minimum needed to establish the diagnosis and extent of spread. Prophylaxis is the best form of treatment. All recurrent ulcerations in scar tissue are best excised and resurfaced.

CASE HISTORY*

A 32 year old male carpenter was referred to the Lahey Clinic in February, 1969, for the treatment of Marjolin's ulcer of the right calf. At nine years of age, both legs were severely burned and allowed to heal by scar formation. A small right calf ulcer developed four years prior to admission and was treated symptomatically by his local physician, despite gradual increase in size, until swelling was noted in the right groin. He was referred to the Lahey Clinic at that time. On admission to the New England Deaconess Hospital in February, a 9 × 18 cm. irregular ulcer of the right inner calf was noted just below the knee (Fig. 41–1). The margin was raised and rolled; the bed was granular with surrounding erythema. The groin nodes were palpable and firm but mobile; the largest measured 3.5 cm. in maximum diameter. The abdomen and chest were normal, as were the laboratory findings. A biopsy of the ulcer and aspiration biopsy of the groin node revealed epidermoid carcinoma with femoral lymph node metastases.

A multidisciplined approach to therapy was prescribed, consisting of intra-arterial infusion of the extremity with methotrexate and FUDR (floxuridine), preoperative radiation to the primary ulcer and right inguinal region, followed by a groin dissection and wide local excision.

Infusion through the right femoral artery was begun in conjunction with external radiation; however, a sharp drop in the

*The case history and photographs were generously contributed by Dr. Blake Cady of the Lahey Clinic Foundation, Boston, Massachusetts.

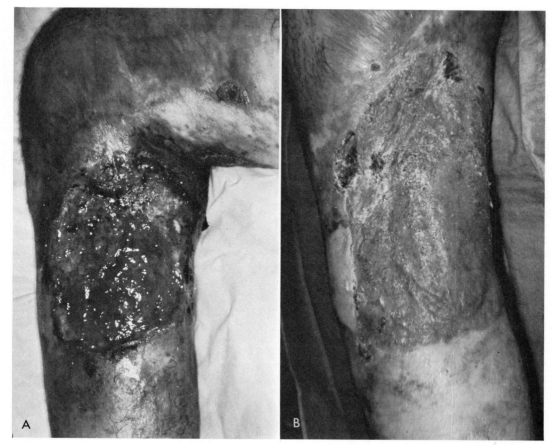

Figure 41-1 *A*, A 9 × 18 cm. Marjolin's ulcer of the right inner calf. The patient was burned 23 years previously, and the wounds were allowed to granulate. *B*, Local lesion following wide excision and split-thickness skin graft. (Courtesy of Dr. Blake Cady, Lahey Clinic Foundation, Boston, Massachusetts.)

white cell count after one week necessitated discontinuance of the FUDR therapy. In late April, following six weeks of methotrexate and 3600 R. to the primary and 4000 R. to the right inguinal region, the patient was readmitted for groin dissection. The nodes had shrunk by 50 percent. A right radical groin dissection was performed; the 31 nodes recovered were free of tumor. The postoperative course was complicated by a superficial wound slough, which healed by second intention. In September the patient underwent a wide excision and split-thickness graft to the primary tumor (Fig. 41–1). The lesion, which was excised down to the underlying muscle, measured 15 × 13 × 0.9 cm. and revealed acute and chronic inflammation within an area of dense fibrosis. The blood vessels showed thickening of the walls consistent with a radiation reaction, but no residual tumor was found. An uneventful recovery ensued.

The patient has been observed periodically at the Lahey Clinic over the past five years and is currently free of tumor.

EXPERIMENTAL OBSERVATION

Since the earliest association between scars and cancer of the skin, research has been oriented toward the development of a laboratory model. The discovery by MacKenzie and Rous in 1941 that certain tars applied to rabbit skin resulted in neoplastic change stimulated an avalanche of studies on the ability of various irritants to produce carcinoma. This stimulus of chronic irritation over a prolonged interval is common both to Marjolin's ulcer and to chemical carcinogenesis.

Sporadic laboratory findings paralleling the clinical observations have been reported. Bang (1925), using only cauterization, was able to forge skin cancer in the mouse. Simpson (1947), combining heat and a carcinogen, produced tumors following a seven-month latent period. Saffiotti and Shubik (1956) also produced tumors in mice following burns and noted an increase from 7 per cent to 47 per cent in animals burned and treated with the cocarcinogen, croton oil. More recently Castillo and Goldsmith (1968) were able to develop scar tumors in rats following the combined irritation of thermal burn and methylcholanthrene.

This two-stage theory is currently invoked to account for Marjolin's ulcer, the burn being the initiating agent and repeated trauma the promoting factor. While this principle has clinical application, experimental Marjolin's ulcer, except for Bang's report, has not been produced without the addition of a chemical adjuvant.

TREATMENT

The therapy of Marjolin's ulcer varies with the three stages of the disease. The premalignant, unstable scar demands wide excision with appropriate soft tissue coverage. In general, a thick split-thickness graft providing minimal contraction and adequate bulk with the least morbidity is selected. Over a compromised bed, a thinner graft, 0.012 inch to 0.014 inch, will increase the percentage of acceptance. If the burn or injury has been full thickness over a gliding or contracting surface, consideration must be given to a flap or pedicle reconstruction. Regardless of the reconstructive measures, the final result must be a healed, minimally scarred surface which can tolerate ordinary functional trauma. A few cases of Marjolin's ulcer arising in previously treated scars have led to the concept of wider excision for long-standing ulcerated burns. This ensures removal of the grossly damaged and adjacent partially injured skin, thereby eliminating all foci of potentially malignant tissue.

Primary treatment of a Marjolin's ulcer confined to the original scar or adjacent tissue is wide surgical excision and skin coverage. A 2-cm. to 4-cm. margin of normal skin with excision of the underlying fascia is desired. A split-thickness skin graft is usually adequate for closure, reserving the more sophisticated procedures for use over moving surfaces. In all doubtful cases, simple split-thickness graft coverage is used initially. Extensive reconstruction, which might mask recurrence, is delayed until tumor control is reasonably certain.

Amputation has been reserved for deep-seated lesions which extend into bone or joint cavities. In selected cases, this more radical approach has been curative. Radium or x-ray therapy, a popular modality in the 1930's, has been supplanted by surgery. The rationale of using radiation alone in poorly vascularized scar tissue is questionable, and surgery appears more efficacious. Preoperative radiation may prove to be beneficial in special cases (see Case History).

The therapy of the end-stage lesions, the metastatic Marjolin's ulcer, usually has poor results, regardless of the approach. The primary lesion is treated by excision extending well into the uninvolved healthy skin below the fascia. Palpable lymph nodes are excised in continuity, if practical, or as a second operative procedure. Prophylactic node dissection has not been generally recommended for these slow-growing tumors. However, should nodes develop after the primary surgery, they are excised. In contrast, Taylor et al. (1941), on the basis of the higher incidence of metastasis in Marjolin's ulcer than in other epitheliomas, advocated prophylactic lymph node excision. With palpable nodes, forearm lesions require both epitrochlear and axillary node dissection, the leg a groin dissection. Preoperative and postoperative radiation have been suggested in the management of nodal diseases and appear to have been life-saving in the case report. Similarly, the merits of intra-arterial infusion are also unproved, but this treatment must be given credit in the successful resuscitation of the patient described. Cases with visceral metastases are sufficiently rare that successful treatment has not been reported.

The current therapy of Marjolin's ulcer has been reached by trial and error. The lesion's rarity has precluded any prospective treatment protocols, and even comparisons between modalities suffer from inadequate numbers for statistical correlation. Since this state is unlikely to change with the ever-decreasing number of Marjolin's ulcer patients, new treatment guides must necessarily be extrapolated from tumors which behave in parallel fashion, the cutaneous epithelioma being the most logical surrogate.

PREVENTION AND PROGNOSIS

The prognosis of scar carcinoma in its advanced stage is sufficiently grave to warrant maximum preventive therapy. Since 75 percent or more of such cancers originate after a burn, attention must be focused on improved management of burn scars. Survival following a major thermal injury has drastically improved in the past 20 years. A measure of this improvement is an apparent decrease in Marjolin's ulcers because of early and sustained burn coverage. It is conceivable, however, that, as patients with greater and greater burns are salvaged, permanent coverage problems will expand, and carcinomatous ulcers may reappear several decades hence. Prevention can only be achieved when scars, regardless of etiology, which are subject to weight-bearing, friction, or stretching and which involve prolonged periods of healing or subsequent reulceration, are widely excised and resurfaced with normal stable tissue.

An ecology-minded culture assumes at least a modest interest in prevention of burns and other physical injuries. Couple this with the aggressive treatment of wounds failing to heal because of repeated trauma, and one has the format for a Marjolin's ulcer prevention campaign.

A patient's survival following carcinomatous degeneration of a scar is related to several predictable and nonpredictable factors. First, the microscopic pathology: basal cell lesions almost never metastasize

and rarely result in death. Second, the stage at which the lesion is first treated is of considerable import (as described under Pathology), as most tumors are slow-growing until they extend beyond the scar barrier. Therapy prior to this event is often curative. Lastly, the larger series of Marjolin's ulcer patients, from which survival figures can be extrapolated, was collected prior to the current regimens of burn scar management, and the numbers are considerably worse than in a comparable population today. Similarly, the available studies are small and all are restrospective, with groupings of treated and untreated patients, early and late cases, which undermine the validity of the survival estimates. With this preamble the figures from the larger reports are presented.

Byrd et al. (1961) reviewed the Vanderbilt experience with Marjolin's ulcer and concluded that the prognosis was more grave than previously reported, their absolute five-year survival being only 62 percent. However, their incidence of basal cell lesions was a low 9.7 percent. Treves and Pack (1930) reported eight deaths in 21 patients with squamous cell ulcers; 7 of the 13 survivors were free of disease for three years or more when reviewed.

MEDICOLEGAL CONSIDERATIONS

The relationship between trauma and scar cancer has medicolegal considerations within industry (Kantor et al., 1970; Julliard, 1932). The literature has established that a cause and effect relationship exists, and despite the inability to identify the inciting factor, compensation boards have taken the position that without the scar the tumor would not have arisen. Thus the scar producing the injury is compensable (Hursthouse, 1969). The largest series reported by Dix (1960) cited 27 cases arising in 25 well-documented patients employed in heavy industry in the Milwaukee area. Most injuries were small burns, resulting from contact with acids or molten metals, in which healing was protracted. Despite the evidence, a latent period of 20 to 30 years introduces a variable about which only individual deliberation between the compensation board, physician, and insurance carrier can decide. As a guide, Ewing's postulate (1940) must be fulfilled before compensation can be considered. This includes the following: (1) there should be no previous injury to the involved area; (2) proof of injury must be established; (3) a definitive time lapse between injury and tumor development should be established; (4) the tumor must be representative, that is, a squamous or a basal cell carcinoma.

REFERENCES

Arons, M. S., Lynch, J. B., Lewis, S. R., and Blocker, T. G.: Scar tissue carcinoma. Part I. A clinical study with special reference to burn scar carcinoma. Ann. Surg., 161:170, 1965.

Bang, F.: Le cancer des cicatrices; étude clinique et expérimental. Bull. Assoc. Fr. Cancer, 14:203, 1925.

Bowers, R. F., and Young, J. M.: Carcinoma arising in scars, osteomyelitis and fistulae. Arch. Surg., 80:564, 1960.

Broders, A. C.: Squamous cell epithelioma of the skin. Ann. Surg., 73:141, 1921.

Browne, H. R.: Marjolin's ulcer. Am. J. Surg., 54:466, 1941.

Byrd, B. F., Munoz, A. J., and Ferguson, H.: Carcinoma of the skin following acute and chronic trauma. South. Med. J., 54:1262, 1961.

Castillo, J., and Goldsmith, H. S.: Burn scar carcinoma. CA, 18:140, 1968.

Conway, H., Hugo, N. E., and Tulenko, J. F.: Surgery of Tumors of the Skin. Ed. 2. Springfield, Ill., Charles C Thomas, Publisher, 1966.

Cornil, L., Paillas, J. E., and Bonneau, H.: Le cancer des brûlures, a propos de 15 observations personnelles. Bull. Assoc. Fr. l'Etude Cancer, 28:359, 1937.

DeBell, P. J., and Stevenson, T. D.: Squamous cell epithelioma of the extremities. Surg. Gynecol. Obstet., 63:222, 1936.

DiPirro, E., and Conway, H.: Carcinoma after frostbite: A case report. Plast. Reconstr. Surg., 38:541, 1966.

Dix, C. R.: Occupational trauma and skin cancer. Plast. Reconstr. Surg., 26:546, 1960.

Dupuytren, G.: Leçons Orales de Clinique Chirurgicale. Ed 2. Paris, Gemer-Baillière, 1839.

Ewing, J.: Neoplastic Diseases. Ed. 4. Philadelphia, W. B. Saunders Company, 1940.

Gardner, A. W.: Trauma and squamous skin cancer. Lancet, 1:760, 1959.

Gaughan, L. J., Bergeron, J. R., and Mullins, J. F.: Giant basal cell epithelioma developing in acute burn site. Arch. Dermatol., 99:594, 1969.

Glover, D. M., and Kiehn, C. L.: Marjolin's ulcer, a preventable threat to function and life. Am. J. Surg., 78:772, 1949.

Goncalves, J. C. A.: Malignant change in smallpox vaccination scars. Arch. Dermatol., 93:229, 1966.

Halliday, J. P.: Squamous carcinoma in a venous ulcer. Med. J. Aust., 1:449, 1968.

Hawkins, C.: On warty tumors in cicatrices. London Med. Gaz., 13:481, 1833.

Horton, C. E., Crawford, H. H., Love, H. G., and Loeffler, R. A.: The malignant potential of burn scar. Plast. Reconstr. Surg., 22:348, 1958.

Hueper, W. E., and Conway, W. D.: Chemical Carcinogenesis and Cancer. Springfield, Ill., Charles C Thomas, Publisher, 1964.

Hursthouse, M. W.: Basal cell carcinomas arising in burn scars: A case report. New Zealand Med. J., 69:157, 1969.

Johnson, F. M.: The development of carcinoma in scar tissue following burns. Ann. Surg., 83:165, 1926.

Josserand, A., Dargent, M., Papillion, J., and Pinet, F.: Les cancers des brulures. Presse Méd., 66:1479, 1957.

Juillard, C.: Cancer à apparition rapide après un traumatisme unique. Marseille Méd., 2:593, 1931. Abs. in Am. J. Cancer, 16:1038, 1932.

Kantor, I., Berger, B. W., and Wilentz, J. M.: Basal cell epithelioma in a thermal burn scar. J. Occup. Med., 12:170, 1970.

Kayabali, I., and Duman, M.: Cancer des brulures. Lyon Chir., 66:29, 1970.

Kennaway, E. L., and Hieger, I.: Carcinogenic substances and their fluorescence. Br. Med. J., 1:1044, 1930.

Lawrence, E. A.: Carcinoma arising in the scars of thermal burns. Surg. Gynecol. Obstet., 95:579, 1952.

MacKenzie, I., and Rous, P.: The experimental disclosure of latent neoplastic changes in tarred skin. J. Exp. Med., 73:391, 1941.

Macomber, W. B., and Traube, J. C.: Marjolin ulcer case reports. Plast. Reconstr. Surg., 7:152, 1951.

Macomber, W. B., Wang, M. K. H., and Sullivan, J. G.: Cutaneous epithelioma. Plast. Reconstr. Surg., 24:545, 1959.

Margolis, M. H.: Superficial multicentric basal cell epithelioma. Arch. Dermatol., 102:474, 1970.

Marjolin, J. N.: Ulcère. Dictionnaire de Med., 21:31, 1828.

Marmelzat, W. L.: Malignant tumors in smallpox vaccination scars. Arch. Dermatol., 97:400, 1968.

Mladick, R. A., Pickrell, K. L., Thorne, F. L., and Hall, J. H.: Squamous cell cancer in discoid lupus erythematosus. Plast. Reconstr. Surg., 42:497, 1968.

Murray, J., and Cannon, B.: Basal-cell cancer in children and young adults. New Engl. J. Med., 262:440, 1960.

Neve, E. F.: Kangri-burn cancer. Br. Med. J., 2:1255, 1923.

Ruffo, A. H., and Gandolfo, A.: Carcinoma desarrollado sobre cicatriz de quemadura. Prensa Med. Argent., 21:351, 1934.

Saffiotti, U., and Shubik, P.: The role of burning in carcinogenesis. Br. J. Cancer, 10:54, 1956.

Schlosser, R. J., Kanar, E. A., and Harkins, H. N.: The surgical significance of Marjolin's ulcer. Surgery, 39:645, 1956.

Schrek, R.: Cutaneous carcinoma. Arch. Pathol., 31:422, 1941.

Simpson, W. L.: An experimental study of single trauma malignancy. Cancer Res., 7:726, 1947.

Stone, N. H., and Montiel, M. M.: Multiple basal cell carcinomas arising in radiated burn scars. Plast. Reconstr. Surg., 46:506, 1970.

Taylor, G. W., Nathanson, I. T., and Shaw, D. T.: Epidermoid carcinoma of the extremities with reference to lymph node involvement. Ann. Surg., 113:268, 1941.

Touraine, A., and Bour, H.: Les cancer post traumatique de la peau. France Méd., 2:5, 1938.

Treves, N., and Pack, G. T.: The development of cancer in burn scars. Surg. Gynecol. Obstet., 51:749, 1930.

Wolbach, S. B.: A summary of the effects of repeated roentgen ray exposures upon the human skin, antecedent to the formation of carcinoma. Am. J. Roentgenol., 13:139, 1925.

42

Melanoma of the Skin

Stephen L. Gumport, M.D., and Matthew N. Harris, M.D.

HISTORY

The description of the melanoma goes far back into antiquity. Hippocrates in the fifth century, B.C., is credited with first describing this lesion. Carswell (1838) first used the term "melanoma." Pemberton (1858) suggested wide local excision of the lesion and the removal of the inguinal lymph nodes for melanoma of the lower extremities. Handley (1907) set forth the concept of lymphatic permeation and discussed how widely the tumor should be resected. Pringle (1908) recommended "in-continuity" removal of the primary site of the tumor with its lymphatic bed. This principle is still valid today, although it is not always possible to accomplish (Urteaga and Pack, 1966; Hovnanian, 1967).

INCIDENCE AND EPIDEMIOLOGY

MacDonald (1948) stated that, in the Connecticut Tumor Registry of 1946, melanoma accounted for almost 1 percent of the total cancer recorded. In males, 1.6 per 100,000 population were treated for the first time each year, and in females, 2.0 per 100,000 population.

Attie and Khafif (1964) reported that the incidence of melanoma in the Armed Forces of the United States among its young adult population was 0.82 per 100,000.

Davis et al. (1966) reported a much higher incidence of melanoma in Queensland, Australia, than elsewhere, with an overall rate of 16.4 per 100,000 population. Booher (1969), commenting on this report from Australia in his excellent review article, believed that this incidence was due not only to an increased awareness of the problem and to a very early diagnosis, but also to the influence of race, complexion, and exposure to excessive amounts of sunlight.

Pack et al. (1963) stated that there was a higher incidence of melanoma in patients who were blond and had blue or hazel eyes and fair skin. He believed the incidence to be much higher in Caucasians than in Negroes.

MacDonald (1963), in Texas, reported that many melanomas were found on the covered parts of the body. Therefore, he was unable to confirm the work of Lancaster and Nelson (1957) in Australia, who reported that sunlight was an important factor in the cause of melanoma. On the other hand, Lee and Merrill (1970)

suggested that, while some types of melanoma may result directly from the trauma
of sunlight, other varieties on the nonex-
posed surfaces of the body may be due to
the effect of substances released by sun-exposed skin which are carried by the circulation, resulting in the production of a
melanoma elsewhere in the body.

MacDonald (1963) stated that in the
Negro the melanoma occurred most often
where pigment deposition was the least,
and the most common sites were the soles
of the feet, the subungual regions, and the
oral cavity (Figs. 42–1 and 42–2). A study
by Lewis and Kiryabwire (1968) revealed
the common sites of incidence of melanoma in the African Negro to be similar to
those found in the American Negro. Shah
and Goldsmith (1971) also stressed the
high incidence of melanoma of the sole of
the foot.

The diagnosis of melanoma has been
made in pure albino patients. This is a rare
occurrence and has been reported only a
few times. Melanoblasts are present in the
usual number in the skin of albinos, but
the defect appears to be one of melano-

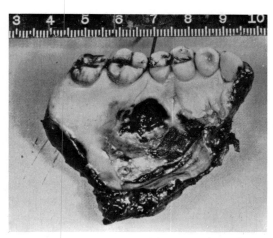

Figure 42–2   L.H., a 35 year old Negro female with
melanoma of the mucous membrane of the hard
palate.

blastic pigment production, resulting in a
negative DOPA and tyrosinase reaction
(Young, 1957). The diagnosis of melanoma can be substantiated by the electron
microscopic demonstration of premelano-
somes and melanosomes. This would indicate that the melanocyte is needed but
that melanin production is not required
for the melanoma to develop (Kennedy
and Zelickson, 1963).

Age

True metastasizing melanomas may
occur at any age from infancy and childhood, in which it is rare, to the nonagen-
arian. In numerous published series of
cases the highest incidence of melanoma
occurred in the fourth, fifth, and sixth decades of life (Meyer and Gumport, 1953;
Charalambidis and Patterson, 1962;
McSwain et al., 1964; Cochran, 1969).

Location

Melanoma occurred at the following
sites in order of frequency, as stated in an
analysis of 1190 cases by Pack et al.
(1952a):

1. Lower extremity, 27 percent
2. Trunk, 24 percent
3. Head and neck, 22 percent
4. Upper extremity, 9.8 percent
5. Subungual region, 2.9 percent

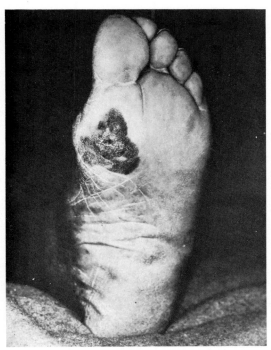

Figure 42–1   H.H., a 58 year old Negro male with
melanoma on the sole of the foot.
(See also Color Plate III-D.)

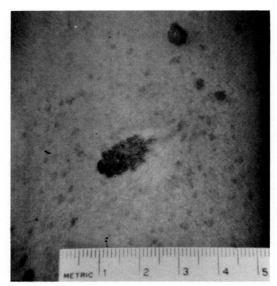

Figure 42–3 R.T., a 39 year old male with a melanoma arising at a previous smallpox vaccination site. (See also Color Plate III-E.)

6. Various unusual sites, 10.9 percent

7. Unknown primary sites, 2.4 percent

Melanomas have been reported as arising at the site of smallpox vaccination scars. Marmelzat (1968) reviewed the literature and reported 24 cases of proven malignant tumors arising in this location. Six of these patients had proven melanoma, and the remainder had either basal cell carcinoma or squamous cell carcinoma. The authors have seen one case of a melanoma arising in this location (Fig. 42–3).

Familial Incidence

The hereditary aspects of melanoma have been shown to exist in many species of animals (Hadwen, 1931; Gordon, 1941). The familial tendency of melanoma has been further substantiated in man. Smith et al. (1966) reported a mother and son, each with melanoma, and said that this was the thirty-third such extraocular melanoma occurrence. Andrews (1968) reported the case of a brother and sister, each with a melanoma. The authors have a patient with a melanoma whose father and paternal great-aunt are said to have died of melanoma.

St. Arneault et al. (1970) reported a set of triplets in which monozygous twins developed cutaneous melanomas simultaneously at nearly identical sites. The third member of this triplet group appeared to be just a fraternal member and did not develop melanoma. It was concluded that the steps leading to the development of these two melanomas "occurred in the conceptus prior to twinning."

Melanoma in Childhood

For many years it was thought that melanoma occurring in childhood had a good prognosis. This erroneous conclusion was reached prior to the work of Spitz (1948) and of Allen and Spitz (1953). They showed that the reason a good prognosis was anticipated was because the benign juvenile melanoma was actually being classified as a true melanoma. Following the classic description of the benign juvenile melanoma by Allen and Spitz, it was found possible to separate this entity from the true melanoma. It was then found that the true melanoma in childhood did not have any better prognosis than a similar lesion in the adult (McWhorter et al., 1954; Skov-Jensen, 1966).

The benign juvenile melanoma often presents as an elevated pink nodule. Pigmentation is minimal. The microscopic picture is characterized by large cells

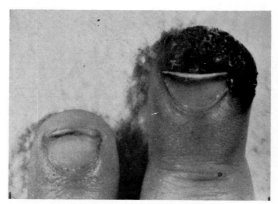

Figure 42–4 R.K., a 12 month old infant born with melanoma of the right middle fingertip. Also had a positive axillary lymph node. Patient alive and well five years after amputation of finger and axillary lymph node dissection. (Courtesy of Dr. David Lyall.) (See also Color Plate III-F.)

which lack anaplastic change. This benign lesion should be treated conservatively.

The true melanoma, although rare, does occur in infancy and childhood (Fig. 42–4). It can metastasize with fatal results. Grossly and microscopically it resembles the adult melanoma. The treatment in infancy and childhood is the same as for older patients.

In a study by Lerman et al. (1970), there were 12 cases of melanoma in children with proven metastases, which may be added to the total of 48 such cases as reported by others up to 1968. Two of these 12 melanomas originated in a nevus pigmentosus giganticus, and both patients subsequently died of their disease.

Pregnancy

Pregnancy has long been thought to affect unfavorably the prognosis of the melanoma patient (Pack et al., 1952a). More recent studies indicate that the prognosis for the pregnant patient with a melanoma is essentially the same as if the patient were not pregnant (George et al., 1960).

It does seem sensible to advise women who have recently been treated for melanoma not to become pregnant until at least several years have passed. They should be reasonably certain of remaining well and able to care for a young child.

If a pregnant woman develops a melanoma, the treatment should be the same as if she were not pregnant. Whether or not the pregnancy should be interrupted depends upon how the prognosis appears to the attending physician.

No description of melanoma in pregnancy would be complete without noting that metastases may occur from the mother to the placenta or to the fetus itself. This is a rare occurrence, but it has been documented (Brodsky et al., 1965; Skov-Jensen et al., 1966).

THE NEVUS AND ITS RELATIONSHIP TO THE MELANOMA

The relationship of the common benign nevus or mole to the relatively uncommon melanoma is a most interesting one. According to Pack et al. (1952b), there is an average of 14.6 nevi per white person, based upon a study of 1000 patients. Whether or not the nevus cell may be of either epidermal or neural origin has not yet been definitely determined. However, a good percentage of patients with melanoma give a history that would indicate the presence of a preexisting nevus at the site of the melanoma. Lane et al. (1958) found that 71 percent of their patients gave such a history.

Allen (1946) is one of the foremost proponents of the theory that the junction nevus is a precancerous forerunner of the melanoma. The term junction nevus means one in which the nevus cells are in contact with the epidermal cells. Junction nevi are grossly smooth, flat, or just slightly elevated in character and from light tan to deep brown in color. Kopf and Andrade (1963) have concluded that, as the junction nevus grows older, its cells lose their epidermal position and migrate into the underlying dermis; these are called intradermal nevi and are not related to the melanoma etiologically.

The melanoma may also arise from other lesions which contain melanocytes. Notably, these are the pigmented freckle of Hutchinson (also called circumscribed precancerous melanosis of Dubreuilh), the nevus pigmentosus giganticus, and possibly the benign cellular blue nevus.

It was thought at one time that the presence of hair in a nevus was indicative of a benign lesion. This is not true (Fig. 42–5). It should be noted that a melanoma may arise in the large hairy nevus called nevus pigmentosus giganticus (Skov-Jensen et al., 1966). This lesion has also been called the bathing trunks nevus.

The benign cellular blue nevus has been a particularly difficult lesion to differentiate from the melanoma, since this nevus has been known to metastasize to the regional lymph nodes. However, the metastases are unusual in that the disease does not become widespread beyond the regional lymph nodes, and the patient does not die. The authors have one such case in which the primary site was removed 27 years before the regional lymph nodes showed the presence of metastases from

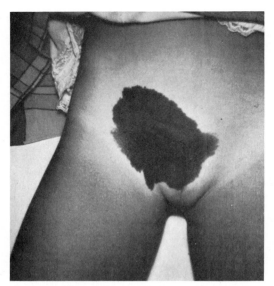

Figure 42–5 J.McA., nevus pigmentosus giganticus on a young female child 6 years of age. (See also Color Plate IV-A.)

EXAMINATION OF PATIENTS WITH MELANOMA

A patient with a possible melanoma has a thorough history taken and then is carefully examined. A search is made for a history of possible previous primary lesions. The family history is investigated for melanoma. On physical examination, using a good light, the patient's entire skin is carefully examined, including the palms and soles, the subungual regions, and the mucous membranes. The vicinity of the primary tumor is examined for satellite lesions. Regional lymph nodes are carefully palpated. The subcutaneous tissues are also examined for the presence of nodules. The abdomen is examined for the presence of a palpable liver and other masses. Rectal and pelvic examinations are performed.

A chest x-ray is taken at the time of the initial visit to be sure that there is no evidence of pulmonary metastases. Despite a negative chest x-ray, if there is any suspicion that there may be distant spread, tomographic studies of the lungs are recommended.

this so-called benign metastasizing cellular blue nevus. This patient is living and well for almost three years following a radical groin dissection, at which operation many of the lymph nodes contained metastases. This course is unusual and certainly not one which is to be expected in the usual melanoma. Rodriguez and Ackerman (1968) reported 14 cellular blue nevi with metastases in the regional lymph nodes. These patients remained well for as long as 16 years following the removal of the regional lymph nodes. None of these patients developed subsequent metastasis to any of the internal organs, and none died of their disease.

MULTIPLE PRIMARY LESIONS

Multiple primary melanomas are not common in occurrence. The various series reported indicate an incidence of between 1.28 and 3.6 percent (Pack et al., 1952c; Allen and Spitz, 1953). The majority of the reported cases showed only two separate and proven primary sites. However, one reported case showed 48 separate, proven primaries removed before death (Kahn and Donaldson, 1970) (Fig. 42–6).

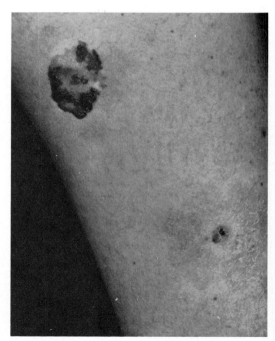

Figure 42–6 J.H., a 30 year old male with two separate primary melanomas on left thigh. (See also Color Plate IV-B.)

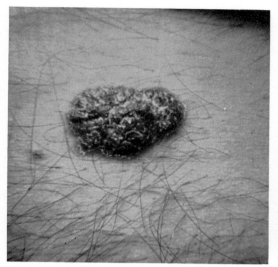

Figure 42–15 F.T., a 34 year old male with invasive melanoma of the right side of the skin of the abdomen.
(See also Color Plate V-E.)

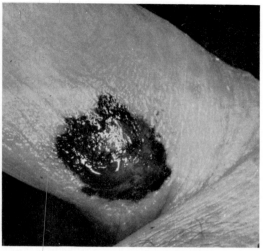

Figure 42–17 R.D., a 40 year old female with invasive melanoma of the right middle finger. (Courtesy of Dr. Robert Beasley.)
(See also Color Plate VI-A.)

regard. On the other hand, the anatomic location of the lesion may require modification of these dimensions. For example, a melanoma on the face may have to be removed with a substantially narrower margin.

The depth of the excision usually in-

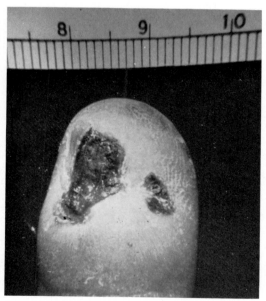

Figure 42–16 H.S., a 60 year old male with subungual melanoma of the left middle finger.
(See also Color Plate V-F.)

cludes the fascia of the underlying muscle. Here, too, there is no complete agreement, and Olsen (1966) preferred to leave the fascia intact.

We prefer not to shift flaps to cover any defects resulting from the excision of malignant tumors. We believe that such flaps may act to conceal the local reappearance of the tumor for an unduly long period. This procedure also has the real disadvantage of shifting the known boundaries of the defect before the pathologist has had a chance to carefully examine all the surgical margins of the specimen.

If the pathologist feels that a melanoma has been inadequately excised and that re-excision is indicated, this can easily be done if only a simple split-thickness or full-thickness skin graft has been used to cover the defect. On the other hand, it is much more difficult to accurately perform a re-excision if a flap has been rotated into the area. Theoretically, the entire flap should then be removed if the tumor has been incompletely excised.

The elective or so-called "prophylactic" removal of the regional lymph nodes for melanoma before they become grossly positive is to be encouraged when done selectively. The methods used have previously been described (Martin et al., 1951; Harris et al., 1972 and 1973). Our contraindica-

TABLE 42–1   ERROR OF CLINICAL
JUDGMENT

232 Cases: Nodes Were Microscopically Negative,
of these, 15 Were Called Positive Clinically

Error 6%

74 Cases: Nodes Were Microscopically Positive,
of these, 41 Were Called Negative Clinically

Error 55%

Total Overall Error 18%

(*From* Gumport and Harris: Results of regional
lymph node dissection for melanoma. Ann. Surg.,
179:1, 1974.)

tions for elective regional lymph node
dissections are:
1. The melanoma which is definitely
classified as superficial (Levels I and II).
2. The melanoma arising in a melanotic
freckle of Hutchinson.
3. The primary site so situated that the
lymphatic drainage may be to several different
groups of regional lymph nodes
4. The presence of serious intercurrent
disease
5. The aged patient
6. Distant metastases
The use of these criteria serves to reduce
the operative mortality, minimize the morbidity,
and increase the frequency with
which microscopically positive nodes are
found at operation.
We are now endeavoring to identify patients
who possess a high resistance to their
melanoma. Attempts are also being made
to grade these tumors on the basis of their
individual aggressiveness. If these factors
can be established, they, too, should aid in
selecting patients for elective lymph node
dissections.

TABLE 42–3   ERROR OF CLINICAL
JUDGMENT BY REGION: AXILLA

87 Cases: Nodes Were Microscopically Negative,
of these, 6 Were Called Positive Clinically

Error 7%

25 Cases: Nodes Were Microscopically Positive,
of these, 16 Were Called Negative Clinically

Error 60%

Since 1949 we have been engaged in a
long-term clinical study of melanoma.
During this period, upwards of 800 patients
with melanoma have been seen; 306
regional lymph node dissections have been
performed. Using the above contraindications
to the procedure, we feel that the
operations have been performed for those
patients in whom the lymph nodes are
most apt to be involved. The morbidity
rate has been low, and the mortality rate,
thus far, has been zero.
It can be seen in Table 42–1 that there
was only a 6 percent preoperative clinical
error in correctly diagnosing those lymph
nodes which were later reported by the
pathologist to be microscopically free of
tumor on random sections. However,
there was a very large error clinically (55
percent) in preoperatively correctly diagnosing
those lymph nodes which were later
reported to contain melanoma on microscopic
examination. It is this latter group
which particularly should have regional
lymph node dissections performed, but
the members of this group cannot be accurately
determined clinically prior to the
removal of their lymph nodes. There have
been reports of similar experiences (Gum-

TABLE 42–2   ERROR OF CLINICAL
JUDGMENT BY REGION: NECK

33 Cases: Nodes Were Microscopically Negative,
of these, 2 Were Called Positive Clinically

Error 6%

14 Cases: Nodes Were Microscopically Positive,
of these, 9 Were Called Negative Clinically

Error 65%

TABLE 42–4   ERROR OF CLINICAL
JUDGMENT BY REGION: GROIN

107 Cases: Nodes Were Microscopically Negative,
of these, 7 Were Called Positive Clinically

Error 7%

40 Cases: Nodes Were Microscopically Positive,
of these, 20 Were Called Negative Clinically

Error 50%

TABLE 42–5   RESULTS OF REGIONAL NODE DISSECTIONS
(185 CASES HAVING OPERATIONS OVER FIVE YEARS AGO)

		L & W	Ill with recur.	Lost	Dead*	Total
Nodes Microscopically Negative	Clin. ⊖	69 (56%)	6 (5%)	12 (10%)	37 (30%)	124
	Clin. ⊕	3 (27%)	0	2 (18%)	6 (55%)	11
Nodes Microscopically Positive	Clin. ⊖	6 (30%)	2 (10%)	1 (5%)	11 (55%)	20
	Clin. ⊕	3 (10%)	0	3 (10%)	24 (80%)	30
						185

*Death from all causes.

(*From* Gumport and Harris: Results of regional lymph node dissection for melanoma. Ann. Surg., 179:1, 1974.)

port and Meyer, 1959; Moore and Gerner, 1971). Our overall results of the clinical assessment of the lymph node status preoperatively are set forth in Table 42–1, and the detailed breakdown by anatomic region is given in Tables 42–2 to 42–4. Our results in 185 regional lymph node dissections performed five or more years ago are set forth in Table 42–5.

When the surgeon thought the regional lymph nodes were negative, and after removal they were reported by the pathologist on random sections to be negative, 56 percent of these patients survived five years or longer.

When the surgeon thought these regional lymph nodes were positive, and after removal they were reported to be negative, 27 percent of these patients survived five years or longer. This lower survival rate might be due to the fact that some of these nodes actually were micro-

scopically positive, for they were reported as microscopically negative only on random sections, and serial sections were not done by the pathologist.

When the surgeon thought the regional lymph nodes were negative, and they were reported as being microscopically positive, 30 percent of these patients survived five years or longer. While this is only half as well as the patients did in the clinically negative–microscopically negative group (56 percent), it is still three times as well as the patients did in the group where the nodes were clinically and microscopically positive (10 percent).

In the last group in which the nodes were clinically positive and microscopically positive, the survival rate was by far the lowest. Only 10 percent of these patients lived for five years or longer after their definitive surgery.

These figures are not substantially dif-

TABLE 42–6   RESULTS OF REGIONAL NODE DISSECTIONS –
30 NECK DISSECTIONS (HAVING OPERATIONS OVER
FIVE YEARS AGO)

		L & W	Ill with recur.	Lost	Dead*	Total
Nodes Microscopically Negative	Clin. ⊖	11 (58%)	3 (16%)	2 (10%)	3 (16%)	19
	Clin. ⊕	0	0	1 (50%)	1 (50%)	2
Nodes Microscopically Positive	Clin. ⊖	0	0	0	4 (100%)	4
	Clin. ⊕	1 (20%)	0	0	4 (80%)	5
						30

*Death from all causes.

TABLE 42–7   RESULTS OF REGIONAL NODE DISSECTIONS —
64 AXILLARY NODE DISSECTIONS (HAVING OPERATIONS
OVER FIVE YEARS AGO)

		L & W	Ill with recur.	Lost	Dead*	Total
Nodes Microscopically Negative	Clin. ⊖	28 (60%)	1 (2%)	5 (10%)	13 (28%)	47
	Clin. ⊕	2 (67%)	0	0	1 (33%)	3
Nodes Microscopically Positive	Clin. ⊖	0	1 (20%)	1 (20%)	3 (60%)	5
	Clin. ⊕	1 (11%)	0	2 (22%)	6 (67%)	9
						64

*Death from all causes.

ferent from those of our previous studies (Gumport and Meyer, 1959; Gumport and Harris, 1974).

Table 42–5, giving overall results, has been broken down to show the results by region and set forth in Tables 42–6 through 42–8. The number of cases in each of these specific regions is too small to say other than that the general results by region are similar to the overall results, as seen in Table 42–5.

While the elective removal of these lymph nodes is encouraged, this does not solve the problem of the hematogenous spread of melanoma.

Others also feel that an elective regional lymph node dissection should be done (Lane et al., 1958; Charalambidis and Patterson, 1962; Conley and Pack, 1963; Fortner et al., 1964; McSwain et al., 1964; Goldsmith et al., 1970). Our present work

continues to indicate that these elective dissections done selectively are of value. However, a controlled study has yet to be published, and there is no unanimity on this point (Polk et al., 1969; Polk and Linn, 1971; Moore and Gerner, 1971). Polk and his colleagues are endeavoring to answer this question using a mathematical model. By this method they feel that they have found little benefit from elective lymph node dissections done routinely. We agree that these procedures should not be done routinely in all cases of melanoma, but we believe that by the careful selection of cases for elective lymph node dissection, the benefit to be derived is considerably greater than they have found.

We do not ordinarily remove either the epitrochlear or the popliteal lymph nodes in melanomas of the extremities. These lymph nodes are seldom involved with

TABLE 42–8   RESULTS OF REGIONAL NODE DISSECTIONS —
91 RADICAL GROIN DISSECTIONS (HAVING OPERATIONS
OVER FIVE YEARS AGO)

		L & W	Ill with recur.	Lost	Dead*	Total
Nodes Microscopically Negative	Clin. ⊖	30 (52%)	2 (3%)	5 (8%)	21 (37%)	58
	Clin. ⊕	1 (17%)	0	1 (17%)	4 (66%)	6
Nodes Microscopically Positive	Clin. ⊖	6 (55%)	1 (9%)	0	4 (36%)	11
	Clin. ⊕	1 (6%)	0	1 (6%)	14 (88%)	16
						91

*Death from all causes.

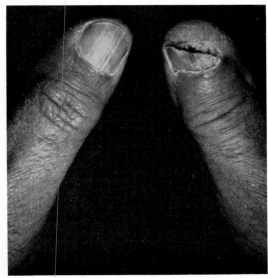

Figure 42–28 D.F., a 63 year old male with an amelanotic melanoma under the right thumbnail. The lesion had been treated for four years as a "fungus infection." After the diagnosis was established as melanoma, the treatment consisted of amputation of the thumb and axillary lymph node dissection.

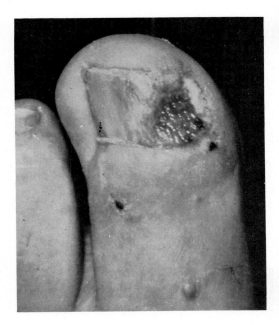

Figure 42–29 J.G., a 70 year old male with amelanotic melanoma under the left great toenail and satellitosis. The lesion had been treated for five years as a "fungus infection" before the diagnosis of melanoma was made.
(See also Color Plate VI-D.)

Figure 42–30 R.M., a 50 year old male with melanoma of the right heel. A recently performed punch biopsy and electrodesiccation of the site of a nearby benign nevus, done before the patient was seen for definitive treatment of melanoma, is seen inferior to the melanoma.
(See also Color Plate VI-E.)

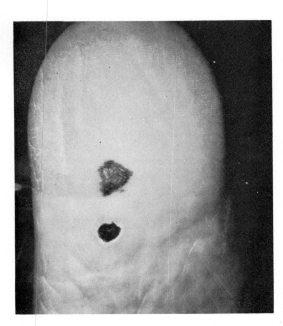

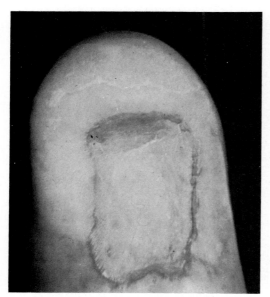

Figure 42–31   Same patient as in Figure 42–30 two months after wide and deep excision of melanoma of the heel, coverage of the defect with a split-thickness skin graft, and radical groin dissection.

method of treatment (Figs. 42–30 and 42–31).

In the treatment of melanoma of the trunk, reference is made to the work of Das Gupta and McNeer (1964) on the regional lymph nodes most likely to be involved. If only one group of these lymph nodes is highly suspect, this group should be removed. If more than one group may be involved theoretically but none appears to be clinically involved, then a choice must be made between multiple prophylactic regional lymph node dissections and careful observation.

Stehlen et al. (1966), in their discussion of melanomas of the extremities, emphasized that these may give rise to metastatic lesions of the skin or subcutaneous tissues between the primary site and the regional lymph nodes. They called these "in-transit metastases" and defined them as "deposits of melanoma which have lodged within the lymphatics between the primary tumor, or its excisional site, and the regional lymph nodes." Stehlen believed that lymphatic obstruction with subsequent lymph stasis was the most important etiologic factor in this regard. These "in-transit metastases" carry an ominous prognosis.

LESS COMMON PRIMARY SITES OF MELANOMA

Primary melanomas may occur whenever melanocytes are present. However, when a melanoma is found in an unusual site for a primary lesion, care must be taken to be sure that it does not represent a metastasis from a more common primary site.

The less common primary sites include the mucous membranes of the oral and nasal cavities, the external ear, the respiratory tract, larynx, esophagus, gallbladder, ovary, vagina, adrenal glands, meninges, and the anal canal (Das Gupta et al., 1969). These are discussed elsewhere in this book.

The appropriate treatment for primary melanoma of either the oral or nasal cavity is a wide and deep excision of the primary site and a cervical node dissection. When the primary site is near the midline of the tongue, a bilateral cervical node dissection should be done in addition to a partial glossectomy (Fig. 42–32). Lesions of the external ear are treated by either total amputation or partial amputation of the ear and a cervical lymph node dissection (Ward and Acquarelli, 1968). Lesions of the esophagus require esophagectomy. Lesions of the anorectal region may require an abdominoperineal

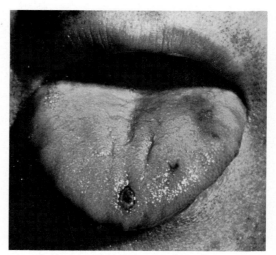

Figure 42–32   A.N., a 36 year old male with melanoma of the tip of the tongue. Note nevus on left side of tongue.
(See also Color Plate VI–F.)

resection and a bilateral groin dissection. Pack and Martins (1960) reported seven such cases of the anorectal region; only two patients were alive 30 and 32 months later, and one already had recurrent disease.

The exact treatment of these unusually located primary lesions is dependent upon the sites involved. They all carry a very poor prognosis, no matter how extensive the surgical resection. This serves to emphasize once again the aggressiveness of this disease and its tendency to spread by means of the blood stream as well as by the lymphatic route.

METASTATIC MELANOMA WITH UNKNOWN PRIMARY SITE

In a number of instances, melanomas may present as metastatic deposits in the regional lymph nodes or more distant regions, and no ascertainable primary site is to be found. At times, on diligent search, the primary site may be discovered by the taking of an extremely careful history or by the most minute examination of the patient. However, there are instances when even this may be unrewarding.

If a primary site cannot be found, and if the disease is limited to one group of regional lymph nodes (stage II), their surgical removal may still yield a long-term survival.

Das Gupta et al. (1963) reported 24 cases with an unknown primary site and a stage II situation out of 922 melanomas studied. Ten of these patients were alive and well five or more years later. Pack and Miller (1961) reported two cases of long-term survival out of 29 cases with an unknown primary site in a group of 1190 melanomas. We have one such case alive and well nine years after a radical groin dissection was performed; a second case is alive and well three years following a similar procedure.

The most likely explanation for a primary site that cannot be found is that the original melanoma was very small and became ulcerated; then this primary site subsequently healed completely with no evidence of any residual tumor. However, before this occurred it had produced metastases.

HEMATOGENOUS SPREAD

The hematogenous spread of the melanoma is the limiting factor in our present methods of treatment. While we may have reasonably good methods of controlling the direct local extension of the disease and its lymphatic type of spread, we have no effective way of preventing the blood-borne spread. In order to minimize this type of metastasis, *total* excisional biopsy is urged for any suspicious lesion, when possible, rather than an incisional biopsy. This also permits accurate classification of the melanoma. The most gentle handling of all involved tissue is also recommended in order to prevent the possible dislodgment of melanoma cells. The administration of prophylactic systemic chemotherapy at the time of the definitive operation does not appear to lessen the incidence of this hematogenous dissemination.

Some observers have even suggested that, prior to biopsy for a suspicious melanoma, very large doses of radiation should be administered to prevent the dislodging of viable melanoma cells into the blood stream.

Romsdahl et al. (1960) studied the blood specimens of their patients for the presence of melanoma cells. They were able to find circulating tumor cells and believed that the available evidence suggested that the host destroyed most of these. They could not find any relationship between the presence of circulating cancer cells and the prognosis. Romsdahl also believed that further experience with the melanoma might indicate a poor prognosis, particularly if peripheral circulating cancer cells were found postoperatively.

GENERALIZED MELANOSIS SECONDARY TO MELANOMA

Generalized melanosis secondary to melanoma is an unusual complication and

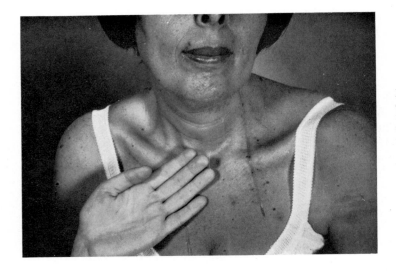

Figure 42–33 A.F., a 44 year old female with generalized melanosis following treatment of melanoma of the right nasolabial fold and right cervical node dissection. Note normal color of observer's hand. (*From* Sohn et al.: Cancer, 24:897, 1969.)

a most dramatic phenomenon when it occurs. The patient may change completely from one of fair complexion to one who appears so deeply pigmented as to be almost blue-black in color from head to foot. This is a terminal event associated with melanuria as well as diffuse melanosis. Apparently, melanin excretion is unable to keep up with the greatly increased production of melanin, and, as a result, large quantities of this pigment are deposited within the macrophages throughout the body (Silberberg et al., 1968; Sohn et al., 1969) (Figs. 42–33 and 42–34).

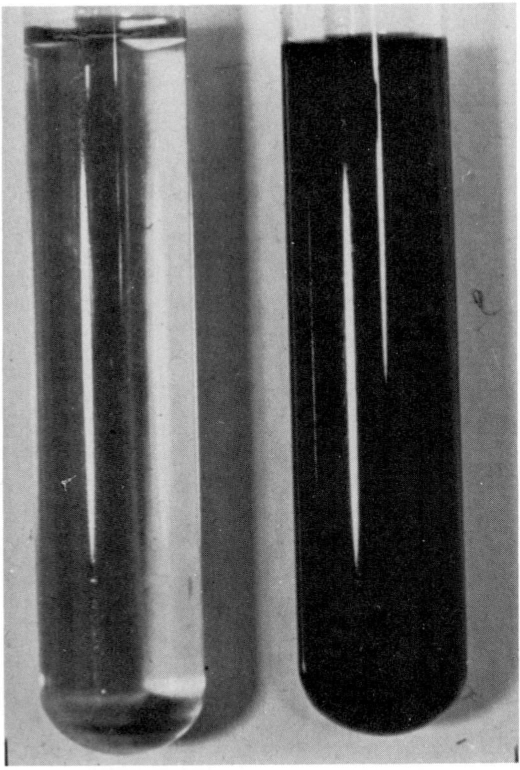

SPONTANEOUS REGRESSION AND IMMUNOLOGIC FACTORS

The melanoma is one of a number of malignant tumors in which spontaneous regression has been documented. Everson (1964) reported 12 such cases of melanoma. Since this is a particularly high number compared with the majority of malignant tumors, it has served to emphasize the possible importance of immunologic factors (Morton et al., 1970; Moore and Gerner, 1971; Krementz et al., 1971). For a detailed discussion of the immunologic features, see Chapter 77.

OCCURRENCE OF OTHER MALIGNANCIES IN PATIENTS WITH MELANOMA

It is our impression that the occurrence of other malignancies in patients with

Figure 42–34 Urine of patient in Figure 42–33 showing melanuria next to a normal urine specimen. (*From* Sohn et al.: Cancer, 24:897, 1969.) (See also Color Plate VII-A.)

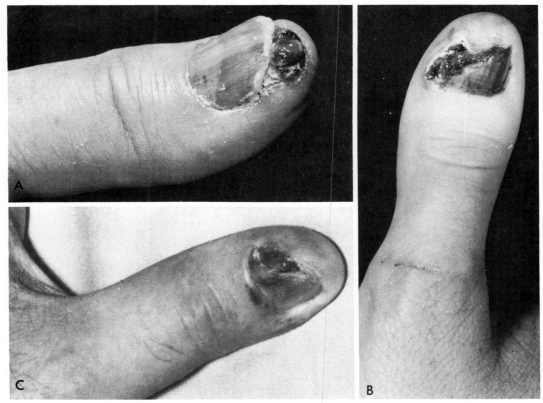

Figure 43–6 Subungual melanomas erroneously diagnosed as inflammatory lesions. *A*, subungual melanoma of the thumb. *B*, Subungual melanoma of the thumb which had been treated as a granuloma. *C*, Subungual melanoma of the thumb erroneously diagnosed as an inflammatory lesion. (*From* Pack and Oropeza: Surg. Gynecol. Obstet., 124:571, 1967. By permission of Surgery, Gynecology and Obstetrics.)

Figure 43–7 Subungual melanoma which had been mistaken for a fungus and treated with iodine salve and radium. A node in the groin had been excised six years previously and reported as being metastatic melanoma of unknown primary site. (*From* Pack and Oropeza: Surg. Gynecol. Obstet., 124:571, 1967. By permission of Surgery, Gynecology and Obstetrics.)

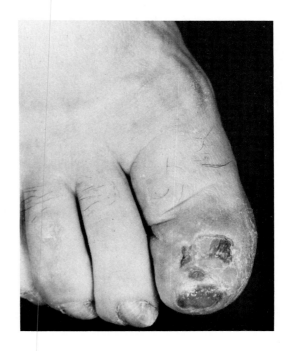

TABLE 43–1 FIVE-YEAR SURVIVAL OF 72 PATIENTS WITH SUBUNGUAL MELANOMA ACCORDING TO STAGE OF THE DISEASE*

Stage of Disease	No. of Patients	Determinate Cases				Indeterminate Cases		
		Living		Dead		Not Treated	Lost to Follow-up	5 Years Not Elapsed
		NED†	With Melanoma	Of Melanoma	Other Causes			
I. No prior treatment of primary melanoma or biopsy only	28	7	2	6	2	6	4	1
Locally recurrent after improper treatment	12	5	–	2	2	–	–	3
II. Primary operable melanoma, lymph node metastases	6	1	–	3	–	1	–	1
Primary melanoma controlled: nodal metastases	7	–	–	4	–	1	–	2
Recurrent primary melanoma; nodal metastases	6	–	–	2	2	1	–	1
III. Distant metastasis	6	–	–	5	–	1	–	–
Satellitosis localized to extremity	5	1	–	2	–	2	–	–
Not classified	2	–	–	–	–	1	–	1
Total:	72	14	2	24	6	13	4	9

*From Pack and Oropeza: Surg. Gynecol. Obstet., 124:571, 1967. By permission of Surgery, Gynecology and Obstetrics.
†No evidence of disease.

Condition of the Primary Melanoma Upon Admission

The primary tumor was either untreated or a biopsy only had been performed in 28 of the 72 patients (Pack and Oropeza, 1967a) (Table 43–1). In the remaining patients, the tumors had been treated for from one month to four years as paronychia, felon, pyogenic granuloma, fungus, and ingrown nail. In several cases the discoloration of the nail was interpreted as being a hematoma, especially if the patient mentioned that it became apparent after trauma. In the majority of patients, proper treatment was delayed because the patients had been previously treated for assumed benign conditions without biopsy from the diseased tissue. This delay caused by previous improper therapy constitutes an important factor in the end results of treatment.

Clinical Status of the Regional Lymph Nodes

In some patients the regional lymph nodes are large and firm; therefore, the clinical suspicion of metastatic involvement is great. In nine patients the initial examination revealed massive involvement of the regional nodes. In 14 patients the nodes were suspected of containing metastases, and pathologic examination confirmed this expectation in 12. Forty patients had no clinically enlarged nodes. A biopsy of the lymph nodes in five patients had been obtained elsewhere prior to our examination and revealed metastases. In one patient, no information regarding the lymph nodes was recorded. Of the 72 patients, 28 (38.8 percent) had enlarged nodes on admission; pathologic examination revealed that in two of these patients the nodes were enlarged but did not contain metastatic deposits, leaving 36 percent positive for metastases (Fig. 43–8).

Treatment

Stage I Subungual Melanoma. There were 40 patients who were without evidence of metastatic disease to the regional lymph nodes or distant spread.

The accepted treatment for subungual melanomas is either a transmetacarpal, transmetatarsal, metacarpocarpal, or metatarsotarsal amputation (Fig. 43–9). More conservative amputations have frequently been followed by local recurrences, because the tumor frequently invades the underlying periosteum and bone (Fig. 43–10). Amputation through either a metacarpophalangeal or metatarsophalangeal joint is not only less adequate but also less functional and more disfiguring.

There is contention as to whether or not elective regional lymph node dissections should be performed for these patients with localized disease, and whether or not this should be carried out at the dissection of the primary melanoma or at a later date. Some surgeons favor performing an elective nodal dissection simultaneously with the amputation in the hope that any microscopic foci of melanoma will be removed at an early stage, that is, before they become clinically evident. However, simultaneous amputation with elective nodal dissection has sometimes been followed by the appearance of melanotic dermal satellites or subcutaneous in-transit metastases in the extremity, possibly due to the blockage, stagnation, hypertension, and backward flow of the lymph and the resultant implantation of tumor cells. On the other hand, when clinically negative regional nodes are removed electively, and even if found to be involved by metastases, the end results are far better than those resulting from waiting until the nodes are grossly involved with metastases when removed.

Some surgeons advocate the performance of elective regional node dissections in a period of from four to six weeks following surgery. The theoretic advantages are that this prevents stagnation of the lymphatic flow immediately after removal of the primary tumor, with incarceration of cancer cells in the intervening lymphatics and lymph nodes, and possibly temporarily leaves the lymph nodes to serve as filters to "catch" melanoma cells in lymphatic transit. It would seem reasonable to assume that only a few days wait may be necessary for the in-transit metastases to

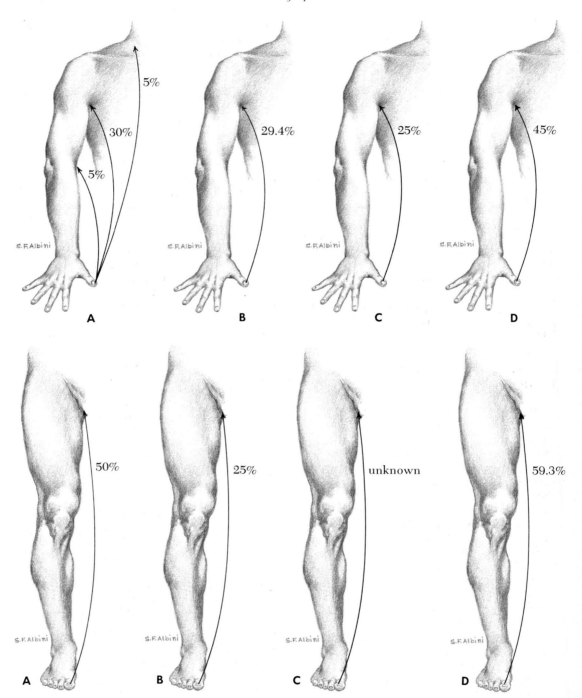

Figure 43–8   *Above,* subungual melanoma of the fingers. *A,* Incidence of greatly enlarged lymph nodes on admission, 12 of 40 patients. *B,* No enlarged nodes on admission; nodal metastases developed after amputation of the primary melanoma only, 5 of 17 patients. *C,* Incidence of metastases in elective nodal dissection, 1 of 4 patients. *D,* Total incidence of metastasis to lymph nodes on admission (*A*) and subsequently (*B*), 18 of 40 patients. *Below,* subungual melanoma of the toes. *A,* Incidence of significantly enlarged nodes on admission, 16 of 32 patients. *B,* Patients with no enlarged nodes on admission in whom nodal metastases subsequently developed after amputation of the primary tumor, 3 of 12 patients. *C,* No elective lymph node dissection performed. *D,* Total incidence of metastasis to lymph nodes on admission (*A*) and subsequently (*B*), 19 of 32 patients. (*From* Pack and Oropeza: Surg. Gynecol. Obstet., 124:571, 1967. Courtesy of Surgery, Gynecology and Obstetrics.)

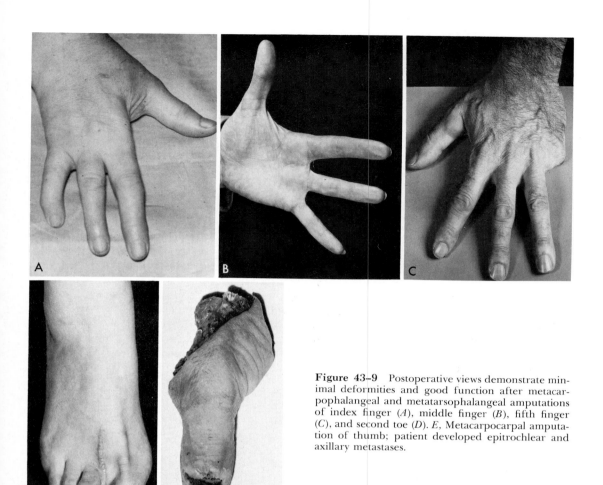

Figure 43–9 Postoperative views demonstrate minimal deformities and good function after metacarpophalangeal and metatarsophalangeal amputations of index finger (*A*), middle finger (*B*), fifth finger (*C*), and second toe (*D*). *E*, Metacarpocarpal amputation of thumb; patient developed epitrochlear and axillary metastases.

Figure 43–10 Surgical specimen of subungual melanoma of thumb with deep invasion of bone. Treatment had been for an inflammatory lesion for a period of three years, and the thumb had been cauterized several times.

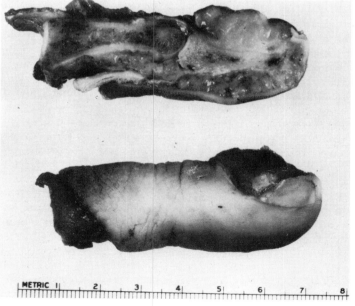

travel to and become lodged in the regional lymph nodes.

Theoretically, the amputation of the involved digit only without lymph node dissection has the advantage of not interfering with the lymphatic flow, but it has the great disadvantage of allowing cancer cells in-transit to the regional lymph nodes to grow, thus impairing to some degree the chance for possible cure in the early stages. As mentioned before, in-transit metastases carry the hazard of melanotic satellitosis following elective groin or axillary dissections. This is important and sometimes quite tragic when the primary melanoma is situated on the distal extremity, but it appears to occur less frequently than we originally believed. If detected early, it may still be curatively treated by high exarticulation above the inguinal or axillary scars. Perfusion therapy is also used for this difficult problem.

Admittedly, the problem has not yet been solved, and new approaches to the treatment of this disease have been tried. Amputation of the digit, followed by or preceded by the intralymphatic administration of radioactive isotopes, is being pursued by Ariel (1964).

Prognosis will depend upon the stage of the disease at the time of the initial definitive treatment. For stage I subungual melanoma without involvement of the regional lymph nodes, the results may be worsened by the delay in performing amputation and by the scope of the operation. Improper treatment by such measures as cautery excision, caustics, or irradiation, as well as procrastination in performing amputation, contributes to early and widespread dissemination of the melanoma. The five-year survival rate, as reported by Pack and Oropeza (1967a), in this stage of the disease was 46.1 percent. Table 43–2 summarizes the treatment received by these patients. As can be seen, there was not sufficient evidence for evaluation of the efficacy of amputation and elective node dissection versus amputation of the digit only. The one patient treated by an incomplete amputation of the digit was free of melanoma at five years, indicating merely that an occasional patient may possibly be cured by a conservative operation, although this is exceptional.

No patient in this early stage of disease was treated by an amputation of the extremity.

Stage II Subungual Melanoma. Nineteen patients in stage II of the disease presented with an untreated primary tumor and lymph node metastases, or a recurrent primary tumor with lymph node metastases, or lymphatic metastases only and the primary melanoma controlled (Table 43–2). The usual method of treating these patients has been by the amputation of the involved digit and therapeutic dissection of the lymph nodes. Due to the degree of malignancy of these tumors, amputation of the entire extremity has been proposed, but few patients will consent to such extensive surgery for what seems to them to be a "slight" skin cancer. Paradoxically, patients with melanomas on the soles of the feet or other soft tissue sarcomas will consent to radical surgical procedures rather readily (Pack and Miller, 1964).

Hemipelvectomy has not been found to be very effective for the control of subungual melanomas or melanomas of the lower extremity with metastasis as high as the iliac lymph nodes, as reported by McPeak and his colleagues (1959). This operative procedure has admittedly been carried out in many patients with in-transit metastases in an attempt to control their disease and pain and to prevent massive bleeding from the femoral vessels due to a fungating lesion. Patients with metastasis to the iliac lymph nodes were all dead within five years (McPeak et. al., 1959). There seemed to be a better salvage rate in patients who had only femoral lymph node involvement and who had hemipelvectomies. Hemipelvectomy or interscapulothoracic amputation is too large a procedure to purely palliate advanced melanomas. As a potentially curative operation, hemipelvectomy or interscapulothoracic amputation should be performed only for those melanomas involving the regional lymph nodes and/or vascular structures to the extremity. However, since vascular grafts and perfusion therapy have been developed there are few occasions to do these procedures.

For patients with an untreated primary lesion and lymph node metastases, or re-

TABLE 43-2 FIVE-YEAR SURVIVAL OF 72 PATIENTS WITH SUBUNGUAL MELANOMA ACCORDING TO TYPE OF TREATMENT*

Stage of Disease On Admission	Treatment	No. of Patients	Living NED†	Living With Melanoma	Dead Of Melanoma	Dead NED†	Dead Cause Unknown	Lost to Follow-up	5 Years Not Elapsed
I. Untreated	Not treated	6	–	–	–	–	–	6	–
	Amputation of digit only	19	6	2	5	–	1	4	1
	Incomplete amputation	1	1	–	–	–	–	–	–
	Amputation of digit, elective nodal dissection	2	–	–	1	1	–	–	–
Locally recurrent after improper treatment	Amputation of digit only	10	5	–	1	1	–	–	3
	Amputation of digit; elective nodal dissection	2	–	–	1	–	1	–	–
	Totals	40	12	2	8	2	2	10	4
II. Primary operable melanoma; nodal metastases	No treatment	1	–	–	1	–	–	–	–
	Amputation of digit; roentgenotherapy to nodes	1	–	–	–	–	–	1	–
	Amputation of digit; therapeutic nodal dissection	4	1	–	2	–	–	–	1
Primary melanoma controlled; nodal metastases	No treatment	2	–	–	1	–	–	1	–
	Amputation of digit; therapeutic nodal dissection	1	–	–	–	–	–	1	–
	Amputation of digit; roentgenotherapy to nodes	1	–	–	1	–	–	–	–
Recurrent primary melanoma; nodal metastases	Nodal dissection only	3	–	–	2	–	–	–	1
	No treatment	1	–	–	–	–	–	1	–
	Amputation of digit; therapeutic nodal dissection	4	–	–	1	–	–	–	3
	Interscapulothoracic amputation (curative)	1	–	–	–	–	–	1	–
	Totals	19	1	–	8	–	–	5	5
III. Distant metastasis	Not treated	1	–	–	1	–	–	–	–
	Palliative nodal dissection	2	–	–	2	–	–	–	–
	Hemipelvectomy (palliative)	1	–	–	1	–	–	–	–
	Other treatment	2	–	–	2	–	–	–	–
Satellitosis localized to extremity	Not treated	2	–	–	2	–	–	–	–
	Amputation of digit; palliative groin dissection	2	–	–	–	–	2	–	–
	Hip joint disarticulation (curative)	1	–	–	–	–	–	1	–
	Totals	11	–	–	8	–	2	1	–
Not classified (NED)† on admission	Not treated	2	1	–	–	–	–	1	–
	Total:	72	14	2	24	2	4	17	9

*From Pack and Oropeza: Surg. Gynecol. Obstet., 124:571, 1967. By permission of Surgery, Gynecology and Obstetrics.

†No evidence of disease.

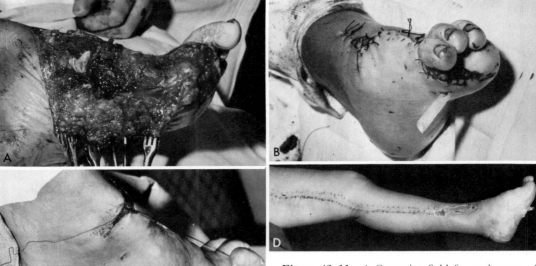

Figure 43–11 *A*, Operative field for melanoma of the first toe. *B*, Postoperative view. *C*, Isotopic lymphogram of the leg. *D*, Postoperative view of removal of the lymphatics of the leg.

current primary tumors with lymph node metastases, or a controlled primary lesion with lymph node metastases, the intralymphatic injection of radioactive isotopes or chemotherapeutic drugs (Ariel and Pack, 1962; Ariel and Resnick, 1964), combined with amputation of the involved digit and dissection of the regional nodes, is under investigation as a possible curative or palliative procedure. The incidence of local recurrences or metastases or both within the extremity may be reduced by perfusing the extremity with chemotherapeutic agents or radioactive isotopes, in addition to surgically excising the primary tumor and its regional node metastases (Fig. 43–11). Conclusive evidence of this improvement in terms of five-year survival awaits further studies with larger groups of patients.

Stage III Subungual Melanoma. In stage III subungual melanoma are those patients with in-transit metastases localized to the extremity. The treatment of patients with more distant metastases is palliative at best. A patient may survive in "mutual coexistence" with the tumor for many years but will eventually die as a result of metastasis to vital organs.

Patients with satellitoses or in-transit metastases localized to the extremity may be treated either by the isolation perfusion of the limb with various chemotherapeutic agents or by the amputation of the extremity. Five patients in this series were admitted with satellitoses or in-transit metastases. All these lesions were located on the lower extremity, without extension to the skin of the buttocks or abdomen. As seen in Table 43–2, although the number of patients is small, it seems more than just a coincidence that the satellites or in-transit metastases in all of the patients involved only the lower extremity, which may be the result of greater lymphatic stasis influenced by gravity, increased venous pressure, or impaired valves of the veins.

Summary

The salient factor in attempting to improve the curative rate for subungual melanomas is an early and accurate diagnosis of the lesion by an incisional biopsy, followed by the proper treatment as soon as possible. Amputations which include either the metacarpal or the metatarsal bones have proved most successful in controlling the primary disease. Patients with clinically apparent regional node metastases should be treated by regional node dissection and perfusion techniques. If the nodes have become fixed, then a palliative radical amputation procedure should be considered if the limb is painful or disabling, or there is diffuse ulceration. The alternative — performing a discontinuous radical groin or axillary dissection in conjunction with perfusion of the extremity with cancer chemotherapeutic drugs or the intralymphatic administration of radioactive isotopes — gives some promise of long-term palliation. It may very well be the treatment of choice for elderly patients or patients who are poor operative risks.

MELANOMAS OF THE ANAL CANAL

Thirty-five years of experience in the management of melanomas of the anal canal are reviewed by Pack and Oropeza (1967b). Accordingly, it is estimated that melanomas of the anus comprise from 0.25 to 1.25 percent of all malignant tumors of this region (Pack et al., 1952; Pack and Martin, 1960).

Material

Twenty patients with melanoma of the anal canal were studied. Because of their location in a region which is infrequently inspected minutely, melanomas of the anal canal are frequently overlooked. The chief symptoms of this group of patients — itching and bleeding — are also common symptoms of such benign conditions as hemorrhoids and anal fistulas. This similarity may mask the true disease and delay the treatment, therefore decreasing the opportunity for possible cure.

Of the 20 patients studied, 14 (70 percent) had melanomas which originated in the anal canal; the remaining six patients (30 percent) had lesions which originated in the perianal skin.

Clinical Diagnosis

When one considers the many proctoscopic examinations which are done annually, it is a significant fact that pigmented nevi are seldom encountered or recognized in the anal canal. An accurate clinical diagnosis of melanoma is rarely made at the first examination because of the common rectal lesions which coexist and the relative rarity of this tumor. The final diagnosis is made by the pathologist, usually unexpectedly after the removal of what appeared to be hemorrhoidal tissue, anal tags, or polyps. *Any pigmented lesion of the anal canal should be considered melanoma until proven otherwise under careful microscopic examination.*

In amelanotic lesions, the differential diagnosis will be between such benign conditions as fissures, anal tags, cysts, papillomas, and dermatitis. The chief lesion that may be confused with and must be differentiated from the amelanotic melanoma is the epidermoid carcinoma. If the lesion is extensive and involves a great portion of the anal canal, it most probably will be an epidermoid carcinoma. Because of the polypoid appearance of these melanomas, as compared with epidermoid carcinomas, patients often noted the appearance of a mass in the rectal outlet (often mistaken for thrombosed hemorrhoids) before seeking medical advice.

The surgeon should be aware of these uncommon lesions, and all patients who appear to have "hemorrhoids" should be thoroughly examined. Accordingly, a biopsy of any doubtful lesion is essential.

Clinical Features

Age. There was no apparent age difference between patients with melanoma of the anus and those patients with melanomas of other regions of the body (Table 43–3).

It is interesting to note that one patient gave a history of associated pregnancy at the time the melanoma became evident.

Complexion. As with melanomas of other anatomic sites, the majority of patients had the characteristic sandy hair, blue eyes, and fair skin.

Sex. In this study the ratio of women to men was 3:1, a disparity attributable to the fact that this was a relatively small series.

TABLE 43–3 MELANOMA OF THE ANAL
CANAL: CLINICAL FEATURES

Total number of patients	20
Age (years)	
Youngest	34
Oldest	75
Mean	53.5
Primary (untreated patients)	8
Secondary (treated patients)	12
Metastasis to lymph nodes	6

TABLE 43–5 MELANOMA OF THE ANAL
CANAL: INITIAL SYMPTOMS

Initial Symptoms	Number of Patients
Bleeding	9
Mass noted by patient	4
Pain	3
Itching	1
Other or unknown	3
Total:	20

Initial Signs and Symptoms. As with subungual melanomas these 20 patients were divided into three groups, according to the clinical stage of the disease when first seen by us. There were 13 patients with stage I melanoma (lesions still limited to primary site). Five patients were untreated, and eight had previous treatment. There were five patients with stage II melanoma (with evidence of metastasis to the regional lymph nodes); two were untreated and three were previously treated). There were two patients in stage III (with evidence of distant metastases) (Table 43–4).

The initial signs and symptoms are summarized in Table 43–5. In the 20 patients with melanomas of the anal canal, bleeding was the most frequent initial manifestation, being present in ten (50 percent), either alone or associated with rectal pressure, pain, itching, or change in bowel habits. Six patients noted a mass, either in the anal canal or in the inguinal region. One patient complained of pain only. The melanomas of three patients

TABLE 43–4 MELANOMA OF THE ANAL
CANAL: PREVIOUS TREATMENT

Previous Treatment	Number of Patients
None	2
Wedge excision or limited biopsy	1
Biopsy (type unstated)	3
Limited excision with local recurrence	6
Limited excision without local recurrence	5
Adequate excision without local recurrence	1
Desiccation and/or administration of caustics and local recurrence	2
Abdominoperineal resection	0
Total:	20

were asymptomatic and were discovered by their family physicians.

The duration of the symptoms ranged from less than one month to 48 months, with an average time of 8.1 months. Nine patients (45 percent) had symptoms for three months or less.'

None of the patients described a history of the presence of a longstanding mole, and this is hardly surprising because of the inaccessibility of this region to inspection. None of the patients reported a family history of melanoma.

Treatment

Conservative Surgery. Junctional and compound nevi of the anal canal should be excised prophylactically and the specimen sent for microscopic diagnosis. When a small pigmented lesion is suspected of being melanoma, a biopsy may be performed under local anesthesia. If the excised lesion proves to be a melanoma, abdominoperineal resection of the rectum with bilateral groin dissections should be considered. Whenever possible, one should consider a less radical procedure because the prognosis with this operation is so poor.

Abdominoperineal Resection and Groin Dissection. Treatment of malignant neoplasms of the anal canal has undergone a transition in the past 25 years, with emphasis being diverted from dependence upon irradiation to the surgical extirpation of the primary tumor and contiguous structures, as well as the lymph nodes draining this area. Anal melanomas are notorious for their tendency to metastasize by means of the lymphatic and blood routes to the systemic and portal systems. The high incidence of metas-

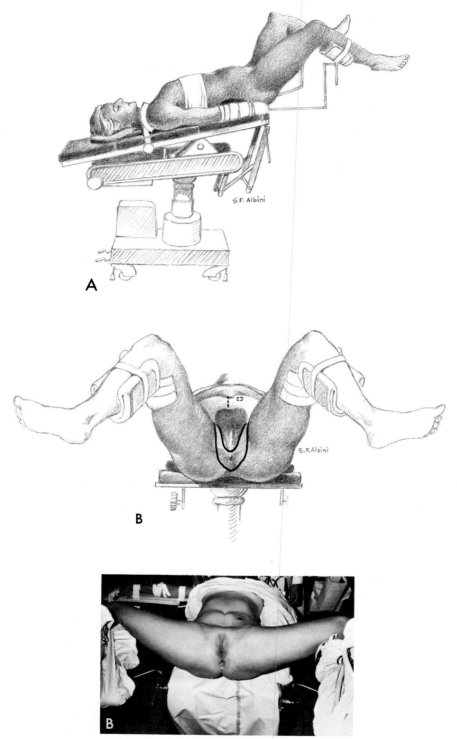

Figure 43–12 *A,* Position of patient for synchronous two-team abdominoperineal resection and groin dissection in-continuity.

B, Perineal exposure (sketch and actual patient) for surgical team performing from below.

Illustration continued on following page.

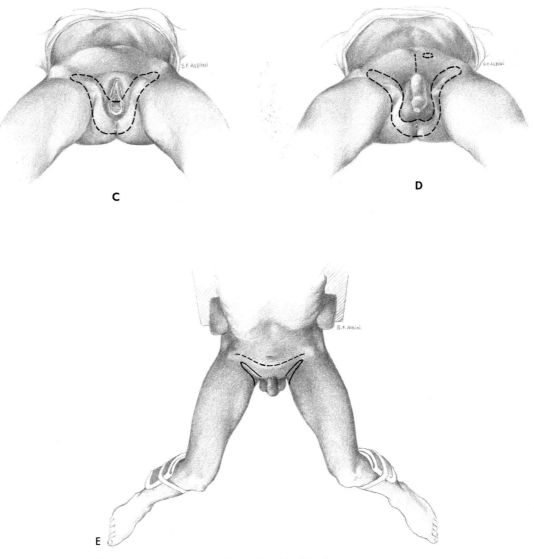

Figure 43–12 *Continued.* *C,* Scope of the inguinoperineal incision in women.
  D, Scope of the inguinoperineal incision in men.
  E, Exposure and circumlinear transverse suprapubic laparotomy incision for surgical team working from above.

Illustration continued on opposite page.

tasis to the lymph nodes of the inguinal, iliac, obturator, rectosigmoid, and aortic regions emphasizes the necessity for removing the primary lesion and the chains of draining lymph nodes, preferably in-continuity. In these melanomas, the frequent route of spread is via the veins of the portal system to the liver.

It should be noted that an elective or therapeutic groin dissection will tend to control the regional metastases, but the prognosis is grave if dissemination by hematogenous routes has occurred.

Synchronous Two-Team Operation. In the performance of these extensive operations, two surgeons are utilized,

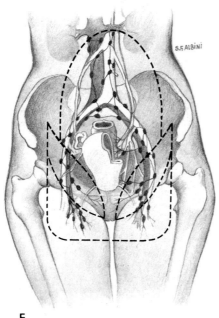

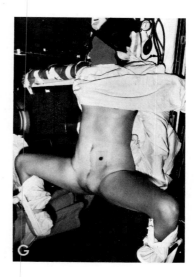

Figure **43-12** *Continued. F*, Schematic outline of the lymph node dissection afforded by approach from above.

G, Actual patient prepared for surgery.

H, Scope of pelvic and perineal resection. (*From* Pack and Oropeza: Dis. Colon Rectum, 10:161, 1967.)

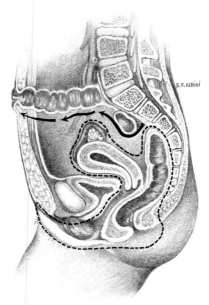

each with an assistant. The patient is placed in the Trendelenburg lithotomy position with the pelvis elevated and with the thighs widely abducted (Fig. 43–12). One team may be operating from above, peforming the bilateral groin dissections, while the second team is resecting the rectum. Another approach is that the rectal resection is performed first, and then each group performs a unilateral groin dissection, thereby cutting the operating time in half.

Irradiation. Irradiation for primary or metastatic melanomas of the anal region has ceased to be employed by the knowledgeable clinician owing to the fact that, in our experience, these lesions have proven to be radioresistant; moreover, the anal region does not tolerate large doses of radiation.

Five-Year End Results

Of the 20 patients with melanoma of the anal canal, only 18 were eligible for five-year surveillance. Of these 18 patients, 5 were lost to observation; therefore, the definitive group consisted of only 13.

From the results obtained, we may conclude that age may affect the prognosis very slightly, as the patient who was without metastases at 10+ years was 68 years of age when she was first treated (Table 43–6).

It appears that both the patients who are first seen with primary or recurrent lesions or both without lymph node metastases and the patients who exhibit primary, controlled, or recurrent lesions with lymph node metastases have a poor prognosis owing to the high degree of malignancy of these melanomas. These highly malignant lesions spread early by means of the rich lymphatic network of the anal region and the blood vessels to the systemic and portal systems (Fig. 43–13).

Prognosis

The prognosis for melanoma of the anal canal is influenced only slightly by the type of treatment, regardless of the stage of the neoplasm (Table 43–7). More often, a palliative result is the most that one should expect. This highly malignant lesion will usually have extended beyond the confines of the pelvis and the regional nodes at the time that treatment is begun.

TABLE 43–6   MELANOMA OF THE ANAL CANAL: FIVE-YEAR SURVIVAL ACCORDING TO AGE

Age (Years)	Number of Patients	No Evidence of Disease
31–40	3	0
41–50	1	0
51–60	6	0
61–70	9	1
71–80	1	0

Although we advocate the performance of a radical operative procedure, meaning the radical removal of the primary lesion by abdominoperineal rectal resection with a bilateral groin dissection as an elective procedure (Fig. 43–14), we believe that its curative value is unpredictable, and the likelihood of failure is great (Table 43–8).

Summary

A study of the natural history, treatment, and prognosis of 20 patients with melanoma of the anal canal has been made.

The early detection and radical removal of the primary lesion by abdominoperineal resection in-continuity with bilateral groin and pelvic lymph node dissection is the preferred treatment for patients with anal melanomas.

Inasmuch as there is no alternative treatment for proper surgical excision, this operation should be done if there is no evidence of distant dissemination. Cures are possible although they do not occur with encouraging frequency.

MELANOMA OF THE VULVA

Melanomas of the vulva occur more frequently than do melanomas of the male genitalia. They are infrequent tumors and represent only 1.5 percent of melanomas of both sexes (Pack et. al., 1952). In melanomas of the female, only about 3 percent are located on the genitalia. It is to be noted that the skin surface of the female genitalia comprises between 1 and 2 percent of the total body area.

Ahumada (1953) reported 164 patients with melanomas of the vulva collected from the world literature.

Material

Forty-one patients with melanoma of the vulva were reported by Pack and Oropeza (1967c). When the melanoma was located at the introitus or in the lower third of the vagina close to the hymenal ring, it was considered to be a melanoma

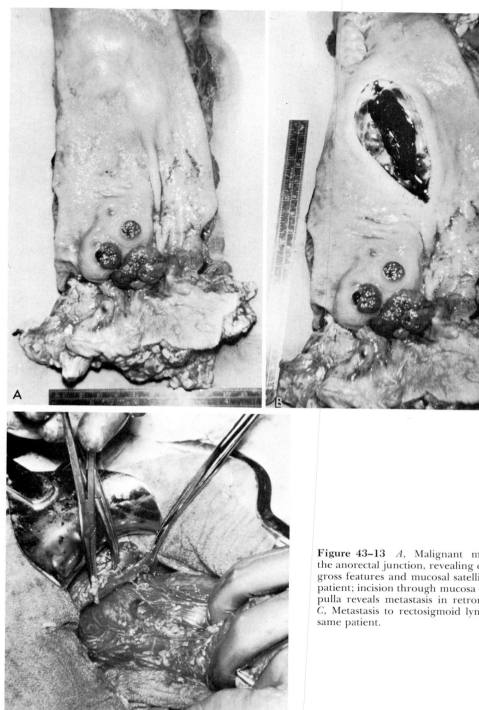

Figure 43–13 *A*, Malignant melanoma of the anorectal junction, revealing characteristic gross features and mucosal satellites. *B*, Same patient; incision through mucosa of rectal ampulla reveals metastasis in retrorectal nodes. *C*, Metastasis to rectosigmoid lymph node in same patient.

TABLE 43–7   MELANOMA OF THE ANAL CANAL: FIVE-YEAR END RESULTS
ACCORDING TO CLINICAL STAGES

Stage	Condition on Admission	Total	Living, NED°	Dead		Not Treated or Lost to Observation	5 Years Not Elapsed
				Of Melanoma	Other Causes		
I. a	Primary melanoma not treated or recent biopsy only	5	1	3		1	
b	Melanoma locally recurrent after improper treatment	8		3	2	1	2
II. a	Primary melanoma not treated; lymph node metastasis	2		1		1	
b	Primary melanoma controlled; lymph node metastasis	1				1	
c	Recurrent primary melanoma; lymph node metastasis	2		1	1		
III. a	Distant metastasis or disease advanced locally	2			1	1†	
	Total:	20	1	8	4	5	2

°No evidence of disease (melanoma).
†Treated but lost to observation.
From Pack and Oropeza: Dis. Colon Rectum, 10:161, 1967.

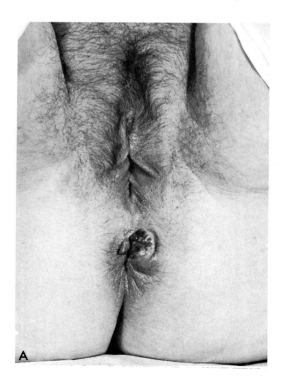

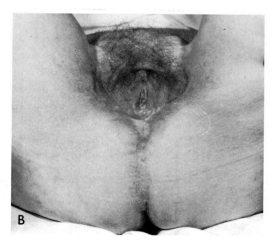

Figure 43–14   *A*, Preoperative view of anal melanoma. *B*, Postoperative result following abdominoperineal resection and bilateral groin dissection.

TABLE 43–8 MELANOMA OF THE ANAL CANAL: FIVE-YEAR SURVIVAL RATE ACCORDING TO TYPE OF TREATMENT (1930 to 1965)

Stage	Treatment	Total	Living, NED*	Dead		Lost to Observation	5 Years Not Elapsed
				Of Melanoma	Other Causes		
I.	No treatment	2				2	
	Wide excision with unilateral groin dissection	2					2
	Abdominoperineal resection	3		3			
	Abdominoperineal resection with bilateral groin dissection	6	1	3	2		
II.	No treatment	2				2	
	Wide excision with bilateral groin dissection	1		1			
	Abdominoperineal resection with bilateral groin	2		1	1		
III.	No treatment; exploratory laparotomy only	1				1	
	Unilateral groin dissection	1			1		
	Total:	20	1	8	4	5	2

*No evidence of disease (melanoma).
From Pack and Oropeza: Dis. Colon Rectum, 10:161, 1967.

of the vulva because of the difficulty in establishing the precise location.

Anatomic Distribution

Of the 41 patients with melanoma of the vulva, relatively few—five of 41 (12.2 percent)—had lesions which originated on the labium majus; most of the tumors—36 of 41 (87.8 percent)—originated on the mucosa of the genitalia (Fig. 43–15).

Clinical Features

Age. The youngest patient with melanoma of the vulva was 15 years old, and

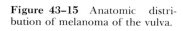

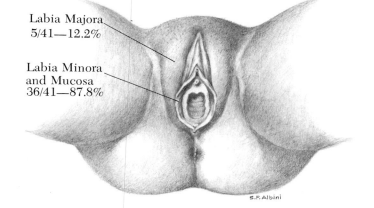

Figure 43–15 Anatomic distribution of melanoma of the vulva.

Labia Majora
5/41—12.2%

Labia Minora and Mucosa
36/41—87.8%

S.F.Albini

TABLE 43–9 MELANOMA OF THE VULVA: FIVE-YEAR SURVIVAL ACCORDING TO AGE

Age (Years)	Number of Patients	NED*
15–39	5	0
40–49	8	2
50–59	10	4
60–69	12	2
70–79	5	1
84	1	0

*No evidence of disease (melanoma).

the oldest was 84 years of age. The mean age was 56 years. There was no apparent difference between the age of these patients and that of patients with melanomas in other anatomic regions (Tables 43–9 and 43–10).

It should be mentioned that none of these patients had an associated pregnancy at the time of diagnosis.

Complexion. As in other melanomas, these patients had the characteristic sandy hair, fair complexions, and blue or hazel eyes. None of these patients was Negro.

Patient's Initial Evidence of Melanoma. Fifteen patients reported that the initial symptom of the disease was bleeding, and six reported pruritus; five had no symptoms and the tumor was discovered by either the patient or the physician. Of two previously treated patients, one complained of bleeding and one of pruritus.

There were 17 patients in stage I in this series who had only a primary lesion which was untreated or locally recurrent without lymph node metastases.

TABLE 43–10 MELANOMA OF THE VULVA: CLINICAL FEATURES

Number of patients	41
Age (years)	
Youngest	15
Oldest	84
Mean	56
Main symptom	bleeding
Primary	
Untreated without lymph node metastases	17/41
Secondary	
Untreated with lymph node metastases	16/41
Previously treated with lymph node metastases	8/41
Metastasis to lymph nodes	24/41

A total of 24 patients in stages II and III had primary lesions or recurrent primary lesions with lymph node involvement and satellitosis. Sixteen of these were previously untreated patients, in whom bleeding was the first sign in six, pruritus in three, and a palpable mass in the groin in four. Of the eight previously treated patients, four complained of bleeding, three had evidence of metastatic disease in the groin, and one had no symptoms.

In summary, bleeding was the most frequent initial evidence of the disease, being present in 15 patients; pruritus was present in ten. In seven patients there was evidence of metastasis to lymph nodes as the presenting manifestation. In four patients there was no information as to symptomatology. One patient had disseminated melanoma on admission, and there was no clear indication as to the onset of the disease. Three patients had satellitosis, and in one there was no evidence of melanoma on admission. None of the patients gave a history of long-standing mole. The duration of symptoms for patients with melanomas of the vulva varied from 1 to 48 months, with a mean of 13.5 months.

Clinical Diagnosis

Any pigmented lesion of the vulva should be considered a melanoma until proven otherwise by excisional biopsy (Figs. 43–16 and 43–17). Nevi in this location are hazardous because of the frequency of the junctional component.

In amelanotic lesions the differential diagnosis will be between such benign conditions as cysts, papillomas, dermatitis extramammary Paget's disease, Bowen's disease, and furuncles, all frequently found in the vulva because of the presence of many hair follicles and sebaceous and sweat glands. The presence of condyloma acuminatum and other granulomas, although less frequent today, can make the diagnosis even more difficult. The main lesion that may be confused with, and which must be differentiated from, the amelanotic melanoma is the epidermoid carcinoma. If the lesion is lo-

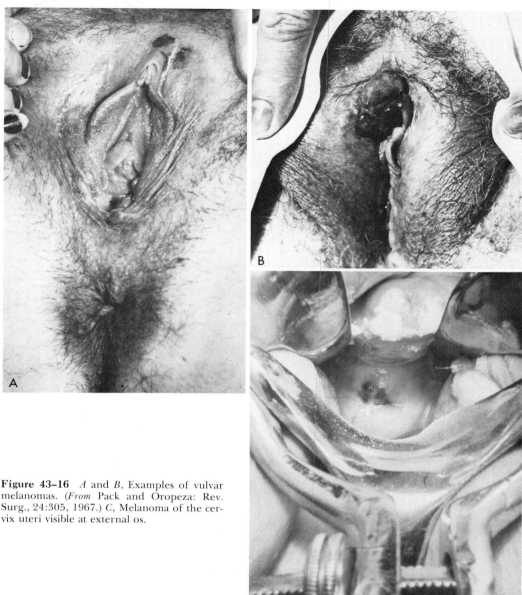

Figure 43–16 *A* and *B*, Examples of vulvar melanomas. (*From* Pack and Oropeza: Rev. Surg., 24:305, 1967.) *C*, Melanoma of the cervix uteri visible at external os.

cated on the labium majus or is very extensive and involves a great portion of the vulva, it will most likely be an epidermoid carcinoma. The bluish black lesion is practically pathognomonic but not necessarily so, because the melanoma may be nonpigmented, and other pigment diseases, such as acanthosis nigricans, cavernous hemangiomas, or freckles may simulate melanoma. A biopsy, either excisional if the lesion is small or incisional if it is ex-

tensive, will provide a precise pathologic diagnosis.

Condition of the Primary Tumor on Admission

The lymph nodes in 15 of the patients were not enlarged on physical examination. Twenty-four of the patients had lymph nodes containing metastatic dis-

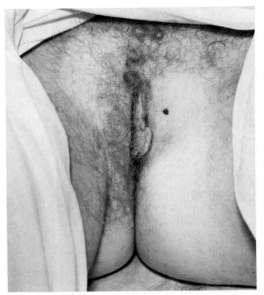

Figure 43–17 Benign junctional nevus in young, red-haired woman; excised for prophylaxis and histologic study.

ease. A previous pathologic analysis of the lymph nodes in 18 of these patients was available, and in every instance but one the metastases were confirmed. In five patients the metastases in the regional lymph nodes were bilateral, in six they were unilateral, and in six the precise location of the metastasis was not reported.

Surgical Treatment

Because these lesions are commonly disseminated through the lymphatics, an important principle in the planning of an adequate operation is the removal of all lymph nodes which are vulnerable to metastasis. The regional lymph nodes which are potentially implicated are the superficial and deep inguinal nodes, the pubic and the medial and lateral external iliac nodes, and rarely the obturator and femoral nodes (the latter probably by retrograde extension from blocked inguinal nodes). The lymph nodes for the labia majora and the clitoris are the medial superficial inguinal group. Other inguinal nodes are rapidly involved by metastasis because of the abundant interconnecting lymphatic channels. Thus the lymphatic

trunks of the right labium may course and empty directly into the left inguinal nodes. The efferent lymphatic vessels traverse upward in the genitofemoral fold and terminate in a horizontal tract of the superficial inguinal nodes. This anatomic fact constitutes the basis for a one-stage, monobloc procedure which encompasses the vulva and lymph nodes in the groin (Fig. 43–18*A*). The lymphatic trunks from the labia minora, hymen, vestibule, and fourchette anastomose with those of the labia majora and therefore drain into the same regional lymph nodes. The lymph vessels of the clitoris are both superficial and deep; the former are sometimes tributary to the femoral nodes (Bartels, 1909). The deep lymph channels from the clitoris may run close to the superior ramus of the pubic bone, along the pubic ligament, cross under the round ligament, and empty into the femoral ring nodes and the node of Cloquet. These anatomic facts provide the indication for including bilateral femoral lymph node dissections in the operation. The lymphatics of the clitoris traverse vertically upward into the fat of the mons veneris and therefore should be routinely excised during the operative procedure (Fig. 18*B, C, D*). The deep efferent lymph vessels from the clitoris penetrate the urogenital diaphragm in the preurethral ligament and terminate in the pelvic lymph nodes. Because of these facts, it follows that a bilateral retroperitoneal pelvic lymph node dissection should be done for cancers of the clitoris and female prepuce as well as for melanomas.

Conservative Surgical Management. Junctional and compound nevi of the vulva should be excised prophylactically. Small, pigmented lesions which are suspected of being melanomas may be removed by total excisional biopsy under local anesthesia. If the excised lesion is proved to be a melanoma, radical vulvectomy with bilateral groin dissections should be performed.

Radical Vulvectomy. Total vulvectomy, with removal of the vulva inward as far as the hymenal ring and including the skin of the genitocrural folds bilaterally, the mons veneris, together with dissection of both groins en bloc should be per-

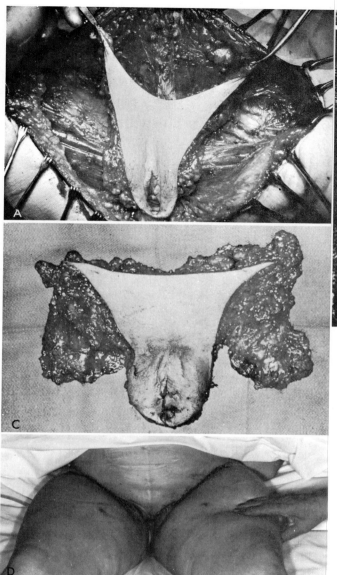

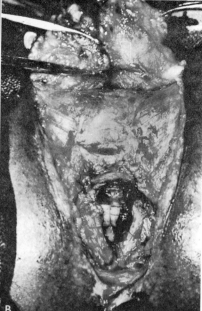

Figure 43–18 Radical vulvectomy for melanoma. *A,* Dissection below fascia; muscles exposed. *B,* Bilateral groin dissections and removal of mons veneris. *C,* Operative specimen. *D,* Wound closure.

formed for all vulvar melanomas (Fig. 43–19). If there is metastatic involvement of the inguinal or femoral nodes or both and the clitoris, then pelvic lymph nodes dissections should be part of the operative procedure. The following structures are exposed prior to skin closure: ischiocavernosus muscles, bulbocavernosus muscle, triangular ligament, superficial transverse perineal muscle, crest of the pubis, ilioinguinal ligament, aponeurosis of the external oblique muscles, sheath of the rectus abdominis muscles, and vessels and structures of the femoral triangles. For lesions located in the labia minora or the lower half of the vagina, panhysterectomy and vaginectomy should be included because of the high incidence of recurrence in these organs.

Synchronous Two-team Operation. As with melanomas of the anal canal, a synchronous two-team operation reduces the operative trauma, blood loss, and operating time.

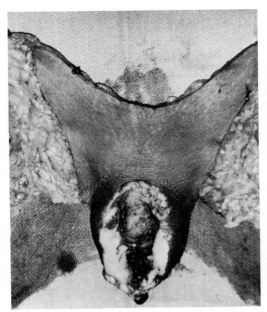

Figure 43–19 Operative specimen of a radical vulvectomy.

Results of Treatment

The lack of uniformity of treatment in this series of patients, because some of the patients were seen as early as 1930 when the management of vulval melanomas differed somewhat from that of today, makes an accurate and meaningful interpretation of the results rather difficult. Table 43–11 shows the five-year end results according to the clinical groupings of the patients on admission; Table 43–12 shows the end results according to the type of treatment.

Patients with disseminated vulval melanoma may also be treated by the systemic administration of cancer chemotherapeutic agents, and vaccines such as BCG may also be tried. Along with the chemotherapy, the immediate administration of autogenous bone marrow infusion probably protects the patient to some degree from severe myeloplasia (Ariel and Pack, 1967).

The overall five-year cure rate for melanoma of the vulva was 29.1 percent.

Prognosis

As with other tumors, a number of variables will influence the prognosis. This includes the tumor-host relationship, the degree of malignancy of the tumor, the stage of the lesion at the initial surgery, and the type of definitive treatment.

It is rather difficult to evaluate the factors influencing the prognosis because of the small number of patients suitable for analysis in this series.

For patients in stage I of the disease with locally recurrent or primary lesions without lymph node metastases, a vulvectomy with an elective bilateral groin dissection is the treatment of choice.

For patients in stage II, their prognosis will be influenced by the type of operation performed. In patients with melanomas of this stage which were treated by modalities other than radical vulvectomy, no cures were obtained. Radiation therapy did not control either the primary lesion or the regional metastases.

Disseminated melanoma (stage III) is invariably fatal, but occasional palliation may be obtained with chemotherapy.

The age of the patient with vulvar melanoma seemed to influence the end results of treatment; no patient between the ages of 15 and 40 years in this series was cured.

Local Recurrence

After the performance of a radical vulvectomy, the incidence of local recurrence is still high, being present in 5 out of 12 patients. This high incidence of recurrence is attributed to the performance of a conservative excision of the vagina; therefore, vaginectomy and hysterectomy should be considered part of the operative procedure, particularly for lesions located around the introitus.

Summary

The effectiveness of radical vulvectomy on the prognosis was particularly evident in those patients who were first seen with lymphatic metastases. The high incidence of local recurrences following radical vulvectomy indicates that a more liberal excision of the vagina, the skin around the primary tumor and its metastases, and the

TABLE 43–11 MELANOMA OF THE VULVA: FIVE-YEAR END RESULTS ACCORDING TO CLINICAL STAGING

Stage	Condition on Admission	Total	Living		Dead			Lost to Follow-up	5 Years Not Elapsed
			NED*	With Melanoma	Of Melanoma	Other Causes	Not Treated		
I.	Primary melanoma not treated or recent biopsy only	15	4	2	2	1	4		2
	Melanoma locally recurrent after improper treatment	2						1	1
II.	Primary melanoma not treated; lymph node metastases	13	3		8		1		1
	Primary melanoma controlled; lymph node metastases	3			1			1	1
	Recurrent primary melanoma; lymph node metastases	5	1		2			2	
III.	Distant metastases with satellitosis	3			3				
	Total:	41	8	2	16	1	5	4	5

*No evidence of disease (melanoma) on first examination.

TABLE 43–12 MELANOMA OF THE VULVA: FIVE-YEAR SURVIVAL ACCORDING TO TYPE OF TREATMENT

Stage	Treatment	Total	Living		Dead		Lost to Follow-up	5 Years Not Elapsed
			NED*	With Melanoma	Of Melanoma	Cause Unknown		
I.	Radical vulvectomy	10	4	1	2	1		2
	Simple vulvectomy	2	1				1	
	Radiation therapy only	1		1				
	No treatment	4					4	
II.	Radical vulvectomy	12	4		6		1	1
	Simple vulvectomy; radiation therapy to nodes	6			4		1	1
	Radiation therapy only	2			2			
	Wide excision and unilateral groin dissection	1					1	
	Total:	38†	9	2	14	1	8	4

*No evidence of disease (melanoma).
†An additional two patients (stage III) received palliative therapy only, and one patient had no evidence of disease when first examined.

underlying subcutaneous tissue, lymph nodes, and fascia should be done. A panhysterectomy and vaginectomy should be done for lesions located around the introitus.

MELANOMAS OF EXTRACUTANEOUS ORIGIN OF THE HEAD AND NECK REGION

Of all anatomic locations, melanomas of the mucous membranes of the head and neck region have the worse prognosis. The most frequent site of origin is either in the nasal cavity or the oral cavity. The tongue is the most unusual location, and the tonsils, lips, larynx, bronchus, conjunctiva, and esophagus are included. About one-half of the lesions are amelanotic, mainly in the white race. The same criteria for histologic diagnosis of primary melanoma of the skin apply to those of the mucous membranes. The presence of a junction nevus is the most important clinical feature (Allen and Spitz, 1953, 1954).

Because these tumors are rare in occurrence, they are often overlooked; therefore, diagnosis and proper treatment may be delayed. Masson (1951) stated that pigmentation in the oral mucosa of the white race was first considered pathologic, but it has been demonstrated so frequently in the mouth and pharynx that it is now considered normal. Laidlaw and Cahn (1932) demonstrated that melanoblasts were a normal and constant constituent of the oral mucosa even in blond, blue-eyed individuals.

Material

Thirty-six patients with melanomas of extracutaneous origin in the head and neck region were available for analysis.

Clinical Features

Age. These melanomas can be present in any age group. The youngest patient reported by Catlin et. al. (1966) was a 4 year old Negro boy with a lesion of the buccal mucosa. The majority of melanomas present during the fifth and sixth decades of life. The majority of patients do not complain of any symptoms other than the eventual appearance of a mass, most probably at the primary site or tributary lymph nodes or both. This one factor accounts for the delay in the proper treatment of this tumor. The majority of patients waited six months or longer before seeking the advice of a physician. A great many of the patients had undergone some previous form of therapy before they were referred for formal treatment.

TABLE 43–13   MELANOMA OF EXTRACUTANEOUS REGIONS OF THE HEAD AND NECK*

Anatomic Location	Number of Patients	Percent	No Evidence of Disease
Palate	10	27.8	1 (with interim recurrence 56 months postoperatively)
Floor of nose and nasal cavity	7	19.4	0
Gingiva	6	16.7	0
Superior alveolus	2	5.5	1 (with interim recurrence)
Tonsil	2	5.5	1
Maxillary antrum	2	5.5	0
Alveolar ridge	1	2.8	0
Mandible	1	2.8	1
Area of epiglottic fold	1	2.8	0
Buccal mucosa	1	2.8	0
Tonsillar fossa	1	2.8	0
Floor of mouth	1	2.8	0
Ethmoid sinus	1	2.8	0
Total:	36	100.0	4

*Unpublished data, reviewed by Ruben Oropeza, M.D., at Pack Medical Group, New York, New York, 1968.

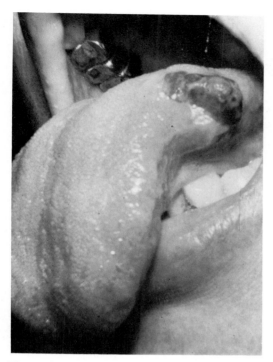

Figure 43-25 Deeply pigmented lesion of tongue. Clinical appearance of melanoma; biopsy proved pyogenic granuloma.

tion of the primary melanoma in-continuity with the lymph nodes of the area, as in the case of melanomas of the gingiva, floor of the mouth, and tonsils, should be carried out. In some of these lesions an exenteration of the orbit, a maxillectomy, and/or excision of the tubinates and discontinuous neck dissection will be required. The importance of treating the lymph nodes electively is stressed by the fact that about 25 percent of the patients admitted for treatment will present metastasis to the lymph nodes, so that it is reasonable to think that a better prognosis might be achieved if the nodes are removed electively before metastases become apparent.

Prognosis

Prognosis for patients with melanomas of the mucous membranes of the head and neck region is very poor, but it is not hopeless, since there are some cases which can be cured. The location of some of these melanomas, such as in the upper turbinates, limits the scope of resectability because of the upward extension of the tumor into the ethmoids and base of the skull. A continuous operation is not possible for lesions of the upper gingiva, sinuses, palate, and nasopharynx. The poor prognosis is due to various other factors, such as the delay in recognition; the ensuing delay in diagnosis; prior improper methods of surgery; the rich network of lymphatics in the region, causing in-transit metastases and satellitosis; and the inherently high degree of malignancy of the melanoma itself.

Summary

Primary melanomas of the mucosa of the head and neck have a predilection for the nasal passages and the palate; primary lesions in the esophagus and the remainder of the gastrointestinal tract are very rare.

Because of the high incidence of local recurrence as well as the high incidence of metastases when a conservative excision has been done, a radical approach should be undertaken, that is, removal of the primary melanoma in a wide en bloc excision with a discontinuous resection of the regional lymph nodes. Unfortunately, control of dissemination is difficult, for hematogenous spread usually takes place.

The radiosensitivity and response to chemotherapy of some of these lesions have been pointed out and should be considered when attempting to obtain palliation.

By the time a melanoma of the mucous membranes is discovered, the disease has usually spread beyond the confines of the head and neck region via the blood stream and the lymphatics. Early diagnosis and proper therapy may improve some of these dismal results.

It is not uncommon for melanomas to metastasize to the gastrointestinal tract with a definite predilection for the mucosa of these organs, presenting the clinical manifestations of intussusception (Fig. 43–26), hemorrhage, anemia, perforation, peritonitis, and bowel obstruction, which may be the initial and only manifestations of the disease.

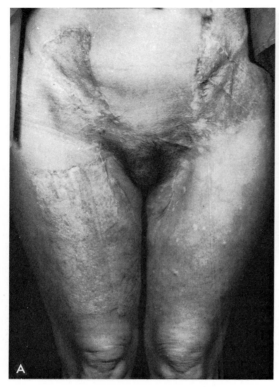

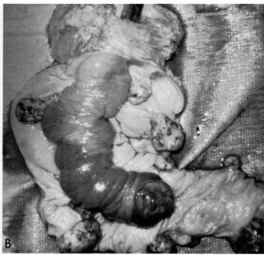

Figure 43–26 *A,* Patient with spontaneous involution of melanoma of the buttocks and thigh, showing leukoderma acquisitum centrifugum in the areas of previous satellitosis. *B,* Same patient presented with metastasis to the ileum and ascending colon two years later, giving the clinical picture of intussusception.

MELANOMA OF THE EXTERNAL EAR

An analysis of melanomas of the external ear was undertaken to determine the best method of management because of its rarity, its unique biologic behavior, and the importance of the ear in the cosmesis of the face. These facts are paramount when considering the type and extent of the surgery to be performed.

Location

In a review by Pack, Conley, and Oropeza (1970), melanoma of the external ear was found to comprise 14.5 percent of all melanomas of the head and neck region, and 6.7 percent of all melanomas. The great majority of melanomas of the external ear were located on the peripheral aspects of the ear. There were 18 (42.8 percent) on the helix, 10 (23.8 percent) on the anthelix, 3 (7.1 percent) on the lobes and the tragus, 2 (4.8 percent) on the posterior aspect of the helix, and 1 (2.3 per-

cent) on the concha (Fig. 43–27). The behavior of these melanomas regarding their lymphatic spread is predetermined by their anatomic location. The type of treatment and the prognosis are also greatly influenced by the location.

Clinical Behavior

Local. The majority of these melanomas begin as superficial lesions in situ and, if left alone, will progress to become invasive. Because of the tightly stretched skin overlying the cartilaginous framework of the ear, the tendency to spread is toward the periphery. The lymphatic drainage is predominantly downward, and this facilitates the permeation of the primary lesion towards the lower part of the ear from a melanoma located in the upper portion (Fig. 43–28).

Regional Dissemination. The invasive melanomas spread early through the lymphatic system to the regional lymph nodes; frequently there is hematogenous spread. The lymphatic system of the

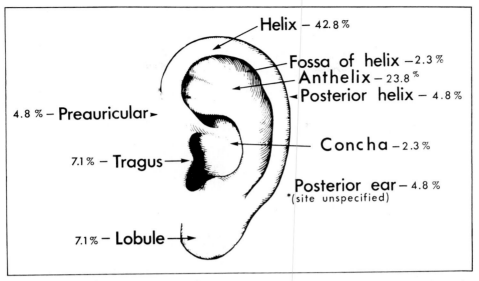

Figure 43–27   Anatomic location on ear of melanomas in 42 patients. (*From* Pack et al.: Arch. Otolaryngol., 92:106, 1970.)

lower portion of the ear drains inferiorly toward the lymph nodes in the upper portion of the neck and parotid gland. Melanomas on the posterior portion of the ear seem to favor drainage to the occipital and mastoid nodes. Lesions which are located on the upper part of the ear may spread to the parotid, mastoid, occipital, spinal accessory, jugular, or submandibular lymph nodes. Lesions which are located on the tragus or the concha may disseminate into the upper portion of the neck as well as into the parotid and lymphatics of the external auditory canal.

Widespread Dissemination.   In the widespread dissemination of a melanoma of the external ear, there is a predilection for certain organs, mainly the liver, brain, peritoneum, and lungs. On postmortem examination, no organ may be found to be immune, including the heart.

Classification

In melanomas of the external ear, several factors must be considered in order to arrive at a meaningful classification.

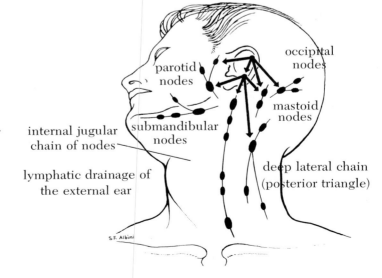

Figure 43–28   Lymphatic drainage of the external ear.

One has to consider the clinical appearance of the primary lesion, the presence or absence of palpable lymph nodes, and the extent of dissemination. In stage I lesions, we refer to melanomas which are localized to the ear only, and for practical purposes they can be classified as (1) primary or non–previously treated superficial melanomas, and (2) infiltrating primary or secondary invasive melanomas. In stage II, we refer to melanomas which have spread to the regional lymph nodes, with or without an active primary melanoma. Stage III refers to melanomas which have disseminated to distant sites.

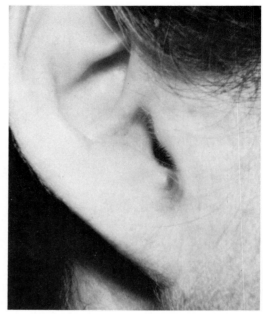

Figure 43–29   Cavernous hemangioma.

Diagnosis

The diagnosis should be established by microscopic examination following either an incisional or excisional biopsy prior to the undertaking of any modality of treatment.

Although pigmented lesions of the ear are rarely seen, differential diagnosis must be made between a melanoma of the external ear and benign lesions, such as a keratosis, cavernous hemangioma (Fig. 43–29), or pigmented basal cell carcinoma. Usually there is no difficulty in arriving at the clinical diagnosis. The amelanotic melanoma of the external ear may be mistaken for a squamous cell carcinoma, a basal cell carcinoma, or a keratoacanthoma.

In the group of 42 patients reported by Pack et al. (1970), 47.5 percent noticed the presence of a melanotic lesion for less than one year (Table 43–14). Eight patients stated that the lesion had been present for from one to five years. Fourteen patients believed that the lesion had been present for more than five years. The majority of patients (33) were in the fourth through the seventh decades of life.

One patient recently seen by the author, a 12 year old male, had a pigmented lesion of the external ear. The pathologist reported it to be a melanoma. On further pathologic consultation, because of the age of the patient, it was believed that this lesion should be considered a "juvenile melanoma" despite its histologic appearance of being a malignant lesion.

The youngest patient in this series of 42 patients was 7 years of age, and the oldest

TABLE 43–14   FIVE-YEAR END RESULTS ACCORDING TO DURATION OF PRIMARY MELANOMA

Duration	Number of Patients	NED°	NED (Interim Local Recurrence)	Died of Melanoma	Lost to Observation	Condition Unknown	5 Years Not Elapsed
<1 mo.	1	1	–	–	–	–	–
1–11 mo.	19	2	1	3	6	1	6
1–2 yr.	5	1	–	2	–	1	1
3–5 yr.	3	–	–	2	1	–	–
<5 yr.	2	–	–	1	–	–	1
Uncertain	12	5	1	3	2	–	1
Total:	42	9	2	11	9	2	9

°No evidence of disease (melanoma).
From Pack et al.: Arch. Otolaryngol., 92:106–113, 1970. Copyright 1970, American Medical Association.

was 81 years; the average age was 49.6 years.

The ratio of males to females was more than 3:1, which is higher than that for melanoma of any other location except the penis and scrotum.

A similar complexion to that observed in patients suffering from melanomas of other anatomic sites was found in these patients. The majority had reddish or blond hair, fair skin, and hazel or blue eyes.

Clinical Features

Six patients had intact melanomas; 17 had excisional biopsies, and one patient had incisional biopsy only. More than one-fourth of the patients had been improperly treated before the definite diagnosis of melanoma was established. Their management consisted of the use of silver nitrate, cauterization, and inadequate excision. This, no doubt, influenced the poor prognosis. The fact that one-third of the patients had metastasis to the regional lymph nodes on admission demonstrates not only the aggressiveness of the melanoma but also the consequence of delay in treatment. This also points out the importance of doing a radical lymph node dissection as an elective or therapeutic operative procedure for those patients who have an infiltrating or recurrent lesion.

Treatment

As in other melanomas, a wide excision of the primary lesion should be performed. In this particular instance, an amputation of the ear with total parotidectomy and radical neck dissection is the most effective plan of management whether or not regional metastases are present. This plan is resisted by many patients because of the aesthetic importance of the external ear and the resultant cosmetic disfigurement in most cases. However, one must balance the latter with the possible eradication of the tumor.

For those patients who have a superficial melanoma of the helix, a wide wedge resection will suffice (Fig. 43–30). These

patients should be followed most carefully to watch for the possibility of local recurrence and regional and distant metastasis. The patient should understand the compromise involved and that there is no assurance that either local recurrence or metastasis will not occur.

For stage I primary or secondary infiltrating melanomas of the helix, the cure rate of approximately 25 percent could be improved by doing a composite resection of the entire ear, that is, an en bloc excision of the primary lesion and tributary nodes. For lesions located on the lower one-half of the ear, the excision of the lower two-thirds of the ear en bloc with a radical neck dissection and parotidectomy should be undertaken (Fig. 43–31). Figure 43–31B demonstrates the presence of a local recurrence on the lower part of the ear after the performance of a simple wedge excision for a recurrent melanoma.

The disease in another patient demonstrated both the capriciousness and lymphatic spread of melanoma. This patient had a pigmented lesion on the ear for 15 years and underwent, unfortunately, cautery excision. Following local recurrence, he was treated by wedge excision. Six years later he developed metastasis to the cervical lymph nodes and underwent radical neck dissection. One year later, a recurrence was noted in the mastoid region, and a mastoid resection was performed. Several months later a total parotidectomy was done for metastasis to the parotid gland. Fifteen years after the initial surgery, the patient was free of melanoma and has remained so to date. This case shows the localization of the melanoma to the lymph nodes of the neck and demonstrates the competency of the regional lymph node depots in the immune mechanism.

In most cases, this type of "piecemeal" surgery will be unsuccessful. The classic initial operation in both cases described above should have encompassed a resection of the lower one-half of the ear en bloc with a superficial parotidectomy and radical neck dissection.

For patients with invasive melanomas located on the upper one-half of the external ear, a complete resection of the ear en bloc with tributary lymph nodes, in-

Text continued on page 1017.

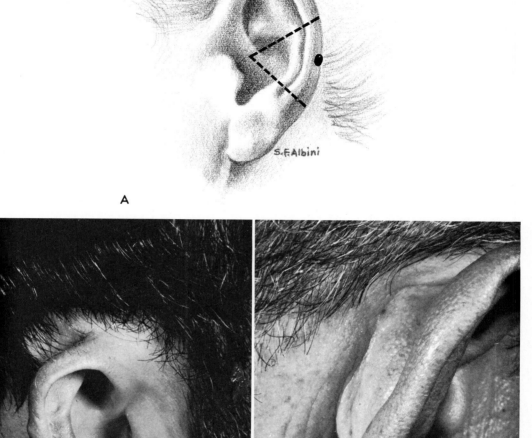

Figure 43–30 *A*, Wedge resection for superficial melanoma of the helix. *B*, Six years following wedge resection for superficial melanoma. *C*, Superficial melanoma of helix.

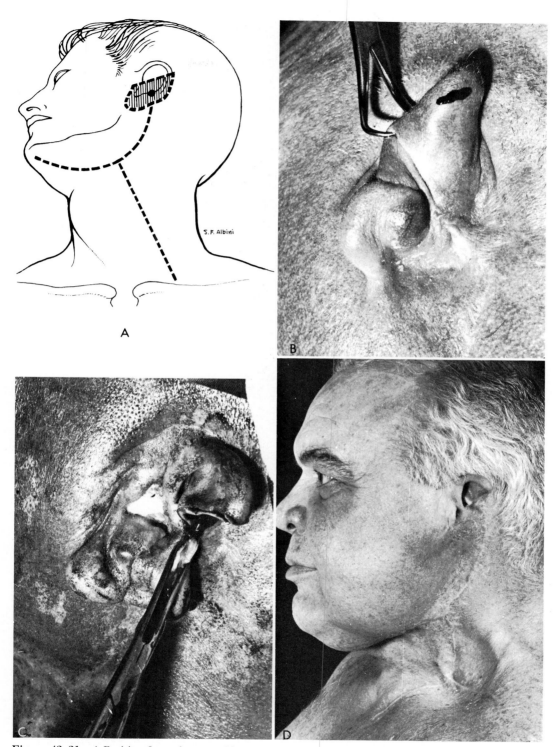

Figure 43–31 *A*, Excision for melanoma of lower one-half of ear. *B*, Recurrent melanoma of lower one-third of ear previously treated by wedge excision. *C*, Operative field. *D*, Postoperative result.

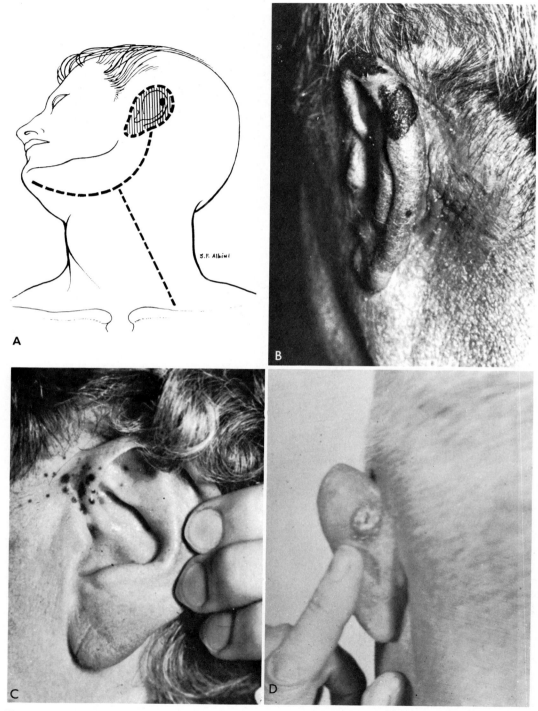

Figure 43–32 *A*, Complete resection for melanoma on upper one-half of ear. *B*, Primary melanoma of upper part of ear with metastasis to mastoid. *C*, Satellitosis in the skin of parotid region. *D*, Melanoma of posterior aspect of concha.

Illustration continued on opposite page.

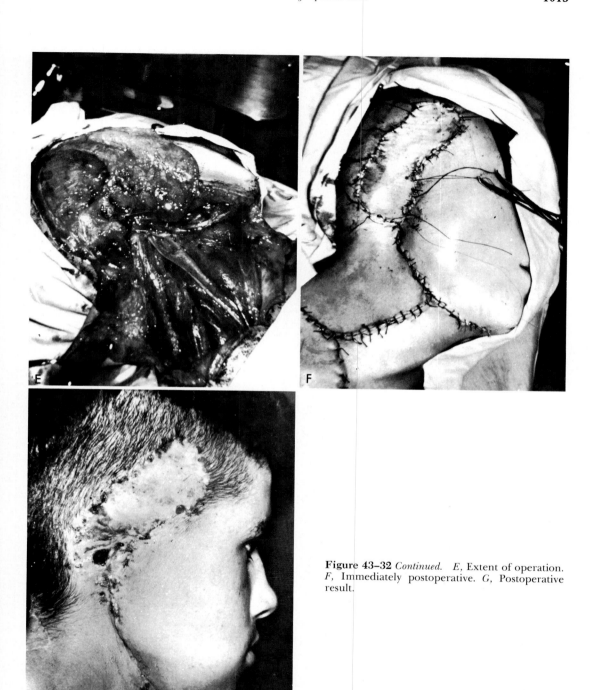

Figure 43–32 *Continued.* *E*, Extent of operation. *F*, Immediately postoperative. *G*, Postoperative result.

TABLE 43-15 FIVE-YEAR END RESULTS ACCORDING TO CLINICAL STATUS

Stage	Condition on Admission	Number of Patients	NED*	NED (Interim Recurrence)	Condition Unknown	Died of Melanoma	Lost to Observation	5 Years Not Elapsed
I	Primary melanoma untreated or recent biopsy only (16)	24	7	–	1	3	2	3
	Melanoma locally recurrent after improper treatment (8)		2	1	–	3	1	1
II	Primary melanoma untreated: lymph node metastases (8)	13	1	–	–	4	1	2†
	Primary melanoma controlled: subsequent lymph node metastases (5)		1	1	1	–	2	–
III	Recurrent melanoma; lymph node metastases (1)	5	–	–	–	–	1	–
	Organic metastases (1)		–	–	–	1	–	–
	Stage indefinite (3)		–	–	–	1	1	1
Total:		42	11	2	2	12	8	7

* No evidence of disease (melanoma).
† Died 4½ years later of heart attack free of evidence of melanoma.

From Pack et al.: Arch. Otolaryngol., 92:106–113, 1970. Copyright 1970, American Medical Association.

TABLE 43-16 FIVE-YEAR END RESULTS ACCORDING TO TREATMENT

Stage	Operative Procedure	Total Number of Patients	NED*	NED (Interim Recurrence)	Condition Unknown	Died of Melanoma	Lost to Observation	5 Years Not Elapsed
I	None	6	1	–	1	1	–	3
	Wide excision; primary closure	9	5	–	–	2	1	1
	Wide excision; graft	5	–	1	–	3	1	–
	Wide excision; nodal dissection in-continuity	3	2	–	–	1	–	–
	Wide excision; subsequent multiple regional node dissection	1	1†	–	–	–	–	–
II	None	4	–	–	1	–	2	1‡
	Wide excision; primary closure	2	–	–	–	–	1	1
	Wide excision; nodal dissection in-continuity	4	–	1	–	2	1	–
	Wide excision; subsequent nodal dissection in-continuity	1	–	–	–	1	–	–
	Wide excision with simultaneous disseparate nodal dissection	1	1	–	–	–	–	–
	Wide excision with disseparate and subsequent nodal dissection	2	1	–	–	1	–	–
III	None	3	–	–	–	1	1	–
	Abdominal surgery for multiple organ metastases	1	–	–	–	1	–	–
Total:		42	11	2	2	13	7	7

* No evidence of disease (melanoma).
† Died 4½ years later of heart attack; NED (melanoma).

cluding the preauricular, parotid, mastoid, and cervical nodes, should be undertaken (Fig. 43–32*A, B*). When the lesion presents satellites close to the skin of the ear, a wide sacrificial excision should be performed (Fig. 43–32*C*). Some of the details of the en bloc excision should be mentioned. The importance of removing the lymph nodes of the mastoid region for lesions of the upper ear or lesions located on the posterior aspect of the ear should be emphasized (Fig. 43–32*D*). The postauricular nodes; the paraparotid, parotid, infralobular, superficial, and deep lymph nodes; the posterior belly of the digastric muscle; and the platysma muscle are all an integral part of the composite resection (Fig. 43–32*E, F, G*). The facial nerve need not be sacrificed; however, resection of the inferior branch of this nerve will facilitate the removal of the infralobular and parotid nodes and the parotid gland, with a minimal amount of weakness of the lower third of the face.

The five-year end results according to clinical stages are shown in Table 43–15; the different modalities of treatment are shown in Table 43–16.

Prognosis

We cannot present a great statistical analysis in this small but significant group of patients; however, we have gleaned many salient and pertinent facts. It is reasonable to state that 70 to 80 percent of the small superficial melanomas have a good prognosis when treated with a conservative excision. Infiltrative and recurrent melanomas have a poor prognosis because of inadequate previous treatment and delay in definitive treatment, plus the not to be forgotten inherent aggressive nature of the lesion. The salvage rate of about 30 percent might be improved by doing a more radical operative procedure at the outset. In melanomas with satellitosis or extensive gross metastases, the cure rate was approximately 14 percent. The prognosis is greatly affected by misdiagnosis and mismanagement, especially with the use of electrodesiccation and caustics.

Summary

As with melanomas located elsewhere in the body, proper diagnosis by means of proper biopsy and adequate treatment in the face of inadequate previous treatment are rules which should be followed for melanoma of the external ear.

REFERENCES

Ahumada, J. C.: El cáncer ginecológico. Vol 2. Buenos Aires, El Atenco, 1953, p. 847.

Allen, A. C., and Spitz, S.: Malignant melanoma: A clinicopathological analysis of the criteria for diagnosis and prognosis. Cancer, 6:1, 1953.

Allen, A. C., and Spitz, S.: Histogenesis and clinicopathologic correlation of nevi and malignant melanomas: Current status. Arch. Dermatol., 69:150, 1954.

Ariel, I. M., and Pack, G. T.: Treatment of disseminated melanoma with phenylalanine mustard (Melphalan) and autogenous bone marrow transplants. Surgery, 51:583, 1962.

Ariel, I. M., and Pack, G. T.: Treatment of disseminated melanoma by systemic melphalan, methotrexate and autogenous bone marrow transplants. Cancer, 20:77, 1967.

Ariel, I. M., and Resnick, M. I.: The intralymphatic administration of radioactive isotopes and cancer chemotherapeutic drugs. Surgery, 55:355, 1964.

Bartels, T.: Das Lymphagesäzsystem. *In* Bardeleben, V.: Handbuch der Anatomie des Menschen. Vol. 3. Jena, 1909, pp. 224, 228, 307.

Bullock, W. K., Thompson, H. L., and Gregory, G.: Primary melanocarcinoma of the esophagus. Cancer, 6:578, 1953.

Catlin, D.: Cutaneous melanoma of head and neck. Am. J. Surg., 112:512, 1966.

Catlin, D., Das Gupta, T., and McNeer, G.: Noncutaneous melanomas. CA, 16:75, 1966.

Curtiss, C., and Kosinski, A. A.: Primary melanoma of the larynx. Cancer, 8:961, 1955.

Grace, C. G.: Malignant melanoma of the nasal mucosa. Arch. Otolaryngol., 46:195, 1947.

Hertzler, A. E.: Melanoblastoma of the nail bed. Arch. Dermatol., 6:701, 1922.

Hutchinson, J.: Melanotic whitlow. Br. Med. J., 1:491, 1886.

Keeley, J. L., Rooney, J. A., Guzauskas, A. C., and Brynjolfsson, G.: Primary malignant melanoma of the esophagus. Surgery, 42:607, 1957.

Laidlaw, G. F., and Cahn, L. R.: Melanoblasts in the gum. J. Dent. Res., 12:534, 1932.

Lewis, M. G., and Martin, J. A. M.: Malignant melanoma of the nasal cavity in Ugandan Africans (relationship of ectopic pigmentation). Cancer, 20:1699, 1967.

McPeak, C. H., McNeer, G. P., Whitley, H. W., and Booher, R. J.: Amputation for melanoma of the extremity. Surgery, 54:426, 1959.

Mason, M., and Friedman, I.: Melanoma of the nose and ear. J. Laryngol., 69:98, 1955.

Masson, P.: Le glomus neuromyoarteriel des regions tactiles et ses tumeurs. Lyon Chir., 21:257, 1934.

Masson, P.: My conception of cellular nevi. Cancer, 4:9, 1951.

Oropeza, R.: Melanomas of extracutaneous origin of the head and neck region. Unpublished data, 1968.

Pack, G. T.: End results in the treatment of malignant melanoma. Surgery, 46:447, 1959.

Pack, G. T., and Adair, F. R.: Subungual melanoma. Surgery, 5:47, 1939.

Pack, G. T., and Martins, F. G.: Treatment of anorectal malignant melanoma. Dis. Colon Rectum, 3:15, 1960.

Pack, G. T., and Miller, T. R.: Extraarticulation of the innominate bone and corresponding lower extremity (hemipelvectomy) for primary and metastatic cancer. J. Bone Joint Surg. (Am.), 46:91, 1964.

Pack, G. T., and Oropeza, R.: Subungual melanoma. Surg. Gynecol. Obstet., 124:571, 1967a.

Pack, G. T., and Oropeza, R.: A comparative study of melanoma and epidermoid carcinoma of the anal canal; a review of 20 melanomas and 29 epidermoid carcinomas (1930–1965). Dis. Colon Rectum, 10:161, 1967b.

Pack, G. T., and Oropeza, R.: A comparative study of melanomas and epidermoid carcinomas of the vulva: A review of 44 melanomas and 58 epidermoid carcinomas (1930–1965). Rev. Surg., 24:305, 1967c.

Pack, G. T., Lenson, N., and Gerber, D. M.: Regional distribution of moles and melanomas. Arch. Surg., 65:862, 1952.

Pack, G. T., Conley, J., and Oropeza, R.: Melanomas of the external ear. Arch. Otolaryngol., 92:106, 1970.

Pomeranz, A. A., and Garlock, J. H.: Primary melanocarcinoma of the esophagus. Ann. Surg., 142:296, 1955.

Rubenfeld, S.: Melanoma of the nasal air passages. Jew. Mem. Hosp. Bull. (N.Y.), 6–7:119, 1962.

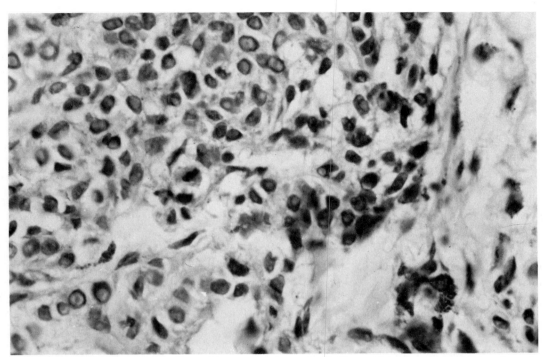

Figure 44–5 Melanoma cells, small nevoid type. This is another field, at a higher power, of the case shown in Figure 44–4. Again from this field alone, a distinction from a benign nevus cannot be made. There is a mitotic figure approximately in the center of the field. Many nuclei are vacuolated, a feature that occasionally can be found in both nevus cells and melanoma cells. *About ×250.*

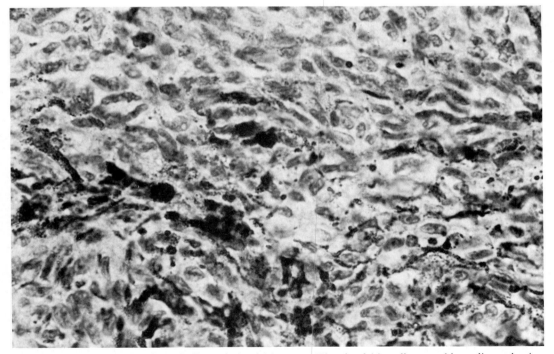

Figure 44–6 Melanoma cells, spindle and dendritic types. The dendritic cells resemble ordinary benign dendritic melanocytes, except that they are larger and have coarser cytoplasmic processes. This is a metastasis of the tumor shown in Figure 44–19, which had a resemblance to a cellular blue nevus. *About ×250.*

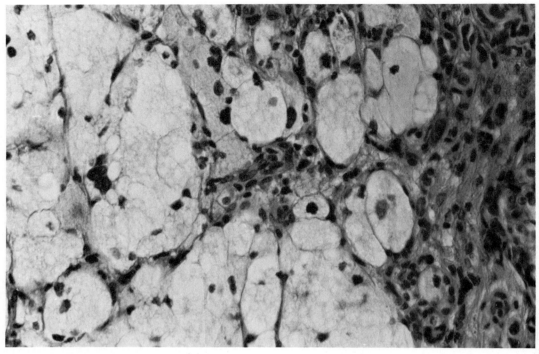

Figure 44–7   Melanoma cells, balloon type. Note the large, pale cells that have a resemblance to xanthoma cells. Special stains showed no lipid, however. The diagnosis of melanoma depends on the characteristics of the remaining predominant cells. Balloon cells were present in both the primary and metastatic tumors in this case. *About ×250.*

nucleus and the amount of intranuclear basophilic material. It does not apply to simple density of stain; a small pyknotic nucleus is not hyperchromatic in this sense. A practical comparative reference in judging the presence of hyperchromatism is the appearance of the normal nuclei of adjacent epidermal cells.

Intranuclear vacuoles are occasionally noted. They are single and often occupy the greater part of a nucleus. They also can be found in benign nevus cells. Their presence suggests a melanocytic tumor, whether benign or malignant, but this is not pathognomonic.

Mitotic figures are usually present in melanomas, but on occasion they may not be demonstrable. They are usually most numerous in the large epithelioid cells and uncommon in the small nevoid cells. Mitotic figures are most abundant in cells in the junctional and intraepidermal part of a primary tumor. It must be stressed that they can also be found in the junctional foci of benign nevi, especially in the nevi of patients in the first and second decade (Lund and Stobbe, 1949). Rarely,

they can be found in deeper cells of such nevi. Mitotic figures have the most significance in the differential diagnosis of malignant melanoma if they are found in all levels of the tumor. Abnormal mitotic figures are occasionally seen. In general, the presence of mitotic figures has little significance in the differentiation of benign juvenile melanomas and malignant melanomas. We believe, however, that abnormal mitotic figures are more commonly noted in the latter.

RELATIONSHIP OF MELANOMA CELLS TO THE EPIDERMIS

Melanomas arise principally in the distribution of epidermal melanocytes, i.e., along the dermoepidermal junction (Figs. 44–8 and 44–9), but origin at the dermo-follicular junction is often seen. Sometimes this feature is quite conspicuous in lentigo maligna. The epidermal involvement is in an extended stratum resembling lentigo, or in theques. The origin is

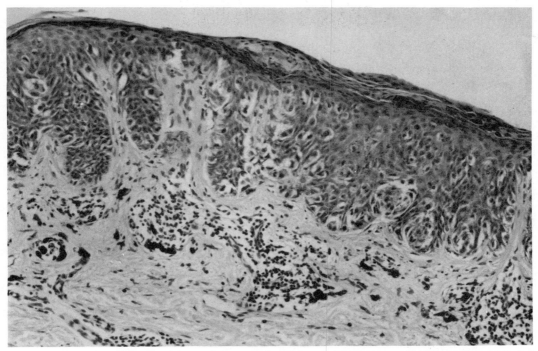

Figure 44–8. Relationship of evolving melanoma to the epidermis. This is a case of lentigo maligna of the face in a 53 year old white woman. Note the proliferation of pigmented and nonpigmented cells singly and in ill-defined groups. Moderate melanocytic atypia is manifested by hyperchromatism of nuclei. There is an infiltration of lymphocytes in the upper cutis. ×*100.*

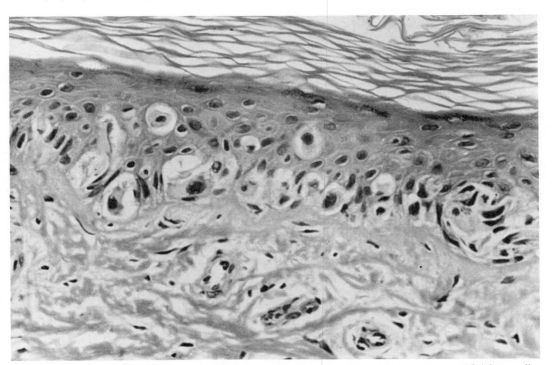

Figure 44–9 Relationship of evolving melanoma to the epidermis. This is a biopsy of a superficial spreading melanoma of the leg in a 39 year old white woman. Note the pigmented and nonpigmented cells at the dermal-epidermal junction and scattered into the upper levels of the epidermis. Nuclei of these cells are distinctly hyperchromatic. The cellular changes here are those of a malignant melanoma, but the lesion is not tumorlike, and there is no invasion demonstrated. This could be designated as superficial spreading melanoma, noninvasive, but this is only a small biopsy of a larger lesion and may not represent the full degree of development of the melanoma. ×*250.*

similar to that of a benign nevus, but in addition to the intrinsic cytologic differences, melanoma cells tend to be less cohesive, theques are more irregular in size and shape, and there is a greater tendency for the melanoma cells to scatter into the upper layers of the epidermis in a pagetoid manner than is seen in benign nevi (Fig. 44–9).

RELATIONSHIP OF MELANOMA CELLS TO THE CONNECTIVE TISSUE

The relationship of melanoma cells to the surrounding connective tissue stroma has diagnostic significance and is to be compared with and contrasted with that of benign nevi. Usually in benign nevi the dermal cells are within a fibrillar syncytium and tend to be grouped or alveolated by the fibrils. Furthermore, the fibrillar stroma of benign nevi often forms neuroid structures which have a resemblance to large tactile corpuscles. Occasionally it is difficult to distinguish neurofibromas from pigmented nevi.

In contrast, the cells of malignant melanomas tend to have a random distribution with a lesser tendency to be grouped by connective tissue or to form neuroid structures. A bulky, expansile growth of cells with comparatively little fibrillar

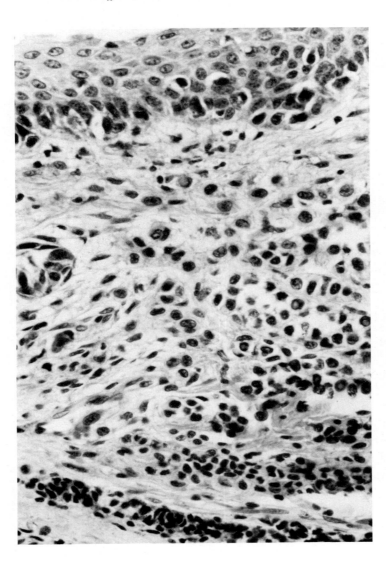

Figure 44–10 Malignant melanoma associated with fibrils. Most malignant melanomas have a random and haphazard hyperplasia of cells without a fibrillar syncytium. This one, however, shows a proliferation of fine fibrils, giving a deceptive resemblance to a benign nevus. Mitoses could be found in this tumor, and there were atypical junctional clumps. Although the malignant nature of this primary tumor was difficult to recognize, it metastasized and caused death of the patient. *About ×250.*

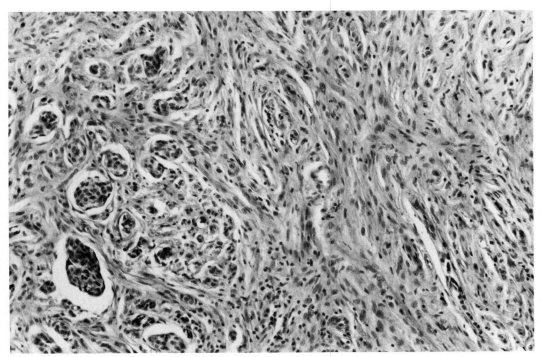

Figure 44–11 Malignant melanoma with a "sclerotic" appearance. This is an unusual variant. Note the close resemblance of the spindle cells to fibrous tissue. This appearance blends with the more obviously nevoid and epithelioid type of tumor in the left half of the picture. *About ×100.*

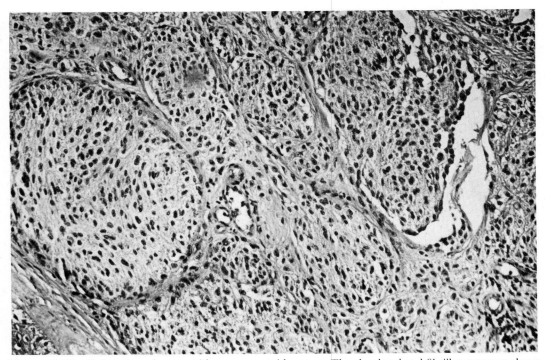

Figure 44–12 Malignant melanoma with a neuromatoid pattern. The alveolated and fibrillar structure shown here has a resemblance to a neural tumor. Elsewhere in the biopsy specimen the cells were more clearly of an epithelioid type. *About ×100.*

stroma may be seen. The presence or absence of reticulin fibers has been stressed by McGovern (1970) as a criterion in differentiating melanomas from pigmented nevi. However, the distinction of benign and malignant on the basis of fibrillar and stromal relationship can be overemphasized. There are occasional malignant melanomas in which the cells are enclosed by fine fibrils, and the pattern resembles that of benign dermal nevi (Fig. 44–10). The resemblance is especially close if the melanoma cells are of the small nevoid type. The presence of nuclear atypia and mitotic figures is helpful in identifying the malignant nature of such tumors.

Again there are occasional spindle cell melanomas that may be associated with abundant connective tissue. Conley et al. (1971) designate these as desmoplastic malignant melanomas. Figure 44–11 shows such a tumor. Sometimes spindle cell melanomas may imitate neural tumors (Fig. 44–12). Melanomas with a neuromatoid appearance have been described by Petersen, Bodenham, and Lloyd (1962). We have encountered at least ten primary and recurrent melanomas in which the cellular proliferation so closely resembled the appearance of neural tissue that the true diagnosis was obscured. Adding to the deceptive appearance was actual involvement of nerves and little epidermal involvement in the skin.

The ultrastructure of melanomas has been described by Clark and Bretton (1971) and by Clark, Ten Heggeler, and Bretton (1972).

HISTOPATHOLOGY OF EVOLVING AND EARLY MALIGNANT MELANOMAS

A frequently recurring problem in diagnostic dermatopathology is the "borderline melanoma." Indeed, there may be more "melanomas in the making" than fully developed, truly aggressive melanomas. These early or evolving lesions have different degrees of cellular atypia and proliferation, which vary not only from lesion to lesion but also from one part to another of the same lesion. Frequently a lesion may exhibit the changes of a fully developed invasive melanoma but away from the obvious tumor may show only minor degrees of melanocytic atypia and proliferation. Early changes are not always distinguishable from certain examples of benign lentigo or benign junctional nevi, but usually there are features that do indicate that these early changes are "melanoma-directed," and recognition of them has obvious prognostic implications.

Evolution of a melanoma is not uniformly progressive and not necessarily inexorable. The slowest and least aggressive type of melanoma, lentigo maligna melanoma, may not evolve to a truly invasive and aggressive tumor for decades or even the lifetime of the patient. Superficial spreading melanomas on the average evolve more rapidly, but this is highly variable. On the other hand, the more aggressive nodular melanomas may evolve rapidly from normal skin to invasive tumor, and evolutionary stages are rarely evident in biopsies.

Terms used to designate early or evolving stages of melanoma vary widely, partly because there are different patterns of evolution and partly because of the ambiguous use of the term "junction nevus." In the recommended terminology presented by McGovern et al. (1973), "Hutchinson's melanotic freckle" (or lentigo maligna) designates one category of evolving melanoma, and "superficial spreading melanoma, noninvasive, "designates another. The terms "Hutchin's freckle" and "lentigo maligna" are adequate for that special type of evolving melanoma, allowing for a wide spectrum of changes from minimal to pronounced. However, the term "superficial spreading melanoma, noninvasive," is not as broad. It points to the far end of the spectrum of evolution and conjures up a picture of advanced cellular changes equivalent to a melanoma except for failure to demonstrate invasion. (Incidentally, many pathologists will not use the term "melanoma" unless at least microinvasion is demonstrated.) Thus, there remains a hiatus for a broad term, not restricted to the lentigo maligna or Hutchinson's freckle category, that designates all pigmented lesions that deviate from the appearance of benign nevi and are likely melanoma-directed. In practice, the earliest changes are frequently referred to as "atypical junction nevus," and in using the term "nevus" for a malignant evolutionary process, we have acceded to custom. We do not imply a benign junction nevus changing over to an evolving melanoma. "Activated junction nevus" is a still less desirable term. More adequate designations of the evolving melanoma are atypical melanocytic hyperplasia, precancerous melanocytic hyperplasia, melanocytic dysplasia, or premalignant melanosis. The term "precancerous melanosis" would be satisfactory if it could be broadened to include more than Hutchinson's melanotic freckle. This appears to be the usage advised by the World Health Organization (Ten Seldam et al., 1974). The term "borderline melanoma" is not elegant, but it is readily understood.

The evolving melanoma, unless it is related to a nevus, appears as a macule without tumorlike growth. It often exhibits irregularity in color and consistency. The histologic findings often give a clue to the type of melanoma that is evolving, whether lentigo maligna melanoma or superficial spreading melanoma.

In the lentigo maligna type of lesion (Hutchinson's melanotic freckle), the appearance is usually widely variable in different parts of the lesion. In places, the appearance is closely similar to that of benign lentigo and may be indistinguishable from it. Elsewhere, definite atypia may be noted in the clear cells along the basal layer of the epidermis, as evidenced by enlarged hyperchromatic nuclei, and cells are occasionally multinucleated (Fig. 44–13). Other cells may be of a small spindle type or a small epithelioid type. Junctional clumps, if present, tend to be small and poorly defined (see Fig. 44–8). There is comparatively little intraepidermal scattering (Fig. 44–13). Occasional small aggregates of spindle cells may be found.

Lesions evolving in the direction of superficial spreading melanoma are more apt to show junctional aggregates (Figs. 44–14 and 44–15) and intraepidermal scattering in a pagetoid manner (Figs. 44–9 and 44–15). Usually the aggregates are more irregular in shape and size and more loosely constructed than in benign

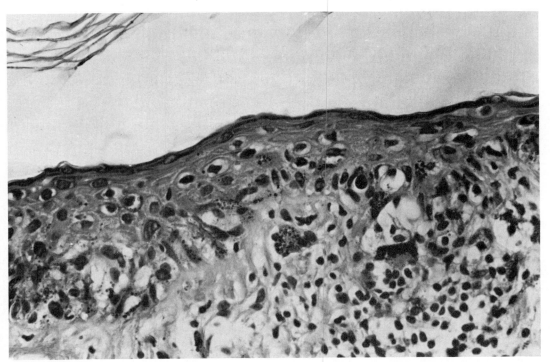

Figure 44–13 Lentigo maligna (Hutchinson's melanotic freckle). Note the irregular proliferation and the pleomorphism of melanocytes. Nuclei are hyperchromatic. There are occasional multinucleated giant cells. Tumorlike growth and invasion are not seen. ×250.

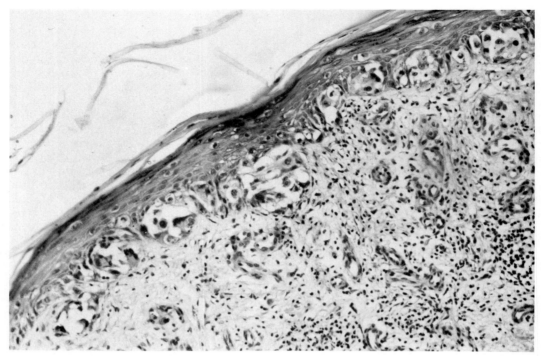

Figure 44–14 Malignant melanoma, noninvasive. Note the clearly atypical cells at the dermal-epidermal junction. They are mostly a small epithelioid type. There are several multinucleated cells. There are junctional clumps which are well delineated by connective tissue. Freely scattered tumor cells are not seen in the papillary dermis. This tumor was not definitely classified as either lentigo maligna or superficial spreading type of melanoma. ×250.

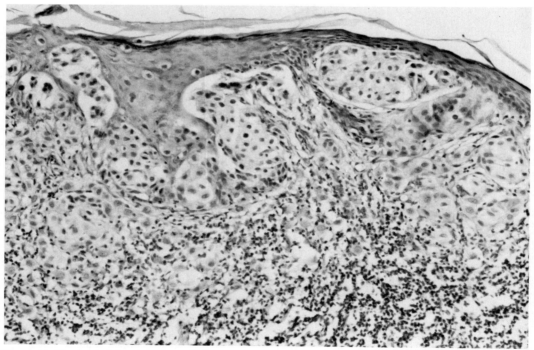

Figure 44–15 Superficial spreading melanoma, invasive. Note the penetration of melanoma cells into the connective tissue. The penetration is characterized by haphazard scattering of melanoma cells not enclosed and alveolated by connective tissue. The penetration was confined to the papillary dermis and designated as level II. The cells are predominantly of an epithelioid type. ×100.

junction nevi. The cells tend to be epithelioid (Figs. 44–9 and 44–15).

Often an evolving or "borderline" melanoma may not be clearly designated as either a lentigo maligna type of melanoma or a superficial spreading melanoma (Fig. 44–14).

In all forms of the evolving melanoma, there are usually a superficial infiltration of lymphocytes and a variable number of melanophages.

As proliferation and atypia become more advanced, the tumor is virtually a melanoma in situ, or noninvasive melanoma (Figs. 44–9 and 44–14). Neither of these terms is popular, however, perhaps because they overemphasize the potential hazards of such lesions.

The appearance of invasion and tumor-like growth completes the evolution to a truly aggressive melanoma.

Early invasion can be difficult to demonstrate, and the lesion may, in comparison with early carcinomas of the cervix, be labeled "microinvasive." Invasion is recognized by the scattering of cells either singly or in irregular small groups (Helwig, 1963b). Their identification as invading cells is most reliable if they are not grouped or alveolated by connective tissue (Fig. 44–15). Cells in the papillary or subpapillary dermis which are alveolated by connective tissue may be junctional aggregates cut in a plane which does not happen to show their association with the epidermis. Alveolation is not, however, a constant indicator of a benign type of proliferation. Occasionally, melanoma cells invading the papillary and even the reticular dermis can be grouped by connective tissue and have a deceptive resemblance to ordinary pigmented nevi. The diagnosis in such cases rests largely on the atypical nature of the cells and the presence of mitotic figures. Expansile growth can cause a pseudoalveolation by compression of the surrounding tissue.

GROWTH PATTERNS OF MALIGNANT MELANOMA

In recent years, melanomas have been divided into three neoplastic systems (Clark et al., 1969; McGovern, 1970). Terminology varies but can be summarized as follows (adapted from McGovern et al., 1973): melanoma, invasive, without adjacent intraepidermal component (nodular melanoma); melanoma, invasive, with adjacent intraepidermal component of superficial type (superficial spreading melanoma); melanoma, invasive, with adjacent component of Hutchinson's melanotic freckle (lentigo maligna melanoma). We will use the parenthetic terms above, those originally proposed by Clark et al. (1969). Each of these tumor systems in its typical form represents a fairly distinctive *gross and histologic appearance*. The classification needs clinical and microscopic correlation. We have found that the system is clearly applicable in most but not all cases. Difficulties are most frequently encountered in the separation of lentigo maligna melanomas and superficial spreading melanomas. Furthermore, there are bizarre melanomas that do not fit neatly into this scheme, e.g., the sclerotic and neurotized types. Melanomas arising in congenital nevi or malignant blue nevi are obviously not part of this classification.

Nodular Malignant Melanoma (see Color Plate VII-B)

This type of tumor is expansile and invasive; occasionally it is pedunculated. It protrudes abruptly from the surface of the skin and is not associated with peripheral macular hyperpigmentation. Often the tumor is ulcerated. Histologically, it appears as an expansile growth of melanoma cells. Any or all types may be present. Invasion into the papillary dermis is constant, and deeper invasion is frequently seen. The lateral margins of the tumor usually shown an abrupt transition to uninvolved epidermis, in contrast to superficial spreading or lentigo maligna melanoma, in which atypical melanocytic proliferation in the junctional zone extends away from the principal tumor.

Superficial Spreading Melanoma (see Color Plate VII-C and Figs. 44–9 and 44–15)

Tumors in this category tend to enlarge and spread in a centrifugal manner, especially in their early stages. The spread is usually intraepidermal or into the adjacent papillary layer. Clinically a raised, irregularly outlined, mottled plaque is formed. The colors include black and brown, but some areas may be depigmented. Parts of the tumor may be macular; others are plaques, and tumorlike nodules may appear. The histologic findings will correspond to the gross appearances. Macular areas may exhibit different degrees of evolution toward a fully developed melanoma. Often there is an in situ pattern, with a diffuse pagetoid distribution of relatively monomorphous atypical cells, predominantly epithelioid. Pigmentation varies in degree and may be absent in places. In plaquelike or nodular areas, there is expansile growth and usually clear-cut invasion. A superficial infiltrate of lymphocytes is present. Necrosis and ulceration, if present, are accompanied by an exudate of serum, fibrin, and neutrophils.

Lentigo Maligna Melanoma (see Color Plate VII-D and Fig. 44–16)

Although the term lentigo maligna has been used occasionally for any precancerous melanocytic proliferation, its usage has come to imply a distinct clinicopathologic entity, often called melanotic freckle of Hutchinson or melanosis circumscripta preblastomatosa of Dubreuilh. Clark and Mihm (1969) refer to the precancerous phase as lentigo maligna and the fully developed tumor as lentigo maligna melanoma. Lentigo maligna melanoma is the most indolent of the three types of melanoma. Clinically the lesion is a slowly evolving, centrifugally spreading, pigmented macule seen most commonly on the sun-damaged skin of elderly individuals. The lesions are mottled brown, black, and bluish black, and there may be depigmented foci. The histologic appearance will depend upon the evolutionary phase

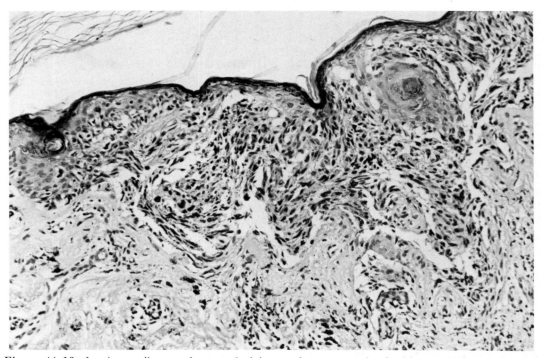

Figure 44–16 Lentigo maligna melanoma (incipient melanoma associated with Hutchinson's melanotic freckle). Note the small tumorlike proliferation of atypical spindle cells. A few foci such as this were found in a large pigmented macule of the face in a 70 year old white man. Almost all parts of the lesion showed only atypical melanocytic proliferation similar to that shown in Figure 44–13. The age, the presence in sun-damaged skin, the predominantly macular nature of the lesion, the small foci of tumorlike growth, and the spindle type of cell indicate the diagnosis of lentigo maligna melanoma. Contrast the appearance of this lesion with that of the lesion in Figure 44–15, in which an epithelioid type of cell predominates and there are distinct intraepidermal nests, features more in keeping with nodular or superficial spreading melanomas. *Approximately ×100.*

of the proliferation, and this varies from place to place in the same lesion. There may be only hyperpigmentation resembling a benign lentigo. In other places, more cellular atypia and proliferative changes are seen. The proliferation of atypical melanocytes is usually in an extended stratum with only a limited tendency to form junctional theques or to manifest pagetoid scattering into the upper epidermis. The atypical cells are of variable types: small nevoid cells, spindle cells, and multinucleated cells. A monomorphous proliferation of epithelioid cells is unusual and is more likely to indicate a melanoma of the superficial spreading type. A superficial infiltrate of lymphocytes and melanophages is invariably present. When truly neoplastic foci arise (lentigo maligna melanoma), they tend to be small. The cells in these are usually of the spindle type. Usually there is only a limited degree of invasion, but there are exceptions.

HISTOPATHOLOGIC EVALUATION OF PROGNOSIS

The diagnosis of a premalignant melanocytic proliferation offers a good prognosis, *granting that the lesion has been adequately sampled.* A biopsy should be sectioned extensively in a "borderline" case in the search for evidence of invasion and tumorlike growth. Furthermore, random biopsy on a large macular tumor may not give a full appreciation of the degree of change. We have had the experience of receiving an initial small biopsy specimen, showing only premalignant melanocytic proliferation, followed by an excision of the entire lesion in which clearly invasive malignant melanoma was found.

In general, lesions showing only premalignant melanocytic proliferation are cured by local excision. Sometimes, however, it is difficult both grossly and microscopically to delineate the exact limits of epidermal involvement, and a narrow excisional clearance may be followed by recurrence.

We believe the odds are good for cure if only a limited focus of microinvasion can be found in the biopsy specimen.

However, we have encountered four or five cases in which metastases occurred from primary lesions with very limited superficial invasion.

Prognosis is closely correlated with depth of invasion (Mehnert and Heard, 1965; Clark et al., 1969; McGovern, 1970). Clark et al. (1969) subdivided melanomas according to five levels of penetration: I, in situ; II, into the papillary layer; III, to the upper margin of the reticular layer; IV, into the reticular layer; V, into the subcutaneous fat. They show a progressively greater incidence of fatalities and a progressively lower incidence of survival with increased depth of invasion. No cases of level I melanomas are listed in the comparative figures. Histologically it is difficult to ascertain depth of invasion if the biopsy specimen is small. Furthermore, atypical melanocytic proliferation may occur at the margins of hair follicles within the stratum reticularis. This is not true invasion but can simulate invasion.

It is important to recognize and separate lentigo maligna melanoma, since in most series the course is slow and death due to metastasis is less common than in other forms of melanoma (Davis et al., 1967; Clark and Mihm, 1969). Our experience coincides with this conclusion, although Jackson et al. (1966) disagreed. It is of interest that cutaneous melanomas of the head and neck have in the past been reported to have a more favorable prognosis (Catlin, 1966); this may well be related to the high percentage of lentigo maligna melanomas in this region.

The complete histologic diagnosis of malignant melanoma takes into account three considerations: (1) the stage of evolution (whether an in situ dysplasia or a truly invasive tumor); (2) the growth pattern (whether nodular, superficial-spreading, or the lentigo maligna type); and (3) the depth of invasion.

Melanomas have many other gross and histologic features, and some of these may have prognostic significance. The subject is discussed by McGovern et al. (1973). The volume of the tumor probably is significant (Breslow, 1970). According to Little [1972 (cited by McGovern et al., 1973)], melanomas composed of small nevoid cells have a more favorable outlook than others.

SPECIAL VARIANTS OF MALIGNANT MELANOMA

Prepubertal Malignant Melanoma

This is rare and is to be distinguished from benign juvenile melanoma, which is discussed elsewhere. Also excluded from this discussion are benign neurocutaneous melanomatoses (Slaughter et al., 1969) and cellular blue nevi with regional lymph node metastasis or local deep invasion.

Cases of prepubertal melanoma with proven metastasis may be placed in three general categories: (1) those secondary to placental metastasis (Dargeon et al., 1950; Brodsky et al., 1965); (2) those arising in giant congenital nevi; and (3) those not related to either of the above. A few cases in this last category are congenital. Melanomas in the last group have the same histologic appearance as melanomas of adults (Skov-Jensen et al., 1966; Lerman et al., 1970), and the prognosis is similar.

The pathology of the tumors arising in giant congenital nevi requires special comment. Estimates of their occurrence range from 2 to 13 percent, but this figure may be high, since many benign lesions are not reported. Occasionally, malignant melanoma arising in giant congenital lesions may not be clinically detected until adult life, and this would technically not be considered prepubertal melanoma.

The benign giant nevi have a mixed pattern of nevocytic nevus and neuroid nevus (Reed et al., 1965). Certain foci may in part resemble blue nevi. Rarely, cartilage is noted. It is to be stressed that giant congenital nevi arise when the skin and subcutaneous tissues are in an undeveloped state, and therefore the tumor is found more deeply than postnatal pigmented nevi. The mere presence of nevus cells in the subcutaneous tissue is not necessarily evidence of invasion. The associated malignant tumors have different appearances. Some are similar to adult melanomas except that occasionally the origin of the tumor appears to be intradermal rather than at the dermoepidermal junction. Other tumors are much more anaplastic (Figs. 44–17 and 44–18) and may have no discernible melanin. They can be confused with neuroblas-tomas or malignant lymphomas. Twelve of 17 tumors histologically reviewed by Reed et al. (1965) were of this anaplastic type.

Malignant Blue Nevus

As used in the literature, the term malignant blue nevus has two meanings. The first is an otherwise characteristic cellular blue nevus attended by foci of similar tissue in the regional lymph nodes. These metastases follow an indolent course. Rodriguez and Ackerman (1968) noted 14 cases, constituting 5.2 percent of the total number of cellular blue nevi reported at that time. This figure must be too high, since cellular blue nevi are well recognized and seldom reported.

The second meaning is a malignant melanoma, usually of a spindle cell type, which resembles a cellular blue nevus. The resemblance is enhanced if junctional proliferation is limited or absent. This group is poorly defined and not clearly separated from the general group of melanomas. Failure to note significant involvement at the dermoepidermal junction is not sufficient reason in itself to relate the melanomas to blue nevi. Usually these tumors have a mixed spindle and epithelial like cell population, with varying degrees of cellular atypia, mitotic activity, and necrosis (Allen and Spitz, 1953; Lund and Kraus, 1962). The case originally illustrated by Lund and Kraus is shown in Figures 44–6 and 44–19. The only cutaneous lesion, taken to be the primary lesion, did have a close resemblance to a blue nevus. Metastases occurred but were indolent over a long period of years. Although metastatic melanoma was found at autopsy, death did not result from melanoma but rather from carcinoma of the pancreas. Certain melanomas metastatic to the skin can be confused with "malignant blue nevi."

Regression of Malignant Melanoma

Focal regression of primary lesions of melanoma is occasionally observed (Clark et al., 1969). However, complete and total

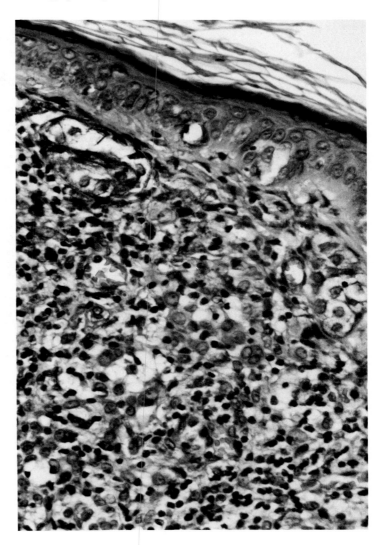

Figure 44–20 Halo nevus. Note the proliferation of nevus cells extending from the dermoepidermal junction into an underlying infiltrate of lymphocytes. This has a superficial resemblance to an early stage of malignant melanoma. *About ×200.*

dominate in a malignant melanoma; however, they can also occur in otherwise characteristic benign juvenile lesions.

As a rule there is less intraepidermal involvement in juvenile melanomas, and there is little or no laterally extending lentiginous or atypical melanocytic proliferation. The cells of juvenile melanomas often tend to show an intimate mixture with the connective tissue of the deep dermis, often making it difficult to decide which cell is a fibrocyte and which is a tumor cell. Fibrous and vascular proliferation and telangiectasis are often seen in juvenile melanomas but can also be found in nodular melanomas.

Clinically, most juvenile melanomas differ from melanomas tending to resemble granulomas or hemangiomas. We have been impressed by their comparatively short history, and usually there is a definite statement of time of onset.

Atypical Fibroxanthoma
(Helwig, 1963a; Fretzin and Helwig, 1973)

Comparable lesions have been designated pseudosarcomatous dermatofibroma (Lever, 1967) and paradoxical fibrosarcoma (Bourne, 1963). This tumor can afford some of the most difficult problems in differential diagnoses (Fig. 44–21). However, it is usually distinguished from melanomas by the lack of junctional pro-

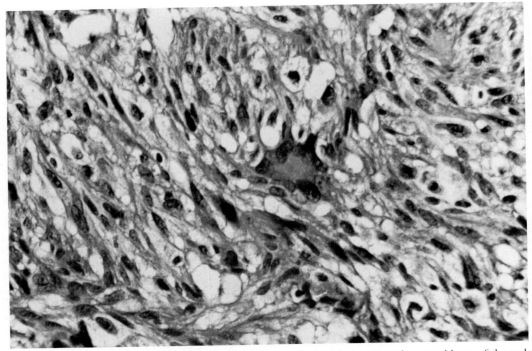

Figure 44–21   Malignant melanoma resembling an atypical fibroxanthoma. Note the resemblance of the melanoma cells to fibrous and histiocytic tissue. The large cell resembles a reactive giant cell. Elsewhere in this biopsy the features of a melanoma were more clear cut. *About ×250.*

liferation; the wide variety of cells, including large bizarre cells and lipid-containing cells; often the presence of hemosiderin; and in most instances the clearly mesenchymal nature of the tissue. These tumors are sharply defined and lack laterally extending lentiginous or junctional changes. Clinically, these tumors are usually nodular and ulcerated, and located in sundamaged or roentgen-damaged skin (Hudson and Winkelmann, 1972).

Squamous Cell Carcinoma

Spindle cell squamous cell carcinomas are often difficult to distinguish from melanomas. Lack of pigment (with exceptions), definite atypia of squamous cells in the overlying epidermis or adjacent epidermis, and focal keratinization help in recognizing this tumor. Pseudoepitheliomatous hyperplasia in melanomas (Fig. 44–22) can lead to a false diagnosis of squamous cell carcinoma. Usually the melanoma cells contrast sharply with the "islands" or pegs of squamous cells. The melanoma cells are anaplastic and lack any evidence of keratinization or intercellular bridges.

Bowen's Disease

This can have a superficial resemblance to an in situ melanoma, especially when the involvement of the epidermis is spotty. Such involvement can resemble junctional theques. However, the cells tend to merge insensibly with the surrounding squamous cells. Usually intercellular bridges and keratinization can be found. Extensive sampling usually shows complete transepidermal cellular atypia somewhere in the lesion.

Paget's Disease

The relative lack of pigmentation, the more extensive suprabasal involvement of the epidermis, focal suggestion of acinus formation, and the demonstration of mucin specifically by mucicarmine or al-

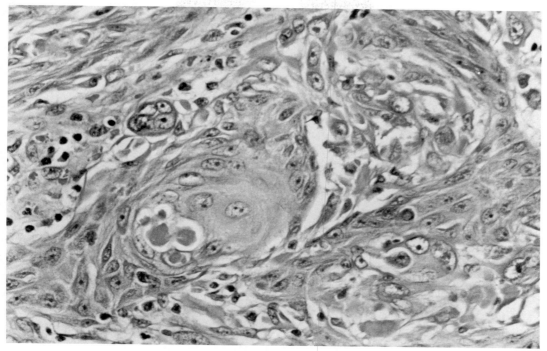

Figure 44-22 Malignant melanoma resembling squamous cell carcinoma. It is very difficult to distinguish melanoma cells from squamous cells in this illustration, and much of the biopsy had this confusing appearance. The two types of cells are of similar size, and they mingle intimately. The largest field of melanoma cells is in the lower right corner. The squamous cells represent pseudoepitheliomatous hyperplasia. *About ×250.*

dehyde fuchsin stains (Helwig and Graham, 1963) help to distinguish this tumor. The distinction, however, can be very difficult in some instances, and it should be kept in mind that Paget's cells can contain pigment.

Primary vs. Metastatic Melanoma

The distinction is not always evident from a histologic standpoint (Olsen, 1966). Contrary to the usual belief, epidermal involvement is not an exclusive feature of primary melanomas. Metastases can involve the epidermis (Fig. 44-23). However, the involvement by metastatic tumor is usually focal and closely associated with an underlying dermal mass of tumor cells. Involvement of the epidermis extending away from the principal neoplastic nodule, especially if it includes incompletely evolved stages of melanoma, is indicative of a primary tumor.

Conversely, occasional primary tumors, especially the nodular type, can have meager epidermal involvement in a given

section, or indeed in step sections, and distinction from a metastatic tumor can be uncertain. The reason for the limited junctional component is not clear. We can speculate that ulceration occurred, and in healing, the epidermis alone regenerated. Alternately, one can speculate that there are trophic disturbances in the stretched-out epidermis overlying an expansile tumor, and epidermal cells survive while melanoma cells undergo atrophy. Finally, melanomas need not arise from the epidermal junction alone. They can arise from dermofollicular junctions or the margins of deeply extending pegs of epidermal cells.

Recurrent Benign Nevi

Occasionally, varying degrees of nodularity and pigmentation may occur at the site of a previously treated benign nevus.

In our preliminary and unpublished review of 100 such lesions, this phenomenon characteristically occurred within one year after the initial surgical procedure, which

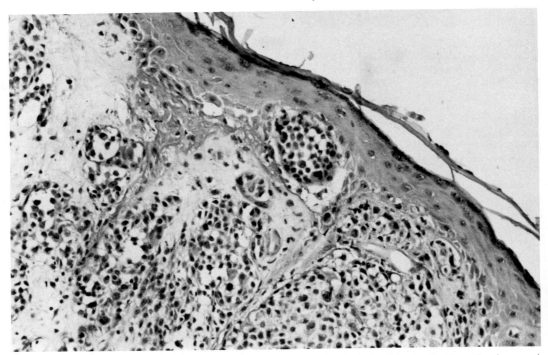

Figure 44–23 Metastatic melanoma with epidermal involvement. Note the cluster of cells at the dermoepidermal junction and the mixture of melanoma cells and cells of the basal layer of the epidermis. This was one of a "shower" of cutaneous metastases at a distance from the primary tumor. *About ×100.*

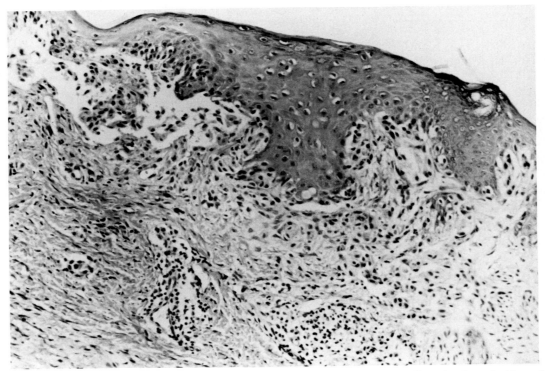

Figure 44–24 Recurrent nevus. Note the irregular proliferation of melanocytic cells at the dermalepidermal junction. There is a loss of cellular cohesion with slight intraepidermal scattering but no significant cellular atypia, and mitoses are not present. In the cutis there is a lymphocytic infiltrate.

The specimen is from a young female who developed pigmentation in a scar following shave biopsy of a typical benign intradermal nevus.

was invariably a shave biopsy. The patients are usually between 10 and 40 years of age. As previously described by Cox and Walton (1965), the recurrent lesions often show an exaggerated junctional component in comparison to the original biopsy.

In addition, a few such lesions demonstrate an irregular junctional growth pattern (Fig. 44–24) with some variation in the size and staining of nuclei of melanocytes. These features in association with fibrosis, a variable inflammatory infiltrate, and history of recurrence have led to an erroneous diagnosis of malignant melanoma.

Awareness of this general problem is important, and it is essential that the pathologist review the original biopsy in all of these cases.

Nevi of Pregnancy

Pigmented nevi of pregnancy may undergo increased pigmentation but nevertheless usually do not offer difficulty in histologic diagnosis should they be biopsied. However, we have repeatedly encountered examples of nevi, usually of the perineal region, removed incidentally during delivery that do offer difficulty in histologic interpretation. They are papillary "compound nevi" with a very active junctional component. However, cellular atypia is not clearly shown, and there is a regular and progressive differentiation of the cells to small typical nevus cells in the depth of the lesion. Rarely, the diagnosis remains in doubt.

REFERENCES

Allen, A. C., and Spitz, S.: Malignant melanoma. A clinicopathological analysis of the criteria for diagnosis and prognosis. Cancer, 6:1, 1953.

Bourne, R. G.: Paradoxical fibrosarcoma of skin (pseudosarcoma); review of 13 cases. Med. J. Aust., 1:504, 1963.

Breslow, A.: Thickness, cross-sectional areas and depth of invasion in the prognosis of cutaneous melanoma. Ann. Surg., 172:902, 1970.

Brodsky, I., Baren, M., Kahn, S. B., Lewis, G., Jr., and Lellem, M.: Metastatic malignant melanoma from mother to fetus. Cancer, 18:1048, 1965.

Catlin, D.: Cutaneous melanoma of the head and neck. Am. J. Surg., 112:512, 1966.

Clark, W. H., Jr., and Bretton, R.: A comparative fine structural study of melanogenesis in normal human epidermal melanocytes and in certain human malignant melanoma cells. *In* Helwig, E. B., and Mostofi, F. K. (Eds.): The Skin. Baltimore, The Williams & Wilkins Company, 1971.

Clark, W. H., Jr., and Mihm, M. C., Jr.: Lentigo maligna and lentigo maligna melanoma. Am. J. Pathol., 55:39, 1969.

Clark, W. H., Jr., From, L., Bernardino, E., and Mihm, M. C., Jr.: The histogenesis and biologic behavior of primary human malignant melanomas of the skin. Cancer Res., 29:705, 1969.

Clark, W. H., Jr., Ten Heggeler, B., and Bretton, R.: Electron microscope observations of human cutaneous melanomas correlated with their biologic behavior. *In* McCarthy, W. H. (Ed.): Melanoma and Skin Cancer. Sydney, N. S. W., Australia, V. C. N. Blight, Government Printer, 1972.

Conley, J., Lattes, R., and Orr, W.: Desmoplastic malignant melanoma (a rare variant of spindle cell melanoma). Cancer, 28:914, 1971.

Cox, A. J., and Walton, R. G. The induction of junctional changes in pigmented nevi. Arch. Pathol., 79:428, 1965.

Dargeon, H. W., Eversole, J. W., and Del Duca, V.: Malignant melanoma in an infant. Cancer, 3:299, 1950.

Davis, J., Pack, G. T., and Higgins, G. K.: Melanotic freckle of Hutchinson. Am. J. Surg., 113:457, 1967.

Echevarria, R., and Ackerman, L. V.: Spindle and epithelioid cell nevi in the adult: Clinicopathologic report of 26 cases. Cancer, 20:175, 1967.

Fretzin, D. F., and Helwig, E. B.: Atypical fibroxanthoma of the skin, a clinicopathologic study of 140 cases. Cancer, 31:1541, 1973.

Helwig, E. B.: Tumor seminar. Case 6. Atypical fibroxanthoma. Texas State J. Med., 59:652, 1963a.

Helwig, E. B.: Malignant melanoma of the skin in man. Natl. Cancer Inst. Monogr., 10:287, 1963b.

Helwig, E. B., and Graham, J. H.: Anogenital (extramammary) Paget's disease. A clinicopathologic study. Cancer, 16:387, 1963.

Hudson, A. W., and Winkelmann, R. K.: Atypical fibroxanthoma of the skin: A reappraisal of 19 cases in which the original diagnosis was spindle-cell squamous carcinoma. Cancer, 29:413, 1972.

Jackson, R., Williamson, G. S., and Beattie, W. C.: Lentigo maligna and malignant melanoma. Can. Med. Assoc. J., 95:846, 1966.

Kopf, A. W., and Andrade, R.: Benign juvenile melanoma. *In* Year Book of Dermatology, 1965-1966. Chicago, Year Book Medical Publishers, 1966.

Lerman, R. I., Murray, D., O'Hara, J. M., Booher, R. J., and Foote, F. W., Jr.: Malignant melanoma of childhood. A clinicopathologic study and a report of 12 cases. Cancer, 25:436, 1970.

Lever, W. F.: Histopathology of the Skin. Ed. 4. Philadelphia, J. B. Lippincott Company, 1967.

Lund, H. Z.: Pigment cell neoplasms. Problems in the diagnosis of early lesions. *In* Proceedings of the Fourth National Cancer Conference. Philadelphia, J. B. Lippincott Company, 1961.

Lund, H. Z., and Kraus, J. M.: Melanotic tumors of the skin. Atlas of Tumor Pathology, Section 1, Fascicle 3. Washington, D.C., Armed Forces Institute of Pathology, 1962.

Lund, H. Z., and Stobbe, G. D.: The natural history of the pigmented nevus; factors of age and anatomic location. Am. J. Pathol., 25:1117, 1949.

McGovern, V. J.: The classification of melanoma and its relationship with prognosis. Pathology, 2:85, 1970.

McGovern, V. J., Mihm, M. C., Jr., Bailly, C., Booth, J. C., Clark, W. H., Jr., Cochran, A. J., Hardy, E. G., Hicks, J. D., Levene, A., Lewis, M. G., Little, J. H., and Milton, G. W.: The classification of malignant melanoma and its histologic reporting. Cancer, 32:1446, 1973.

Mehnert, J. H., and Heard, J. L.: Staging of malignant melanoma by depth of invasion. Am. J. Surg., 110:168, 1965.

Olsen, G.: The malignant melanoma of the skin. Acta Chir. Scand. (Suppl.), 365:1, 1966.

Peterson, N. C., Bodenham, D. C., and Lloyd, O. C.: Malignant melanomas of the skin. Br. J. Plast. Surg., 15:49, 1962.

Reed, W. B., Becker, S. W., Sr., Becker, S. W., Jr., and Nickel, W. R.: Giant pigmented nevi, melanoma and leptomeningeal melanocytosis. Arch. Dermatol., 91:100, 1965.

Rodriguez, H. A., and Ackerman, L. V.: Cellular blue nevus. Cancer, 21:393, 1968.

Schrader, W. A., and Helwig, E. B.: Balloon cell nevi. Cancer, 20:1502, 1967.

Shapiro, L., and Kopf, A. W.: Leukoderma acquisitum centrifugum. Arch. Dermatol., 92:64, 1965.

Skov-Jensen, T., Hastrup, J., and Lambrethsen, E.: Malignant melanoma in children. Cancer, 19:620, 1966.

Slaughter, J. C., Hardman, J. M., Kempe, L. G., and Earle, K. M.: Neurocutaneous melanosis and liptomeningeal melanomatosis in children. Arch. Pathol., 88:298, 1969.

Smith, J. L., Jr., and Stehlin, J. S., Jr.: Spontaneous regression of primary malignant melanoma with regional metastases. Cancer, 18:1399, 1965.

Strum, S. B., Park, J. K., and Rappaport, H.: Observation of cells resembling Sternberg-Reed cells in conditions other than Hodgkins disease. Cancer, 26:176, 1970.

Ten Seldam, R. E. J., and Helwig, E. B., with Sobin, L. H., Torloni, H., et al.: Histologic Typing of Skin Tumours. Geneva, World Health Organization, 1974.

Wayte, D. M.: Pathology of nevi and melanomas. *In* Helwig, E. B., and Mostofi, F. K. (Eds.): The Skin. Baltimore, The Williams & Wilkins Company, 1971.

45

Adnexal Skin Carcinomas

Jean Civatte, M.D., and
Georges Tsoïtis, M.D.

Adnexal carcinomas of the skin represent a special group of very rare skin cancers. This chapter deals only with skin tumors which have the structures resembling that of the skin appendages and which are really malignant, leading to metastases.

The leading characteristic of these tumors is their adnexal differentiation. The word "adnexal" may have two different meanings: it may refer either to the origin or to the differentiation. Lack of absolute proof of the origin of a tumor and the concept of pluripotentiality and equipotentiality of adult cells of both epidermis and appendages (Pinkus, 1953) are responsible for the difficulty of giving a precise definition of an adnexal tumor. As a matter of fact, there are tumors originating from the appendages but losing their adnexal differentiation, whereas others, originating from the epidermis, evidence an adnexal differentiation. Obviously, adnexal origin does not necessarily imply an adnexal differentiation and vice versa. However, the only criterion that is to be kept in mind while defining an adnexal tumor is differentiation, whereas the adnexal origin of these

tumors is very likely but cannot be demonstrated.

The second point that should be emphasized is the malignancy of these adnexal carcinomas, as proved by occurrence of metastases. It is now generally accepted that the criterion of malignancy is the presence of metastases, and the word "carcinoma" should apply exclusively to really malignant epithelial tumors. Formerly, the group of malignant adnexal tumors of the skin was very general: it comprised not only the real malignant carcinomas, as previously defined, but also many other tumors, such as basal cell epithelioma* and squamous cell carcinoma with adnexal differentiation and also adnexal origin; adenoacanthoma of sweat glands (Lever, 1947); and tumors of low grade malignancy presently considered as being benign, such as sweat gland adenoma or nodular hidradenoma and its variants, eccrine spiradenoma, sudoriferous adenoepithelioma of Grynfeltt and

---

*In this chapter this tumor is referred to as basal cell epithelioma. It should be mentioned that it is also referred to in the literature as basal cell carcinoma.

Aimes (1922), trichoepithelioma, calcifying epithelioma of Malherbe, and cylindroma.

Disagreement on the term "epithelioma" may also lead to some misunderstanding. Presently, the word "epithelioma" applies only to the tumors which exhibit the lowest degree of differentiation amongst the benign adnexal tumors (Lever, 1948; Mehregan and Pinkus, 1963; McMullan, 1963). According to this, the basal cell epithelioma is not really malignant, because it leads only exceptionally to metastases; it has a strictly local malignancy, as already noticed by Dubreuilh in 1893. It should also be mentioned that Foot (1947) first suggested that the word "adnexal carcinoma" be applied to the basal cell epithelioma. General agreement on the notion of adnexal carcinoma has not yet been obtained. Abulafia (1963) included in this group the basal cell epitheliomas (fetal adnexal epitheliomas), the true metastasizing adnexal carcinomas (adult adnexal epitheliomas), and intermediate epitheliomas. Panja (1969) included in the group of adnexal carcinomas not only the real adnexal carcinomas but also basal cell and squamous cell epitheliomas with adnexal differentiation, as French authors do. Others used the term "adnexal carcinoma" as synonymous to metatypical carcinoma. The biologic malignancy of the adnexal carcinomas does not always correspond to a precise histologic malignancy, and histologic differentiation is sometimes very difficult to establish between a real adnexal carcinoma and a benign adnexal tumor.

According to the type of differentiation, the adnexal carcinomas may be classified under three different headings: pilar, sebaceous, and sweat gland carcinomas.

PILAR CARCINOMAS

Publications on the pilar carcinomas are very rare. Loos, in 1936, published a case and, reviewing the literature, considered as true pilar carcinomas only two other cases (Hedinger, 1925; Picard and Liégeois, 1931). Our personal feeling is that these two cases and the one of Loos may be of pilar origin but do not represent true pilar carcinomas. In 1949, Liu reported four cases of a tumor which he called clear cell papillary carcinoma and which he considered to have originated in the hair follicle; however, it is now widely accepted that this tumor is a clear cell hidradenoma. Several cases have been reported of a benign tumor of the hair follicle called tricholemmoma by Headington and French in 1962. These authors believed that a tricholemmoma could become malignant, and they considered the three cases of clear cell hidradenomas with metastases published by Keasbey and Hadley in 1954 as malignant tricholemmomas. The first case of malignant tricholemmoma was reported by Mehregan in 1967. Holmes, in 1968, proposed the term trichochlamydocarcinoma for solid, noncystic tumors of the scalp, which are mostly seen in old women and are usually nonaggressive, but which may produce metastases. Holmes identified these tumors with the proliferating epidermoid cysts of Wilson-Jones (1966) and, on the basis of histologic and histochemical criteria, suggested that they derive from the lower outer root sheath of the hair follicle, which normally contains glycogen and lipids. In trichochlamydocarcinoma, Sudan and PAS stains are both positive, and in some instances one may find large areas of clear cells similar to those of the anagen phase of the hair follicle, as well as vitreous membranes surrounding the primary and metastatic tumor masses. We believe that the last three cases of trichochlamydocarcinoma of Holmes may represent malignant tricholemmomas. In consequence, from the recent publications, one may not exclude the existence of pilar carcinomas of the malignant tricholemmoma type which, however, are exceptional.

The clinical data of these cases are not always available. In the last three cases of Holmes, the tumors were solid, ulcerated or nonulcerated, 3 to 12 cm. in diameter, and located on the scalp, and they occurred in old women. They were only slowly growing; recurrences occurred as well as lymph node metastases (one case).

(Masson and Géry, 1922; Gay and Ortiz Picón, 1927; Lund, 1957; Castelain and Spitalier, 1962; Cabanne et al., 1965).

Diagnosis

Diagnosis of sebaceous carcinoma is impossible on a clinical basis only and has to be established histologically. Several other tumors are to be considered in the differential diagnosis: basal cell epithelioma with sebaceous differentiation, squamous cell carcinoma with sebaceous differentiation, cutaneous metastases of a carcinoma of the kidney, malignant clear cell hidradenoma or clear cell hidradenocarcinoma, malignant tricholemmoma and some cases of trichochlamydocarcinoma, and malignant melanoma.

Almost all the published cases of sebaceous epitheliomas are in fact basal cell epitheliomas with sebaceous differentiation, or basosebaceous epitheliomas (Fig. 45–3). The differential criteria established by Beach and Severance (1942) and later by Lever (1948) are as follows: in the sebaceous carcinoma, there are no cells of the basal type; the sebaceous cells, whether well-differentiated or undifferentiated, exhibit a considerable amount of atypicality. The cytoplasm of the undifferentiated cells is more eosinophilic than the cytoplasm of the cells of the basal type. Absence of connection with the epidermis in the sebaceous carcinoma is of less value. According to Pinkus (1953), the stroma-dissociated invasiveness in sebaceous carcinoma contrasts to the stroma-associated proliferation in sebaceous epithelioma. Also noteworthy is the fact that the malignancy of the basosebaceous epithelioma is only a local one without any metastases.

The group consisting of squamous cell carcinoma with sebaceous differentiation is not clear-cut. The published cases are exceptional (Leroux and Cornil, 1923; Dupont, 1938; Degos et al., 1960; Urban and Winkelmann, 1961; Cabanne et al., 1965). Some authors deny its existence (Laffargue et al., 1962); others do not mention it (Lever, 1948; Pinkus, 1953). Still others accept it as an existing tumor (Urban and Winkelmann, 1961; Zackheim, 1964; Cabanne et al., 1965; Miller

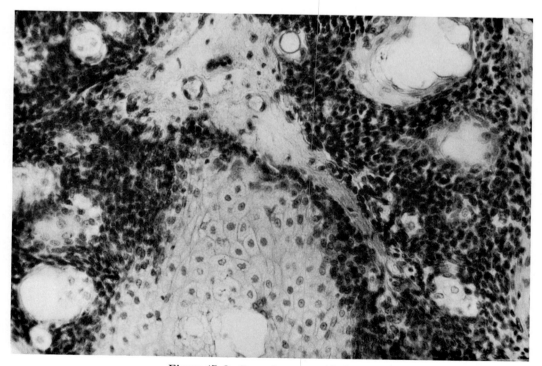

Figure 45–3 Basosebaceous epithelioma.

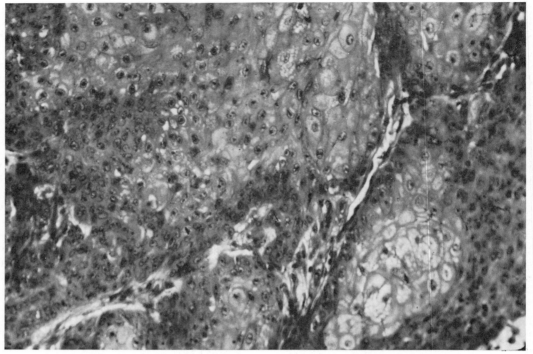

Figure 45–4   Squamous cell carcinoma with sebaceous differentiation.

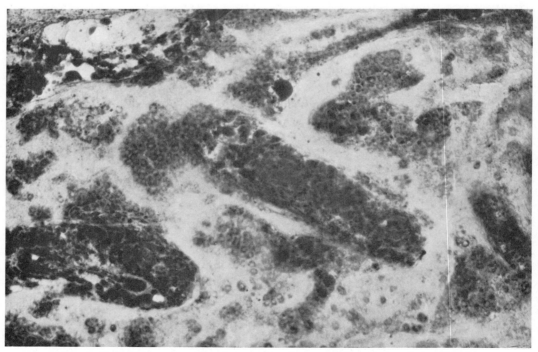

Figure 45–5   Squamous cell carcinoma with sebaceous differentiation. *Sudan IV stain.*

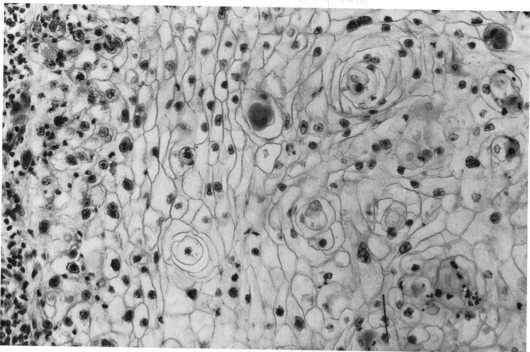

Figure 45–6 Pseudosebaceous squamous cell carcinoma.

and White, 1967; Constant and Leahy, 1968). Our personal feeling is that squamous cell carcinomas with sebaceous differentiation do exist but are extremely rare. The general structure is that of a squamous cell carcinoma with groups of sebaceous cells (Figs. 45–4 and 45–5). These tumors are to be differentiated from squamous cell carcinomas with unusual keratinized lesions, leading to pseudosebaceous pictures with particularly clear keratinized cells (Fig. 45–6). There may be a lipid deposit in these cells, as could be evidenced on frozen sections, but because of the lack of foam cells, this is not a real sebaceous differentiation. However, in some instances, differential diagnosis may be very difficult. The other diagnoses to be considered include cutaneous metastases of carcinoma of the kidney, clear cell hidradenocarcinoma, malignant tricholemmoma, trichochlamydocarcinoma, and malignant melanoma.

SWEAT GLAND CARCINOMAS

Sweat gland carcinomas represent the best known group of carcinomas of the skin appendages. They have been known for a long time, but they were misdiagnosed with various benign sweat gland tumors, or with adenoid basal cell epithelioma and adenoid squamous cell carcinoma. In the bibliographic studies of Loos (1936), Gates et al. (1943), and Puente Duany (1950), the collected cases have been considered carcinomas because of their histologic structures; however, only a small number of these cases evidenced metastases. The sweat gland origin and the real malignancy of most of these cases are doubtful. Lever (1948) and especially Puente Duany (1950) clearly distinguish a group of rare sweat gland carcinomas leading to metastases in the regional lymph nodes and in the internal organs. The structure of these carcinomas is generally glandular and anaplastic and resembles that of carcinomas of the breast, stomach, bowel, and so forth. Stout and Cooley (1951), reporting 11 personal cases, six of which metastasized, stressed the difficulty of establishing reliable histologic criteria on which diagnosis of true sweat gland carcinoma can be based. In their cases, either metastasizing or not, there was a similar histologic picture, characterized by an infiltrative growth with varying degrees of cellular anaplasia, these features sometimes being found at a less advanced stage in some benign sweat gland tumors. The authors wanted to keep the term sweat gland carcinoma only for the rare cutaneous, glandular, infiltrating, and metastasizing tumors. This problem, later studied by many others (Keasbey and Hadley, 1954; Teloh, 1955; Moran and Horn, 1958; Miller, 1967), remains unsolved, and the absence of reliable histologic criteria makes the differentiation of true sweat gland carcinomas and benign sweat gland tumors difficult. For this reason, in the recent literature, most of the bibliographic reviews (Smith, 1955; Teloh et al., 1957; Jacobson et al., 1959; Wilde and Bader, 1963) and publications are dealing with metastatic sweat gland carcinomas, whereas reports on nonmetastasizing sweat gland carcinomas are rare.

According to Miller (1967), the total number of confirmed cases of sweat gland carcinomas is only 39, 28 of which metastasized. On the other hand, Damsgaard-Sørensen and Søeborg Ohlsen (1969) felt that the number of cases of metastatic sweat gland carcinomas was 39. In reviewing the literature, we found 48 cases of metastatic sweat gland carcinoma, apart from the cases of extramammary Paget's disease and of carcinomas of ceruminous glands and Moll's glands which are not included in this study. As far as cases of nonmetastatic sweat gland carcinomas are concerned, it is very difficult to know their exact number and whether they are malignant or not, because of the lack of clear histologic criteria in this group of tumors.

Some of the true sweat gland carcinomas have a peculiar histologic picture. On the basis of this particularity and the fact that these variants of sweat gland carcinomas are not very well known, they will be studied separately: these variants are the *clear cell malignant hidradenoma or hidradenocarcinoma,* the *malignant mixed tumor,* and the *eccrine porocarcinoma.*

Some authors divide the sweat gland carcinomas into eccrine and apocrine varieties and describe them separately. Moreover, Morioka and Mishima (1968) subdivide the eccrine sweat gland carcinomas into three groups: porocarcinomas, ductocarcinomas, and spirocarcinomas. We feel that the division of sweat gland carcinomas into eccrine and apocrine groups is suitable, but it is impossible to classify the published cases in these two subvarieties and to study them separately, because this distinction is not made in most of the publications.

Clinical Study

Sweat gland carcinomas are to be seen in both males and females with about the same frequency. They are predominantly seen in elderly people, especially in those around the age of 55, but they may occur in those between 23 and 84 years of age. However, as far as age of onset is concerned, younger people, around 40, may be affected. The tumor has no particular clinical features. The appearance is generally that of a firm, nodular mass, hard, ulcerated or nonulcerated, often red or purple in color; usually, it is unique and exceptionally multiple (Darier, 1889; Damsgaard-Sørensen and Søeborg Ohlsen, 1969). The size varies from 0.5 to 10 cm. in diameter, with an average size of 2 to 3 cm. The most common location is the head, particularly the scalp, but it also occurs on the upper limbs, axilla, lower limbs, and trunk. Exceptional sites may be the groin (Calissano, 1926), the vulva (Eichenberg, 1934), and the perianal area (Shenoy, 1961). The duration varies from 2 months to 25 years. The course may be rapid, leading to death within a period of a few months (Crosti, 1931) to two years after onset (Teloh, 1955; Damsgaard-Sørensen and Søeborg Ohlsen, 1969; Wilde and Bader, 1963; Morini and Montagnani, 1921; Stout and Cooley, 1951). However, in most cases the course is progressive: the tumor grows slowly or may not increase in size for a rather long period of time, then suddenly increases in volume and invades the underlying tissues; subsequently metastases occur, mostly to the regional lymph nodes, skin, bones (vertebrae, ribs), lungs, and rarely to the brain (Mincy and Lee, 1966; Damsgaard-Sørensen and Søeborg Ohlsen, 1969), pelvis (Shenoy, 1961), and kidneys (Mincy and Lee, 1966). Of the 48

1963; Matz et al., 1969); one was histologically malignant (Desorgher and Saout, 1968); and the last two were more doubtful as far as malignancy is concerned (Hirsch and Helwig, 1961; Sharvill, 1962). As a matter of fact, these last two cases had been considered malignant because of the presence of islands of tumor cells far away from the main tumor and possibly within lymphatic vessels; however, there was neither pleomorphism, atypical cells, nor mitoses. Moreover, the case of Sharvill (1962) recurred once. The case published by Desorgher and Saout (1968) showed histologic invasion with many mitoses and atypical cells. Postoperative follow-up in these cases is too short to give a real idea about their future behavior.

In the three confirmed cases, the tumor appeared in women aged 25, 80, and 83, and exhibited no clinical features of particular interest. The tumor was located on the sole, arm, or scalp, was 3 to 5 cm. in diameter, was not ulcerated but was painful in two cases, and lasted for 5 to 10 years. After having been slowly growing, there was a rapid evolution, characterized by recurrences and metastases to the skin (Gubareva, 1963; Matz et al., 1969), the lymph nodes (Rosborough, 1963; Matz et al., 1969), and the lungs (Matz et al., 1969). One of these patients died seven years after onset (Matz et al., 1964); the postoperative survey of the second patient lasted only six months (Rosborough, 1963); there was no follow-up of the other patient.

The histologic structure is that of a mixed tumor of the skin, well-circumscribed and lobulated, composed of epithelial cells, which form tubuloalveolar or ductal structures, and of chondroid, myxoid, or even osteoid matrix (Rosborough, 1963). However, in some areas there is an intense proliferation of epithelial cells with a considerable amount of mitoses and a tendency to deep invasion (Rosborough, 1963). In the case of Matz et al. (1969), there were cellular pleomorphism and bizarre multinucleated and vacuolized cells with occasional mitoses. Gubareva's (1963) case showed a structure similar to that of a benign mixed tumor, but the tumor cells were arranged along the large blood vessels. The recurring and metastasizing lesions may be histologically similar to the primary tumor. However, tendency toward tubuloalveolar and sweat duct differentiation is less evident, whereas cellular pleomorphism is prominent (Matz et al., 1969). In the case of Rosborough (1963), the structure of the metastases was polymorphic and quite different from that of the primary tumor: in the same tumor, one may see a well-differentiated squamous cell carcinoma close to areas of clear or undifferentiated cells.

ECCRINE POROCARCINOMA

Mishima and Morioka (1968 and 1969) have described epitheliomatous and carcinomatous tumors derived from the intraepidermal part of the eccrine sweat ducts (acrosyringium) and proposed the names eccrine poroepithelioma and porocarcinoma, respectively. In 1963, Pinkus and Mehregan had already reported a case under the name of epidermotropic eccrine carcinoma which probably represented a malignant eccrine poroma. In 1968, Miura et al., at the same time as Mishima and Morioka, published another case of epidermotropic eccrine carcinoma which they considered as very close to the case of Pinkus and Mehregan and as being a malignant eccrine poroma or eccrine porocarcinoma.

The eccrine poroepithelioma, considered by Mishima and Morioka as identical to the dermal duct tumor of Winkelmann and McLeod (1966), is a less mature tumor than the eccrine poroma and is characterized by a tendency to invade the underlying and surrounding tissues and by the presence of inflammatory reaction of the stroma, but without noticeable atypical cells: for this reason, it will not be studied here.

Clinical information about Mishima and Morioka's case of porocarcinoma is partly lacking; there was an extensive and proliferative plaque situated in the inguinal area in a 51 year old woman, but date of occurrence and duration are not known. The clinical features on the two other cases may be summarized as follows: ulceration below the ankle of an 82 year old woman (Pinkus and Mehregan, 1963);

pedunculated tumor with a granulated and eroded surface, 5 × 6 cm. in diameter on the leg of a 69 year old man (Miura et al., 1968); the affected limb was lymphedematous in both cases. Evolution is progressive and marked by recurrences and metastases to lymph nodes and to the skin, especially on the lower limbs and on the lower part of the trunk. Death occurred six years (Pinkus and Mehregan, 1963) or 13 years (Miura et al., 1968) after onset. Autopsy (Miura et al., 1968) disclosed diffuse superficial cutaneous metastases and lymph node metastases without any other visceral involvement.

The histologic structure of the eccrine porocarcinoma, as described by Mishima and Morioka (1968 and 1969), is characterized by an intraepidermal proliferation of cells, sometimes isolated but usually arranged in nests with ductlike or irregular clefts, especially in the central part of the lesion. Most of the nests are directly in contact with the basement membrane and, in some places, invade the dermis or the granular layer and sometimes the horny layer. The cells of the nests are large and not keratinized; their cytoplasm is clear and finely granular; and they show great atypicality and numerous mitoses. Some of them resemble Paget's cells. There is a large amount of glycogen in the cytoplasm, but the content of acid mucopolysaccharide is poor; the intercellular tonofibrils are not significant. The lesion and the normal epidermis are sharply demarcated. In the stroma there is a round cell inflammatory infiltrate.

In the cases of Pinkus and Mehregan (1963) and Miura et al. (1968), the metastatic cutaneous lesions exhibited the same histologic aspect: nests of cells in the epidermis and in the dermis situated often within the lymphatic vessels. Grouping of the tumor cells in nests is also seen in the lymph node metastases (Miura et al., 1968).

The eccrine porocarcinoma has to be diagnosed from the metastatic epidermotropic carcinomas, which are rare (Pinkus, 1968; Kawamura et al., 1968), and from extramammary Paget's disease. The main differential criterion is the presence not only of glycogen but also of mucin in Paget's cells, whereas there is much glycogen but little mucin in the porocarcinoma cells.

ETIOPATHOGENESIS

It is known that cancer inducing substances (aromatic amines) may lead to experimental sebaceous carcinomas in animals (Skoryna et al., 1951; Tannenbaum et al., 1962), but the etiologic factors of these tumors in men remain unknown. The sebaceous carcinomas are mostly located on the uncovered parts of the body (face), where there are a considerable number of sebaceous glands. Twort and Bottomley (1932), on the basis of experimental studies done in mice, noticed that oleic acid is a good irritant of the sebaceous cells and felt that it probably induces increasing sensitivity of the cells to carcinogenic agents. The eventual occurrence of sebaceous carcinomas on areas having been given x-rays (Justi, 1958; Urban and Winkelmann, 1961; Constant and Leahy, 1968) suggests the possibility of an etiologic relationship between radiation and sebaceous carcinomas. Boniuk and Zimmerman (1968) also reported two cases of carcinomas of meibomian glands occurring in patients who had received x-ray therapy for a bilateral retinoblastoma. However, experimental studies performed in rabbits irradiated in the area of anal sebaceous glands (Kuznitzky, 1946) and in the area of the orbital sebaceous glands or Harder's gland (Cogan et al., 1955) led to negative results.

Györkey and Shimamura's (1967) electron microscopic study of lymph node metastases of a sweat gland carcinoma disclosed the presence of viruslike particles located in the nucleus of the tumor cells.

As far as pathogenesis is concerned, Pinkus (1966) felt that adnexal carcinomas are similar to adenocarcinomas of other organs and respond to the same mechanisms as those which probably are involved in experimental cancer. It is likely that the epithelial cells turn into strains of stable and autonomous cancer cells that can produce metastases and be developed in tissue culture and in foreign hosts.

TREATMENT

In most cases, patients were initially given surgical treatment, consisting of a limited or wide excision of the primary tumor. In the case of recurrence or of skin or lymph node metastases, a very wide excision of the recurring or metastasizing tumor has been performed, as well as excision of the lymph nodes.

Radiotherapy has been used in some cases as initial, postoperative, or palliative treatment when there are recurrences and metastases.

Chemotherapy using cytotoxic agents [Cytoxan, nitrogen mustard, triethylenemelamine, triethylenethiophosphoramide (TEPA), cyclophosphamide] have also been used in sebaceous carcinomas (Constant and Leahy, 1968) as well as in sweat gland carcinomas (Moran and Horn, 1958; Wilde and Bader, 1963; Paine, 1965; Miura et al., 1968). It is difficult to get a good idea of the value of these therapeutic procedures, because the number of patients was very small, and most of them had only a short follow-up.

Antimitotic substances have been given to patients, who then developed generalized metastases and rapidly died.

Radiotherapy seems to prove ineffective. Constant and Leahy (1968) felt that sebaceous carcinomas are radioresistant. On the other hand, Shapiro et al. (1953) expressed the opinion that these tumors are extremely radiosensitive: they had excellent results in the irradiated tumor, but several months later the patient developed skin and bone metastases. Radioresistance of sweat gland carcinomas, as generally accepted, is particularly emphasized by Keasbey and Hadley (1954), Moran and Horn (1958), and Wilde and Bader (1963).

Surgical procedure (early initial wide local excision and dissection of involved regional lymph nodes) is considered the best treatment, which, however, does not prevent recurrences and metastases. Lack of sufficient experience with radiotherapy and chemotherapy and the real malignancy of adnexal carcinomas may in some instances justify the combined use of these three methods.

REFERENCES

Adnexal Skin Carcinomas

Abulafia, J.: Epitheliomas cutâneos. Ensayo de clasificación histogenética. An. Brasil. Dermatol., 38:14, 1963.

Andrade, R.: Die präcanceröse und canceröse Wucherung von Epidermis und Anhangsgebilden. *In* Jadassohn's Handbuch der Haut- und Geschlechtskrankheiten. I, 2:344, Berlin, Springer-Verlag, 1964.

Civatte, A.: Tumeurs des annexes épidermiques. Bull. Soc. Fr. Dermatol. Syphiligr., 48:155, 1941.

Civatte, J.: Les épithéliomas cutanés annexiels. *In* Xe Congrès des Dermatologistes et Syphiligraphes de Langue Française, Alger, 1959. Paris, Masson et Cie, Ed., 1961, p. 281.

Civatte, J.: Histopathologie Cutanée. Paris, Editons Médicales Flammarion, 1967.

Dubreuilh, W.: De l'ulcus rodens. II. Internationaler Dermatologischer Congress, Wien, 1892. Wien, Druck von Friedrich Jasper, 1893, p. 377.

Foot, N. C.: Adnexal carcinoma of the skin. Am. J. Pathol., 23:1, 1947.

Grynfeltt, E., and Aimes, A.: Etude histopathologique de deux tumeurs des glandes sudoripares. Bull. Assoc. Fr. Cancer, 11:91, 1922.

Lever, W. F.: Adenoacanthoma of sweat glands. Carcinoma of sweat glands with glandular and epidermal elements; report of four cases. Arch. Dermatol. Syph. (Berl.), 56:157, 1947.

Lever, W. F.: Pathogenesis of benign tumors of cutaneous appendages and of basal cell epithelioma. Arch. Dermatol. Syph. (Berl.), 57:679, 1948.

Lever, W. F.: Histopathology of the Skin. Ed. 4. Philadelphia, J. B. Lippincott Company, 1967.

Lund, H. Z.: Atlas of Tumor Pathology. Tumors of the Skin, Section I, Fascicle 2. Washington, D.C., Armed Forces Institute of Pathology, 1957.

McMullan, F. H.: Basal cell tumors. Classification based upon histogenesis. Pillsbury, D. M., and Livingood, C. S. (Eds.): Proceedings of the XII International Congress of Dermatology, Washington, D.C., 1962. Vol. II. Amsterdam, Excerpta Medica Foundation, 1963, p. 1595.

Mehregan, A. H., and Pinkus, H.: Organoid tumors of the skin. *In* Pillsbury, D. M., and Livingood, C. S. (Eds.): Proceedings of the XII International Congress of Dermatology, Washington, D.C., 1962. Vol. II. Amsterdam, Excerpta Medica Foundation, 1963, p. 1597.

Montgomery, H.: Dermatopathology. Vol. 2. New York, Hoeber Medical Division, Harper and Row, Publishers, 1967.

Panja, S. K.: Adnexal carcinomas. Indian J. Dermatol., 14:76, 1969.

Pinkus, H.: Premalignant fibroepithelial tumors of skin. Arch. Dermatol. Syph. (Berl.), 67:598, 1953.

Pinkus, H., and Mehregan, A. H.: A Guide to Dermatohistopathology. Appleton-Century-Crofts, Publishing Division of Prentice-Hall, Inc., Englewood Cliffs, N.J., 1969.

Pilar Carcinomas

Headington, J. T., and French, A. J.: Primary neoplasms of the hair follicle. Histogenesis and classification. Arch. Dermatol., 86:430, 1962.

Hedinger, E.: Zur Lehre der Hautcarcinome (Das Carcinom der äusseren Haarwurzelscheide). Virchows Arch., 254:321, 1925.

Holmes, E. J.: Tumors of lower hair sheath. Common histogenesis of certain so-called "sebaceous cysts," acanthomas and "sebaceous carcinomas." Cancer, 21:234, 1968.

Jones, E. W.: Proliferating epidermoid cysts. Arch. Dermatol., 94:11, 1966.

Liu, Y.: The histogenesis of clear cell papillary carcinoma of the skin. Am. J. Pathol., 25:93, 1949.

Loos, H. O.: Die Carcinome der Anhangsgebilde der Haut. Arch. Dermatol. Syph. (Berl.), 174:465, 1936.

Mehregan, A. H.: Clear celled epithelial tumors of the skin. *In* Jadassohn, W., and Schirren, C. G. (Eds.): XIII Congressus Internationalis Dermatologiae, München, 1967. Vol. 1. Berlin, Springer-Verlag, 1968, p. 68.

Picard, E., and Liégeois, P.: Epithéliomas pilaires. Cancer (Brux.), 8:121, 1931.

Wilson-Jones, E.: Proliferating epidermal cyst. Arch. Dermatol., 94:11, 1966.

Sebaceous Carcinomas

Beach, A., and Severance, A. O.: Sebaceous gland carcinoma. Ann. Surg., 115:258, 1942.

Boniuk, M., and Zimmerman, L. E.: Sebaceous carcinoma of the eyelid, eyebrow, caruncle and orbit. Trans. Am. Acad. Ophthalmol. Otolaryngol., 72:619, 1968.

Cabanne, F., Dusserre, P., and Michiels, R.: Carcinomes sébacés. J. Med. Lyon, 46:1635, 1965.

Castelain, P. Y., and Spitalier, J. M.: Epithélioma sébacé sur naevus sebaceus de Jadassohn. Bull. Soc. Fr. Dermatol. Syphiligr., 69:436, 1962.

Constant, E., and Leahy, M. S.: Sebaceous cell carcinoma. Plast. Reconstr. Surg., 41:433, 1968.

Degos, R., Civatte, J., and Guilaine, J.: Epithélioma sébacé. Bull. Soc. Fr. Dermatol. Syphiligr., 67:32, 1960.

Dupont, A.: Epithéliomas sébacés multiples à point de départ épidermique. Bull. Soc. Fr. Dermatol. Syphiligr., 45:704, 1938.

Favre, M., Josserand, A., and Martin, J. F.: Cancers des glandes annexes de la peau. Epithéliomas sudoripares et sébacés. *In* Nouvelle Pratique Dermatologique, Tome VI. Paris, Masson et Cie, Ed., 1936, p. 768.

Gay, and Ortiz Picón: Epitelioma baso-espino celular de origen sebáceo. Act. Dermo-sifiliogr. (Madr.), 19:256, 1927.

Ginsberg, J.: Present status of meibomian gland carcinoma. Arch. Ophthalmol., 73:271, 1965.

Justi, R. A.: Sebaceous carcinoma. Report of case developing in area of radiodermatitis. Arch. Dermatol., 77:195, 1958.

Laffargue, P., Mussini-Montpellier, J., Ferrand, B., Smadja, A., Belaïch, S., and François, H.: Étude histologique des tumeurs annexielles. Algérie Méd., 66:325, 1962.

Leroux, R., and Cornil, L.: Epithélioma sébacé. Bul. Mem. Soc. Anat. Paris, 93:352, 1923.

Masson, P., and Géry, L.: L'épithélioma sébacé. Bull. Assoc. Fr. Cancer, 11:284, 1922.

Miller, R. E., and White, J. J.: Sebaceous gland carcinoma. Am. J. Surg., 114:958, 1967.

Parreira, H.: Sôbre tumores das glândulas cutâneas. Arq. Patol., 7:244, 1935.

Puente Duany, N.: Epithéliome récidivant de la nuque, de différenciation sébacée. Ann. Dermatol. Syphiligr. (Paris), 87:618, 1960.

Santini, R., and De Panfilis, G.: Adenocarcinoma sebaceo metastatizzante. Rilievi clinici ed istopatologici. Minerva Dermatol., 44:279, 1969.

Shapiro, M. P., Keen, P., Cohen, L., and Murray, J. F.: Skin cancer in the South African Bantu. Br. J. Cancer, 7:45, 1953.

Urban, F. H., and Winkelmann, R. K.: Sebaceous malignancy. Arch. Dermatol., 84:63, 1961.

Warren, S., and Warvi, W. N.: Tumors of sebaceous glands. Am. J. Pathol., 19:441, 1943.

Zackheim, H. S.: The sebaceous epithelioma. A clinical and histologic study. Arch. Dermatol., 89:711, 1964.

Sweat Gland Carcinomas

Ackerman, L. V.: Surgical Pathology. St. Louis, Mo., The C. V. Mosby Company, 1953, p. 90.

Calissano, G.: Adenocarcinoma delle ghiandole sudoripare. Arch. Ital. Chir., 15:578, 1926.

Crosti, A.: Sul carcinoma delle ghiandole sudorifere. Arch. Ital. Dermatol. Venereol., 7:91, 1931.

Damsgaard-Sørensen, P., and Søeborg Ohlsen, A.: Multiple metastasizing sweat gland carcinoma. Acta Derm. Venereol. (Stockh.), 49:314, 1969.

Darier, J.: Contribution à l'étude de l'épithéliome des glandes sudoripares. Arch. Med. Exp. Anat. Pathol., 1:115, 267, 1889.

Degos, R., Civatte, J., and Baptista, A.: Aspect pseudo-glandulaire d'épithéliomas spinocellulaires dyskératosiques (discussion de l'adénoacanthome des glandes sudoripares de Lever). Bull. Soc. Fr. Dermatol. Syphiligr., 65:578, 1958.

Delacrétaz, J., Madjedi, A. S., and Loretan, R. M.: Epithelioma spino-cellulare segregans. Hautarzt, 8:512, 1957.

Eichenberg, H. E.: Hidradenoma vulvae. Z. Geburtshilfe Gynaekol., 109:358, 1934.

Elliott, G. B., and Ramsay, D. W.: Sweat gland carcinoma. Ann. Surg., 144:99, 1956.

Freeman, R. G., and Winkelmann, R. K.: Basal cell tumor with eccrine differentiation (eccrine epithelioma). Arch. Dermatol., 100:234, 1969.

Fresen, O.: Über das Carcinom der Hautdrüsen am Beispiel eines Schweissdrüsenkrebses der Hohlhand. Hautarzt, 11:15, 1960.

Gates, O., Warren, S., and Warvi, W. N.: Tumors of sweat glands. Am. J. Pathol., 19:591, 1943.

Grant, R. A.: Sweat gland carcinoma with metastases. J.A.M.A., 173:490, 1960.

Hedinger, E.: Zur Frage des Plasmocytoms (Granulationsplasmocytom in Kombination mit einem krebsig umgewandelten Schweissdrüsenadenom des behaarten Kopfes). Frankfurt. Z. Pathol., 7:343, 1911.

Horn, R. C.: Malignant papillary cystadenoma of sweat glands with metastases to the regional lymph nodes. Surgery, 16:348, 1944.

Hufschmitt, G., and Diss, A.: Epithélioma sudoripare. Bull. Soc. Fr. Dermatol. Syphiligr., 36:503, 1929.

Jablonska, S., and Chorzelski, T.: Dyskeratoma and epithelioma (carcinoma) dyskeratoticum segregans. Dermatologica, 123:24, 1961.

Jacobson, Y. G., Rees, T. D., Grant, R., and Fitchett, V. H.: Metastasizing sweat-gland carcinoma. Arch. Surg., 78:574, 1959.

Johnson, W. C., and Helwig, E. B.: Adenoid squamous cell carcinoma (adenoacanthoma). A clinicopathologic study of 155 patients. Cancer, 19:1639, 1966.

Kipkie, G. F., and Haust, M. D.: Carcinoma of apocrine glands. Report of case. Arch. Dermatol., 78:440, 1958.

Kreibich, K.: Ein Fall von Adenocarcinoma lenticulare capillitii. Dermatol. Z., 14:651, 1907.

Maier, T.: Autoptisch gesichertes metastasierendes Schweissdrüsenkarzinom auf dem Boden eines Naevus syringo-adenomatosus papilliferus. Zentralbl. Allg. Pathol., 85:377, 1949.

Miller, W. L.: Sweat-gland carcinoma. A clinicopathologic problem. Am. J. Clin. Pathol., 47:767, 1967.

Mincy, J. E., and Lee, L. C.: Intracranial metastasis of sweat gland carcinoma. Case report. J. Neurosurg., 25:564, 1966.

Moran, J. J., and Horn, R. C.: Carcinoma of sweat gland origin. Report of a case of 30 years' duration with autopsy findings. Surgery, 44:683, 1958.

Moriconi, L.: Adenocarcinoma delle ghiandole sudoripare. Policlinico [Chir.], 38:634, 1931.

Morini, L., and Montagnani, P.: Circa un caso di carcinoma del corion ad andamento maligno, iniziato dai tubuli sudoriferi. G. Ital. Mal. Vener., 62:733, 1921.

Morioka, S., and Mishima, Y.: Oncogenic differentiation of intradermal eccrine sweat duct and gland: Benign, epitheliomatous and carcinomatous tumors. Jap. J. Dermatol., 78:237, 1968.

Muller, S. A., Wilhelmj, C. M., Harrison, E. G., and Winkelmann, R. K.: Adenoid squamous cell carcinoma (adenoacanthoma of Lever). Arch. Dermatol., 89:589, 1964.

Neely, J. M.: Rep. Proc. Lincoln Hosp. Tumour Cong. Nebraska Med. J., 37:193, 1952. Cited by Smith, C. C. K.

Paine, C. H.: Very late recurrence of a previously excised sweat gland carcinoma: Case report with review of the literature. Br. J. Cancer, 19:263, 1965.

Pinkus, H.: Adnexal tumors, benign, not-so-benign, and malignant. *In* Montagna, W., and Dobson, R. L. (Eds.): Advances in Biology of Skin. Vol. VII. Carcinogenesis. New York, Pergamon Press, 1966, p. 255.

Puente Duany, N.: Epiteliomas de las glándulas sudoríparas. Arch. Cuba. Cancer., 9:44, 97, 205, 1950.

Puente Duany, N.: Imágenes glandulares verdaderas y falsas en los epiteliomas espino-celulares (adeno-acantoma de W. Lever, epitelioma malpighiano disqueratósico o acantolítico). Arch. Cuba. Cancer., 15:83, 1956.

Seitchik, M. W.: Adenocarcinoma of eccrine origin. J. Albert Einstein Med. Center, 13:71, 1965. Cited by Damsgaard-Sørensen, P., and Søeborg Ohlsen, A.

Shenoy, Y. M. V.: Malignant perianal papillary hidradenoma. Arch. Dermatol., 83:965, 1961.

Smith, C. C. K.: Metastasizing carcinoma of the sweat-glands. Br. J. Surg., 43:80, 1955.

Stout, A. P., and Cooley, S. G. E.: Carcinoma of sweat glands. Cancer, 4:521, 1951.

Suzuki, S.: Ein Beitrag zur Kenntnis des Schweissdrüsencarcinoms, mit besonderer Berücksichtigung seiner histologischen Einteilung. Jap. J. Med. Sci., Dermatol. Urol., 2:165, 1941.

Teloh, H. A.: Sweat-gland carcinoma. Cancer, 8:1003, 1955.

Teloh, H. A., Balkin, R. B., and Grier, J. P.: Metastasizing sweat-gland carcinoma. Report of a case. Arch. Dermatol., 76:80, 1957.

Wilde, J., and Bader, G.: Zur Klinik und Morphologie des metastasierenden Schweissdrüsenkarzinoms. Bruns Beitr. Klin. Chir., 206:436, 1963.

Wolfe, J. J., and Segerberg, L. H.: Metastasizing sweat gland carcinoma of the scalp involving transverse sinus. Report of a case. Am. J. Surg., 88:849, 1954.

Zink, H. K.: Ein Fall von maligner Degeneration bei einem Syringom. Strahlentherapie, 81:419, 1950.

Clear Cell Hidradenocarcinomas

Kay, S., and Hall, W. E. B.: Sweat-gland carcinoma with proved metastases. Report of case. Cancer, 7:373, 1954.

Keasbey, L. E., and Hadley, G. G.: Clear-cell hidradenoma. Report of three cases with widespread metastases. Cancer, 7:934, 1954.

Kersting, D. W.: Clear cell hidradenoma and hidradenocarcinoma. Arch. Dermatol., 87:323, 1963.

Mackenzie, D. H.: A clear-cell hidradenocarcinoma with metastases. Cancer, 10:1021, 1957.

Santler, R., and Eberhartinger, C.: Malignes Klarzellen-Myoepitheliom. Dermatologica, 130:340, 1965.

Malignant Mixed Tumors of the Skin

Desorgher, G., and Saout, J.: Tumeur mixte maligne du pouce. J. Sci. Med. Lille, 86:457, 1968.

Gubareva, A. V.: Mixed tumours of the skin. Arch. Patol., 25:17, 1963.

Hirsch, P., and Helwig, E. B.: Chondroid syringoma. Mixed tumor of skin, salivary gland type. Arch. Dermatol., 84:835, 1961.

Matz, L. R., McCully, D. J., and Stokes, B. A. R.: Metastasizing chondroid syringoma: Case report. Pathology, 1:77, 1969.

Rosborough, D.: Malignant mixed tumours of skin. Br. J. Surg., 50:697, 1963.

Sharvill, D. E.: Mixed salivary-type tumour of the skin with malignant recurrence. Br. J. Dermatol., 74:103, 1962.

Porocarcinomas

Kawamura, T., Ikeda, S., Mori, S., Mizutani, H., and Funabashi, T.: Three cases of epidermotropic carcinoma. Jap. J. Dermatol., 78:239, 1968.

Mishima, Y., and Morioka, S.: Oncogenic differentiation of the intraepidermal eccrine sweat duct unit: Eccrine poroma, poroepithelioma and porocarcinoma. Jap. J. Dermatol., 78:231, 1968; Dermatologica, 138:238, 1969.

Miura, Y.: Epidermotropic eccrine carcinoma. Jap. J. Dermatol., 78:226, 1968.

Miura, Y., Akano, A., Nakagawa, T., and Kikuchi, Y.: Epidermotropic eccrine carcinoma. *In* Jadassohn, W., and Schirren, C. G. (Eds.): XIII Congressus Internationalis Dermatologiae, München, 1967. Vol. 1. Berlin, Springer-Verlag, 1968, p. 84.

Pinkus, H.: Epidermotropism in sweat apparatus tumors. Jap. J. Dermatol., 78:244, 1968.

Pinkus, H., and Mehregan, A. H.: Epidermotropic eccrine carcinoma. A case combining features of eccrine poroma and Paget's dermatosis. Arch. Dermatol., 88:597, 1963.

Winkelmann, R. K., and McLeod, W. A.: The dermal duct tumor. Arch. Dermatol., 94:50, 1966.

Etiopathogenesis

Cogan, D. G., Fink, R., and Donaldson, D. D.: X-ray irradiation of orbital glands of the rabbit. Radiology, 64:731, 1955.

Györkey, F., and Shimamura, Y.: Virus-like particles observed in a human sweat gland carcinoma. Yokohama Med. Bull., 18:1, 1967.

Kuznitzky, E.: Cancer-like epithelial structure as a result of mesothorium radiation of the sebaceous glands of the rabbit (anaplasia or regeneration?). J. Invest. Dermatol., 7:1, 1946.

Skoryna, S. C., Ross, R. C., and Rudis, L. A.: Histogenesis of sebaceous gland carcinomas produced in rats by 2-acetylaminofluorene. J. Exp. Med., 94:1, 1951.

Tannenbaum, A., Vesselinovitch, S. D., Maltoni, C., and Mitchell, D. S.: Multipotential carcinogenicity of urethan in the Sprague-Dawley rat. Cancer Res., 22:1362, 1962.

Twort, C. C., and Bottomley, A. C.: The aetiology of breast cancer. Lancet, 2:776, 1932.

46

Dermatofibrosarcoma Protuberans

Lewis Shapiro, M.D., and Martin H. Brownstein, M.D.

DEFINITION

Dermatofibrosarcoma protuberans (DFSP) is a slowly growing, locally aggressive, frequently recurrent, rarely metastatic neoplasm of the dermis. The characteristic clinical appearance is that of a multinodular, protuberant mass overlying a firm dermal plaque; histologically it displays areas with uniform, closely aggregated spindle-shaped cells arranged in a storiform (L. *storia*, plaited covering or straw mat) pattern.

HISTORY

Darier and Ferrand (1924), in a classic communication, reported four patients with similar tumors and described an entity which they called "dermatofibromes progressifs et récidivants ou fibrosarcomes de la peau." Although it is almost certain that DFSP existed before 1924 and that some earlier authors reported individual cases, credit for the delineation of the entity clearly belongs to Darier and Ferrand. Review of several of the earlier

descriptions and original pictures leaves some doubt about the nature of the conditions described.

The following year Hoffmann (1925) reported three additional patients, referred to the work of Darier and Ferrand, and used the title "knollentreibends Fibrosarkom der Haut (Dermatofibrosarkoma protuberans)." While such terms as Darier-Ferrand's dermatofibrosarcoma, fibrosarcoma, dermatofibroma, tumor, or disease are now usually employed by French-speaking physicians, "dermatofibrosarcoma protuberans" has become almost universally understood and accepted.

More than one hundred examples of DFSP were published between 1925 and 1950, but these usually consisted of individual or small numbers of patients with only short periods of follow-up. Many of the cases were reported under other titles; several authors did not realize they were describing a previously defined condition; and some of the tumors reported as DFSP would appear to be other entities. Emphasis in diagnosis was usually placed on the cllinical appearance and course. Histologic descriptions added little to that of

1069

Darier and Ferrand. It was generally considered that the microscopic picture did not differ from that of other sarcomas; the essential difference was thought to be clinical.

A number of advances in the knowledge of DFSP have taken place since 1950. Notably, several large series of patients have been reported; there has been gradual appreciation of the importance of typical histologic appearances of the tumor; and recent electron microscopic studies have helped to clarify the histogenesis of the disorder. The challenge for the future is the elucidation of the basic nature of the lesion, increased awareness of the entity by physicians, and earlier diagnosis and definitive therapy.

INCIDENCE

DFSP is an uncommon tumor despite the fact that, during the past 25 years, series of 39 (Pack and Tabah, 1951), 115 (Taylor and Helwig, 1962), 56 (Burkhardt et al., 1966), 86 (McPeak et al., 1967) and 33 (Smith, 1971) cases have been reported from this country; 38 from Sweden (Gentele, 1951); and 30 from Canada (Tremblay et al., 1970). In comparison to other malignant tumors of the skin, DFSP is rare. For example, approximately six new patients with DFSP have been seen annually at Memorial Hospital in New York (McPeak et al., 1967), compared with about 60 new cases of malignant melanoma (McNeer and Cantin, 1967). In our private practice of dermatopathology, the ratio of DFSP to melanoma is less than 1:100. Multiple cases of DFSP have apparently not been documented in the same family.

CLINICAL DESCRIPTION

DFSP usually begins as a sclerodermoid plaque in the cutis; for a long time the lesion grows slowly by peripheral extension and the development of small, firm, nontender, blue or red dermal nodules (Fig. 46–1), which increase in size and number. Protuberant nodules eventually develop on the surface. The fully evolved

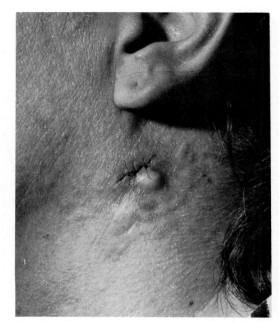

Figure 46–1 Sclerodermoid plaque with central nodule.

lesion is a multilobulated mass (Fig. 46–2) fixed to the overlying skin, which is thin, smooth, and shiny. The tumor rests upon a firm, irregularly shaped dermal plaque, which is usually movable over the deeper tissues. The condition is characteristically asymptomatic, but pain or tenderness was noted in 16 out of 56 (29 percent) patients reported from the Mayo Clinic (Burkhardt et al., 1966) and in 30 out of 115 (26 percent) of those reported from the Armed Forces Institute of Pathology (Taylor and Helwig, 1962). The protuberant portions may ulcerate, bleed, or become infected after minor injury. Occasionally there is a period of rapid growth. Local trauma sometimes precedes the development of the tumor (Taylor and Helwig, 1962; Tremblay et al., 1970). DFSP is almost invariably solitary; approximately eight examples of multiple primaries have been reported (Groetschel and Cramer, 1967).

In most of the larger series there has been a slight predilection for male patients. In a report from Radiumhemmet in Stockholm (Gentele, 1951), 21 out of 38 (55 percent) patients were men; at the Mayo Clinic (Burkhardt et al., 1966), 32 out of 56 (57 percent); at Memorial Hospital (McPeak et al., 1967), 48 out of 82

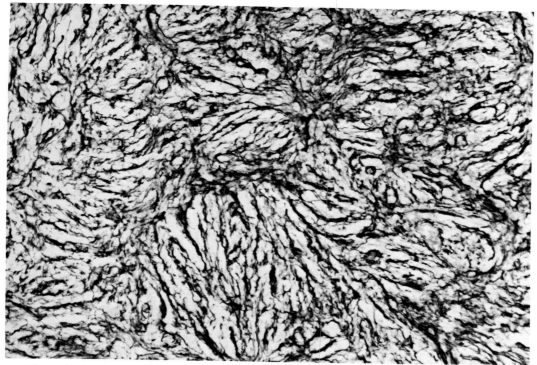

Figure 46–9 Well-developed reticulum displaying storiform configuration. *Laidlaw silver stain, ×220.*

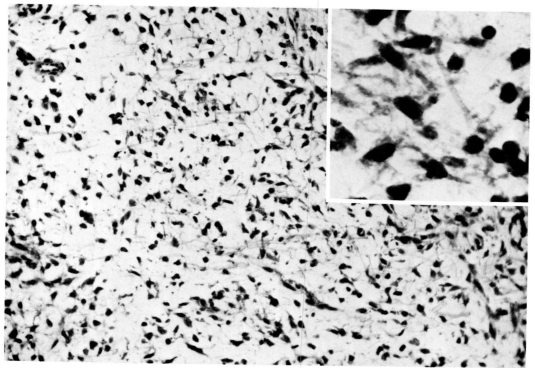

Figure 46–10 Myxomatous pattern. *H & E, ×220; inset ×700.*

present in one case. Large quantities of sudanophilic lipid were observed in one tumor—a highly aggressive one. Acanthosis of the overlying epidermis was present in two specimens.

Electron microscopic studies (Fisher and Vuzevski, 1968; Tremblay et al., 1970) have usually included only one or two cases and have been inconclusive in regard to histogenesis. A recent report of seven cases (Hashimoto et al., 1974) suggests origin from a modified neural supporting cell, either endoneural or perineural. The tumor cells show elaborately convoluted nuclei, extensive cytoplasmic processes, few profiles of rough surfaced endoplasmic reticulum and Golgi lamellae, and spotty basal lamina-like material.

DIFFERENTIAL DIAGNOSIS

The correct diagnosis can usually be made on the basis of the clinical picture of a firm, protuberant, multinodular lesion with a subjacent, irregular, fibrous plaque that has grown slowly and displays the histologic pattern of a dermal tumor with spindle-shaped cells arranged in storiform configuration. Early lesions may be misinterpreted by the clinician as histiocytoma (dermatofibroma), localized scleroderma, keloid, or other fibromatoses. Well-developed lesions have been confused with metastatic tumors, fibrosarcoma, Kaposi's sarcoma, and malignant melanoma.

The main problem for the histopathologist is to differentiate DFSP from histiocytoma (dermatofibroma), fibromatoses, and fibrosarcoma. The microscopic hallmark of DFSP is the storiform pattern. Histiocytomas not infrequently display storiform features, but the fully developed picture is distinctly uncommon. The demonstration of groups of lipid- or hemosiderin-laden histiocytes is strong evidence in favor of histiocytoma rather than DFSP. Fibrosarcoma, malignant schwannoma (neurofibrosarcoma), and even fibrous meningioma (Smith, 1971) may show a similar pattern, but these arise in deeper structures. DFSP, particularly recurrent lesions with mucinous foci, may be confused with myxoid neurofibroma, myxoma, and myxoid liposarcoma.

In reviewing the literature dealing with DFSP and related entities, one encounters the following more or less synonymous terms: fibrous xanthoma, fibroxanthoma, xanthogranuloma, fibrous histiocytoma, and histiocytoma. The adjectives atypical or malignant may precede any of these. In general, the authors wish to convey the impression that there is a spectrum of hyperplastic and neoplastic lesions, composed of histiocytes, fibroblasts, or both, located in the skin, soft tissues, or elsewhere, varying from small, quiescent, intracutaneous nodules to large, deep, potentially metastasizing tumors. On histologic grounds alone—and at times even with detailed clinical information as well—it is often impossible to separate them into distinct entities or predict their biologic behavior. To some who use such nomenclature, DFSP is merely a subgroup within the broader category. We agree there is a continuum of pathologic changes encompassed by these terms and admit there are a number of cases that do not lend themselves to precise categorization. Nevertheless, we believe that, with adequate clinical information and a representative pathologic specimen of sufficient size, the more meaningful diagnosis of DFSP can be established most of the time.

TREATMENT

The treatment of choice is surgical excision. Since the tumor microscopically almost invariably extends well beyond what appear to be adequate surgical margins, conservative excision is often followed by recurrence. At tumor hospitals, the cure rate for primary treatment has been 24 out of 27 (89 percent) (McPeak et al., 1967) and 13 out of 15 (87 percent) (Smith, 1971).

McPeak et al. (1967) adopted the attitude that therapy is inadequate unless a margin of at least 3 cm. of normal-appearing tissue, plus the deep fascia, is excised. With rare exception, skin grafts have been required to repair the defects. Although the failure rate of primary treatment at *general* hospitals is not known, it would appear to be greatly in excess of the 12 percent reported from tumor hospitals.

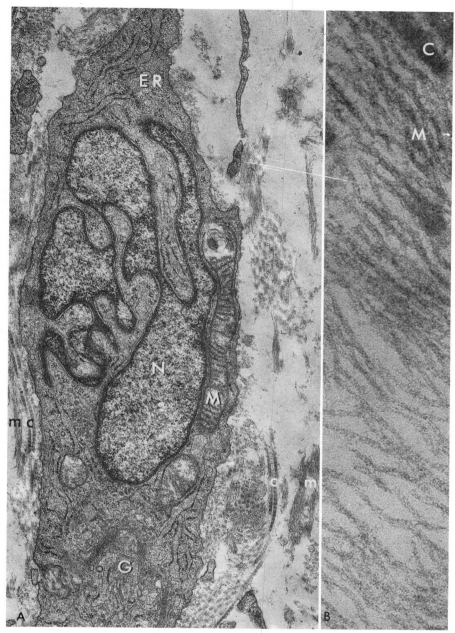

Figure 46–11 Tumor cell characterized by extensively lobulated nucleus *(N)*, Golgi apparatus *(G)*, rough-surfaced endoplasmic reticulum *(ER)*, and mitochondrion *(M)*. Outside the tumor cell, many microfibrils *(m)* are admixed with collagen fibrils *(c)*. ×25,000. *B*, Enlargement of microfibrils *(M)* and a collagen fibril *(C)* shows that the dimension of the former is about one-third of the latter. ×*175,000.* (Courtesy of Dr. Ken Hashimoto.)

PROGNOSIS

DFSP is commonly recurrent, rarely metastatic, and occasionally fatal. Among 21 patients who had their primary treatment at Mayo Clinic (Burkhardt et al.,

1966) and were followed for at least five years, recurrences developed in seven (33 percent). Two patients died, possibly with metastases. In another series (McPeak et al., 1967), recurrences developed in three of 27 patients who received their primary treatment at Memorial Hospital; neither metastases nor fatalities were reported. Recurrences occurred in two of 15 patients treated initially at M.D. Anderson Hospital (Smith, 1971); there were no metastases or fatalities.

By contrast, patients previously treated elsewhere and referred to tumor hospitals with clinical recurrences followed a much more aggressive course. In a group of 42 patients (McPeak et al., 1967) reoperated on because of recurrent tumor, subsequent recurrences developed in 12 (29 percent). Five of these manifested only local tumor, two died from intracranial extension, and five died with metastases. Eighteen patients with recurrent DFSP were referred for retreatment to another oncologic hospital (Smith, 1971). Subsequent recurrences appeared in 13; one patient died from metastases.

The natural history of the disease in patients treated in general hospitals is unknown, but it presumably falls somewhere between the relatively good results of those operated on initially in tumor hospitals and the poor results of those subsequently referred there because of treatment failure.

The incidence of metastases in reported series ranges from 0 out of 37 (Taylor and Helwig, 1962) to 5 out of 82 (6 percent) patients who had at least three years of follow-up (McPeak et al., 1967). In reviewing the literature, Burkhardt et al. (1966) found eight cases of histologically documented metastases in DFSP.

The prognosis depends upon the stage at which the correct diagnosis is made and appropriate therapy instituted, as well as the intrinsic potential for aggressiveness of the particular tumor in a given patient. Increased awareness by clinicians of the nature of the lesion, wider recognition by pathologists of its histologic features, and greater understanding by surgeons of its biologic behavior and tendency for microscopic invasion beyond the main tumor masses might improve the outlook in this condition.

REFERENCES

Burkhardt, B. R., Soule, E. H., Winkelmann, R. K., and Ivins, J. C.: Dermatofibrosarcoma protuberans. Study of 56 cases. Am. J. Surg., 111:638, 1966.

Darier, J., and Ferrand, M.: Dermatofibromes progressifs et récidivants ou fibrosarcomes de la peau. Ann. Dermatol. Syphiligr. (Paris), 5:545, 1924.

Degos, R., Touraine, R., and Préaux, J.: Deux cas de dermato-fibrosarcome de Darier-Ferrand chez l'enfant. Bull. Soc.. Fr. Dermatol. Syphiligr., 70:134, 1963.

Fisher, E. R., and Vuzevski, V. D.: Cytogenesis of schwannoma (neurilemoma), neurofibroma, dermatofibroma, and dermatofibrosarcoma as revealed by electron microscopy. Am. J. Clin. Pathol., 49:141, 1968.

Gentele, H.: Malignant, fibroblastic tumors of the skin. Acta Derm. Venereol (Stockh.), Suppl. 27, 31:1, 1951.

Groetschel, H., and Cramer, H. J.: Multilokulär-symmetrisches Dermatofibrosarkoma protuberans. Dermatol. Wochenschr., 153:574, 1967.

Hashimoto, K., Brownstein, M. H., and Jakobiec, F. A.: Dermatofibrosarcoma protuberans: A tumor with perineural and endoneural cell features. Arch. Dermatol., 110:874, 1974.

Hoffmann, E.: Uber das knollentreibends Fibrosarkom der Haut (Dermatofibrosarkoma protuberans). Dermatol. Z., 43:1, 1925.

McNeer, G., and Cantin, J.: Local failure in the treatment of melanoma. Am. J. Roentgenol. 99:791, 1967.

McPeak, C. J., Cruz, T., and Nicastri, A. D.: Dermatofibrosarcoma protuberans: An analysis of 86 cases—five with metastasis. Ann. Surg., 166:803, 1967.

Pack, G. T., and Tabah, E. J.: Dermatofibrosarcoma protuberans: A report of 39 cases. Arch. Surg., 62:391, 1951.

Smith, J. L., Jr.: Tumors of the Corium. In Helwig, E. B., and Mostofi, F. K. (Eds.): The Skin. Baltimore, The Williams & Wilkins Company, 1971.

Taylor, H. B., and Helwig, E. B.: Dermatofibrosarcoma protuberans: A study of 115 cases. Cancer, 15:717, 1962.

Tremblay, M., Bonenfant, J-L., and Cliche, J.: Le dermatofibrosarcome protubérant étude clinicopathologique de trente cas avec l'ultrastructure de deux cas. Union Med. Can., 99:871, 1970.

47

Pseudosarcomatous Lesions of Skin and Superficial Tissues

Raffaele Lattes, M.D.

The term pseudosarcoma has been used by different authors and by practicing pathologists for such a wide spectrum of conditions, benign and malignant, that it is necessary to start this chapter by defining clearly our own understanding and limitations of the term and by listing then those lesions which we consider as pseudosarcomatous for the purpose of this discussion. We shall deal here with a group of tumors and pseudotumors of mesenchymal origin, involving either skin or the superficial soft tissues, which are benign biologically, but which, as a common denominator, exhibit a microscopic morphology which is often erroneously interpreted as malignant. For some of these lesions, the pathogenesis is known. For many others, it is uncertain. Most of them belong in that twilight zone which borders on one side on true neoplastic conditions, and on the other side on the so-called reactive and/or reparative processes.

The following lesions will be defined, described, and illustrated:

1. Atypical fibroxanthoma
2. Pseudosarcoma and postradiation fibromatosis of skin following irradiation
3. Pseudosarcomatous fasciitis
4. Proliferative myositis
5. Infantile digital fibromatosis
6. Fibrous hamartoma of infancy

We shall also list, but not describe, a small number of other better known lesions which can be mistaken for true sarcoma but are now generally recognized as benign.

We do not intend to include in this chapter either those pseudoneoplastic lesions which will be covered elsewhere in this book (i.e., benign lymphoid infiltrations of the skin) or those *definitely malignant epithelial* tumors exhibiting a spindle cell metaplasia which can lead the pathologist toward an erroneous diagnosis of "sarcoma" (Sims and Kirsch, 1948; Martin and Stewart, 1935). Among these are squamous cell carcinomas of the skin with predominant spindle cell pattern, some rare desmoplastic variants of malignant melanoma (Conley et al., 1971), and some unusual polypoid tumors of the mucous membranes near the body orifices which are sometimes classified as carcinosarcoma because of a neoplastic spindle cell population in the stroma (Lane, 1957). These malignant lesions are "pseudosarcomatous" only insofar as the neoplastic *epithelial* cells are sarcoma-like.

By necessity, it is expected that there will be overlapping between some of the entities discussed in this chapter and similar lesions covered in other parts of this book.

ATYPICAL FIBROXANTHOMA

This is a tumor or tumorlike lesion which occurs predominantly in exposed parts of the skin of patients of advanced age. The head and neck region is most frequently but not exclusively involved. They are generally superficial nodular lesions which can be slightly pigmented. They vary in size, but most are 2 to 4 cm. in diameter when diagnosed and have a definite tendency to ulcerate (Fig. 47–1). For all these reasons (age, topography, tendency to ulceration, pigmentation), it is understandable that the initial clinical impression is often in favor of one of the common malignant skin tumors (basal or

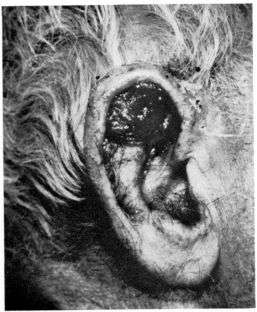

Figure 47–1 Atypical fibroxanthoma of external ear in an 85 year old man. It has not recurred after excision.
(See also Color Plate VII–F.)

squamous cell carcinoma, malignant melanoma).

Histologically this is a pleomorphic lesion which certainly belongs to the family of histiocytic or fibrohistiocytic proliferations (Figs. 47–2 to 47–4). The cell population includes giant cells whose multiple nuclei may have conspicuous nucleoli and whose cytoplasm may contain lipid vacuoles or phagocytosed hemosiderin. The remainder of the cellular components consists of polygonal or elongated cells with considerable variation in size and in nuclear-cytoplasmic ratio. The nuclei may be bizarre, and the mitotic activity may be considerable, with occasional atypical mitoses. Typical storiform arrangement of the elongated cells is seldom seen. The amount of collagen and of argyrophilic reticulin fibrils is patchy as it is in the majority of the histiocytic tumors.

These lesions, which are grossly nodular and apparently well circumscribed, are never encapsulated, but their cell population interdigitates with the accessory skin structures and may extend into the subcutaneous fat. There is almost always an infiltration of inflammatory cells.

There are now several good articles on this lesion. The term "atypical fibroxanthoma" was originally suggested by Helwig. One of the best reviews is that published by Kempson and McGavran in 1964. We agree with these authors that the entity described by Bourne in 1962 as "paradoxical fibrosarcoma" is most probably the same lesion as that which was just discussed.

As implied earlier in this discussion, we feel that this lesion is a member of the family of histiocytic tumors and pseudotumors. It is important to learn how to differentiate it from malignant lesions, whether epithelial or mesenchymal. The absence of junctional changes, the absence of melanin (the only pigment occasionally present is hemosiderin), and the obvious phagocytic and histiocytic nature of the cells rule out malignant melanoma. Squamous carcinomas with spindle and pleomorphic cell metaplasia likewise do not exhibit the features already mentioned and in addition would show neoplastic changes in the epidermis. More difficult may be the differentiation from malignant

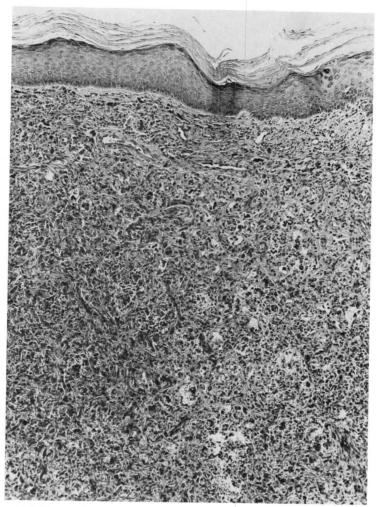

Figure 47–2   Atypical fibroxanthoma of the skin. Note the pleomorphism and hyperchromatism of the nuclei. There are scattered foam cells, some of which also contain phagocytized hemosiderin. *H & E, ×63.*

mesenchymal tumors. Diagnoses of pleomorphic liposarcoma and rhabdomyosarcoma have been occasionally made for these lesions, but the differentiation is easy. Rhabdomyosarcoma should not be diagnosed if no myofibrils and preferably cross-striations are seen. Liposarcomas should have recognizable lipoblasts with signet-ring morphology, myxoid areas, and typical vascular pattern. In addition, these two sarcoma types do not start as skin lesions as a rule.

The only real problem is in differentiating the benign atypical fibroxanthoma from malignant fibrohistiocytoma or malignant fibroxanthoma of the pleomorphic type. Their occurrence on the exposed

skin surface of elderly individuals rather than in the deep soft tissues, the absence of definitely "fibrosarcomatous" areas and generally of storiform arrangement of the spindle cells, the lack of definite histologic agressiveness, even though they lack circumscription, are of great help in making the final decision.

Whether these are true tumors or tumorlike reactive proliferations of histiocytic nature has not been solved. Most of them occur in sun-damaged skin; some have occurred in previously irradiated areas. Kempson and McGavran (1964) mention one case which occurred at the site of a previous surgical procedure and suggest that some of the postirradiation

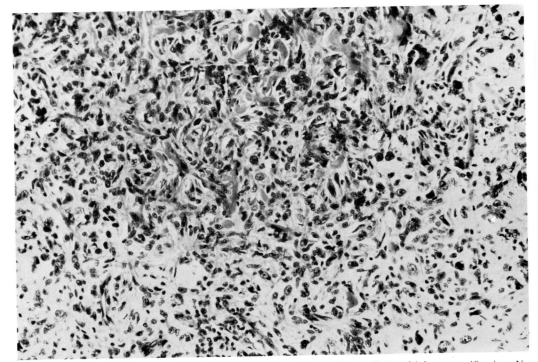

Figure 47–3 Atypical fibroxanthoma of the skin. Same case as in Figure 47–2 at higher magnification. Note suggestion of storiform arrangement of the elongated fibroblast-like histiocytes. In this field, bizarre nuclei and mitoses are rare. *H & E*, ×*160.*

lesions reported by Rachmaninoff et al. (1961) may belong to this category. These features would be consistent with, but not necessarily decisive for, a pseudoneoplastic reactive nature of these lesions. We are not aware that any of the reported cases showed evidence of spontaneous regression, which would be a very convincing argument in favor of their non-neoplastic nature.

The most important point is that the atypical fibroxanthoma is considered by most as a recognizable benign lesion. It is therefore imperative that the pathologists learn its distinguishing features, so that it can be treated by limited local excision.

One hears occasionally of an exceptional instance of malignant behavior of an atypical fibroxanthoma. This writer is not personally familiar with any such case but has observed true malignant fibroxanthomas originating deep to the skin but invading it very early, so as to be occasionally interpreted as a primary skin lesion.

PSEUDOSARCOMATOUS LESIONS FOLLOWING IRRADIATION

Pseudosarcoma Associated With Radiodermatitis

Not infrequently, the dermis and superficial subcutaneous tissues of previously irradiated areas can exhibit either diffuse or nodular thickenings which histologically may contain varying concentrations of anaplastic and bizarre cells (Fig. 47–5). It is easy, therefore, to understand that these lesions are frequently classified as malignant, i.e., some variant of sarcoma, especially if the history of previous irradiation is not available to the pathologist. However, true instances of postirradiation fibrosarcoma have also occasionally been observed (Pettit et al., 1954).

It is generally stated that these lesions are rare, but probably that is not true.

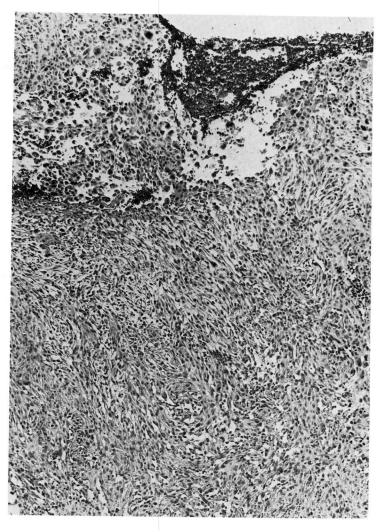

Figure 47–4 Atypical fibroxanthoma of skin of external ear (same case as Figure 47–1). Note the ulcerated surfaces, the predominantly elongated shape of the cells, and the scattered nests of more definitely histiocytic cells with lack of cohesiveness and bizarre nuclei. *H & E, ×63.*

The reason for the discrepancy between the scanty literature and their actual incidence is probably that this entity is still poorly known to the practicing pathologist.

The time interval between irradiation and diagnosis of postirradiation pseudosarcoma varies but is seldom less than five to six years. The doses given vary from small doses intended to treat various benign skin conditions, such as acne or hypertrichosis, to larger doses adequate for the treatment of true skin tumors, such as basal or squamous cell carcinoma, or deep-seated tumors, during which skin damage had occurred.

The diagnosis can be suspected clinically when there is a known history of irradiation associated with the classic signs of radiodermatitis, such as telangiectasia, atrophy of the skin, or hyperkeratosis, and the lesion is detectable as a nodule or a diffuse thickening of the dermis. There are, however, cases in which, even when the history of irradiation, with or without the findings of radiodermatitis, is present, no dermal thickening is palpable. In these instances, the diagnosis can be made only microscopically.

Pathology. When gross changes are present, they consist essentially of more or less discrete fibrous thickenings which can extend toward the subcutaneous tissues and which can resemble hypertrophic scars or keloids. Occasionally, they may result in ulcerated lesions (Fig. 47–6).

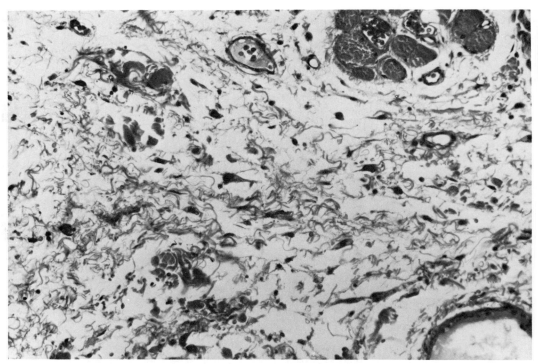

Figure 47–5 Pseudosarcomatous changes in radiated skin. The dermis is edematous and contains irregularly shaped cells with bizarre hyperchromatic nuclei. *H & E, ×160.*

The histologic findings consist essentially of a desmoplastic process associated with bizarre cells with hyperchromatic nuclei. It is probable that these cells are abnormal fibroblasts. There are enormous quantitative variations. At one end of the spectrum only occasional bizarre fibroblasts are found in the damaged, fibrosed, and atrophic skin. At the other end, true "tumors" can be found which are composed of bundles of fibroblastic-like cells, the majority of which are bizarre in shape and vary in size. Stellate-shaped cells are frequent, the nuclei are hyperchromatic, and mitoses are either rare or absent. The ground substance is generally dense collagen, but it might have patchy myxoid areas (Figs. 47–5 and 47–7).

The differential diagnosis with true sarcoma is generally possible, but it is difficult to draw a line between pseudosarcomatous changes in irradiated skin and postirradiation fibromatosis, which is a slowly infiltrating tumor (see next section).

In addition, the problem occasionally arises of differentiating a postirradiation spindle cell carcinoma from a pseudosarcoma. When the overlying epidermis shows no anaplasia, and there is no evidence of a transition between the epidermal cells and the dermal lesion, the differential diagnosis can be made without too much difficulty.

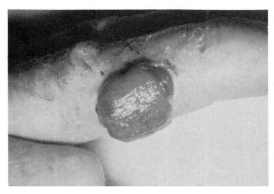

Figure 47–6 Postirradiation pseudosarcomatous ulcerated lesion of lateral aspect of finger in a dentist who used x-ray in his practice for a number of years. It did not recur for four years after excision, at which time he died of unrelated disease. (Courtesy of Dr. R. G. Freeman, Dallas, Texas, and Dr. L. G. Owen, Louisville, Kentucky.) (See also Color Plate VII–E.)

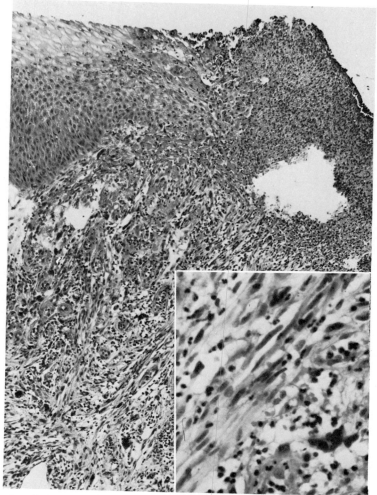

Figure 47-7 Postirradiation pseudosarcoma of skin of finger (same case as in Figure 47-6). Note the hyperplastic epithelium at the margin of the ulcerated lesion. This is essentially granulation tissue containing large numbers of bizarre fibroblasts. *H & E* ×76. Detail at higher magnification. *H & E*, ×240. (Courtesy of Dr. R. G. Freeman, Dallas, Texas, and Dr. L. G. Owen, Louisville, Kentucky.)

The presence of postirradiation pseudosarcomatous dermal changes does not, of course, protect the patient from developing a radiation-induced squamous cell carcinoma. This possibility has been suggested by Rachmaninoff et al. (1961) in their Cases No. 2 and 3. In the Surgical Pathology files of Columbia Presbyterian Medical Center, we have a well-documented example of this possibility. A young physician who had received radiation to the face during adolescence for acne developed a diffuse dermal thickening of the upper lip at age 30, about 11 years postirradiation. This was examined by biopsy and then excised with a nonradical procedure when recognized as a post-irradiation pseudosarcoma (Figs. 47-8 and 47-9). Eight years later, an infiltrating, moderately differentiated, squamous cell carcinoma developed from the skin surface which in the original partial excision showed no neoplastic change.

Postirradiation Fibromatosis

We have discussed the pseudosarcomatous changes associated with radiodermatitis. There is another group of more definitely neoplastic lesions which can occur in the superficial soft tissues, generally just beneath the skin, in areas which have been subjected to irradiation at an

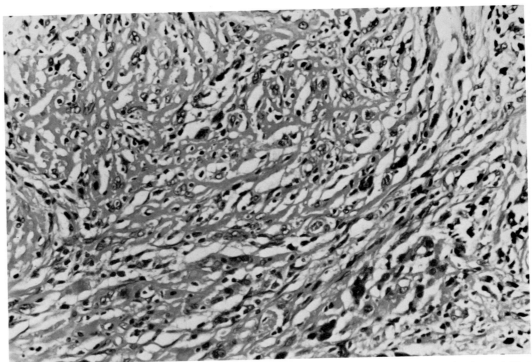

Figure 47–8   Postirradiation pseudosarcomatous fibromatosis of upper lip (clinical information in text). Note the intense collagenization and the bizarre hyperchromatic nuclei. *H & E, ×240.*

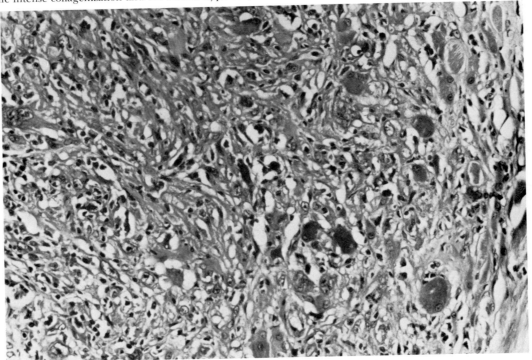

Figure 47–9   Postirradiation pseudosarcomatous fibromatosis of upper lip (same case as in Figure 47–8). The large elements are remnants of skeletal muscle fibers engulfed and replaced by the pseudosarcomatous process. *H & E, ×230.*

the muscular tissues, but frequently palpable as superficial nodules. Swelling and reddening of the overlying skin may occur. According to Enzinger and Dulcey (1967, 33 cases), the median age of the patients was 50 years, and there was a slight predominance of males. One third of Enzinger's cases had a history of trauma. The most common sites are the shoulder and thigh.

Pathologic Findings

Grossly these are poorly circumscribed areas resembling fibrosis of the involved muscle. Histologically (Figs. 47–14 and 47–15) there appears to be an infiltration of the septa between the bundles of striated muscle fibers by a highly cellular proliferation of immature mesenchymal cells, resembling fibroblasts, associated with clusters of large polygonal or elongated cells with basophilic cytoplasm, large nuclei, and prominent nucleoli. Enzinger compares these large cells with ganglion cells or rhabdomyoblasts. Some-

times these cells are so conspicuous in size and number that it is easy to mistake this process for a malignant tumor, such as rhabdomyosarcoma. We have never observed distinct myofibrils or cross-striations in these lesions. Important features which help in the differential diagnosis are: (a) the absence of destruction of the muscle by these proliferating elements, and (b) the resemblance of the fibroblastic-like proliferation to the cellular population seen in the pseudosarcomatous fasciitis. The origin of the ganglion-like or rhabdomyoblast-like cell is uncertain. Enzinger expresses skepticism about their possible rhabdomyoblastic nature, partly because he has also observed them in 12 similar lesions of his series, which were located in the subcutaneous tissue and which he considered "a link with nodular fasciitis." Kern (1960), on the other hand, believes in the rhabdomyoblastic origin of these elements.

In some of the cases which we have observed, there were microscopic fields suggesting a possible origin from the cells of the striated muscle fibers. In addition,

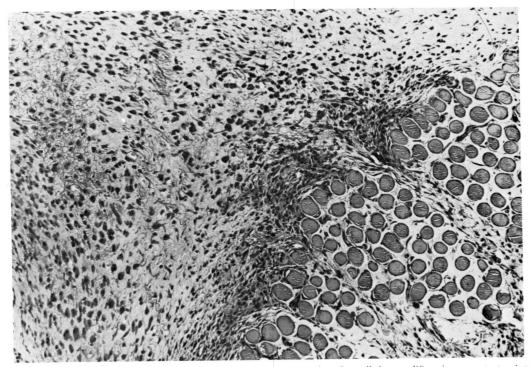

Figure 47–14 Pseudosarcomatous proliferative myositis. Note that the cellular proliferation penetrates into the septa but seldom between individual muscle fibers. The cellular population includes fibroblast-like cells and larger basophilic cells. *H & E, ×90.*

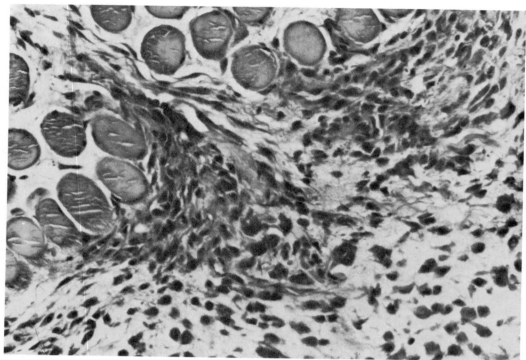

Figure 47–15   Pseudosarcomatous proliferative myositis. Same case as in Figure 47–14 at higher magnification. Note that the large basophilic cells are often concentrated about the sarcolemma of the muscle fibers. *H & E, ×240.*

we have observed microscopic findings in previously traumatized muscular tissue (re-excised biopsy sites) which in our opinion were indistinguishable from proliferative myositis (Fig. 47–16). There is not yet a satisfactory electron microscopic study, which might help in determining the histogenesis of the basophilic cells.

Pathogenesis

It seems highly probable that proliferative myositis is a reaction to injury (trauma, infection, ischemia, and so forth).

Treatment

Limited excision or even partial excision is necessary to establish the diagnosis. The lesion appears to be self-limited, and it probably tends to spontaneous regression.

INFANTILE DIGITAL FIBROMATOSIS

This term and equivalent ones (i.e., recurring digital fibrous tumour of childhood) refer to a rare lesion which, however, has been apparently observed for many years (Sakurane, 1924). The lesion is clinically benign; it occurs in the fingers and toes of infants and young children (Fig. 47–17), presents itself as sometimes conspicuous nodules of fibrous consistency which can be multiple, and has the general histologic pattern of infantile fibromatosis (Fig. 47–18). However, it has the unique feature of containing intracytoplasmic round inclusion bodies, which stain red with methyl green–pyronine stains, and which have been considered by some authors possibly to be of viral origin (Fig. 47–19). These inclusions were first observed by Reye in 1956 and subsequently confirmed by other authors (Shapiro, 1969; Burry et al., 1970). By electron microscopic study (Burry et al.,

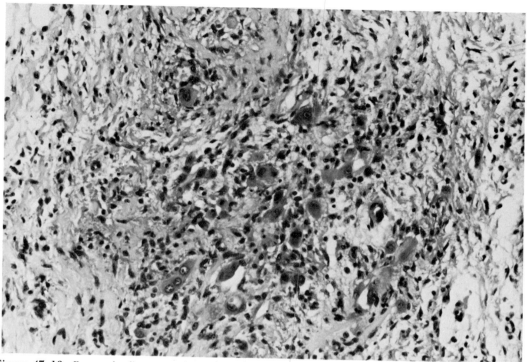

Figure 47–16 Recent healing wound in face, about one week following previous surgery. The large, ganglion-like cells are remnants of striated muscle fibers of the platysma, distorted and engulfed by the reparative process. Note resemblance to proliferative myositis. *H & E, ×160.*

1970), the inclusions within the tumor fibroblasts could be of viral origin, but viral particles were not definitely identified. In addition, these cells contain crystalline bodies of uncertain significance.

Some of these tumors have recurred locally following limited excision, but no cases of metastases are recorded to our knowledge. These clinical pathologic features therefore justify the term fibromatosis.

This rare and interesting tumor has

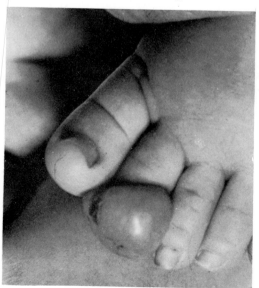

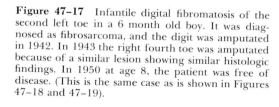

Figure 47–17 Infantile digital fibromatosis of the second left toe in a 6 month old boy. It was diagnosed as fibrosarcoma, and the digit was amputated in 1942. In 1943 the right fourth toe was amputated because of a similar lesion showing similar histologic findings. In 1950 at age 8, the patient was free of disease. (This is the same case as is shown in Figures 47–18 and 47–19).

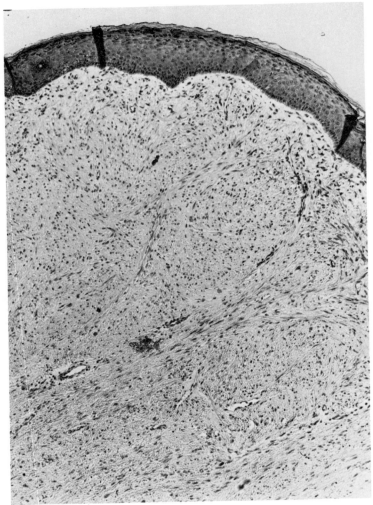

Figure 47–18 Infantile digital fibromatosis (same case as Figure 47–17). Low power view of the fibroma-like tumor. *H & E, ×160.*

been included in this discussion of pseudosarcomatous lesions in order to warn the pathologists and the clinician that, in spite of occasional areas of immaturity in the cell population, its behavior is not that of a true fibrosarcoma, and therefore it should be treated with conservative limited excisions.

FIBROUS HAMARTOMA OF INFANCY

This term was introduced by Enzinger in 1965 to designate a peculiar tumor of uncertain histogenesis, which is generally discovered at birth or during the first year of life, and which presents itself as a palpable mass covered by intact skin and often involving the lower dermis. The most common sites appear to be the axilla and trunk.

These tumors are lobulated and grossly may be mistaken for lipomas or neurofibromas. Some of these tumors at the time of discovery had reached large sizes (up to 8 cm.).

The microscopic features are characteristic (Figs. 47–20 and 47–21). Enzinger described three distinct components: (a) trabeculae of dense fibrous tissue; (b) highly cellular, immature-looking areas,

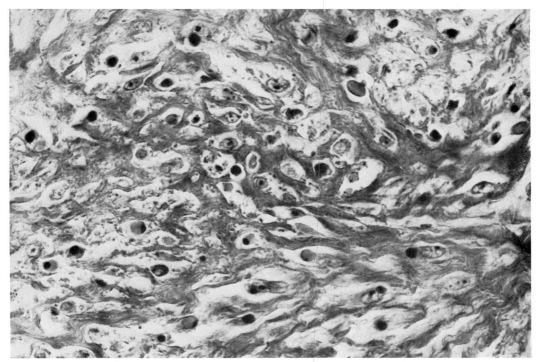

Figure 47–19 Infantile digital fibromatosis (same case as in Figure 47–18) at higher magnification, stained with PTAH. Note the darkly staining spherical bodies, most of which are intracytoplasmic. ×600.

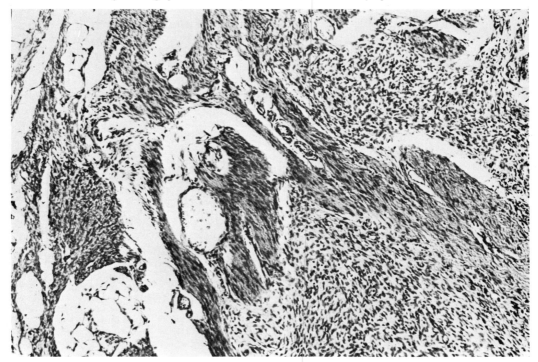

Figure 47–20 Fibrous hamartoma of infancy. Note the bundles of apparently undifferentiated spindle cells, some of which suggest a palisade arrangement of their nuclei. Some fat lobules are seen at left. There were no myofibrils. *H & E*, ×94.

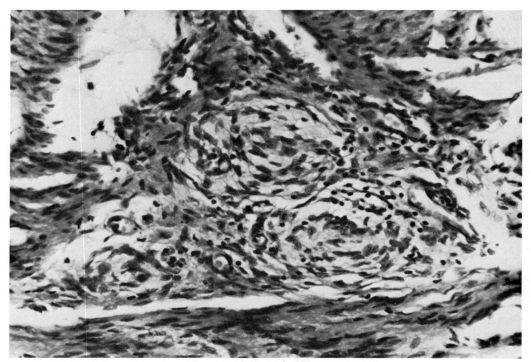

Figure 47–21 Fibrous hamartoma of infancy. Same case as in Figure 47–20. Note the concentric whorls, characteristic of most of these lesions. *H & E, ×240.*

featuring bundles or concentric whorls of undifferentiated small spindle cells of mesenchymal type; and (c) lobules of mature fat. It is the undifferentiated areas which may mislead the pathologist into a diagnosis of malignancy (fibrosarcoma, neurogenic sarcoma, embryonal rhabdomyosarcoma, and so forth). Probably more often "benign" diagnoses, such as neurofibroma, neurolipoma, and benign mesenchymoma, have been suggested in the past. The histogenesis of these lesions is obscure. We agree with Enzinger that it is unlikely that these are just an expression of a reparative phenomenon. Whether they are true neoplasms or congenital malformations (where do we draw the line?) is probably a question of semantics.

These are rare lesions but probably not exceptional. Most likely in the past they were classified either among the infantile fibromatoses (Stout, 1954, Case No. 28) or as infantile fibrosarcoma, neurofibroma-like lesions, or benign mesenchymomas (Reye, 1956; Mackenzie, 1970, p. 101, Ref. 41; Lattes and Enzinger, 1968).

The most important point is that this is a characteristic lesion, easy to recognize, and absolutely benign. Of the 30 cases analyzed by Enzinger, 25 were followed for from eight months to nine years. The treatment apparently was always a limited, and sometimes incomplete, excision. Four cases required re-excision, apparently because of original inadequate removal. Since these lesions are apparently exclusive of infancy and childhood, it is interesting to speculate on the possibility of their spontaneous regression in older age groups. There is, however, no documented proof, because all the cases studied had been excised rather than diagnosed by incisional biopsy.

SUMMARY

In this chapter the writer has discussed in some detail a few lesions of the skin and superficial soft tissues, which are biologically and clinically benign but which, because of their apparent microscopic immaturity or anaplasia, are still mistakenly

Text continued on page 1101.

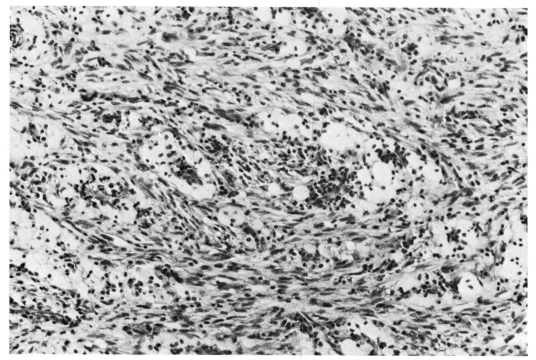

Figure 47–22 Subcutaneous xanthogranuloma surrounding a large abscess in the thigh. The "tumor" disappeared after surgical drainage. Note the fibrosarcoma-like bundles associated with giant cells, some of which have foamy cytoplasm and collections of inflammatory cells. *H & E, ×160.*

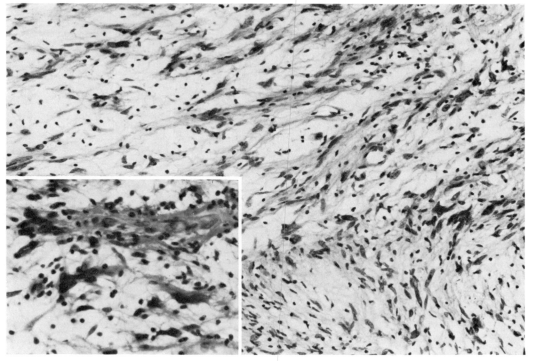

Figure 47–23 Subcutaneous neurofibroma, showing bizarre nuclei associated with myxoid changes in ground substance. *H & E, ×160.* Insert shows details of bizarre Schwann cell nuclei. *×240.*

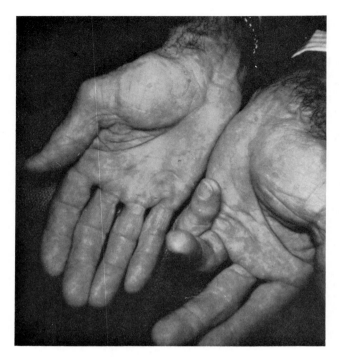

Figure 47–24 Palmar fibromatosis in a case of Dupuytren's contracture. Pseudo-neoplastic nodules in the palmar aponeurosis can become adherent to the overlying dermis. This is a lesion which seldom, if ever, extends beyond the palmar aponeurosis. Analogous lesions occur in the plantar aponeurosis. (Courtesy of Dr. R. Lagier, Geneva, Switzerland.)

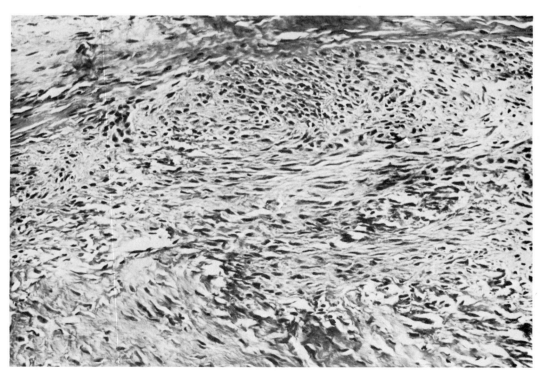

Figure 47–25 Pseudosarcomatous area in palmar fibromatosis in a case of Dupuytren's contracture (see also Fig. 47–24). Note the focus of active fibroblastic proliferation surrounded by mature aponeurotic tissue. *H & E, ×160.*

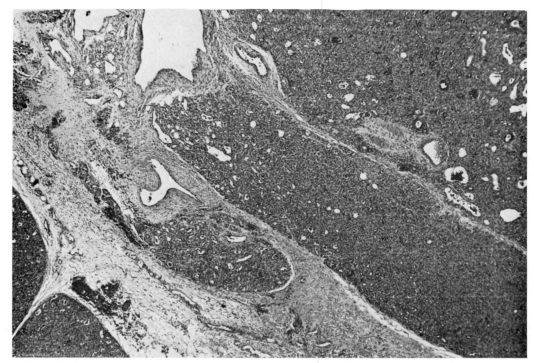

Figure 47–26   Benign infantile hemangioendothelioma of parotid region. Note the pseudoinvasive pattern of this diffuse vascular proliferation. *H & E*, *×30*.

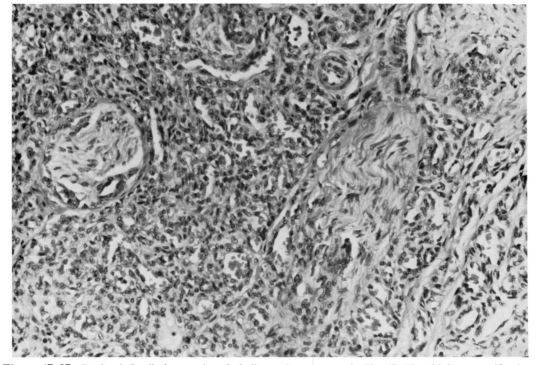

Figure 47–27   Benign infantile hemangioendothelioma. Same case as in Fig. 47–26 at higher magnification. Note the nerve trunks surrounded by the benign capillary proliferation. This is not to be confused with angiosarcoma. *H & E*, *×180*.

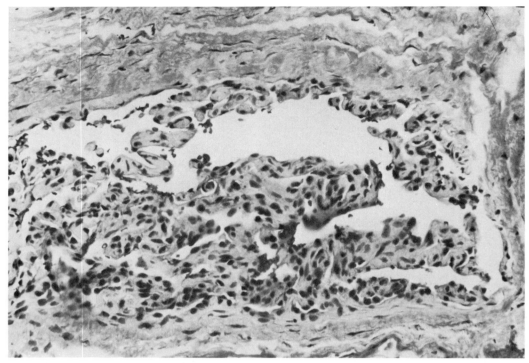

Figure 47–28   Pseudoneoplastic endothelial proliferation in traumatized blood vessel in palm of hand (see Masson, 1923). *H & E, ×224.*

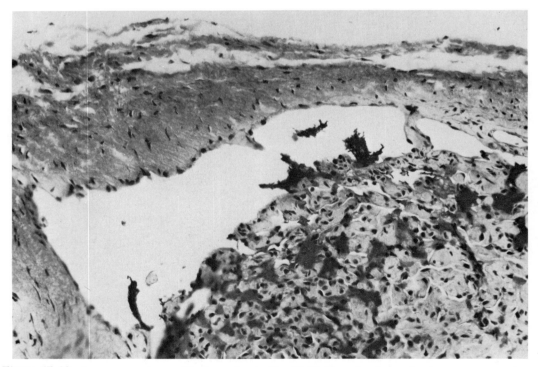

Figure 47–29   Same case and same blood vessel as in Fig. 47–28. Note the obvious benign appearance of the hyperplastic cells in the organizing thrombus. *H & E, ×160.*

diagnosed as "sarcomatous" with a certain frequency. They were selected among a larger number of analogous problems because in our experience, based on our consultation practice, they are those which most frequently mislead the hospital pathologist and occasionally the clinician.

There are of course other better known benign tumors and pseudotumors which may exhibit proliferation of immature or bizarre cells or infiltrative behavior or both, and for this reason they might be referred to as "pseudosarcoma."

Among them we will list briefly the "reticulohistiocytic granuloma" of the skin (Purvis and Helwig, 1954); the xanthogranulomatous lesions of the subcutaneous tissues (Oberling, 1935; Smetana and Bernhard, 1950) (Fig. 47–22); the benign neurofibromas with bizarre hyperchromatic nuclei (Fig. 47–23); the plantar and palmar fibromatosis (Figs. 47–24 and 47–25); the benign infantile hemangioendotheliomas (Figs. 47–26 and 47–27); and the pseudohemangioendotheliomatous proliferations in thrombosed superficial veins (Masson, 1923) (Figs. 47–28 and 47–29). The reader can easily find adequate discussions of the lesions listed above in the references which follow this chapter.

In closing, it is well to re-emphasize that, even though we still do not understand adequately the etiology and pathogenesis of the majority of these conditions, we have now acquired the empirical knowledge which enables us to recognize them as benign or outright harmless lesions. A correct diagnosis will save many patients from unnecessary radical procedures and mental anguish, while at the same time reducing the number of miraculous "cures" of "sarcomas" in some surgical or radiotherapeutic series.

REFERENCES

Benatre, A., Brizon, J., Pelletier, J., and Johard, P.: Fibroxanthome atypique de la peau et des parties molles. Arch. Anat. Pathol. (Paris), 15:242, 1967.

Bourne, R. J.: Paradoxical fibrosarcoma of the skin. Med. J. Aust., 1:504, 1963.

Burry, A. F., Kerr, J. F. R., and Pope, J. H.: Recurring digital fibrous tumour of childhood; an electronmicroscopic and virological study. Pathology, 2:287, 1970.

Caro, M., and Stubenrauch, C. H.: Hemangioendothelioma of the skin. Arch. Dermatol. Syph. (Berl.), 51:295, 1945.

Conley, J., Orr, W., and Lattes, R.: Desmoplastic malignant melanoma (a rare variant of spindle cell melanoma). Cancer, 28:914, 1971.

Enzinger, F. M.: Fibrous hamartoma of infancy. Cancer, 18:241, 1965.

Enzinger, F. M., and Dulcey, F.: Proliferative myositis: Report of 33 cases. Cancer, 20:2213, 1967.

Enzinger, F. M., Lattes, R., and Torloni, H.: Histologic Typing of Soft Tissue Tumors (International Classification of Tumours #3). Geneva, World Health Organization, 1969.

Finlay-Jones, L. R., Nicoll, P., and Ten Seldam, R. E. J.: Pseudosarcoma of the skin. Pathology, 3:215, 1971.

Fritsch, P., and Schellander, F.: Zum Problem der Malignitat histiocytarer Tumoren "fibrous xanthoma." Hautarzt, 21:107, 1970.

Gordon, H. W.: Pseudo-sarcomatous reticulohistiocytoma. Arch. Dermatol., 90:319, 1964.

Harkin, J. C., and Reed, R. J.: Tumors of the peripheral nervous system. Atlas of Tumor Pathology, Second Series, Fascicle 3. Washington, D. C., Armed Forces Institute of Pathology, 1969.

Helwig, E. B., and Hackney, V. C.: Juvenile xanthogranuloma (naevo-xanthoendothelioma). Am. J. Pathol., 30:625, 1954.

Hoede, N., and Karting, G. W.: Pseudosarcomatoses xanthofibrom. Arch. Klin. Exp. Dermatol., 232:119, 1968.

Hutter, R. V. P., Stewart, F. W., and Foote, F. W., Jr.: Fasciitis: a report of 70 cases with follow-up proving the benignity of the lesion. Cancer, 15:992, 1962.

Kay, S.: Subcutaneous pseudosarcomatous fibromatosis. Am. J. Clin. Pathol., 33:433, 1960.

Kempson, R. L., and McGavran, M. H.: Atypical fibroxanthoma of the skin. Cancer, 17:1463, 1964.

Kern, W. H.: Proliferative myositis—A pseudo-sarcomatous reaction to injury. Arch. Pathol., 69:209, 1960.

Konwaler, B. E., Keasbey, L., and Kaplan, L.: Subcutaneous pseudosarcomatous fibromatosis (fasciitis). Am. J. Clin. Pathol., 25:241, 1955.

Kroe, D. J., and Pitcock, J. A.: Atypical fibroxanthoma of the skin. Am. J. Clin. Pathol., 51:487, 1969.

Lane, N.: Pseudo-sarcoma (polypoid sarcoma-like masses) associated with squamous cell carcinoma of the mouth, fauces and larynx. Cancer, 10:19, 1957.

Lattes, R., and Enzinger, F.: Tumors and tumor-like lesions of soft tissues. Accademia Nazionale dei Lincei 367, Quad. #135, 390–429, 1968.

Levan, N. E., Hirsch, P., and Kwong, M. Q.: Pseudosarcomatous dermatofibroma. Arch. Dermatol., 88:908, 1963.

Mackenzie, D. H.: The Differential Diagnosis of Fibroblastic Disorders. Oxford, Blackwell Scientific Publications, 1970.

Martin, H. E., and Stewart, F. W.: Spindle cell epidermoid carcinoma. Am. J. Cancer, 25:273, 1935.

Masson, P.: Hemangioendothelioma vegetant intravasculaire. Bull. Soc. Anat. Paris, 93:517, 1923.

Oberling, C.: Retroperitoneal xanthogranuloma. Am. J. Cancer, 23:477, 1935.

Pettit, V. D., Chamness, J. T., and Ackerman, L. V.: Fibromatosis and fibrosarcoma following irradiation. Cancer, 7:149, 1954.

Pickren, J. W., et al.: Fibromatosis of the plantar fascia. Cancer, 4:846, 1951.

Pohjanpelto, P., Ahlquist, J., Hurme, K., and Hjelt, L.: Recurrent digital fibrous tumor of childhood. 2: Isolation of a cell transforming agent. Acta Pathol. Microbiol. Scand., 70:297, 1967.

Purvis, W. E., III, and Helwig, E. B.: Reticulohistiocytic granuloma ("reticulohistiocytoma") of the skin. Am. J. Clin. Pathol., 24:1005, 1954.

Rachmaninoff, N., McDonald, J. R., and Cook, J. C.: Sarcoma-like tumors of the skin following irradiation. Am. J. Clin. Pathol., 36:427, 1961.

Reye, R. D. K.: Considerations on certain subdermal "fibromatous tumors" of infancy. J. Pathol. Bacterial., 72:149, 1956.

Rosai, J., and Akerman, L . R.: Intravenous atypical vascular proliferations. Arch. Dermatol., 109:714, 1974.

Rose, A. G.: An electron microscopic study of the giant cells in proliferative myositis. Cancer, 33:1543, 1974.

Sakurane, K.: A case of fibroma durum multiplex in the tip of fingers and toes of an infant. Jap. J. Dermatol., 24:8, 1974.

Samitz, M. H.: Pseudosarcoma—Pseudomalignant neoplasm as a consequence of radiodermatitis. Arch. Dermatol., 96:283, 1967.

Shapiro, L.: Infantile digital fibromatosis and aponeurotic fibroma. Arch. Dermatol., 99:37, 1969.

Sims, C. F., and Kirsch, N.: Spindle cell epidermoid epithelioma simulating sarcoma in chronic radiodermatitis. Arch. Dermatol. Syph. (Berl.), 57:63, 1948.

Smetana, H. F., and Bernhard, W.: Sclerosing lipogranuloma. Arch. Pathol., 50:296, 1950.

Stout, A. P.: Juvenile fibromatosis. Cancer, 7:953, 1954.

Stout, A. P.: Pseudosarcomatous fasciitis in children. Cancer, 14:1216, 1961.

Stout, A. P., and Lattes, R.: Tumors of the Soft Tissues. Atlas of Tumor Pathology, Second Series Fascicle #1. Washington, D.C., Armed Forces Institute of Pathology, 1967.

Tapernoux, B., et al.: Atypical fibroxanthoma. Dermatologica, 142:93, 1971.

Toker, C.: Pseudo-sarcomatous fasciitis—Further observations indicating the aggressive capabilities of this lesion, and justifying the inclusion of this entity within the category of the fibromatoses. Ann. Surg., 174:994, 1971.

Von Moss, F.: Hautsarkom nach Roentgen-bestrahlung. Schweiz. Med. Wochenschr., 82:179, 1952.

Warren, S.: The pathological effects of small doses of radiation. Bull. N.Y. Acad. Med., 34:633, 1958.

48

Less Common Malignant Skin Tumors

Howard J. Kesseler, M.D., and Charles F. Schetlin, M.D.

Any one of the soft somatic tissue tumors demands a critical evaluation of all factors relating to the tumor and the patient before embarking upon a therapeutic plan.

The soft somatic tissues constitute over 50 percent of the body weight and are composed of connective tissue, blood and lymphatic vessels, smooth and striated muscles, fat, fascia, synovial structures, and reticuloendothelium.

Of the great numbers and different varieties of these tumors, both benign and malignant, this discussion will include the following six less commonly found malignant skin tumors: the leiomyosarcoma, the neurofibrosarcoma, the malignant granular cell myoblastoma, the liposarcoma, the hemangioendothelioma, and the lymphangiosarcoma (postmastectomy).

LEIOMYOSARCOMA

Malignant smooth muscle tumors of the skin are, indeed, rare in occurrence. Of 1567 cases of primary superficial malig-
nant tumors of the skin studied at Columbia University, only 2.3 percent were leiomyosarcomas (Stout and Hill, 1958). Therefore, during the course of a busy tumor surgeon's experience, he may see this lesion only once or twice.

Leiomyomas of the skin occur four times as frequently as do the leiomyosarcomas. The benign tumor may mimic the malignant variety, and therefore the important differential diagnosis must be made.

Clinical Features

Age. Stout and Hill (1958) collected 35 cases of superficial leiomyosarcoma. The youngest patient was a 5 month old girl; the oldest patient was a woman, aged 84. The age distributions for both leiomyoma and leiomyosarcoma are similar, with the peak incidence occurring in the third decade.

Sex. The leiomyosarcoma is found slightly more frequently in females, although the number of cases is small.

1103

Clinical Description

Leiomyosarcomas can occur anywhere on the skin surface of the body. There is some tendency for the tumors to appear in greater numbers in those areas where the leiomyoma may occur; however, this is not necessarily a feature of the tumor.

Several points in the differential diagnosis between the leiomyoma and the leiomyosarcoma should be made for a clearer understanding of both.

The *leiomyoma* occurs primarily on the exposed surfaces of the body, where the hair distribution is greatest (Montgomery and Winkelmann, 1963). The tumors also occur in the folds of the skin of the groin, genitalia, and axilla (Fox, 1960). The leiomyoma is characteristically painful and sometimes pruritic (Saunders and Fitzpatrick, 1956).

The lesions are frequently multiple, and they are found in groups rather than being scattered. The multiple nodules occur most commonly on the extensor surfaces of the body. The tumors of the scrotum, genitalia, breast, and axilla are usually single and may be nodular. The tumor arises directly in the corium and presents as a slightly raised nodule, usually less than 2.5 cm. in diameter, which is sometimes reddish in hue. Vermiform movements have been noted in these lesions.

The leiomyosarcoma is typically single (Levack and Dick, 1955; Kilgour, 1955). The tumor is hard in consistency and is generally larger than 2.5 cm. in diameter. It arises chiefly within the subcutaneous tissue. The lesion is usually neither painful nor tender and, therefore, essentially asymptomatic unless there has been invasion of the deeper structures of the area.

Color changes are not a characteristic of the malignant tumor. Clinically, it is difficult to differentiate the leiomyosarcoma from other superficial soft tissue sarcomas.

The most important gross feature of the leiomyosarcoma which differentiates it from the leiomyoma is that the tumor is larger than 2.5 cm. in diameter; if it is less than 2.5 cm., it is most likely benign.

Four cases of leiomyosarcomas were noted in Negroes in the 35 cases studied by Stout and Hill (1958).

Pathology

The leiomyosarcoma presents as an irregular nodule, which lies primarily under the corium and has no true capsule.

Microscopically, the leiomyosarcoma resembles the leiomyoma. They both show myofibrils and palisading. In the leiomyosarcoma there is frequently blunting of the nuclei, bizarre cells are seen, and anaplasia appears to be a feature. The presence of mitosis is considered to be the most important differentiation between the leiomyosarcoma and the leiomyoma (Stout and Lattes, 1967b). If mitoses are seen at an average rate of one or more in every five high-power fields, then the tumor must be considered malignant (Fig. 48–1).

The histochemical reaction is of some importance in the differentiation of the smooth muscle tumors from tumors of neurogenous origin; however, the staining techniques are not pathognomonic. Montgomery and Winkelmann (1963) found that the Gomori resorcinol-fuchsin stain for leastic tissue and the Gomori re-

Figure 48–1 Leiomyosarcoma. This 80 year old male was first seen on 3/9/70 with a two-year history of a painless, growing mass located in the posterior left mid-thoracic region. Also noted was a small mass in the left axilla. Physical examination revealed a 10 × 10 cm. mass in the left mid-thoracic region, and a 2.5 cm. lymph node in the left axilla, considered metastatic. On 4/28/70, an incisional biopsy was performed with a proved diagnosis of leiomyosarcoma. On 5/5/70, a wide excision of the left thoracic area was performed with a split-thickness skin graft. On 5/22/70, a radical left axillary dissection was performed. In January, 1971, there was widespread metastasis to the lungs, pleura, and bones. The patient died 2/28/71.

A, Clinical photograph demonstrating the mass in the mid-thoracic region.

B, Leiomyosarcoma invading the dermis. × 50. *Inset*, Bizarre nature of the tumor. The cells show their smooth muscle origin in some areas; bizarre hyperchromatic and pleomorphic nuclei are apparent in other areas. × 260. (Courtesy of Dr. Sheldon Sommers.)

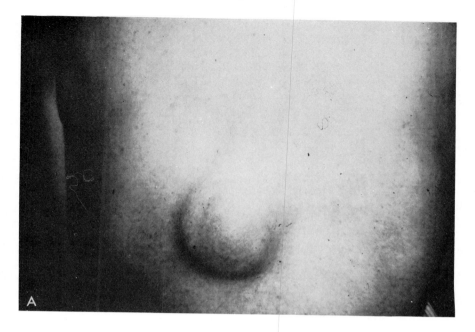

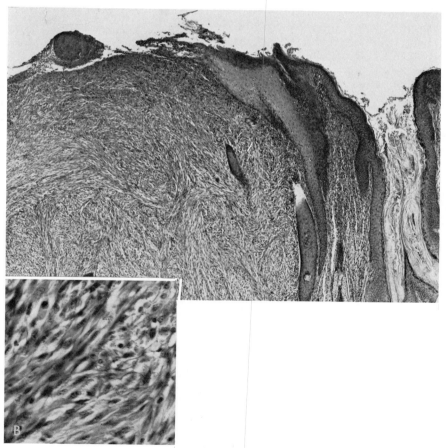

Figure 48–1.

ticulum stain were of some use in the above differentiation. Niemi and colleagues (1964) demonstrated the value of determining the phosphorylase activity in the neoplastic smooth cells, and found this activity to be much greater in the leiomyoma than in the neurogenic tumor.

Clinical Course

Approximately one-third of the leiomyosarcomas have a history of less than six months in duration (Stout and Hill, 1958). Some of the leiomyosarcomas have a long relatively slow growth, with a lapse of from two to three years between the onset of the disease and the first treatment. Local recurrences are frequent because the tumors usually have been treated initially by conservative excision. Metastasis occurs primarily via the blood stream and to the lungs rather early in the course of the disease.

In a series of 35 cases, 58 percent of the patients had generalized metastases at death (Stout and Hill, 1958). There may be metastasis to the regional lymph nodes in the larger lesions, but this is not a clinical feature of most of the malignant tumors (Rising and Booth, 1966).

Treatment

Wide local excision is the preferred method of treatment after adequate diagnosis of leiomyosarcoma has been established by biopsy. A wide local excision must be carried out to prevent local recurrence. A regional lymph node dissection is not done routinely unless the lymph nodes are clinically evident and no distant metastases are demonstrated. If the tumor is in a node-bearing area, such as the neck or axilla, a regional dissection may be included in the initial excisional therapy of the tumor. Amputation may be considered necessary if a wide local excision necessitates the sacrifice of bone.

Summary

The results of therapy are difficult to evaluate since the number of patients is small. These tumors are aggressive and metastasize early in approximately 60 percent of cases. Treatment must be early and adequate.

NEUROFIBROSARCOMA

The neurofibrosarcoma is a malignant tumor of nerve sheath origin. It is derived from the Schwann cell and not from the nerve cell itself. Because the Schwann cell can dedifferentiate into many forms, much confusion as to terminology has existed in the literature. Malignant neurilemoma, malignant schwannoma, fibrosarcoma of nerve sheath, malignant peripheral glioma, myxosarcoma of nerve sheath, neurilemosarcoma, and secondary malignant neuroma are all synonyms for the neurofibrosarcoma (Harken and Reed, 1969).

The neurofibrosarcoma is most commonly associated with preexisting multiple neurofibromatosis (von Recklinghausen's disease). However, there are some malignant nerve sheath tumors which are thought to be derived from isolated, benign tumors of the sheath, or to arise from nerves where no previously existing tumor has been demonstrated. The malignant transformation of benign nerve sheath tumors remains a subject of controversy because of the association of the two diseases, particularly in the multiple neurofibromatosis group. However, this transformation has not been proved and has been questioned by many authors (D'Agostino et al., 1963). It is probable that the neurofibrosarcoma begins as a malignant tumor, which may demonstrate increasing differentiation as either the clinical course progresses or metastases develop.

Clinical Features

The incidence of neurofibrosarcoma is about 5 percent in all cases of neurofibromatosis (Stout, 1949).

Age and Sex. The neurofibrosarcoma associated with multiple neurofibromatosis is a tumor of the young adult, occurring at a mean age of 28 years, as noted in

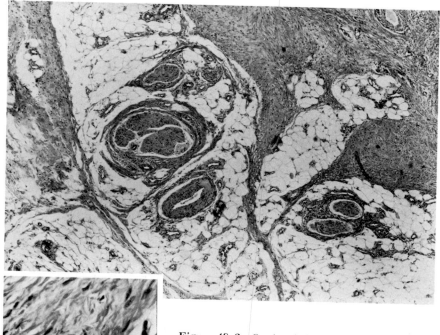

Figure 48–3 *Continued. B,* Well-differentiated neurofibrosarcoma invading dermal fat with perineural involvement. *×50. Inset,* Well-differentiated nerve sheath cells with palisading, occasional bizarre cells with hyperchromatic nuclei. *×500.* (Courtesy of Dr. Sheldon Sommers.)

were studied and reclassified as either nonchromaffin paragangliomas or rhabdomyosarcomas. The histologic differentiation of these tumors is, at best, difficult. The clinical course is more definitive and serves to help identify the malignant granular cell myoblastoma.

Clinical Features

Age and Sex. The distinct rarity of these lesions mitigates any accurate appraisal of age and sex incidence. The tumors occur in young adults with about equal sex distribution.

Clinical Description

The malignant granular cell myoblastoma occurs most frequently in the head and neck region (Crawford and DeBakey,

1953; Allkek et al., 1968). The malignant form of the disease appears to have no predilection for any site. The tumors have been located anywhere on the skin and adnexae, as well as in the bladder, the breast, the vulva, and the gastrointestinal tract. Most malignant granular cell myoblastomas are seen in the subcutaneous tissue. The tumor is frequently painful. The borders are somewhat ill-defined, and attachment to the skin is common (Sadler and Dockerty, 1951; Ross et al., 1952; Svejda and Horn, 1958; Sobel and Churg, 1964; Salvadori and Talamazzi, 1967; Radman and Bhagavan, 1969).

There appear to be two distinct types of malignant granular cell myoblastomas (Gamboa, 1955). The first group, taken from the literature from 1945 to 1955, was classified as "clinically malignant and histologically benign." The average age in this group of patients was 31 years. These tumors were generally about 9 cm. in diameter. Of the six cases in this group, five were females. Four patients were Negroes and two were white. These tumors were not encapsulated and were fixed to the surrounding structures early in the course of the disease. Generally, the patient was asymptomatic. Extensive metastasis occurred within three years after onset of the disease, even though the tumors were histologically benign, proving their malignant tendency.

The second group of five patients, taken from the literature from 1948 to 1952, was classified as "clinically and histologically malignant" (Gamboa, 1955). The average age in this group was 47 years. Two were male and three were female. The average size of the tumors was 3.6 cm. in diameter. The tumors were not encapsulated, and the cut surface was firm and grayish white, similar to the first group. The lesions were found to be locally infiltrating and sometimes painful. The clinical course may be aggressive with early metastasis.

Histogenesis

The histogenesis of the granular cell lesion is controversial. Abrikossoff (1926) first described the lesion and proposed its origin from striated muscle. This thesis was borne out by tissue culture techniques performed by Murray (1951), who demonstrated the morphologic similarity of the tumor cells to striated muscle. Further investigation suggested that the granular appearance of the cell might be degenerative rather than myoblastic, and that these tumors were not of muscle origin. This impression gained support by the fact that the majority of the myoblastomas occurred in the skin, breast, gallbladder, and gastrointestinal tract. None of these areas has striated muscle. Considerable evidence accumulated which suggested that the granular cell was of nerve origin (Fust and Custer, 1949; Ashburn and Rodger, 1952). The histogenesis of the granular cell myoblastoma has been studied by numerous investigators who have demonstrated that the lesion arises

frequently in peripheral nerves (Bangle, 1953). Bangle (1952) also demonstrated, by histochemical techniques, that the granules in the cells were similar to those seen in degenerating myelin. Fisher and Wechsler (1962) studied the myoblastoma both histochemically and by electron microscopy. Their studies further substantiated the theory of the Schwann cell derivation of this tumor.

The clinical course of these tumors has been noted to be similar to that of the fibrous xanthomas and histiocytomas (Kauffman and Stout, 1961a). Gamboa (1955) also found the similarity and separated the group of tumors which he termed "clinically malignant, histologically benign." The preponderance of evidence suggests that the cell origin of the malignant granular cell myoblastoma is either neural or fibrocytic, and that it is not a tumor derived from striated muscle.

Pathology

The gross appearance of the malignant granular cell myoblastoma shows that it is neither encapsulated nor locally infiltrating. It arises within the subcutaneous tissues and quickly involves the deep structures. The cut surface of the tumor usually shows no evidence of necrosis, and is solid, firm and grayish white. Microscopically, the "clinically malignant, histologically benign" type of tumor shows a pattern of cells indistinguishable from the granular cell myoblastoma. On close inspection, however, mytoses and bizarre cells are occasionally seen, and the cytoplasm is extensively granular. In this group of tumors the diagnosis of malignancy is made by the establishment of metastasis to the lymph nodes via the blood stream.

The appearance of the "clinically and histologically malignant" type of tumor is similar to that of the benign granular cell myoblastoma. However, the presence of pleomorphism, mitotic figures, bizarre cells, depolarization of cells, and lack of granularity in the cytoplasm of many of the cells serves to differentiate this lesion from the benign variety (Fig. 48–4).

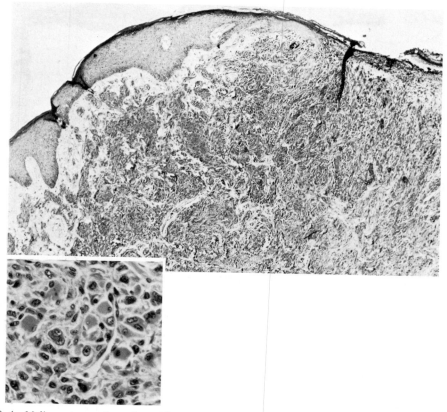

Figure 48–4   Malignant granular cell myoblastoma. This section demonstrates ulceration of the skin by a tumor growing through the top. Dermal fat is invaded by the tumor under the intact skin with some proliferation of the epithelium over the tumor, as noted with granular cell myoblastomas. ×50. *Inset,* Bizarre cells with notably variable granular cells, some with atypical giant nucleoli and mitoses. ×500. (Courtesy of Dr. Sheldon Sommers.)

Treatment

After excisional biopsy is performed as the initial procedure, the treatment of choice is wide local excision of the primary tumor plus dissection of the regional lymph nodes when early metastasis is suspected. This may be done in continuity with the primary lesion if the location of the tumor is favorable. Radiation therapy has virtually no effect on either the primary tumor or on metastatic spread.

Summary

In histologically benign and malignant granular cell myoblastomas, the prognosis is the same; the patients are dead of generalized metastases within five years. Metastasis to the regional lymph nodes, the lungs, the liver, and the bones occurs in that order.

LIPOSARCOMA

The liposarcoma is not a true tumor of the skin but rather a tumor of the soft somatic tissues. Although the liposarcoma is not the most common malignant soft tissue tumor, it is, perhaps, the most important, since prompt diagnosis and adequate therapy should result in a relatively high salvage rate. The presence of multiple lipomas appears to have no relationship to the incidence of liposarcoma.

Clinical Features

Age and Sex.   The liposarcoma occurs primarily after the age of 40, although

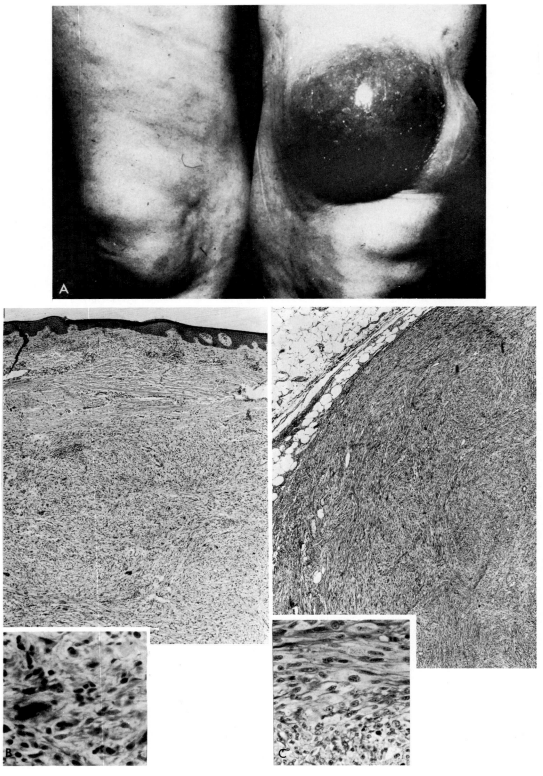

Figure 48–5   *Illustration and legend continued on opposite page.*

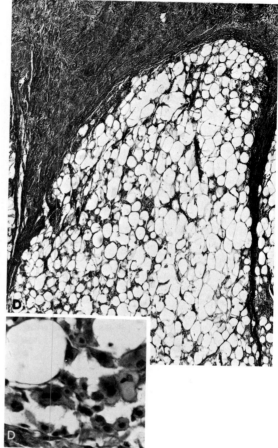

Figure 48–5 Liposarcoma.

A, Liposarcoma of skin just above the knee, present for two years. Note hemorrhage into skin and necrosis in tumor. Deep component of lesion is apparent laterally.

B, Section of skin showing invasion of dermal fat by the tumor with stretching of the overlying epidermis. ×50. *Inset*, Section of the tumor with extremely undifferentiated cells, a few of which are vacuolated, indicating lipoblastic origin. ×500.

C, The tumor at its periphery invading the neighboring subcutaneous tissue. The pseudocapsule of the lesion is evident, within which is a solid cellular proliferation. ×50. *Inset*. The cells in this lesion are well differentiated for the most part. Cytoplasmic vacuoles are present in some areas of the tumor. ×500.

D, Section within the tumor demonstrating mature cells and lipoblasts. ×50. *Inset*, Lipoblasts in various stages of partial or complete maturation with abundant, slightly granular cytoplasm. ×500. (Courtesy of Department of Dermatology, New York University Medical Center.)

tumors have been reported in children (Kauffman and Stout, 1959). The tumor occurs more frequently in males than in females.

Clinical Description

The liposarcoma presents a large asymptomatic mass. It is more firm in consistency than the lipoma, and local infiltration is present early, as is fixation to the skin. The tumor is among the largest recorded, with lesions of 32 kg. in weight being reported; the majority weighed 3 kg. (Wells, 1940). The largest tumors have been found in the retroperitoneum. The tumors of the thigh and gluteal region tend to be smaller in size, probably because they are diagnosed and treated earlier.

Pathology

The gross pathology of the liposarcoma is characterized by the large size of the tumor surrounded by a pseudocapsule. The tumor infiltrates locally. On cut surface, the tumor is predominantly yellow in color, with areas of necrosis and hemorrhage being evident in the more aggressive lesions.

Microscopically, there are two types of lesions. One is the well-differentiated tumor which is either embryonal or myxoid in type, and the other is the poorly differentiated lesion composed of mixed lipoblastic cells, round cells, and bizarre cells (Fig. 48–5).

Clinical Course

Liposarcoma can occur anywhere in the body. Stout (1944) found the most common site to be the lower extremity, especially the thigh. The skin over the lesions becomes secondarily involved. The tumor is asymptomatic until there is invasion of the deep structures. The rate of growth is variable. When rapid growth does occur, there may be metastasis and death within six months of diagnosis. However, the majority of the liposarcomas have a slow, asymptomatic growth which may extend over a period of 16 years, with excision of multiple recurrences during this period (Stout and Lattes, 1967a).

Some liposarcomas are multicentric in origin (Enterline et al., 1960). When dealing with liposarcomas located in several areas of the body at one time, one must differentiate between lesions of multicentric origin and metastases (Ackerman, 1944). Experience has shown the lesions of multicentric origin to have a better prognosis than those which are metastatic. Metastasis may be to the lungs, the liver, and the pleura, and it occurs in 40 percent of the cases. Metastasis in children is a rare occurrence.

Treatment

Incisional biopsy should be used to establish the diagnosis in the suspected case, and then definitive wide local excision should be done as the initial curative procedure. Regional lymph node metastases are uncommon; therefore, lymph node dissections are not recommended. The amputation of an affected limb should be performed in those clinical situations where the wide local excision requires the sacrifice of bone. Radiation therapy has yielded some results insofar as palliation is concerned, but it is not recommended as a primary mode of therapy. To date, chemotherapy has demonstrated no role in the treatment of liposarcoma.

Summary

In the series of 53 cases of liposarcoma (Enterline et al., 1960), the overall survival without evidence of residual tumor was 32 percent at five years and 28 percent at 10 years. Survival was much higher for patients with the purely myxoid type (57 percent and 66 percent) than for those with the nonmyxoid and mixed types (12.5 percent and 8.3 percent). Many patients with the myxoid type have survived many years with known tumor.

HEMANGIOENDOTHELIOMA

The classification of tumors of blood vessel origin has been confusing, stimulated entirely by the multiplicity of clinical characteristics of these lesions. Some of the tumors are primary in the blood vessels, such as the hemangioma and the hemangioendothelioma. Some of the tumors involve the blood vessels secondarily, such as Kaposi's hemorrhagic sarcoma, the hypernephroma, and the choriocarcinoma.

The hemangioendothelioma, first described by Mallory (1908), is a malignant tumor of the blood vessels featuring a proliferation of the vascular endothelial cells. The clinical characteristics of the tumor are varied, with the tumor appearing in many forms. The microscopic appearance is pathognomonic. If the strict criteria, as detailed by Stout (1943), are applied, then identification is positive and excludes lesions which may be clinically similar.

In reviewing 118 lesions which were said to be malignant vascular tumors, only 65 percent were truly vascular in origin (Stout, 1943).

Clinical Features

Age and Sex. The great majority of the lesions developed in adults, and only nine cases were in children under the age of 16 (Kauffman and Stout, 1961b). In 1967, Stout personally reviewed 155 hemangioendotheliomas; no sex preponderance was noted in this group. The lesions in children appeared to be less malignant than the ones in adults (Liebner, 1961). The tumor may be present at birth and may be multicentric in origin (Watson-Jones, 1964; Svane, 1966).

Clinical Description

The hemangioendothelioma presents as a subcutaneous mass in approximately 50 percent of the cases, with or without color changes. Sometimes there is a history of related injury. This history of injury appears in the literature enough times to be of significance (Downing and Mallory, 1930; Bardwil et al., 1968). Most of the lesions are bluish red in color, suggestive of their vascular etiology, but some have no visible color changes. The hemangioendotheliomas seen in adults can occur in any organ of the body; the lesions in children are in the skin and liver.

The tumor varies from 0.5 cm. to lesions of great size. For example, the entire breast may be involved and contain over one liter of blood upon resection (Stout, 1943). Growth of the tumor is slow, although occasionally the clinical course is fulminating. Metastasis by the blood stream or the lymphatics occurs, involving the liver, bone, kidneys, adrenals, lungs, and skin (Caro and Stubenrauch, 1945; Cormie, 1956).

Differential Diagnosis

The differential diagnosis cannot be made on clinical characteristics alone but must await microscopic interpretation. Clinically, Kaposi's sarcoma involves the hands and feet first, and later the thighs and viscera are affected. The hemangioma is most frequently seen in children, whereas the hemangioendothelioma is less commonly found in children. The pyogenic granuloma occasionally creates some confusion in the differential diagnosis of the hemangioendothelioma, but the former usually gives a history of infection prior to the onset of the lesion; both lesions can give a history of injury prior to onset. The hemangiopericytoma, metastatic hypernephroma, and choriocarcinoma are lesions which, on gross examination, simulate the hemangioendothelioma and can only be differentiated microscopically.

Pathology

The gross appearance of the hemangioendothelioma, which is usually a bluish red in color, suggests its type of histology. If it appears blue, then there is usually a preponderance of veins within the lesion. If the tumor is largely composed of lymphatic channels, then it appears whitish in color. If the capillaries or endothelium are the main feature of the tumor, then the lesion usually appears reddish in color. Local hemorrhage is a common finding within the tumor. If the corium is invaded, the tumor will frequently show ulceration. The tumor varies in size from 0.5 to 15 cm. in diameter.

Microscopically, according to Stout and Lattes (1967), the tumor must satisfy two specific criteria: "First, the formation of atypical endothelial cells in greater numbers than are required to line the vessels with a simple endothelial membrane; and, second, the formation of vascular tubes within a delicate framework of reticulum fibers and a marked tendency for the lumen to anastomose. No tumor should be considered a hemangioendothelioma unless these criteria are present." There is a budding of endothelial cells, much as is seen in granulation tissue, with a great proliferation of endothelial cells within the lumen of the vessels (Braverman and Lerner, 1961). Many of these cells are hypochromatic and polygonal. Silver staining techniques serve to differentiate the hemangioendothelium from other vascular tumors, demonstrating the vascular channels, anastomosing capillaries, and proliferating endothelial cells (Fig. 48–6). The silver stain also differentiates the hemangiopericytoma from the hemangioendothelioma (Ramsey, 1966). In the hemangiopericytoma, the endothelial cell lies outside the reticulum, whereas in the hemangioendothelioma, the proliferation of the endothelial cell lies within the reticulum sheath of the vessel. The silver stain also differentiates the hypernephroma, Kaposi's sarcoma, and choriocarcinoma from tumors of the blood vessels.

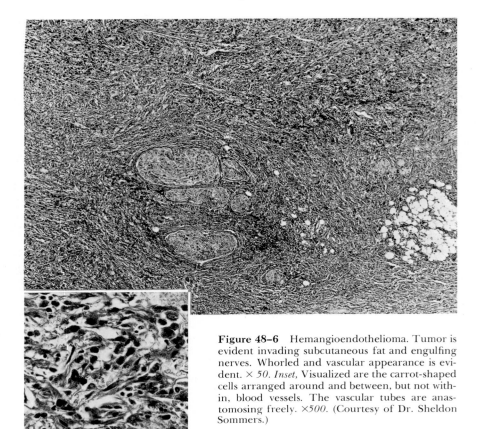

Figure 48–6 Hemangioendothelioma. Tumor is evident invading subcutaneous fat and engulfing nerves. Whorled and vascular appearance is evident. × 50. *Inset,* Visualized are the carrot-shaped cells arranged around and between, but not within, blood vessels. The vascular tubes are anastomosing freely. ×500. (Courtesy of Dr. Sheldon Sommers.)

Clinical Course

The clinical course of the disease may be protracted, or death may ensue rapidly. The tumors in infants and children are slow-growing with either local recurrences or the appearance of lesions in other parts of the body occurring over a period of 20 years (Smith, 1938). In adults, the lesions are much more malignant, the interval between clinical onset and death from disease being from one to two years. Metastasis usually takes place via the blood stream to the liver, lungs, bone, and brain (Weidman, 1950). Occasionally, metastasis to the regional lymph nodes does occur via lymphatic channels.

Treatment

The treatment of choice for hemangioendothelioma is that of wide local excision of the primary lesion after excisional biopsy to establish the diagnosis, since the classification of the tumor is most important to prognosis (Stout and Lattes, 1967c). The margins of the tumor are usually ill-defined, and infiltration is not easily appreciated because of the vascular and spongy nature of the tumor. For this reason, local recurrences are common. A regional lymph node dissection may be considered in the head and neck region, particularly if the lesion arises in the scalp (Bardwil et al., 1968). Radiation therapy has been reported as relatively ineffective (Drucker, 1947). The hemangioendothelioma is considered the least radiosensitive of all vascular tumors. Chemotherapy has not been used on enough cases to render judgment.

Summary

The hemangioendothelioma is a malignant tumor of the blood vessel endothe-

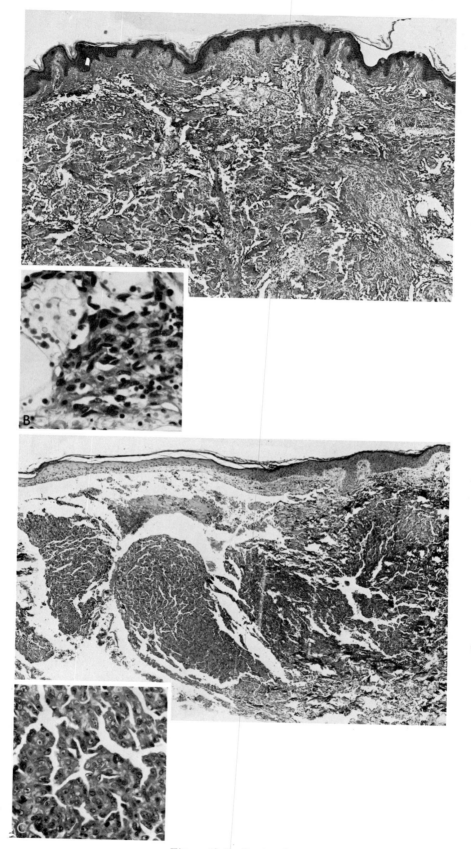

Figure 48–8 *Continued.*

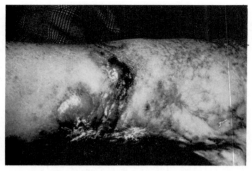

Figure 48–9 Lymphangiosarcoma, postmastectomy. This 54 year old white female had a radical mastectomy followed by radition therapy. Lymphedema of the arm developed immediately postoperatively. Seven years later, the lymphangiosarcoma developed on the medial aspect of the arm. Irradiation to the tumor was ineffective. Note axillary involvement of the tumor. An upper arm amputation was done; the patient died six months postoperatively. (Courtesy of the Department of Dermatology, New York University Medical Center.)

(See also Color Plate VIII-C.)

Summary

The prognosis of the patient with lymphangiosarcoma is grave, with few five-year survivors (Taswell et al., 1962). In a group of 83 patients treated by various modalities, the mean survival was 18.6 months (Herrmann, 1965); the mean duration of life after surgery was 16.8 months in 32 patients. Surgery plus irradiation offered a somewhat longer survival period.

REFERENCES

Abrikossoff, A.: Über Myome, ausgehend von der quergestreiften willkürlichen Muskulatur. Virchows Arch. Pathol. Anat., 260:215, 1926.

Ackerman, I. V.: Multiple primary liposarcomas. Am. J. Pathol., 20:789, 1944.

Allkek, D. S., Johnson, W. C., and Graham, J. H.: Granular cell myoblastoma. Arch. Dermatol., 98:543, 1968.

Ashburn, L. L., and Rodger, R. C.: Myoblastomas, neural origin; report of six cases, one with multiple tumors. Am. J. Clin. Pathol., 22:440, 1952.

Bangle, R., Jr.: Morphological and histochemical study of granular-cell myoblastoma. Cancer, 5:950, 1952.

Bangle, R., Jr.: An early granular-cell myoblastoma confined within a small peripheral myelinated nerve. Cancer, 6:790, 1953.

Bardwil, J. M., Mocega, E. E., Butler, J. J., and Russin, D. J.: Angiosarcomas of the head and neck region. Am. J. Surg., 116:548, 1968.

Barnett, W. O., Hardy, J. D., and Hendrix, J. H.: Lymphangiosarcoma following postmastectomy lymphedema. Ann. Surg., 169:960, 1969.

Braverman, I. M., and Lerner, A. B.: Diffuse malignant proliferation of vascular endothelium; a possible new clinical and pathological entity. Arch. Dermatol., 84:22, 1961.

Caro, M. R., and Stubenrauch, C. H., Jr.: Hemangioendothelioma of the skin. Arch. Dermatol., 51:295, 1945.

Chu, F. C. H., and Treves, N.: Value of radiation therapy in post-mastectomy lymphangiosarcoma. Am. J. Roentgenol., 89:64, 1963.

Cormie, R. L.: Hemangioendothelioma. Arch. Dermatol., 74:144, 1956.

Crawford, E. S., and DeBakey, M. E.: Granular-cell myoblastoma; two unusual cases. Cancer, 6:786, 1953.

D'Agostino, A. N., Soule, E. H., and Miller, R. H.: Sarcomas of the peripheral nerves and somatic soft tissues associated with multiple neurofibromatosis (von Recklinghausen's disease). Cancer, 16:1015, 1963.

Di Simone, R. N., El-Mahdi, A. M., Hazra, T., and Lott, S.: The response of Stewart-Treves syndrome to radiotherapy. Radiology, 97:121, 1970.

Downing, J. G., and Mallory, G. K.: Cavernous hemangioma and trauma. Arch. Dermatol., 22:414, 1930.

Drucker, V.: Hemangioendothelioma; a rare malignant tumor. Radiology, 49:231, 1947.

Eby, C. S., Brennan, M. J., and Fine, G.: Lymphangiosarcoma; a lethal complication of chronic lymphedema; report of two cases and review of the literature. Arch. Surg., 94:223, 1967.

Enterline, H. T., Culberson, J. D., and Rochlin, D. B.: Liposarcoma; a clinical and pathological study of 53 cases. Cancer, 13:932, 1960.

Fisher, E. R., and Wechsler, H.: Granular-cell myoblastoma—a misnomer; electron microscopic and histochemical evidence concerning its Schwann cell derivation. Cancer, 15:936, 1962.

Fox, S. R., Jr.: Leiomyomatosis cutis. New Engl. J. Med., 263:1248, 1960.

Fust, J. A., and Custer, R. D.: On neurogenesis of so-called granular-cell myoblastoma. Am. J. Clin. Pathol., 19:522, 1949.

Gamboa, L. G.: Malignant granular-cell myoblastoma. Arch. Pathol., 60:663, 1955.

Harken, J. C., and Reed, R. J.: Tumors of the peripheral nervous system. Atlas of Tumor Pathology, 2nd Series, Fascicle 3. Washington, D.C., Armed Forces Institute of Pathology, 1969, pp. 107–136.

Herrmann, J. B.: Lymphangiosarcoma of the chronically edematous extremity. Surg. Gynecol. Obstet., 121:1107, 1965.

Herrmann, J. B., and Ariel, I. M.: Therapy of lymphangiosarcoma of the chronically edematous limb; five year cure of a patient treated by intra-arterial radioactive yttrium. Am. J. Roentgenol., 99:393, 1967.

Kauffman, S. L., and Stout, A. P.: Lipoblastic tumors of children. Cancer, 12:912, 1959.

Kauffman, S. L., and Stout, A. P.: Histiocytic tumors (fibrous xanthoma and histiocytoma) in children. Cancer, 14:469, 1961a.

Kauffman, S. L., and Stout, A. P.: Malignant hemangioendothelioma in infants and children. Cancer, 14:1186, 1961b.

Kettle, E. H.: Tumors arising from endothelium. Proc. R. Soc. Med., 11:19, 1918.

Kilgour, C. S.: Cutaneous leiomyosarcoma. Br. J. Plast. Surg., 8:144, 1955.

Kurwa, A., and Waddington, E.: Post-mastectomy lymphangiomatosis. Br. J. Dermatol., 80:840, 1968.

Levack, J., and Dick, A.: Cutaneous leiomyosarcoma with lymphatic spread; report of 2 cases. Scott. Med. J., 36:337, 1955.

Liebner, E.: Hypertrophic hemangioendothelioma of infancy. Am. J. Roentgenol., 86:587, 1961.

McConnell, E. M., and Haslam, P.: Angiosarcoma in post-mastectomy lymphoedema; a report of 5 cases and a review of the literature. Br. J. Surg., 46:322, 1959.

Mallory, F. B.: The results of the application of special histological methods to the study of tumors. J. Exp. Med., 10:575, 1908.

Marshall, J. F.: Lymphangiosarcoma of the arm following radical mastectomy. Ann. Surg., 142:871.

Montgomery, H., and Winkelmann, R. K.: Smooth muscle tumors of the skin. Arch. Dermatol., 88:510, 1963.

Murray, M. R.: Cultural characteristics of 3 granular-cell myoblastomas. Cancer, 4:857, 1951.

Nemoto, J., Stubbe, N., Gaeta, J., and Dao, F.: Pathogenesis of lymphangiosarcoma following mastectomy and irradiation. Surg. Gynecol. Obstet., 128:489, 1969.

Niemi, M., Levonen, E., and Mustakallio, K. K.: Histochemical studies on cutaneous leiomyomatosis. Br. J. Dermatol., 76:341, 1964.

Radman, H. M., and Bhagavan, B. S.: Granular-cell myoblastoma of vulva. Obstet. Gynecol., 33:501, 1969.

Ramsey, H. J.: Fine structure of hemangiopericytoma and hemangioendothelioma. Cancer, 19:2005, 1966.

Rawson, A. J., and Frank, J. L., Jr.: Treatment by irradiation of lymphangiosarcoma in post-mastectomy lymphedema; report of a cure. Cancer, 6:269, 1953.

Rising, J. A., and Booth, E.: Primary leiomyosarcoma of the skin with lymphatic spread; case report. Arch. Pathol., 81:94, 1966.

Ross, R. C., Miller, J. R., and Foote, F. W., Jr.: Malignant granular-cell myoblastoma. Cancer, 5:112, 1952.

Sadler, W. P., and Dockerty, M. B.: Malignant myoblastoma vulvae. Am. J. Obstet. Gynecol., 61:1047, 1951.

Salm, R.: The nature of the so-called post-mastectomy lymphangiosarcoma. J. Pathol. Bacteriol., 85:445, 1963.

Salvadori, B., and Talamazzi, F.: Malignant granular-cell myoblastoma. Tumori, 53:645, 1967.

Saunders, T. S., and Fitzpatrick, T. B.: Cutaneous leiomyoma; classification and report of solitary angioleiomyoma. Arch. Dermatol., 74:389, 1956.

Schirger, A.: Postoperative lymphedema; etiologic and diagnostic factors. Med. Clin. North Am., 46:1045, 1962.

Smith, C.: Massive cervical hemangioendothelioma in a newly born infant. Am. J. Dis. Child., 55:124, 1938.

Sobel, H. J., and Churg, J.: Granular cells and granular cell lesions. Arch. Pathol., 77:132, 1964.

Stewart, F. W., and Treves, N.: Lymphangiosarcoma in post-mastectomy lymphedema. Cancer, 1:64, 1948.

Stout, A. P.: Hemangioendothelioma; a tumor of blood vessels featuring vascular endothelial cells. Ann. Surg., 118:445, 1943.

Stout, A. P.: Liposarcoma; the malignant tumor of lipoblasts. Ann. Surg., 119:86, 1944.

Stout, A. P.: Tumors of the peripheral nervous system. Atlas of Tumor Pathology, 2nd Series, Facicle 6. Washington, D.C., Armed Forces Institute of Pathology, 1949.

Stout, A. P., and Hill, W. T.: Leiomyosarcoma of the superficial soft tissues. Cancer, 11:844, 1958.

Stout, A. P., and Lattes, R.: Tumors of the soft tissues. Atlas of Tumor Pathology, 2nd Series, Facicle 1. Washington, D.C., Armed Forces Institute of Pathology, 1967a, p. 116.

Stout, A. P., and Lattes, R.: Tumors of the soft tissues. Atlas of Tumor Pathology, 2nd Series, Fascicle 1. Washington, D.C., Armed Forces Institute of Pathology, 1967b, p. 127.

Stout, A. P., and Lattes, R.: Tumors of the soft tissues. Atlas of Tumor Pathology, 2nd Series, Fascicle 1. Washington, D.C., Armed Forces Institute of Pathology, 1967c, p. 145.

Svane, S.: Foetal exsanguination from hemangioendothelioma of the skin. Acta. Paediatr. (Stockh.), 55:536, 1966.

Svejada, J., and Horn, V.: Disseminated granular-cell pseudotumour; so-called metastasizing granular-cell myoblastoma. J. Pathol. Bacteriol., 76:343, 1958.

Taswell, H. F., Soule, E. H., and Coventry, M. B.: Lymphangiosarcoma arising in chronic lymphedematous extremities. J. Bone Joint Surg. (Am.), 44-A:277, 1962.

Tragus, E. T., and Wagner, D. E.: Current therapy for post-mastectomy lymphangiosarcoma. Arch. Surg., 97:839, 1968.

Watson-Jones, E.: Malignant angioendothelioma of the skin. Br. J. Dermatol., 76:21, 1964.

Weidman, A. I.: Hemangioendothelioma of skin with metastasis to liver, lungs and lymph nodes. Arch. Dermatol., 62:655, 1950.

Wells, H. G.: Adipose tissue; a neglected subject. J.A.M.A., 114:2177, 1940.

49

Pathology of Malignant Soft Tissue Tumors

Jorge Albores-Saavedra, M.D., Arcelia Mora-Tiscareño, M.D.,
and Hector A. Rodríguez-Martinez, M.D.

Soft part sarcomas correspond to approximately 1 percent of all malignant tumors in man (Albores-Saavedra, 1967). In spite of their low incidence, they constitute an important and heterogeneous group of neoplasms which give rise to formidable diagnostic and therapeutic problems (Stout and Lattes, 1967; Ackerman and Rosai, 1974). The majority of them develop in the deep soft parts, a smaller number in subcutaneous tissue, and very few in the dermis (Enzinger, 1969b). Nonetheless, both those orginating in the deep soft parts and those springing from the subcutis often attain sufficient size to cause direct invasion of the overlying skin. Consequently, it is important that both the dermatologist and the dermatopathologist become well acquainted with this group of neoplasms. This chapter is dedicated to a discussion of the principal clinicopathologic features of these tumors. Since dermatofibrosarcoma protuberans and Kaposi's sarcoma are included in Chapters 46 and 52, they will not be touched upon in the present discussion.

LIPOSARCOMA

Since liposarcomas show such wide variations in their microscopic structure and their clinical evolution, we are compelled to subdivide them. Today most pathologists agree that there are four principal types: myxoid, well-differentiated, round cell, and pleomorphic (Enzinger and Winslow, 1962). The first two are favored by a far better prognosis than the third and fourth. In some liposarcomas one can identify mixtures of the different histopathologic types.

Among all the malignant soft part tumors, the liposarcomas are those which attain the greatest size. They are the most common soft part sarcomas in adults and are rarely found in children (Enterline et al., 1960; Enzinger and Winslow, 1962; Reszel et al., 1966). Almost without exception they spring from the deep soft parts. Generally they are multilobular and surrounded by a fibrous capsule of varying thickness. Their color varies from a grayish-white to bright yellow. In the well-differentiated variety, the large fat content makes the yellow predominate. In the round cell and pleomorphic varieties, since there is very little lipogenesis, the grayish white color is more evident. On sectioning the tumor one observes fibrous tissue bands that divide the neoplastic mass in nodules of variable size, which may reveal areas of cystic degeneration, hemorrhage, calcification, and even osseous spicules. In the myxoid variety of liposarcoma, the nodules frequently have a mucinous or gelatinous aspect.

The myxoid liposarcoma is the most common type and is made up of neoplastic lipoblasts, a prominent capillary network, and a myxoid ground substance (Fig. 49–1). Lipoblasts are stellate or spindle-shaped cells with poorly defined borders and one or multiple intracytoplasmic vacuoles which contain acid mucopolysaccharides and fat droplets. Once in a while one sees large or giant lipoblasts with hyperchromatic nuclei. The capillaries are collapsed but their prominent endothelial cells make them easily indentifiable. The endothelial cells are often seen back to back with the lipoblasts. The ground substance contains large amounts of acid mucopolysaccharides which are digested by testicular hyaluronidase (Winslow and Enzinger, 1960). In some tumors the myxoid substance is deposited in "pools" which flatten out the surrounding cells and give the impression of dilated lymphatic vessels (Fig. 49–2). The round cell liposarcoma often also contains an element of lipoblasts of the type already described. Nonetheless, the stroma has fewer capillaries and less myxoid material than that seen in the myxoid liposarcoma. The round cells have vesicular or hyperchromatic nuclei, and the eosinophilic cytoplasm is vacuolated or granular (Figs. 49–3 and 49–4). Generally these cells form solid masses or trabecular configurations. Sometimes one sees an adenoid pattern. The well-differentiated or lipomatous liposarcoma is basically made up of adult fat and precisely for this reason is often confused with a lipoma. In its sclerosing form the adipose tissue is infiltrated by thick bands of fibrous tissue which contain lipoblasts with characteristic neoplastic properties (Fig. 49–5).

In the other histopathologic variety, the

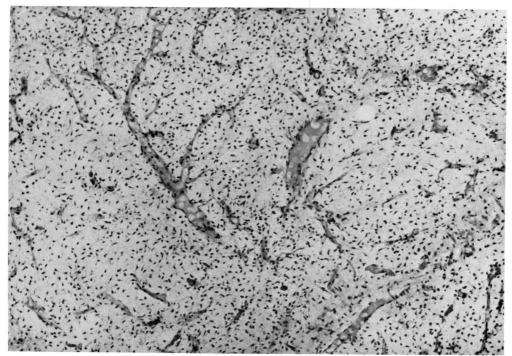

Figure 49–1 The three elements characteristic of myxoid liposarcoma are clearly seen: stellate lipoblasts, a prominent capillary network, and a myxoid ground substance.

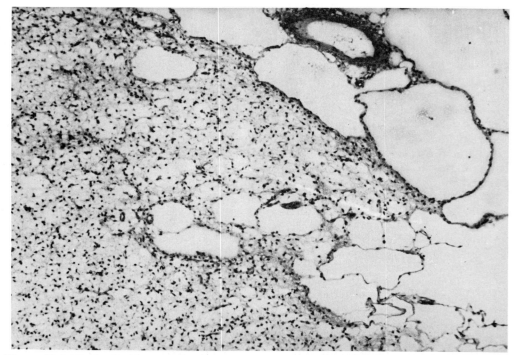

Figure 49–2   Pools of acid mucopolysaccharides resembling lymphatic vessels in a myxoid liposarcoma.

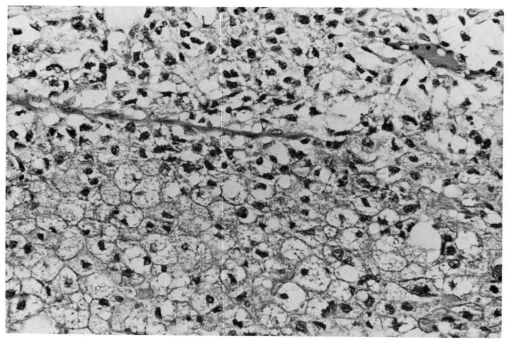

Figure 49–3   Round cell liposarcoma. The cells in the upper portion are small and poorly differentiated, while those of the lower part are large with well-defined borders and granular and vacuolated cytoplasm.

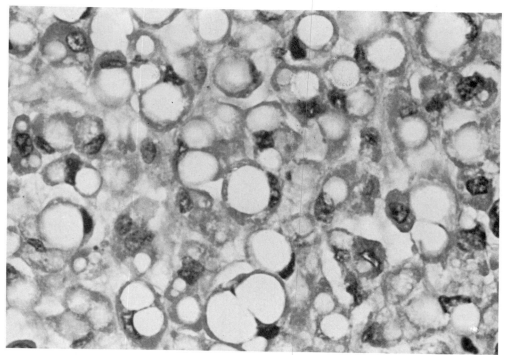

Figure 49–4   Signet ring cells in round cell liposarcoma.

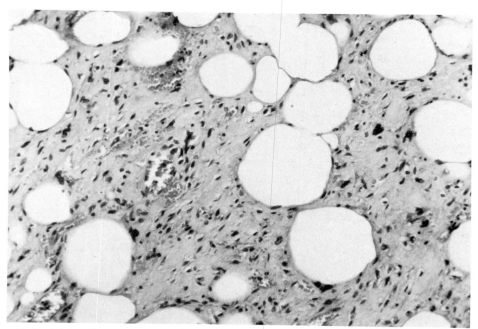

Figure 49–5   Adult adipose tissue infiltrated by irregular fibrous bands, which contain neoplastic lipoblasts and spindle-shaped cells with hyperchromatic nuclei in lipomatous liposarcoma.

thick fibrous bands are not seen but the fat cells show atypical nuclear changes and among them there are occasional lipoblasts. In pleomorphic liposarcoma there is no special histopathologic pattern. As the name implies, cellular pleomorphism is one of its attributes. There are abundant multinucleated giant cells with vacuolated or eosinophilic cytoplasm and prominent nucleoli. In some of these tumors there are little areas made up of small lipoblasts deeply embedded in the myxoid ground substance.

RHABDOMYOSARCOMA

Guided by their clinical and pathologic characteristics but to a greater degree by their microscopic pattern, one can divide rhabdomyosarcomas into three types: embryonal, alveolar, and pleomorphic. Of these, the most common type is the embryonal, which frequently is found in children less than 10 years of age. It responds to radiotherapy and is found principally in the soft parts of the head and neck and especially in the orbit (Horn and Enterline, 1958; Porterfield and Zimmerman, 1962; Masson and Soule, 1965; Nelson,

1968). The alveolar variety is predominantly a tumor of adolescents and young adults and is just as frequently found in the limbs as in the head and neck. It has the worst prognosis of the rhabdomyosarcoma group; survival at five years is less than 10 percent (Riopelle and Theriault, 1956; Enterline and Horn, 1958; Enzinger, 1969b). Pleomorphic rhabdomyosarcoma is the least frequent variety. Found mostly in the lower extremities and in persons past middle age, it does not respond to radiotherapy and apparently has the best prognosis of the three types (Albores-Saavedra, 1965; Linscheid et al., 1965; Keyhani and Booher, 1968; Stout, 1946).

The microscopic pattern of embryonal rhabdomyosarcoma varies from one tumor to another and even from one zone to another within the same tumor. The predominant cells in the well-differentiated tumors are similar to those observed in the striated muscle of 7 to 10 week old human embryos. That is, they are elongated and have one central nucleus which is vesicular or hyperchromatic and contains one or more nucleoli. There is abundant brightly eosinophilic, ribbonlike cytoplasm (Fig. 49–6). These cells are

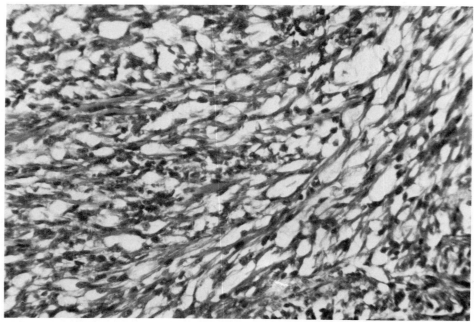

Figure 49–6 Interlacing fascicles of long spindle-shaped cells with abundant eosinophilic cytoplasm in well-differentiated embryonal rhabdomyosarcoma.

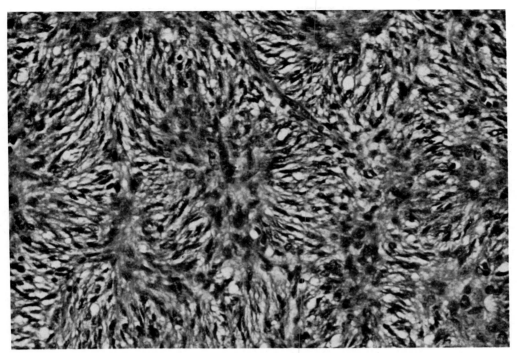

Figure 49–13 Characteristic "cartwheel" pattern in dermatofibrosarcoma protuberans. Compare with Figure 49–12.

coma, epithelioid sarcoma, proliferative myositis, atypical fibroxanthosarcoma, and desmoid (Pritchard et al., 1974). In our experience this tumor is less common than liposarcoma, rhabdomyosarcoma, and synovial sarcoma. It can be found at any age but is more common between the third and fifth decades. It originates in the deep soft tissues, especially in tendons and aponeuroses of the extremities and above all in the legs. Sometimes it is also found in other areas, such as the shoulder, head and neck, and abdominal and thoracic wall. Only exceptionally does a fibrosarcoma originate in the dermis.

In the gross examination one notes one or more well-circumscribed nodules which, however, are not encapsulated. They have a pale gray or whitish color and a firm consistency. Microscopically they are made up of spindle-shaped cells which can be identified as fibroblasts (Stout, 1948; van der Werf-Messing and van Unnik, 1965). They show anaplastic changes and many mitoses, and the cells are arranged in parallel bundles or form basket-weave patterns (Fig. 49–12). The "cartwheel" formation characteristic of

dermatofibrosarcoma protuberans is not found (Fig. 49–13). In the less differentiated tumors there is only scanty collagen production, but one sees an abundant reticulum network and many mitoses; in the well-differentiated variety collagen deposits are prominent, and there are only few mitoses.

The prognosis depends on the anatomic site of the lesion and its degree of differentiation. The five-year survival rate is close to 60 percent (Pritchard et al., 1974). Neoplastic spread is via the bloodstream.

FIBROXANTHOSARCOMA (MALIGNANT FIBROUS HISTIOCYTOMA)

This tumor belongs to the histiocytic group and is formed by a mixture of histiocytes, fibroblasts, and giant cells and can originate in practically any part of the organism (Kempson and Kyriakos, 1972; O'Brien and Stout, 1964; Merkow et al., 1971). Even though it has been reported in all age groups, the majority of the patients in which it occurs are 40 years of age or older. There is a slight male predominance, and perhaps it is found more frequently in the leg and thigh. According to its site of origin, this tumor is divided into superficial and deep types. The first type affects subcutaneous fat and fascia and generally are small in size, while the deep type is found in the body of skeletal muscle, may invade the periosteum or bone, and tends to be a larger tumor. Nonetheless, its size can vary from 1.5 to more than 20 cm. Most of these tumors appear as grayish white, pale gray, brown, or yellow nodules with variable degrees of hemorrhage and necrosis. Microscopically they are made up of a mixture of histiocytes, fibroblasts, multinucleated giant cells, vacuolated macrophages, and a fibrous stroma rich in collagen deposits and reticulum fibers (Figs. 49–14 and 49–15). At least in some places, the fibroblasts and the collagen fibers form whorls (storiform fibroblastic pattern). The proportions of the several cellular elements vary from one tumor to another and even from place to place in the same tumor. In addition, one commonly identifies inflammatory cells, above all lymphocytes, mixed with the neoplastic cells. Reed-Sternberg–like cells are also found. Mitotic activity is variable, since in some of these tumors there are many mitoses and in others very few. The same may be said of nuclear pleomorphism. This tumor tends to recur locally, and in Kempson's and Kiriakos' series 15 percent metastasized to distant sites via the blood stream. Rarely one finds lymphatic metastases.

EPITHELIOID SARCOMA

This neoplastic process was given its definitive description by Enzinger in 1970. Both clinically and microscopically it is often confused with granulomatous inflammations or other tumors, such as synovial sarcoma and carcinoma. It is usually seen in young adults and adolescents and predominates in males. It is especially located in the upper extremities and the fingers; the palms and the forearm are the most frequently affected sites. In the lower extremities this tumor can be found in the leg, thigh, and gluteal region. Only rarely is it found in the

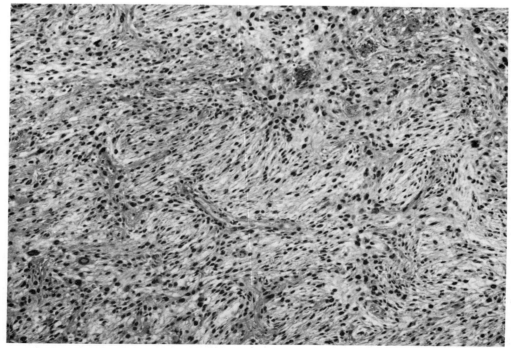

Figure 49–14　Fibroxanthosarcoma. The cells tend to radiate toward central acellular areas, producing the so-called storiform fibroblastic pattern. In other places they radiate toward blood vessels.

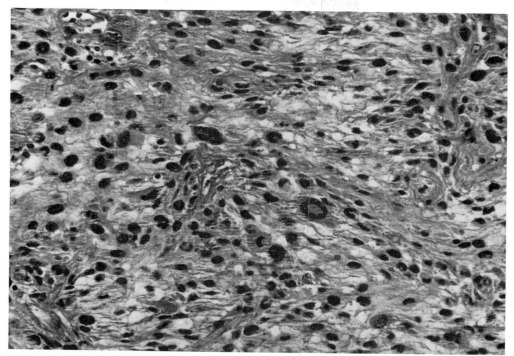

Figure 49–15 Higher magnification of the tumor shown in Figure 49–14. Mononuclear histiocytes with hyperchromatic nuclei and a few multinucleated giant cells are present.

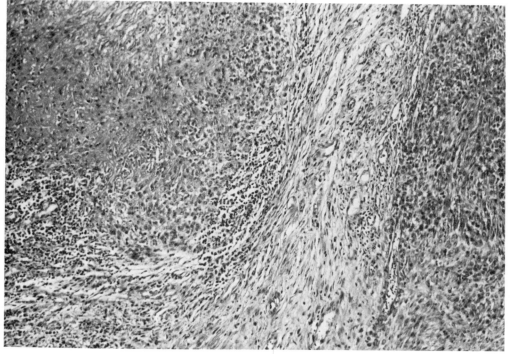

Figure 49–16 Epithelioid sarcoma. Two well-demarcated nodules, one with central necrosis, are separated by a thick fibrous band infiltrated with lymphocytes.

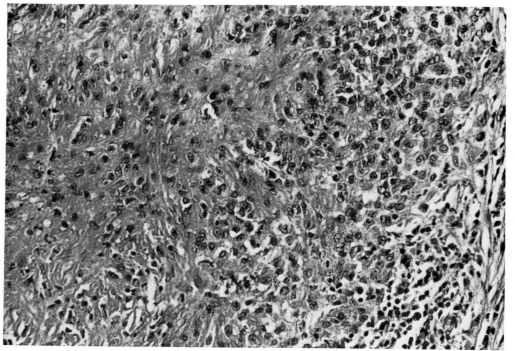

Figure 49–17 Higher magnification of one of the nodules, showing increased cellularity at the periphery. The neoplastic cells are very similar to histiocytes.

head, foot, or abdominal wall (Soule and Enriquez, 1972).

Clinically, when this tumor is found in the dermis, it appears as one or several nodules, with a diameter which varies from one or several millimeters to several centimeters, which produce excrescence and eventually ulceration of the skin. As a result they are frequently diagnosed as abscesses, hard ulcers, or infected warts. The deeper lesions, which are found adjacent to aponeuroses or tendons, generally are somewhat larger. They are also nodular and are mobile with movements of the extremity.

Grossly they appear in the form of one or several firm, grayish white nodules which measure from 0.5 to 6 cm. and which are surrounded by fibrous tissue and fat. Nonetheless, the great majority are less than 2 cm. in their greatest diameter. The neoplastic cells are formed in nodules which show central necrosis or fibrosis with hyalinization (Figs. 49–16 and 49–17). The majority are polygonal or elongated, and their abundant intensely eosinophilic cytoplasm gives them a certain similarity to epithelioid or neoplas-

tic epithelial cells. Infrequently one sees multinucleated giant cells. Generally there is little cellular pleomorphism and there are few mitoses. In some places the neoplastic cells are arranged in long single cell rows, which are separated one from another by bands of dense connective tissue. Reed-Sternberg–like cells and gland-like structures may also be observed (Santiago et al., 1972). The tumor stroma is strongly desmoplastic.

This tumor tends to recur locally, and frequently this takes place several times. However, at least one-half of the patients can be cured by radical surgical procedures. The tumor is spread by the bloodstream, and the lung is the most frequent site of metastases.

MALIGNANT GIANT CELL TUMOR OF SOFT TISSUES

The malignant giant cell tumor of soft tissues is a rarely occurring neoplasia with a microscopic image much akin to that seen in the giant cell tumor of bone (Guccion and Enzinger, 1972; Salm and Sissons, 1972). These tumors are divided arbitrarily into superficial and deep types. Both are seen more frequently in adults between 40 and 80 years of age and are slightly more common in females.

The superficial type principally affects the subcutaneous fat tissue and the low-lying aponeuroses of the leg, while the deep tumors are more commonly seen in the body of skeletal muscles or in tendons and fascias of muscle.

Clinically they are noted as a nontender mass with a diameter of from 1.5 to 30 cm. The superficial tumors are smaller than the deeply located ones. In the gross description one sees pseudoencapsulated whitish gray masses which may have some pale brown areas with hemorrhage and necrosis. The microscopic picture is characterized by a marked proliferation of multinuclear giant cells, mononuclear histiocytes, and fibroblasts arranged in nodules separated one from the other by fibrous tissue bands (Fig. 49–18). In some of these tumors one sees minimal foci of osteoid; mitotic figures and nuclear pleomorphism are more often seen in those tumors which are going to produce metastases. At times there is blood or lymph vessel invasion.

The five-year survival rate in patients with the superficial type of this tumor is considerably greater than that in those who have the deep variety.

MALIGNANT SCHWANNOMA

The malignant tumors formed by cells of the nerve sheath, or Schwann cells, are also known by the terms neurofibrosarcoma, neurogenic sarcoma, and malignant neurilemoma. Since the Schwann cell has the capability of producing collagen fibers, cartilage, bone, and striated muscle, these tumors may present a most varied architectural and cellular pattern. It is estimated that from 5 to 15 percent of patients with von Recklinghausen's disease eventually develop one or more malignant schwannomas (D'Agostino et al., 1965a). Nonetheless, von Recklinghausen's disease is also known to be accompanied by rhabdomyosarcoma and liposarcoma (D'Agostino et al., 1965b). In general, schwannomas are intimately associated

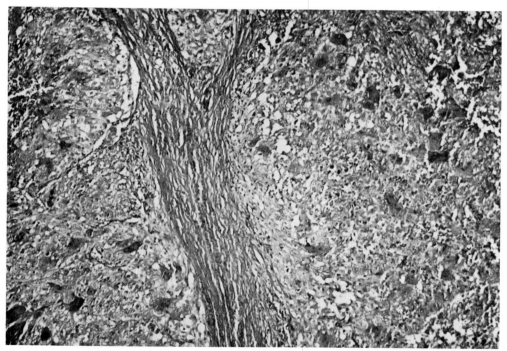

Figure 49–18 Mononuclear and multinucleated giant cells are divided into various-sized nodules by dense fibrous tissue bands.

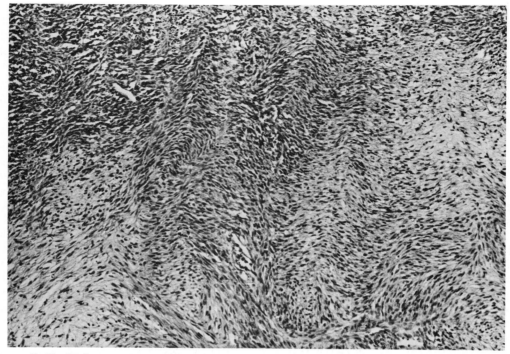

Figure 49–19   Malignant schwannoma in a patient with multiple neurofibromatosis. The "herringbone" pattern is clearly illustrated. Myxoid areas are also seen.

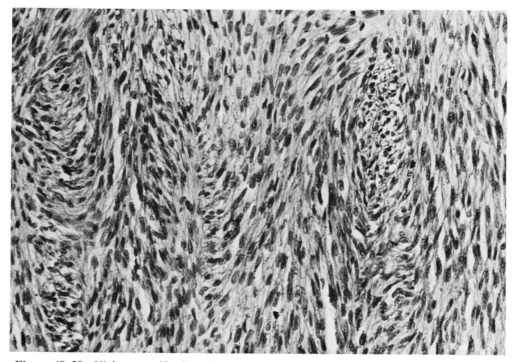

Figure 49–20   Higher magnification of the tumor shown in Figure 49–19. Cell detail is illustrated.

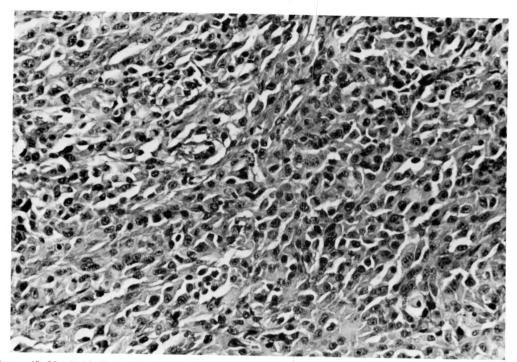

Figure 49–21 Epithelioid malignant schwannoma. The cells are round and polyhedral and are arranged in solid nests. In some places they exhibit loss of cohesion and resemble melanoma cells.

with a peripheral nerve, and this is one of the macroscopic features used in their diagnosis. On the other hand, the fact that a tumor invades a nerve trunk or is run through by a nerve is not sufficient itself to classify it as a malignant schwannoma, since occasionally these relationships are noted in almost any soft tissue sarcoma. At any rate some schwannomas do not have their origin in a visible nerve trunk. Microscopically the tumor is made up of tapered or ovoid cells arranged in compact bundles, which are distributed in a parallel pattern or at times haphazardly, forming whorls or establishing the design which has been called the "herringbone pattern" (Fig. 49–19). Cell palisading and pseudopalisading, the latter due to necrosis, are common phenomena. The neoplastic cells have hyperchromatic nuclei which are either ovoid or elongated (Fig. 49–20). Between the cells are variable amounts of collagen and reticulum fibers which run parallel and adjacent to the cell cytoplasm. In some tumors the stroma reveals myxoid areas, foci of osteoid, or plaques of cartilage. We, as well as others, have even found striated muscle (Woodruff et al., 1973). The epithelioid variety

of malignant schwannoma is made up of round, polyhedral, or fusiform cells which are arranged in compact nests or small alveoli. The neoplastic elements have vesicular or hyperchromatic nuclei, prominent nucleoli, and abundant eosinophilic cytoplasm (Fig. 49–21). Since schwannomas frequently grow towards both the distal and the proximal segments of the nerve in which they originate, their complete surgical excision is often a most difficult task. This, of course, results in a high incidence of local recurrence. This tumor spreads by the bloodstream, and survival rates are poor.

Other primary malignant tumors which have been described in association with peripheral nerves are the neuroepithelioma and the neuroblastoma, which supposedly originate in neuroepithelium (Abell et al., 1970). Since these tumors so rarely occur, their natural history cannot as yet be commented upon.

LEIOMYOSARCOMA

The majority of the superficial leiomyosarcomas arise in subcutaneous tissue

(Stout and Hill, 1958; Phelan et al., 1962). Nonetheless, some originate in the dermis and later on invade adjacent tissues. They are most frequently found in the thigh, the head and neck, and the thoracic and abdominal wall. In general, the superficial leiomyosarcomas are smaller than the deep and visceral variety, perhaps only because they are discovered and diagnosed more promptly. Their size has varied from 1 to 10 cm., and they are nodular, solid, and of a firm consistency. The majority of them are well delimited, but they are not encapsulated. They are made up of grayish white or brown-yellow tissue. On occasions the cut surface reveals a fascicled pattern such as that seen in leiomyomas. In contrast with the deep variety of leiomyosarcoma, the superficial type generally does not show degenerative phenomena, such as necrosis, hemorrhage, or cyst formation. Microscopically they are made up of bundles of smooth muscle fibers which show variable degrees of anaplasia (Figs. 49–22 and 49–23). Nonetheless, the most important factor in their differentiation from leiomyomas is their elevated number of mitoses. Frequently these tumors recur locally one or more times and finally are spread to distant sites by the bloodstream.

ANGIOSARCOMA

Angiosarcoma of the skin is a rarely encountered entity. When it does appear, it is almost always in patients who are less than 20 or more than 60 years old. The lesions are usually found in the skin of the face or scalp but once in a while in the extremities, abdomen, or thoracic wall. They are usually multiple lesions and appear as elevated red or purple nodules. Frequently they recur locally, and only after several years some begin to be disseminated by both blood and lymph vessels. Microscopically the angiosarcoma of a low grade of malignancy is formed by freely anastomizing vascular spaces lined by endothelial cells which occasionally have large or hyperchromatic nuclei (Fig. 49–24). Mitotic figures are rarely seen. At least in a few microscopic fields, one sees papillary projections with hyalinized stroma which have the appearance of chorionic villi. There are also small papillary projections which grow toward the

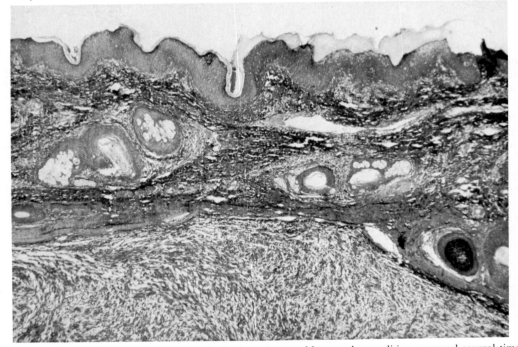

Figure 49–22   Leiomyosarcoma of the scalp from a 48 year old man; the condition recurred several times. The tumor apparently arose in the subcutis and later invaded the deep dermis.

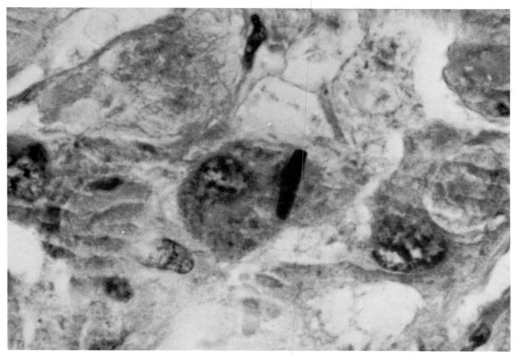

Figure 49–28   Intracytoplasmic, rectangular, PAS-positive crystal in alveolar soft part sarcoma.

of cells, but on a few occasions one finds them completely filled with neoplastic cells. These latter have abundant eosinophilic cytoplasm, which is either vacuolated or finely granular. After long and patient searching, one may find intracytoplasmic rectangular crystals which are PAS-positive in about 20 percent of these tumors (Fig. 49–28). The nuclei are vesicular or hyperchromatic and contain one or two prominent nucleoli. The majority of the cells show a finely granular cytoplasm, which is Schiff-positive and resistant to diastase or saliva, which can also be stained with alcian blue and colloidal iron, and which has been identified as a glycoprotein.

OSTEOGENIC SARCOMA

This is a very rarely occurring soft tissue tumor, and its exact incidence is unknown. Some non-neoplastic lesions which produce bone, such as myositis ossificans, are still frequently confused with osteogenic sarcoma, even by experienced pathologists. In contrast with those os-

teogenic sarcomas found in skeletal bone, the soft tissue variety are found more commonly in middle-aged or older adults, often in the fifth decade of life (Allan and Soule, 1971). They are more common in the extremities, and their microscopic picture is similar to that seen in skeletal osteosarcomas. Their spread is by the bloodstream. Five-year survival is as poor as that seen in skeletal osteosarcoma.

CLEAR CELL SARCOMA OF TENDONS AND APONEUROSES

This rare tumor is of unknown histogenesis but does have a characteristic microscopic picture (Enzinger, 1965). It is usually found in young adults and is frequently adherent to tendons and aponeuroses. It is more common in the foot and in the knee region. Grossly it is a well-defined, whitish gray, firm mass, which makes a crackling sound when cut. It is made up of groups and bundles of round or elongated cells with clear cytoplasm and a vesicular nucleus containing promi-

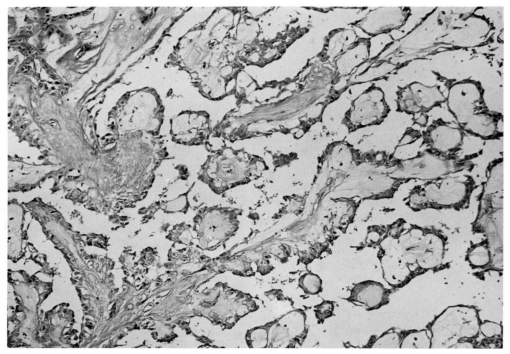

Figure 49–29 Myxopapillary ependymoma of the soft tissues of the sacrococcygeal region.

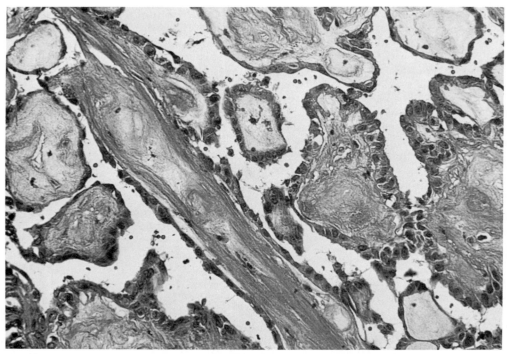

Figure 49–30 Higher magnification of the tumor shown in Figure 49–29. Some papillae show myxomatous changes, while others are hyalinized. They are lined by a low cuboidal epithelium.

nent nucleoli. This tumor usually recurs one or several times locally before spreading via the bloodstream.

MALIGNANT GRANULAR CELL TUMOR (MALIGNANT GRANULAR CELL MYOBLASTOMA)

Since the histogenesis of this tumor is still unknown, we prefer the term granular cell tumor. Up until very recently, alveolar soft part sarcoma was considered to be the malignant equivalent of this tumor. At the present time, we know that this interpretation is incorrect, since these tumors are entirely independent with no interrelationship. The great majority of granular cell tumors are benign. Nonetheless, recently we have seen very thoroughly documented reports of cases which have given rise to metastases (Al-Sarraf et al., 1971). The malignant variety differs from the benign tumor in that there is nuclear pleomorphism and mitotic activity. We now know that the granular aspect of the cytoplasm is due to its high lysosomal content.

EPENDYMOMA

In the subcutaneous and soft tissues of the sacrococcygeal area, one can identify ependymomas which have no connection with the medullary canal (Anderson, 1966). As a result of their anatomic situation, they are confused clinically with pilonidal cysts or sinuses. Even though in general terms this tumor is very slow growing, local recurrences and late metastases are not unusual. Grossly the tumor is lobular with precise limits and is even partially encapsulated. Its color is pale gray, and there are various degrees of hemorrhage. Microscopically the tumor shows all the features of the myxopapillary ependymomas, with papillary projections of varying size covered by a single row of columnar or cuboid cells (Figs. 49–29 and 49–30). The stroma of many of the papillary projections shows myxomatous changes, and the mucoid material stains positively with PAS and alcian blue. In other stromal papillary projections, there is complete hyalinization.

REFERENCES

Abell, M. R., Hart, W. R., and Olson, J. R.: Tumors of the peripheral nervous system. Hum. Pathol., 1:503, 1970.

Ackerman, L. V., and Rosai, J.: Surgical Pathology. Ed. 5. St. Louis, Mo., C. V. Mosby Company, 1974.

Albores-Saavedra, J.: Sarcomas y lesiones seudosarcomatosas de partes blandas. Prensa Med. Mex., 1967.

Albores-Saavedra, J., Buttler, J. J., and Martin, R. G.: Rhabdomyosarcoma: Clinicopathologic considerations and report of 85 cases. *In* Tumors of Bone and Soft Tissue. Chicago, Year Book Medical Publishers, 1965.

Allan, C. J., and Soule, E. H.: Osteogenic sarcoma of the somatic soft tissues. Cancer, 27:1121, 1971.

Al-Sarraf, M., Loud, A. V., and Vaitkevicius, V. K.: Malignant granular cell tumor; histochemical and electron microscopic study. Arch. Pathol., 91:550, 1971.

Anderson, S. M.: Myxopapillary ependymomas presenting in the soft tissue over the sacrococcygeal region. Cancer, 19:585, 1966.

Cadman, N. L., Soule, E. H., and Kelly, P. J.: Synovial sarcoma. An analysis of 134 tumors. Cancer, 18:613, 1965.

Crocker, E. W., and Stout, A. P.: Synovial sarcoma in children. Cancer, 12:1123, 1133, 1959.

D'Agostino, A. N., Soule, E. H., and Miller, R. H.: Primary malignant neoplasms of nerves (malignant neurilemomas) in patients without manifestations of multiple neurofibromatosis (von Recklinghausen's disease). Cancer, 16:1002, 1965a.

D'Agostino, A. N., Soule, E. H., and Miller, R. H.: Sarcomas of the peripheral nerves and somatic soft tissues associated with multiple neurofibromatosis (von Recklinghausen's disease). Cancer, 16:1015, 1965b.

Enterline, H. G., and Horn, R. C.: Alveolar rhabdomyosarcoma; a distinctive tumor type. Am. J. Clin. Pathol., 20:356, 1958.

Enterline, H. T., Culberson, J. D., Rochlin, D. B., and Brady, L. W.: Liposarcoma: A clinical and pathological study of 53 cases. Cancer, 13:932, 1960.

Enzinger, F. M.: Clear-cell sarcoma of tendons and aponeuroses; an analysis of 21 cases. Cancer, 18:1163, 1965.

Enzinger, F. M.: Alveolar rhabdomyosarcoma; an analysis of 110 cases. Cancer, 24:18, 1969a.

Enzinger, F. M.: Histological typing of soft tissue tumours. International histological classification of tumours, No. 3, Geneva. World Health Organization, 1969b.

Enzinger, F. M.: Epithelioid sarcoma: A sarcoma simulating a granuloma or a carcinoma. Cancer, 26:1029, 1970.

Enzinger, F. M., and Shiraki, M.: Extraskeletal myxoid chondrosarcoma. An analysis of 34 cases. Hum. Pathol., 3:421, 1972.

Enzinger, F. M., and Winslow, D. J.: Liposarcoma; a study of 103 cases. Virchows Arch. Pathol. Anat., 335:367, 1962.

Fisher, E. R., and Reidbord, H.: Electron microscopic evidence suggesting the myogenous derivation of the so-called alveolar soft part sarcoma. Cancer, 27:150, 1971.

Gabbiani, G., Kaye, G. I., Lattes, R., and Majno, G.: Synovial sarcoma, electron microscopic study of a typical case. Cancer, 28:1031, 1971.

Girard, C., Johnson, W. C., and Graham, J. H.: Cutaneous angiosarcoma. Cancer, 26:868, 1970.

Guccion, J. G., and Enzinger, F. M.: Malignant giant cell tumor of soft parts; an analysis of 32 cases. Cancer, 29:1518, 1972.

Guccion, J. G., Font, R. L., Enzinger, F. M., and Zimmerman, L. E.: Extraskeletal mesenchymal chondrosarcoma. Arch. Pathol., 95:336, 1973.

Haagansen, C. D., and Stout, A. P.: Synovial sarcoma. Ann. Surg., 120:826, 1944.

Horn, R. C., and Enterline, H. T.: Rhabdomyosarcoma; a clinicopathological study and classification of 39 cases. Cancer, 11:181, 1958.

Kempson, R. L., and Kyriakos, M.: Fibroxanthosarcoma of the soft tissues; a type of malignant fibrous histiocytoma. Cancer, 29:961, 1972.

Keyhani, A., and Booher, R. J.: Pleomorphic rhabdomyosarcoma. Cancer, 22:956, 1968.

Lieberman, P. H., Foote, F. W., Stewart, F. W., and Berg, J. W.: Alveolar soft part sarcoma. J.A.M.A., 198:1047, 1966.

Linscheid, R. L., Soule, E. H., and Henderson, E. D.: Pleomorphic rhabdomyosarcomata of the extremities and limb girdles. J. Bone Joint Surg. (Am.), 47:715, 1965.

Mackenzie, D. H.: Synovial sarcoma; a review of 58 cases. Cancer, 19:169, 1966.

Masson, J. K., and Soule, E. H.: Embryonal rhabdomyosarcoma of head and neck: Report of 88 cases. Am. J. Surg., 110:585, 1965.

Merkow, L. P., Frich, J. C., Jr., Slifkin, J., Kyreages, C. G., and Pardo, M.: Ultrastructure of a fibroxanthosarcoma (malignant fibroxanthoma). Cancer, 28:372, 1971.

Nelson, A. J., III: Embryonal rhabdomyosarcoma; report of 24 cases and study of the effectiveness of radiation therapy upon the primary tumor. Cancer, 22:64, 1968.

O'Brien, J. E., and Stout, A. P.: Malignant fibrous xanthomas. Cancer, 17:1445, 1964.

Phelan, J. T., Sherer, W., and Perez-Mesa, C.: Malignant smooth-muscle tumors (leiomyosarcomas) of soft-tissue origin. New Engl. J. Med., 266:1027, 1962.

Porterfield, J. F., and Zimmerman, L. E.: Rhabdomyosarcoma of the orbit. A clinicopathological study of 55 cases. Virchows Arch. Pathol. Anat., 335:329, 1962.

Pritchard, D. J., Soule, E. H., Taylor, W. F., and Ivins, J. C.: Fibrosarcoma. A clinicopathologic and statistical study of 199 tumors of the soft tissues of the extremities and trunk. Cancer, 33:888, 1974.

Reszel, P. A., Soule, E. H., and Coventry, M. B.: Liposarcoma of extremities and limb girdles: Study of 222 cases. J. Bone Joint Surg. (Am.), 48:229, 1966.

Riopelle, J. L., and Theriault, J. P.: Sur une forme méconnue de sarcome des parties molles; le rhabdomyosarcome alvéolaire. Ann. Anat. Pathol. (Paris), 1:88, 1956.

Salm, R., and Sissons, H. A.: Giant-cell tumours of soft tissues. J. Pathol., 107:27, 1972.

Salvador, A. H., Beabout, J. W., and Dahlin, D. C.: Mesenchymal chondrosarcoma: Observations on 30 new cases. Cancer, 28:605, 1971.

Santiago, H., Feinerman, L. K., and Lattes, R.: Epithelioid sarcoma; a clinical and pathologic study of nine cases. Hum. Pathol., 3:133, 1972.

Shipkey, F. H., Lieberman, P. H., Foote, F. W., and Stewart, F. W.: Ultrastructure of alveolar soft part sarcoma. Cancer, 17:821, 1964.

Soule, E. H., and Enriquez, P.: Atypical fibrous histiocytoma, malignant histiocytoma, malignant fibrous histiocytoma and epithelioid sarcoma; a comparative study of 65 tumors. Cancer, 30:128, 1972.

Soule, E. H., Geitz, M., and Henderson, E. D.: Embryonal rhabdomyosarcoma of the limbs and limb-girdles; a clinicopathologic study of 61 cases. Cancer, 23:1336, 1969.

Stewart, F. W., and Treves, N.: Lymphangiosarcoma in postmastectomy lymphedema: A report of six cases in elephantiasis chirurgica. Cancer, 1:64, 1948.

Stout, A. P.: Rhabdomyosarcoma of the skeletal muscles. Ann. Surg., 123:447, 1946.

Stout, A. P.: Fibrosarcoma—The malignant tumor of fibroblasts. Cancer, 1:30, 1948.

Stout, A. P., and Hill, W. T.: Leiomyosarcoma of the superficial soft tissues. Cancer, 11:844, 1958.

Stout, A. P., and Lattes, R.: Tumors of the soft tissues. *In* Atlas of Tumor Pathology, Fascicle I, Second Series. Washington, D.C., Armed Forces Institute of Pathology, 1967.

Van der Werf-Messing, B., and van Unnik, J. A.: Fibrosarcoma of the soft tissues—A clinicopathologic study. Cancer, 18:1113, 1965.

Winslow, D. J., and Enzinger, F. M.: Hyaluronidase-sensitive acid mucopolysaccharides in liposarcomas. Am. J. Pathol., 35:497, 1960.

Woodruff, J. M., Chernik, N. L., Smith, M. C., Millett, W. B., and Foote, F. W.: Peripheral nerve tumors with rhabdomyosarcomatous differentiation (malignant "triton" tumors). Cancer, 32:426, 1973.

Wooldward, A. H., Ivins, J. C., and Soule, E. H.: Lymphangiosarcoma arising in chronic lymphedematous extremities. Cancer, 30:562, 1972.

50

Angioendotheliomatosis Proliferans Systemisata (Diffuse Malignant Proliferation of Vascular Endothelium)

Josef Tappeiner, M.D., and Lilly Pfleger, M.D.
translated by Helen O. Curth, M.D.

SYNONYMS

Angioendotheliomatosis proliferans systemisata has also been called systemic endotheliomatosis of the cutaneous blood vessels, reticuloendotheliosis (Pfleger and Tappeiner, 1959), diffuse malignant proliferation of the vascular endothelium (Braverman and Lerner, 1961), systemic endotheliomatosis (Haber, 1962), intravascular endothelioma, endothelioma in situ (Haber et al., 1964), and neoplastic angioendotheliosis (Strouth et al., 1965).

DEFINITION

Angioendotheliomatosis proliferans systemisata (APS) is a rare vascular disease of unknown etiology with a variable course and signs which vary in every case. It is characterized by pathognomonic histologic changes in the form of multifocal, tumorlike, endotheliomatous proliferations within dilated, tortuous capillaries and blood vessels of the skin or the central nervous system or both, as well as other organs.

HISTORY

In 1959 Pfleger and Tappeiner reported for the first time, under the title "Zur Kenntnis der systemisierten Endotheliomatose der cutanen Blutgefässe (Reticuloendotheliose?)" [About systemic endotheliomatosis of the cutaneous blood vessels (reticuloendotheliosis?)], on a peculiar, chronic, apparently benign dermatosis with unusual histopathologic changes. This dermatosis so far had not been described in the literature, and the

1151

authors cautiously suggested that they were dealing with a new disease entity.

In 1961, Braverman and Lerner, referring to the above report, published a second case which showed the same histologic changes but which ended fatally with "diffuse malignant proliferation of vascular endothelium." These authors had also searched the literature and had not been able to find a similar description under disorders such as reticulum cell sarcoma, reticuloendotheliosis, hemangioendothelioma, and tumors of the blood vessels. They therefore concluded that these two cases represented a new disease entity, which occurred either in a benign chronic form or in a malignant acutely fulminating form.

Haber reported a third case. In a letter dated February 26, 1962, to J. Tappeiner, he sent a short manuscript under the title "systemic endotheliomatosis" and histologic sections of his female patient. After Haber's death in 1964 his collaborators published this case as "intravascular endothelioma (endothelioma in situ, systemic endotheliomatosis)."

At the Twelfth International Dermatological Congress in September, 1962, in Washington, Braverman showed an exhibit of the clinical and histologic findings of his female patient. He referred to the cases of Pfleger and Tappeiner and Haber and stated that "the purpose of this exhibit is to call attention to a new clinical and pathological entity."

Based on the new data by Braverman and Lerner (1961) and Haber (1962), Tappeiner and Pfleger in 1963 revised their original opinion of the benign character of the disorder and the exclusive cutaneous manifestation of the pathologic changes. They called the clinically and histologically new disorder "angioendotheliomatosis proliferans systemisata."

By 1969, only four additional cases were published. Midana and Ormea (1965) and Abulafia et al. (1969) described one case each with cutaneous manifestations under the name introduced by Tappeiner and Pfleger—angioendotheliomatosis proliferans systemisata. Strouth et al. (1965) described two cases with signs limited to the nervous system without cutaneous involvement. The authors chose the name "neoplastic angioendotheliosis," because they believed the concept of "angioendotheliomatosis" falsely implied the presence of a tumor.

Since the first report appeared on APS, therefore, only six additional cases—altogether seven cases—were published in the literature accessible to us. Since the signs and course vary in the seven patients, abbreviated summaries of the individual histories are given.

OBSERVATIONS OF PATIENTS

Case No. 1: 31 Year Old Greek Nurse *(Pfleger and Tappeiner, 1959)*

The disorder started in 1951, when the patient was in her 25th year, with high fever and the eruption of inflammatory-red moderately pruritic macules of about fingernail size on the trunk and extremities. The macules changed in the course of a few weeks into livid-red palm-sized infiltrations. After treatment with 2.4 million units of penicillin and 3 g. of streptomycin, the patient reported complete regression. In subsequent years similar eruptions, which remained stationary from the end of 1956 on, occurred with increasing frequency and with chills and fever. Since that time continuous fever and edematous swellings of the legs were present. Therapeutic trials with antibiotics, tuberculostatics, and cortisone preparations remained unsuccessful. In 1952, only once, paratyphoid B was demonstrated in the blood culture. All other examinations were negative.

On July 13, 1957, the patient was admitted to the I. University Skin Hospital in Vienna. She was found to be in good physical condition. On the trunk and extremities numerous predominantly annular or serpiginous, moderately firm, tuberous infiltrations were present, which were of fingernail to palm size and protruded over the level of the skin. The lesions were only slightly movable on the base, slightly tender, of livid-red to brown-red color, and surrounded by a finger-wide inflammatory-red margin (Figs. 50–1 and 50–2). The legs were

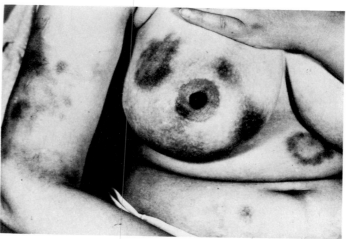

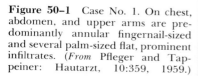

Figure 50-1 Case No. 1. On chest, abdomen, and upper arms are predominantly annular fingernail-sized and several palm-sized flat, prominent infiltrates. (*From* Pfleger and Tappeiner: Hautarzt, 10:359, 1959.)

moderately edematous. Face, scalp, and mucous membranes were free of disease. The palpable lymph nodes were not enlarged. The temperature was elevated at 38.5° C.

Findings. Internally normal. EKG normal, BP 105/90, urinalysis normal, sedimentation rate 65/94 Westergren. CBC: erythrocytes 3.5 million, Hb 72 percent, color index 1.02, leukocytes 7.200. Differ-

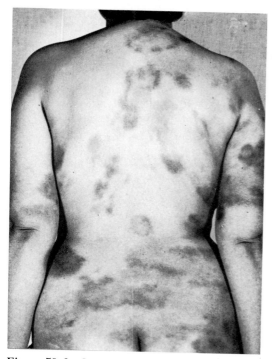

Figure 50-2 Case No. 1. Exanthematous eruption of annular and gyrate infiltrates on back and arms. (*From* Tappeiner and Pfleger: Hautarzt, 14:67, 1963.)

ential count: unsegmented 1 percent, segmented 63 percent, eosinophils 4 percent, monocytes 2 percent, lymphocytes 30 percent, thrombocytes 250,000. A sternal puncture was refused. Coagulation time normal, blood sugar 95 mg. per 100 ml.; Weltmann's serum test: 0.40 percent, Takata 50 mg.; cadmium positive. Thymol: 13.3, zinc sulfate 21.3. Bromsulphalein test: 8.9 percent. Potassium in serum: 8.8 mg. per 100 ml., sodium in serum 597 mg. per 100 ml., urea nitrogen 98 mg. per 100 ml. Total protein: 7.53 g. per 100 ml., albumin–globulin ratio 3.93. Electrophoresis: albumin 43 percent, Alpha-1: 2 percent, Alpha-2: 16.4 percent, Beta, 7.6 percent, Gamma 51 percent. Gastric acid: normal values. X-ray findings: stomach hypotonic, slight hypersecretion; barium enema normal. Skeleton: spina bifida sacralis, otherwise normal. Gynecologic findings: hypoplastic uterus, ovarian insufficiency, oligomenorrhea. Ear, nose, and throat findings: otitis media chronica dextra. Eyes normal. Vascular findings: pulse palpable on both feet; oscillometric values of the anterior feet the same on both sides. The values of the ankles show a slight difference between right and left. A tendency to vasospasms exists. Organic vascular damage could not be ascertained. Lymphography: cutaneous lymph nodes are visualized as normal, electrocardiogram chest leads VI, V, and IV negative. Histologic findings: repeated biopsies of infiltrated lesions of the right arm and thigh show a histologic picture characteristic of APS. Considerably dilated capillaries of the dermis and subcutis are arranged in coils and show intravascular proliferations of atypical cells, derived from the endothelium, and formations of numerous thrombi.

Course and Therapy. Cortisone therapy with 50 mg. prednisone daily and penicillin prophylaxis resulted in a return of the temperature to normal and caused transitory normal values of the ESR. When prednisone was reduced to 30 mg., however, the ESR rose again to 60/87 Westergren. The nodular infiltrates appeared somewhat flatter in places but were still distinctly palpable; however, they were not tender any more. The fading of the inflammatory border zone was conspicuous. X-ray therapy of a few lesions did not result in any difference between treated and untreated lesions. After eight weeks of treatment the patient wished to return to Greece. Half a year later we received a letter informing us that, without any further treatment, she had no complaints. Since that time we have been unable to learn anything further about her fate.

Case No. 2: 66 Year Old Woman
(Braverman and Lerner, 1961)

Onset of the disease was in March, 1959, with weakness, feeling ill, perception of spots (right eye), diminution of vision of the right eye and, 10 days later, of the left eye. The vision improved spontaneously in the right eye after eight days, and in the left eye after four weeks. Ophthalmologic examination showed a granulomatous iridocyclitis with cellular exudate in the vitreous, where a tubular area remained uninvolved. Change of position of the cell-free area caused the vision to improve or deteriorate. Concomitant with the ocular changes, tinnitus and deafness of the right side developed. About two to three weeks after the onset of the ocular and auricular changes, an eruption appeared on the trunk and thighs. It consisted of bluish, 1 to 4 cm., flat or minimally elevated, slightly tender infiltrates. Most of these lesions showed superficially tortuous vessels. Two months after the onset of the disease, some of the cutaneous lesions changed in character.

They looked like the typical picture of poikiloderma atrophicans vasculare. In the seventh month of illness firm subcutaneous nodes appeared on the upper extremities. Vision diminished on both eyes again. With the right eye the patient was able to distinguish only between light and dark; with the left eye she could vaguely see outlines. She was deaf in both ears. Gradually loss of weight, extreme weakness, and generalized myalgia developed. The patient died eight months after the onset of the disease.

None of the therapeutic trials (prednisone, nitrogen mustard, or irradiation of the entire body) had influenced the course.

General examination did not reveal conspicuous changes. There were never any signs of pathologic changes of the kidneys, liver, spleen, lymph nodes, or gastrointestinal tract. All laboratory tests, including punctures of the liver and sternal marrow, were normal.

Repeated biopsies of superficial infiltrates showed the picture of APS. In the histologic section of a firm subcutaneous node, endovascular cell proliferations and a massive extravascular infiltrate of similar cells were present.

The autopsy showed proliferations of the endothelium of dilated vessels of many organs. Infiltration of tissue was present as well in the heart, brain, eye, thyroid gland, skull, and petrous portion of the temporal bones.

Case No. 3: 48 Year Old Woman
(Haber et al., 1964)

In August, 1960, the patient noticed on the extensor surface of both legs nontender plum-colored swellings, which she believed to be insect bites. In spite of antihistamines the nodes became larger and more numerous. No loss of weight was noted; the appetite remained good.

Findings. The patient gives the impression of being perfectly healthy. The thyroid gland shows nodular enlargement without signs of malignancy or thyrotoxicosis. On deep inspiration the spleen is barely palpable; the liver and lymph nodes are not enlarged. Bilaterally, but less frequently the other organs—eyes, heart, lungs, thyroid gland, adrenals, kidneys, and bones. In our patient (Case No. 1) and in the 13 year old girl from Italy (Case No. 4), only cutaneous lesions without involvement of other organs were present. Two male patients, on the other hand, showed neurologic involvement exclusively; cutaneous changes were not present. In the remaining three cases (Cases Nos. 2, 3, and 7), the skin as well as other organs were affected.

Dermatologic Signs

The cutaneous changes have a predilection for the trunk and the extensor surface of the extremities. A few or numerous cutaneous or subcutaneous fingernail- to palm-sized nodular infiltrates are present, which are firmly adherent to the skin and only slightly moveable on the base. They are plaquelike or slightly elevated, moderately firm, and of brownish red to livid-red cyanotic color, surrounded by a light red halo. The tumor shows no or little tenderness.

Aside from these "typical" lesions, each of the five cases with cutaneous manifestations shows individual peculiarities. In Tappeiner and Pfleger's patient, a tendency to annular or gyrate distribution of nodes was observed. Braverman and Lerner described transformation of the infiltrates into poikiloderma-like changes. Haber's patient had "disfiguring" nodes, of which several centrally showed deeply dark atrophic depressions with superficial exfoliation. In Midana's and Ormea's case, extensive necroses existed in a tumor on the lower lid and in a giant tumor above the right breast. Abulafia et al.'s patient had phlegmasia cerulea dolens on the legs, with edema, cyanosis, gangrene, and mummification. The livid lesions on the arms and thighs broke down with ulcerations. No patient had involvement of the mucous membranes or lymph nodes.

Neurologic Signs

The two patients of Strouth and colleagues exhibited numerous signs which did not fit into any known disorder. The signs of each differed from those of the other. Increasing paralysis appeared in Case No. 5 on the right and in Case No. 6 on the lower half of the body. In addition, Case No. 5 became blind in the right eye and developed speech disturbances, somnolence, spasms, headaches, and progressive dementia. He was disoriented. Case No. 6 was lethargic, irritable, and stuporous before his death.

The patient of Haber et al. developed right hemiplegia 10 months after the onset of the disease as a sign of a lesion of the central nervous system.

General Signs

Prodromally or accompanying the main signs, uncharacteristic signs, such as weakness, feeling ill, loss of weight, and fever, were occasionally observed. In Case No. 2 specific signs pointing to involvement of certain organs were disturbed vision and hearing, and myalgia; in Case No. 3 such signs were tachycardia and generalized edema, and in Case No. 7 they were pulmonary edema and right bundle branch block.

Histopathology and Histochemistry

The essential changes are the same in all patients and in all their affected organs. They consist of intravascular proliferations of atypical cells or groups of cells. The proliferation derives from the vascular endothelium and takes place in dilated capillaries and in small and large arteries and veins.

In the biopsies of the cutaneous changes,* the epidermis is usually inconspicuous. In the dermis and sbucutis there is a considerable amount of maximally dilated, tortuous ("glomerulus-like") aggregates of capillaries or thin-walled precapillaries. Abulafia et al. were

---

*Haber and Braverman were kind enough to send us sections from their patients so that we could convince ourselves of the identity of the pathologic picture.

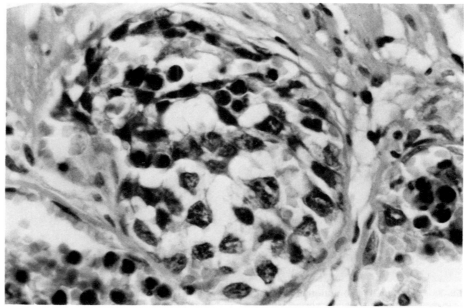

Figure 50–9   Case No. 1. The intravascular polymorphous cells are in close contact with each other and with the cells of the endothelial lining by elongations of the cytoplasm so that a reticulum-like network is formed. Empty spaces surrounded by elongated cells simulate formations of new vessels. (Case of Tappeiner and Pfleger.)

mistaken for newly formed small vessels. In places, the reticulum-like network is torn, so that cell groups or individual cells have become detached (Fig. 50–10) lying in the lumen.

Another characteristic of APS is the fibrin- or hyalin-like thrombi observed in various stages of development or organization. Either alone or together with the tumor formations, they fill the vascular lumen (Figs. 50–6 and 50–11).

Besides these very impressive changes, we find both in our sections and in Braverman's and Haber's sections, predominately

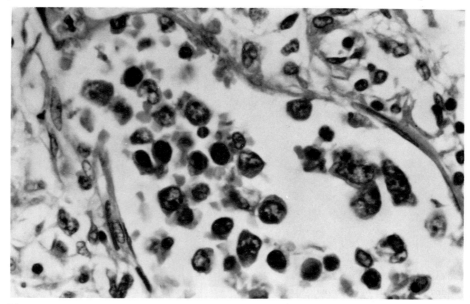

Figure 50–10   Case No. 2. In the capillary lumen, a group of detached tumor cells. (Case of Braverman and Lerner.)

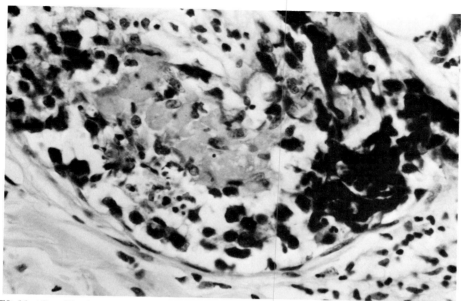

Figure 50–11   Case No. 1. Next to fibrinous thrombi and nuclear remnants are degeneratively changed tumor formations. The cellular nuclei are often elongated, deformed, and clumped. (Case of Tappeiner and Pfleger.)

in the papillary body but also in the subcutis, inconspicuous looking, slightly dilated capillaries which show one or a few atypical cells in normal endothelium. Such enlarged cells exhibit a shift of the nuclear or cytoplasmic ratio in favor of the nuclei, which are darkly stained, irregularly formed, and possess little structure (Figs. 50–12 and 50–13). In some capillaries the endothelial lining consists almost exclusively of such anaplastic cells,

from which the intravascular growth starts (Figs. 50–14 and 50–15).

The striking tumorlike cell proliferations are found only inside the vessels. At no place is the wall of the vessel penetrated. Only in Braverman and Lerner's case was there an extravascular infiltration of the tissue with tumor cells (Fig. 50–16). This occurred in subcutaneous nodes before the patient's death.

The glomerulus-like vascular convolu-

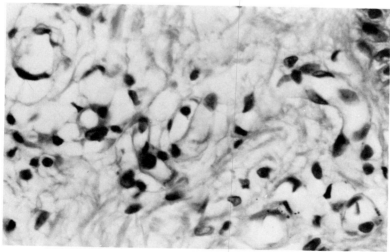

Figure 50–12   Case No. 2. Some cells of the endothelial lining of the capillaries in the papillary layer are strikingly enlarged. (Case of Braverman and Lerner.)

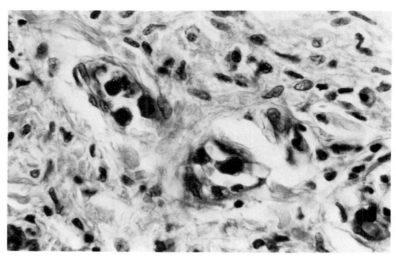

Figure 50–13   Case No. 1. Anaplastic endothelial cells in slightly dilated capillaries. (Case of Tappeiner and Pfleger.)

tions are partly lying without reaction in the connective tissue and are partly surrounded perivascularly by various dense infiltrates made up of lymphocytes and histiocytes. In the subcutis these infiltrates may also contain foam cells.

The connective tissue in the upper corium is inconspicuous; in the deeper layers it is clumped and homogenized. In sections of the elastic tissue stained with Weigert's stain, the elastic fibers are absent in the area of the vascular tortuosities. In the upper corium the elastic tissue is essentially unchanged. In the deep layers the fibers are swollen and fragmented. Silver impregnation (Gomori)

shows the affected vessels to be predominantly capillaries, since the vessel walls consist only of a thin, silvery stained basement membrane, which is connected with the perivascular argyrophilic reticulum fibers (Fig. 50–17). Inside the vessels in the areas of cellular proliferation, the *reticulum fibers* are completely absent. With the Prussian blue stain there is a variable amount of hemosiderin present perivascularly. The intravascular cells fail to show blood pigment.

Stains with van Gieson, Gram, Masson, Ziehl-Neelsen, PAS, and Astra blue show nothing abnormal.

The inner organs in Braverman's and

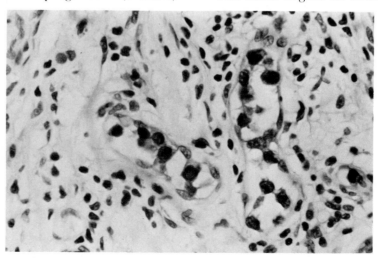

Figure 50–14   Case No. 3. The endothelial lining of the capillaries consists predominantly of atypical cells. (Case of Haber, Harris-Jones, and Wells, 1964.)

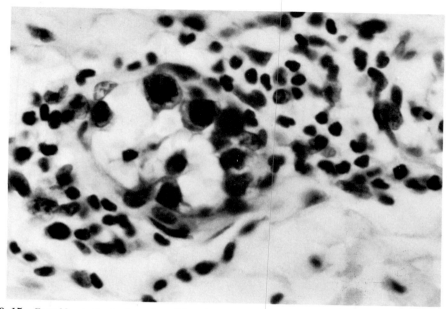

Figure 50–15 Case No. 1. Beginning of proliferation of the atypical endothelial cells. (Case of Tappeiner and Pfleger.)

Lerner's case showed dilated vessels filled with tumor cells in the myocardium, thyroid gland, uveal tract, and brain. In these organs, however, there also existed extravascular tissue infiltrations with "undifferentiated, mononuclear cells of an unclassifiable type." Both in petrous bones and in several osteoporotic parts of the skull, similar tumor cell infiltrates were present. Tumor cells without tissue infil-

tration occurred in the bone marrow, blood, and lymph vessels of almost all organs. Liver, spleen, and lymph nodes were free of tumor cells. In the cerebellum, focal atrophies were present. Acute ballooning degeneration of neurons was demonstrable in the entire brain.

In Case No. 5 of Strouth et al., pathologic changes were present exclusively in the adrenals and the brain. In the adre-

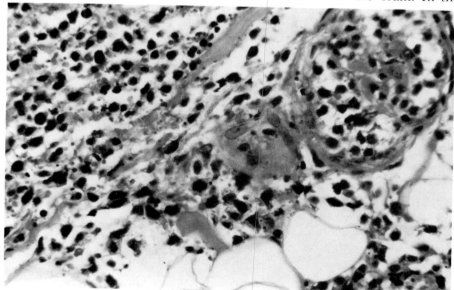

Figure 50–16 Case No. 2. Extravascular infiltration of the tissue with atypical mononuclear cells. (Case of Braverman and Lerner.)

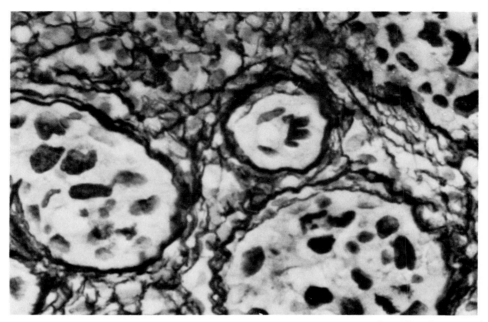

Figure 50–17   Case No. 1. Structure of reticulum fibers in a capillary conglomeration. Silver impregnation according to Gomori. (Case of Tappeiner and Pfleger.)

nals and surrounding adipose tissue, numerous sinuous, dilated capillaries were present, many of which contained neoplastic cells (Fig. 50–18); other capillaries showed new thrombi about to be organized or already organized. In addition, fresh or healed infarcts were observed in the tissue. In the vascular conglomerates a few tumor cells seemed to lie perivascularly. In the brain small and medium-sized arteries and veins were completely filled with neoplastic cells (Figs. 50–19 to 50–21). These were located in places which were in contact with the vascular wall and formed a continuous endothelial lining of the lumen. The lining was con-

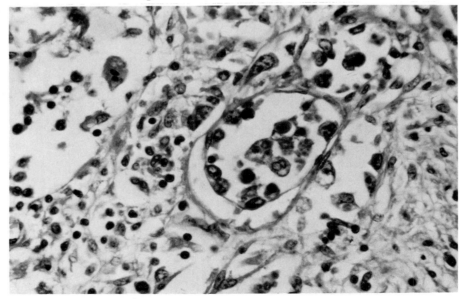

Figure 50–18   Case No. 5. Proliferation of tumor cells in capillaries of the adrenal. (Courtesy of Dr. Wolfgang Zeman.) (Case of Strouth et al.)

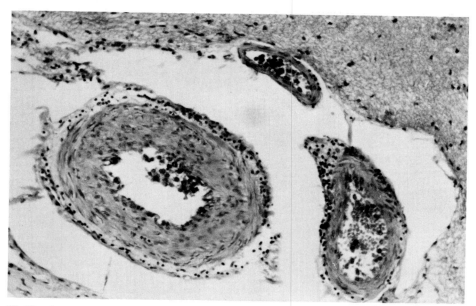

Figure 50–19 Case No. 5. Proliferation of endothelial cells in vessels of the leptomeninges. (Courtesy of Dr. Wolfgang Zeman.) (Case of Strouth et al.)

nected with the cells lying in the lumen by close continuity with the *cytoplasm.* The small arteries showed thickening of the *media;* the medium-sized arteries showed fibrosis of the intima without inflammatory signs. The numerous foci of softening in the brain, having a diameter of a few millimeters, contained macrophages and proliferating astrocytes. In addition, circumscribed areas of neuronal necrosis existed in the grey matter, and areas of demyelinization existed in the white matter. In the patient (Case No. 6) of Strouth et al., neoplastic cells were present in dilated, tortuous capillaries and medium-sized vessels of the brain, lung, kidney, and heart. In the brain, foci of softening existed similar to those seen in the pre-

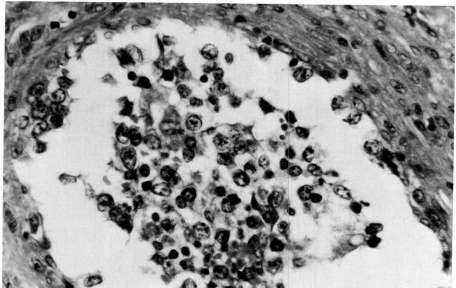

Figure 50–20 Case No. 5. The endothelial lining of an artery consists of atypical cells. In the lumen a syncytium of proliferating cells originating in the endothelium. (Courtesy of Dr. Wolfgang Zeman.) (Case Strouth et al.)

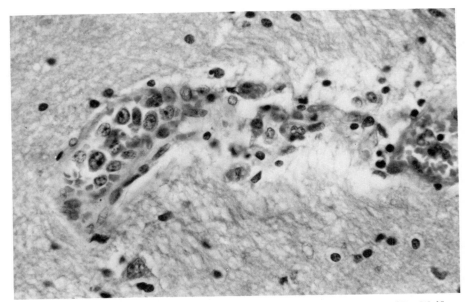

Figure 50–21. Case No. 5. Atypical cell proliferations in a cerebral vessel. (Courtesy of Dr. Wolfgang Zeman.) (Case of Strouth et al.)

ceding case. In the lung signs of edema and stasis were seen.

The descriptions of tumor cells in sections from the autopsies of the patients of Braverman and Lerner and Strouth et al. are almost identical; the atypical cells are about the size of a monocyte. The nuclei are pleomorphic and show irregular distribution of the chromatin. Nucleoli are distinctly visible. The cytoplasm is sparse, pink to pale grey, and in some areas syncytial. Numerous mitoses are present.

The enzymatic activity of the atypical cells was histochemically studied by Strouth et al. The intravascular cells did not contain any fat and were PAS-negative. They did not contain acid phosphatase and did not show cathepsin C activity. Alkaline phosphatase of the neoplastic cells was negative in the larger vessels and positive in the capillaries. These findings confirm the hypothesis of the multifocal origin of the cell proliferations. Since the neoplastic cells in the large vessels, as well as the endothelial cells of the large vessels, do not contain any alkaline phosphatase, it can be assumed that the neoplastic cells originated in situ and were not carried and transported there. The same is true of the capillaries. Alkaline phosphatase is positive in the endothelial cells of the capillaries as well as in the neoplastic cells in the lumen of the capillaries. The

dehydrogenases, particularly NADH and NADPH — diaphoresis, succino-dehydrogenase, beta-hydroxybutyrate, and lacto-dehydrogenase, were, in contrast to normal endothelial cells, only slightly positive. It can be assumed that the weak reaction can be explained by the neoplasia of the cells.

Laboratory Findings

The result of the investigations was neither consistent nor characteristic. In two patients (Case Nos. 2 and 7), the ESR was moderately or considerably increased. In Case No. 1 the electrophoresis showed a distinct increase of the alpha-2 and gamma globulin fractions. The liver function tests were slightly abnormal. In Case No. 1 paratyphoid B was found once in the blood culture. In Case No. 3 thrombocytopenia of 90,000 was observed, and in Case No. 7 a positive Machado-Guerreiro reaction was observed.

DIAGNOSIS AND DIFFERENTIAL DIAGNOSIS

The clinical picture of the disease was considered by all authors, dermatologists and neurologists, as unusual. Up to now it has been impossible to arrive at a diagnosis solely from the clinical manifestations or the neurologic signs. Dermatologists considered the following conditions in the differential diagnosis: tuberous syphilid, sarcoidosis, leprosy, mycosis fungoides, leukemic infiltrates, reticulum cell sarcoma, metastatic reticulum cell sarcoma, vascular tumors, Kaposi's sarcoma, Pfeiffer-Weber-Christian febrile nonsuppurative panniculitis.

The diagnosis of APS is based exclusively on the histologic findings. The microscopic picture, by now well known and generally accepted, is so characteristic that it can hardly be confused with another disorder. In the first case described by Tappeiner and Pfleger, however, considerable difficulties arose in the classification of the unusual findings. Numerous well known pathologists and dermatohistopathologists (see Pfleger and Tappeiner, 1959) arrived at diagnoses such as reticulum cell sarcoma, reticuloendotheliosis, hemangioendothelioma, lymphoblastoma, undifferentiated metastatic carcinoma, metastatic sarcoma, melanoma, seminoma, or dysgerminoma. In any case, all experts whom we consulted considered the disorder a malignant process because of the immaturity and atypia of the proliferating cells and the presence of numerous mitoses. Braverman and Lerner considered the histologic picture of the first biopsies of their case compatible with a disorder of the lymphoma group, i.e., a reticulum cell sarcoma. Now, however, the concept of this unusual disorder as a special disease entity is above doubt.

APS differs histologically from solitary vascular tumors, the hemangioendothelioma or angiosarcoma, by the absence of new formations of blood vessels as well as of solid extravascular tumor formations similar to an undifferentiated sarcoma.

Disorders of the so-called "lymphoma group," i.e., reticuloendotheliosis, lymphoblastoma, or reticulum cell sarcoma, which originate in the perivascular or periglandular indifferent zones, are easily differentiated from the intravascular endothelial proliferation of APS because of their extension in the connective tissue. Difficulties in the diagnosis were encountered only in the sections showing massive tissue infiltrations in Braverman's and Lerner's case. The authors cited as proof of the diagnosis of APS (1) the fact that the tumor cells had overwhelmingly remained in the vessels where they originated, and (2) the striking absence of reactivity in the reticuloendothelial system of liver, spleen, and lymph nodes.

Against the diagnosis of an intravascular metastatic tumor is the fact that in APS an endothelial lining differing from the proliferating cells does not exist.

The differential diagnosis of the microscopic picture of APS and the vascular changes described by Gottron and Nikolowski (1958) and by Ruiter (1964) in subacute bacterial endocarditis can be difficult. (The clinical manifestations of this disease are very characteristic. Symmetrically on the cheeks, the border of the helices of both ears, and the extensor surface of the upper extremities erythematous, flat, oozing, easily bleeding, crusted or eroded lesions are present.) Histologically, dilated vessels arranged in coils are present, as they are in APS. These are filled with or separated by hyalin-like thrombi. The thrombi are covered by proliferating normal (not atypical) endothelial cells, however. In places the proliferating endothelial cells form multiple cell layers encroaching on the lumen or extending plugs into the lumen. Superficially, this is indeed reminiscent of APS. Since Ruiter kindly sent us a section, we could convince ourselves of the resemblance of the histologic pictures. In Ruiter's sections, however, the atypical and polymorphic proliferating cells, the abundant mitoses, and the syncytial cell groups filling the whole vascular lumen are absent. On the other hand, in APS changes of the vascular walls typical of allergic vasculitis, such as fragmented collagen and the presence of metachromatic substances, are not demonstrable. We cannot agree with Lever who, in 1967 in the fourth edition of *Histopathology of the Skin*, considered APS Tappeiner-Pfleger a benign, reversible form of allergic vasculitis and who believed it to be the same condition as that in Gottron's and Nikolowski's and in Ruiter's cases. Lever separates Tappeiner-Pfleger's APS from malignant angioendotheliomatosis (Braverman-Lerner, Midana-Ormea).

ETIOLOGY AND PATHOGENESIS

Braverman and Lerner satisfactorily defined APS by stating that it is "a diffuse multicentric malignant proliferation of the vascular endothelium." The disorder, therefore, represents a neoplasia.

Analysis of the histologic picture permits the conclusion that the process starts with the transformation of single cells or groups of cells within the otherwise intact vascular endothelium. Islands of atypical cells develop multifocally in the capillaries as well as in the larger arteries and veins and seem to spread superficially by pathologic transformation of contiguous cells. From these centers of anaplastic endothelial cells, plugs of tumor cells develop, which expand the lumen of the vessels by closing them partly or completely. As a reaction to the pathologic cell formations thrombi develop, a process favored by the stagnation of the blood stream. The vessels, which can widen only so far, also start to extend longitudinally and form glomuslike tortuosities. The perivascular lymphocytic-histiocytic infiltrates occurring especially near the thrombi may be induced by histolytic processes of decomposition in the tissue of the tumor, since, as Hamperl (1957) remarked in a personal note, "the cancerous cells suffocate in the embrace of the fibrin."

The invasion of the tissue with tumor cells before death is unexplained. Probably, the extensive vascular obliterations are causing ischemia of the tissue and changes in the metabolism with lowering of the defense mechanism. This permits migration of the tumor cells out of the vessels. Braverman and Lerner suspected increasing degrees of malignancy. The collaborators of Haber are of the opinion that the stage of intravascular growth of APS is comparable to the stage of preinvasive carcinomatous growth within the epithelium. The terminal stage in the case of Braverman and Lerner would then correspond to the invasive phase of epithelial neoplasias.

COURSE AND PROGNOSIS

The course of APS is essentially dependent on the location of the affected vessels. As long as the cutaneous vessels exclusively are affected, the disorder does not take a disastrous turn and may by necrosis of the proliferating cells show transitory regressive tendencies. On the one hand, segments of vessels may be recanalized; on the other hand, enough functioning anastomoses—favored by the chronicity of the process—may develop. If, however, the vascular changes are located in vital organs, such as the brain and heart, the blocking of vessels leads to ischemia of the tissue and consecutively to degenerative changes in these organs with severe loss of function and eventually death.

Among the cases observed so far, the first patient survived for seven years. Nothing of what happened to her afterward is known. The question of the "benignity," therefore, remains open. In the last patient (Case No. 7), the follow-up period was too short to allow an opinion on the course. In all other patients the disease ended fatally within 2 to 21 months. The prognosis of this treacherous disease is, therefore, generally poor, since it cannot be foreseen if and when vessels of vital organs will become affected.

THERAPY

The therapeutic measures tried so far have remained without effect. Antibiotics, tuberculostatics, cytostatic drugs, and x-ray irradiation did not influence the course of the disease. Cortisone preparations seemed to be only of temporary benefit. Immunosuppressive drugs have not yet been tried.

REFERENCES

Abulafia, J., Cigorraga, J., Saliva a., J., and Molfino, J. C.: Systemic proliferating angioendotheliomatosis. Dermatol. Ibero Lat. Am. 11:23, 1969.

Braverman, J. M.: Malignant proliferation of vascular endothelium. *In* Pillsbury, D. M., and Livingood, C. S. (Eds.): Proceedings of the XII International Congress of Dermatology. Vol. II. Amsterdam, Excerpta Medica Foundation, 1963.

Braverman, J. M., and Lerner, A. B.: Diffuse malignant proliferation of vascular endothelium. A possible new clinical and pathological entity. Arch. Dermatol., 84:22, 1961.

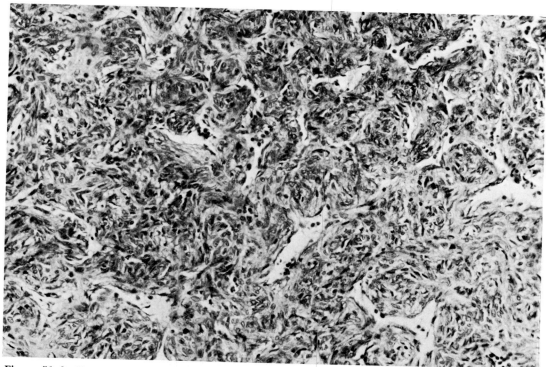

Figure 51–3 Hemangiopericytoma of pelvic region in a middle-aged man; it recurred locally after excision and was definitely invasive. Note the organoid, pseudoendocrine pattern of the neoplastic tissue. *H & E, × 160.*

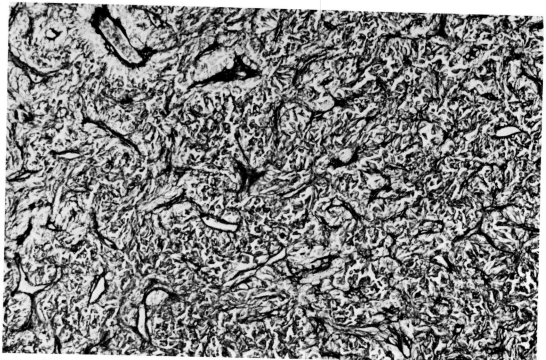

Figure 51–4 Same case as in preceding figure, stained with Masson's trichrome technique, which demonstrates scanty collagen, limited to the perivascular zones. No myofibrils were seen. ×*160.*

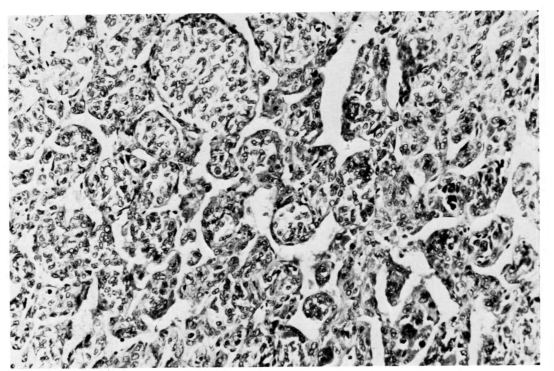

Figure 51–5 Hemangiopericytoma of the back (subcutaneous) in a 62 year old man. *H & E, × 160.*

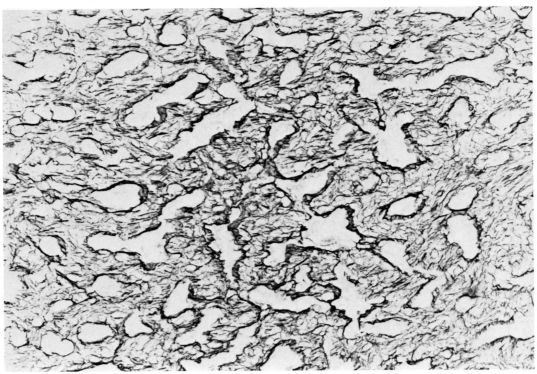

Figure 51–6 Same case as in preceding figure, stained with Laidlaw's technique for reticulin fibrils. Note the regular distribution of the sinusoidal blood vessels and the presence of reticulin fibrils around the individual tumor cells. *×160.*

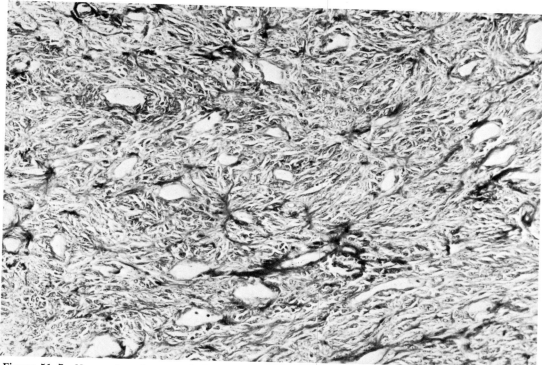

Figure 51–7 Hemangiopericytoma of gluteal region in a 64 year old man. This was a multinodular mass which appeared well circumscribed but not encapsulated. This trichrome stain shows scanty collagen, mostly perivascular, and no myofibrils. The tumor cells, however, somewhat resemble smooth muscle cells. ×160.

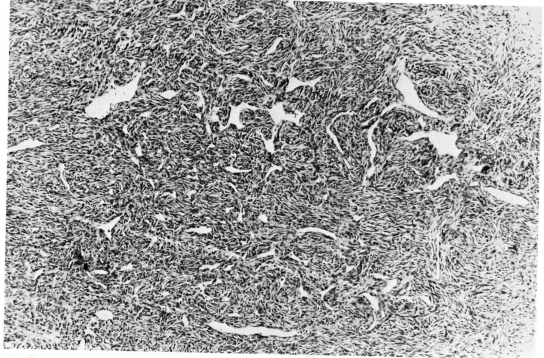

Figure 51–8 Malignant hemangiopericytoma of vulva in a 44 year old woman; it was removed in 1965 by a radical vulvectomy. *H & E*, ×69.

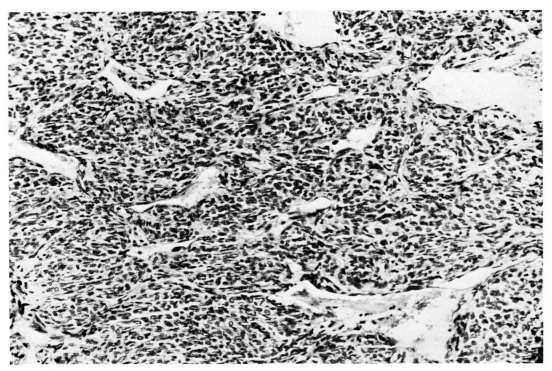

Figure 51–9   Same patient as in preceding figure. This illustration shows a metastasis to the femur four years after vulvectomy. There was neither cytologic anaplasia nor unusual mitotic activity in this case. *H & E, ×160.* (Courtesy of Dr. Edlow, Department of Pathology, Johns Hopkins Medical School.)

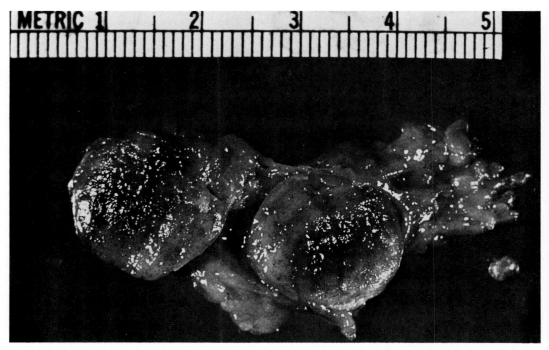

Figure 51–10   Hemangiopericytoma of subcutaneous vein of dorsum of hand in a 48 year old man. This was a well-circumscribed nodule attached to the wall of a superficial vein. The patient has had no recurrences for at least 15 years.

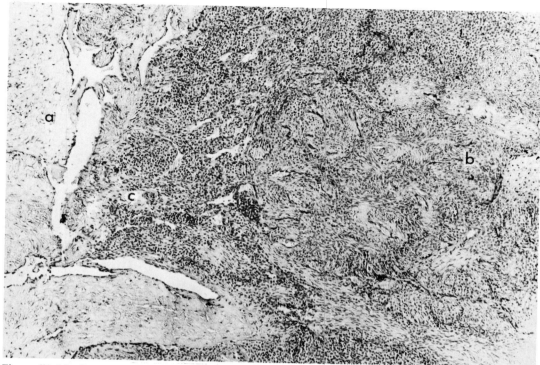

Figure 51–11 Same case as in Figure 51–10. Low-power photomicrograph, showing *(a)* remnants of the vein wall, *(b)* a typical hemangiopericytomatous pattern, and *(c)* a glomangioma-like area. *H & E, ×63.*

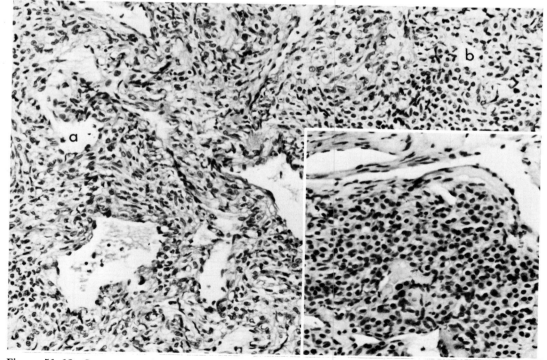

Figure 51–12 Same case as in Figures 51–10 and 51–11. Note the association of the hemangiopericytomatous pattern *(a)* and the glomangioma-like area *(b)* with clear epithelioid cells. No myofibrils were detected in the spindle cells. *H & E, ×160. Insert,* Details of the glomangiomatous area. *×160.*

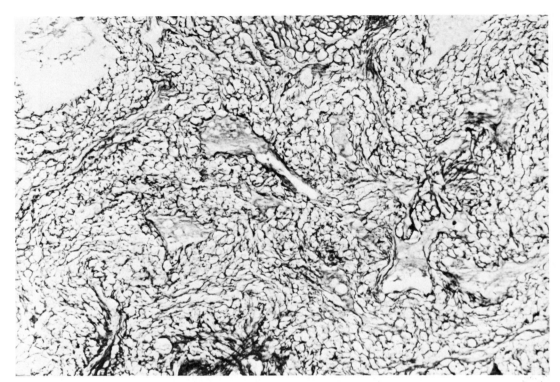

Figure 51–13   Same case as in Figures 51–10, 51–11, and 51–12. Laidlaw's stain for reticulin, showing the characteristic vascular sinusoids and reticulin fibrils distributed regularly around the tumor cells. ×*160.*

never show myofibrils with the usual staining techniques. These cells are generally surrounded individually by reticulin fibrils, but these can be extremely thin and difficult to demonstrate. In addition, stains for reticulin fibrils generally bring out more strikingly the regular vascularity of these tumors and show that the tumor cells are always *outside* the reticulin membrane which supports the vascular endothelium. The basic angioblastic origin of these tumors is further proved by their not infrequent occurrence in association with the walls of vessels, generally veins.

Stout and Murray (1942), using tissue culture techniques, concluded that the cells of these tumors resembled those of the glomus tumor and were also analogous to the normal pericapillary cells described by Zimmermann (1923) as pericytes. Fisher et al. (1952) studied a recurrent hemangiopericytoma in tissue culture and concluded that there was resemblance with the cells of the glomus tumor.

Some electron microscopic studies on tumors diagnosed and acceptable as hemangiopericytomas are available and lead to apparently contradictory conclusions. Murad et al. (1968), studying the ultrastructure of a characteristic hemangiopericytoma of the lateral cervical region and comparing it with a typical glomus tumor of the finger, found no apparent similarity between the cells of these two neoplasms. The cells of the hemangiopericytoma were mesenchymal cells containing no filaments and were not associated with basement membranes, while the glomus cells resembled modified smooth muscle cells, with intracytoplasmic filaments. Apparently similar observations were made by Ramsey (1966) in an electron microscopic study of a so-called meningeal hemangiopericytoma (this is a peculiar variant of vascular meningeal neoplasm, resembling morphologically the hemangiopericytoma of the soft somatic tissues). Essentially, he felt that the perivascular tumor cell is not necessarily the same cell as Zimmermann's pericyte and that it is "cytologically unspecialized." Another interesting ultrastructural study was published by Kuhn et al. (1969) on a tumor which had features of both glomus tumor and hemangiopericytoma. The light microphotographs are convincing, and the authors conclude that in their case there were transition forms between neoplastic glomus cells (modified smooth muscle in type) and other tumor cells consistent with a pericytic origin. These cells contained scanty cytoplasmic fibrils in an arrangement similar to that found in normal pericytes and were associated with basement membrane material.

From these studies it would seem that the mesenchymal cells of the hemangiopericytoma are of uncertain histogenesis. Probably, however, they are basically of angioblastic nature, somewhat related to the normal pericyte and at least in some cases able to differentiate further toward the morphology of the glomus cell, which in turn is a modified smooth muscle cell.

This writer can confirm, on the basis of at least three personal observations, that there are vascular tumors which, with conventional light microscopy, appear to represent a transition between hemangiopericytoma and classical glomus tumor (Figs. 51–10 to 51–13). If these observations are correct, then the only reasonable explanation is that there is a family of angioblastic tumors, featuring periendothelial mesenchymal cells ranging from the highly specialized glomus cells (a modified smooth muscle cell) to cells resembling but not identical to smooth muscle cells (no myofibrils), and finally to an apparently nonspecific mesenchymal spindle cell which, however, still exhibits an affinity to the periendothelial zone of blood vessels, that is, a pericytic arrangement.

This view is also in keeping with the conclusions reached by Rhodin (1968) in his beautiful studies on the ultrastructure of venous capillaries. He stated that the pericyte is the precursor of the smooth muscle cells of the venules and that there are demonstrable transitions from the pericyte to a primitive smooth muscle cell to a "real" smooth muscle cell.

This concept seems to be in agreement with the well-known variations in clinical behavior of these tumors. In fact, a benign course can be expected in those which present as fairly circumscribed, small, superficial nodules, and in which the morphology of the neoplastic cells seems to approach closely the morphology of smooth muscle (and/or glomus cells). Malignant behavior is generally associated with rapidly growing, deeply situated, poorly circumscribed tumor masses which exhibit a high cellularity and in which the cell population, while always arranged in the typical pericytic fashion, consists of more immature-appearing elongated cells. In some of these malignant tumors, only a good reticulin stain will demonstrate the basic vascularity of the tissue, because the vascular spaces may be inconspicuous and collapsed due to crowding by the tumor cells. Mitotic activity has not always been a reliable criterion in the evaluation of the malignant potential of these tumors. For the reasons already stated, however, it is extremely difficult to evaluate statistically the histologic criteria of malignancy and its frequency on the basis of published cases.

DIAGNOSIS

There are no specific clinical features to differentiate these tumors from other superficial or deep soft tissue tumors. Only a histologic study of well-fixed tissue by an experienced pathologist can lead to a correct diagnosis. The pitfalls of confusing these tumors with other tumor entities exhibiting areas of high vascularity histologically have already been pointed out.

THERAPY

As in other tumors, especially of soft tissues, proper therapy can be planned only after obtaining an exact knowledge of the histologic type and the probable biologic potential of the lesion.

Small, superficial nodules will, of course, be studied by excisional biopsy. On the other hand, it is generally wiser to study the nature of a sizable mass by incisional wedge biopsy and decide only then on the extent of the surgical excision to be performed. Radiation therapy of postoperative recurrences or of metastatic deposits, in general, cannot be expected to be more than palliative (Friedman et al., 1960).

REFERENCES

Battifora, H.: Hemangiopericytoma: Ultrastructural study of five cases. Cancer, 31:1418, 1973.

Dotti, G. C., et al.: Su un caso di emangiopericitoma maligno. Minerva Chir., 23:559, 1968.

Enzinger, F. M., Lattes, R., and Torloni, H,: Histologic Typing of Soft Tissue Tumors. Fascicle #3. Geneva, World Health Organization, 1969.

Farr, H. W.: Malignant vascular tumors of the head and neck. Am. J. Surg., 120:500, 1970.

Fisher, E. R., et al.: Hemangiopericytoma: Histologic and tissue culture study. Am. J. Pathol., 28:653, 1952.

Friedman, M., et al.: Irradiation of hemangiopericytoma of Stout. Radiology, 74:721, 1960.

Gensler, S., et al.: Giant benign hemangiopericytoma functioning as an arterio-venous shunt. J.A.M.A., 198:203, 1966.

Hahn, M. J., et al.: Hemangiopericytoma: An ultrastructural study. Cancer, 31:255, 1973.

Kauffmann, S. L., et al.: Hemangiopericytoma in children. Cancer, 13:695, 1960.

Kuhn, C., III, et al.: Tumors arising from pericytes. Ultrastructure and organ culture of a case. Arch. Pathol., 88:653, 1969.

Lidholm, S. O.: Hemangiopericytoma. Acta Pathol. Microbiol. Scand., 38:186, 1956.

Muller, J., et al.: Hemangiopericytoma versus angioblastic meningioma. J. Neuropathol. Exp. Neurol., 26:140, 1967.

Murad, T. M., et al.: Ultrastructure of a hemangiopericytoma and a glomus tumor. Cancer, 22:1239, 1968.

Murray, M. R., and Stout, A. P.: The classification and diagnosis of human tumors by tissue culture methods. Texas Rep. Biol. Med., 12:898, 1954.

Ramsey, H. J.: Fine structure of hemangiopericytoma and hemangio-endothelioma. Cancer, 19:2005, 1966.

Rhodin, J. A. G.: Ultrastructure of mammalian venous capillaries, venules, and small collecting veins. J. Ultrastruct. Res., 25:452, 1968.

Saunders, T. S., et al.: Multiple hemangiopericytomas; their distinction from glomangioma. A.M.A. Arch. Dermatol., 76:731, 1957.

Stout, A. P.: Hemangiopericytoma: A study of twenty five new cases. Cancer, 2:1027, 1949.

Stout, A. P.: Hemangiopericytoma. Mikroskopie, 5:9, 1950.

Stout, A. P.: Tumors featuring pericytes — Glomus tumor and hemangiopericytoma. Lab. Invest., 5:217, 1956.

Stout, A. P.: Tumors of the blood and lymphatic vessels: General considerations. *In* Pack, G. T., and Ariel, I. M. (Eds.): Treatment of Cancer and Allied Diseases. Ed. 2. New York, Hoeber Medical Division, Harper and Row, Publishers, 1964, pp. 130–154.

Stout, A. P., and Lattes, R.: Tumors of Soft Tissues. Atlas of Tumor Pathology, Second Series, Fascicle #1. Washington, D. C., Armed Forces Institute of Pathology, 1967.

Stout, A. P., and Murray, M. R.: Hemangiopericytoma: A vascular tumor featuring Zimmermann's pericytes. Ann. Surg., 116:26, 1942.

Toker, C.: Glomangioma: An ultrastructural study. Cancer, 23:487, 1969.

Tulenko, J. F.: Congenital hemangiopericytoma: Case report. Plast. Reconstr. Surg., 41:276, 1968.

Venkatachalam, M. A., et al.: Fine structure of glomus tumor: Similarity of glomus cells to smooth muscle. Cancer, 23:1176, 1969.

Zimmermann, K. W.: Der feiner Bau der Blut Capillaren. Anat. Entwicklungsgesch., 68:29, 1923.

52

Kaposi's Sarcoma

A.C. Templeton, M.D.

SYNONYMS

There are at least forty synonyms for this condition, most of which represent attempts at defining the cell of origin, which remains unknown, or at describing the clinical appearances, which are many and variable. Multiple idiopathic hemorrhagic sarcoma, idiopathic multiple pigmented sarcoma of the skin, cutaneous angioendothelioma, telangiectatic pseudosarcoma, and angioreticulomatosis are among the more commonly used terms. Lists of synonyms may be found in the publications of Bluefarb (1957) or Lothe (1963). Since the etiology, cell of origin, and nature of process are all subjects under debate, an eponymous term seems justified. Kaposi's sarcoma is a term more widely used than Kaposi's hemorrhagic sarcoma. The use of the word "sarcoma" is hallowed by tradition and follows the majority opinion, though many would hold that the disease is not a true malignant tumor.

DEFINITION

Kaposi's sarcoma is a tumorlike condition characterized by a proliferation of a mixture of spindle cells and vascular structures. This proliferation typically occurs in multiple sites, most frequently in the dermis, and results in the production of nodules or plaques possessing a characteristic violaceous appearance.

HISTORY

First described by the Hungarian dermatologist Moricz Kaposi from Vienna in 1872 as "Idiopathisches multiples Pigmentsarkom der Haut" (Kaposi, 1872), the disease was renamed by Kaposi himself, who set a dangerous precedent by calling it "sarcoma idiopathicum multiplex haemorrhagicum" (Kaposi, 1894). The original description of the disease has seldom been improved upon and reads as follows:

Nodules ranging from the size of a peppercorn to that of a pea or a hazel nut, and brownish red or blueish red in colour, appear in the skin without any apparent cause, either local or general. They are smooth on the surface, elastic in consistency and very often resemble blood blisters. They may occur singly or in plaquelike groups. . . . The nodules generally develop first on the sole or dorsum of the foot, thereafter spreading rapidly to the hands. Most of them appear on these parts.

1183

During the course of the disease, single or multiple tumours may also develop although in lesser numbers, on the legs, arms, face and trunk. The nodules sometimes atrophy, and may ulcerate at a later stage. . . . It (the disease) occurs predominantly in males over 40 years of age. The histological structure consists of foci of fusiform spindle cells and a rich new growth of capillaries, between which pigmentation occurs.

A few years after the original description, the entity had been recognized in many countries (Kaposi, 1887), and the most important facets of the disease were well described, most notably by Kaposi himself and by de Amicis (1882) in a paper rediscovered by Ronchese (1958). Thus it was known that the disease occurred most often in males of mature years, and that it involved the skin most frequently and usually pursued a slow, progressive course punctuated by relapses and remissions. The association with edema was also noted, though not apparently by Kaposi himself. Kaposi (1887) described disseminated disease with a postmortem examination, and de Amicis (1882) described a rapidly fatal form of the disease occurring in a 5 year old child.

The literature for the next 60 or 70 years consists largely of anecdotal case reports and the occasional rediscovery of facts well-described many years before. Reviews of the disease, particularly by Dörffel (1932), Kren (1933), and Aegerter and Peale (1942), attempted to summarize the large number of theories of etiology and cell of origin. Otherwise publications were mainly concerned with descriptions of the histologic and clinical aspects of the disease. Most authors agreed that this disease appeared in Jewish subjects more frequently than in other ethnic groups, but Dörffel (1932) argued that the distribution appeared to be geographically rather than genetically determined. A particularly full review of the development of ideas about the disease is to be found in the monograph by Bluefarb (1957).

The next development of importance was the realization that the disease was very common in Africa. The first case recorded seems to have been that of Hallenburger (1914), but the frequency of the disease was not widely appreciated until much later when reviews of experience with cancer in various parts of Africa were published (Smith and Elmes, 1934; Hennessey, 1942; Chaboeuf, 1945; Kaminer and Murray, 1950). The extraordinary prevalence in some areas was fully brought out by the studies of Thijs (1957) in the Congo. In view of these discoveries, a conference on Kaposi's sarcoma was held in Kampala, Uganda, in 1961, under the auspices of the International Union Against Cancer and the presentations were later published (Ackerman and Murray 1962). This monograph remains a most useful source of reference. Since that time papers on the histochemical, electron microscopic, and tissue culture studies of the disease have attempted to define the pathogenesis but have failed convincingly to demonstrate the cell of origin. Regrettably, it remains largely true that little more is known about this perplexing and variable disease today than was apparent to the original author a hundred years ago.

EPIDEMIOLOGY AND INCIDENCE

The total number of cases now recorded amounts to some 4000, the majority from tropical Africa. In most parts of the world Kaposi's sarcoma is a rare disease. It is unlikely that an average dermatologist working outside central or southern Africa would see more than four or five cases in a lifetime's practice unless working in a referral center. For example, only 70 cases were seen at the Mayo Clinic in 38 years (Reynolds et al., 1965), that is 0.067 percent of tumors diagnosed at that institution (Moertel, 1966). Many authors have commented upon the apparently greater incidence among laborers and persons with outdoor occupations than among white collar indoor workers (van Cleve and Hellwig, 1935). McCarthy and Pack (1950) found an association with occupations entailing long periods of standing. It is widely agreed that this disease is much more common in Eastern Europe (Dörffel, 1932) and tropical Africa than in other parts of the world, and cases reported from elsewhere often trace their ancestry back to one of these regions.

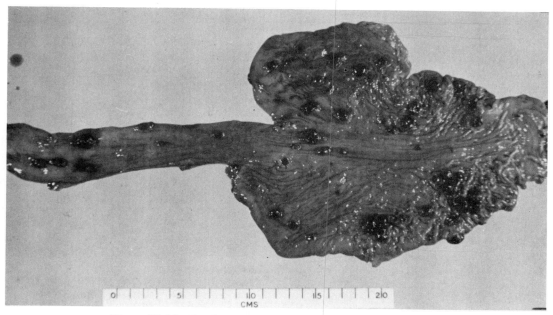

Figure 52–10   Esophagus and stomach showing numerous nodules.

progress is often punctuated by relapse and remission of some or even all nodules. Some cases have shown no visceral lesions after many years of cutaneous disease. The majority of cases show a tendency toward slow erratic spread over a period of many years.

The lower limbs are almost always involved, the upper limbs often, and the trunk, head, and internal organs sometimes (Reynolds et al., 1965). Section of involved skin will often reveal tiny tumor deposits in the dermis in clinically normal skin (Fig. 52–9). Spread is probably not a result of metastases, although there does appear to be some tendency for the nod-

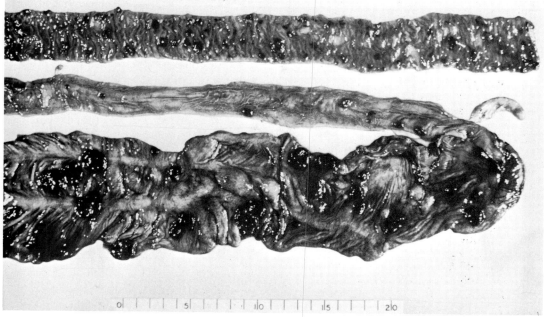

Figure 52–11   Involvement of colon and small intestine.

ules to follow the course of the neurovascular trunks of the limb (Lothe, 1963). It is very doubtful that metastatic disease could produce the pattern of generalized disease, and it is more likely that each nodule at each site develops separately. Metastases undoubtedly do occur from time to time but are very rare and usually are associated with aggressive lesions.

Lesions in the bowel are seen almost invariably in patients who die of disseminated disease (Figs. 52–10 and 52–11) and may cause hemorrhage, perforation, or intussusception (Aegerter and Peale, 1942; Tedeschi et al., 1947; Pelissier, 1953; White and King, 1964). Diagnosis of intestinal lesions may be achieved by gastroscopy, sigmoidoscopy, or barium studies (Seagrave, 1948; Rajan et al., 1969), but in most cases the extent of gastrointestinal involvement is only apparent at postmortem examination. Other sites frequently involved by tumor include adrenals, pericardium, nodes, liver, and mouth (Lothe and Murray, 1962). It is difficult to be certain of the proportion of cases having visceral involvement. A much quoted figure is 10 percent of cases (Ecklund and Valaitis, 1962). Autopsy studies indicate a much greater proportion in excess of two-thirds of patients (Cox and Helwig, 1959), and review of data from published accounts shows that visceral lesions were found in 96 of 102 cases at necropsy. A large proportion of these lesions gave rise to no symptoms, and it is impossible to state at which stage of the disease they developed. It is quite possible that in many cases the disease may even start in the small intestine. Experience in Uganda would indicate that this happens quite frequently. Such nodules in the terminal ileum could remain undetected for many years. It is important to try to discover the frequency of visceral involvement for a number of reasons. If it occurs in many cases, then the rationale of therapy for nonaggressive disease will have to be reconsidered. At present these lesions are usually only discovered at autopsy and have therefore achieved a sinister reputation which is probably undeserved.

Plaque Formation. In this pattern the tumor spreads laterally along the dermis at the level of the sweat glands and produces induration of the skin over quite large areas. The plaque is a combination of tumor tissue itself with induration of the overlying skin, resulting from lymphatic obstruction.

Ulceration of Nodules. This is seen very frequently in Africans but is much more unusual in whites. Ulceration may be a result of invasion of the epidermis by tumor, and in such cases the nodule becomes fixed because of involvement of the deep fascia. Ulceration of smaller nodules may occur without invasion, for example, following trauma or circulatory disorders. When this occurs a hemorrhagic proliferation similar to granuloma pyogenicum develops on the surface (Lee, 1968). An ulcerated nodular lesion may be misdiagnosed as aggressive disease unless attention is paid to the deep aspect of the lesion. It is important to separate these processes, since the treatment of each type is different (Kyalwazi, 1968). Furthermore, biopsy of such a lesion must be excisional rather than incisional if mistakes in histologic diagnosis are to be avoided.

Edema. Patients with Kaposi's sarcoma often exhibit a woody firm edema of the limbs and sometimes of the trunk. This is not due to central obstruction of lymphatics or blood vessels but is a result of peripheral lymph channel obstruction and possibly leakage of lymph from the tumor itself. Many authors have quoted cases in which Kaposi's sarcoma has developed in an edematous limb and have thought that this factor might be important in the etiology. In view of the long history of certain cases, it is sometimes difficult to separate cause from effect.

Regression of Tumor. A careful history taken from a patient with long-standing nodular lesions will almost always reveal that at least one nodule has shown regression at some time during the course of the disease. In some cases spontaneous regression of all nodules, resulting in apparent cure, has been noted. Remissions may last for many years, and such histories are by no means rare and probably occur in excess of 2 percent of cases. It is difficult to be certain of the cause of such remissions, and particularly in Africa it is quite possible that some effective home-brewed medicine may have been taken.

Regression of lesions seems to take

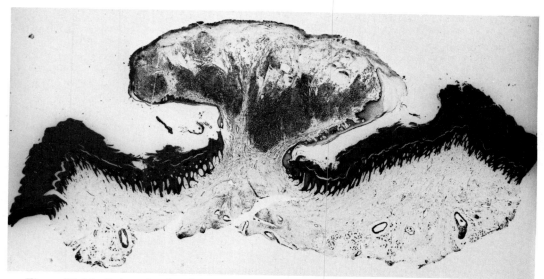

Figure 52–12 Pedunculated nodule of Kaposi's sarcoma closely mimicking granuloma pyogenicum.

place by one of three methods. Autoamputation of pedunculated lesions may occur. It is a characteristic feature of Kaposi's sarcoma that nodules frequently show undermining of the tumor tissue by epithelium (Fig. 52–12), and when extrusion of the nodule has taken place, a depressed, usually depigmented scar remains. Alternatively the nodule may become gradually firmer, smaller, and paler and be transformed into a scar. The cause of this pattern of regression has usually been ascribed to autoinfarction following thromboses in sclerotic vessels (Murray and Lothe, 1962), and it seems certain that it must be due to some local factor, since one nodule may regress as another is growing larger. Browne (1966) has de-

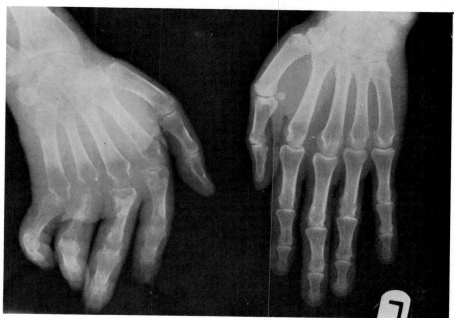

Figure 52–13 Radiograph showing bone cysts and cortical notching in the bones of the hand (same case as in Fig. 52–4). (Courtesy of Dr. John Taylor.)

scribed a third method, which he described as hemorrhagic regression, in which it appears that the nodule becomes fibrotic after hemorrhage into its substance, a pattern also noted by Symmers (1941) and by Kaposi himself (1894). Browne's patient displayed an extraordinary progression with spontaneous universal hemorrhagic regression occurring on a number of occasions, leaving the patient apparently disease-free for a period after each episode.

Involvement of Bone. Hansson (1940) found no lesions of the bone in 23 Scandinavian patients, all of whom had an x-ray skeletal survey. Palmer (1962), on the other hand, claimed that bone lesions are to be found in all African cases if carefully sought. Basset and Payet (1962) stated that bone lesions are seen more

frequently in African cases. Davies (1956) described the x-ray changes as showing generalized osteoporosis, "rubbing out" of the cortical pattern, cortical notching, bone cysts (Fig. 52–13), or complete destruction of bone matrix. The first of these changes is probably a result of the increased blood supply to the limb, but the others are due to tumor actually in the bone (Fig. 52–14) or in the neighboring periosteum (Taylor et al., 1971b). Bone changes are seen more frequently in patients with aggressive lesions than in those with nodular disease. The presence of bone lesions appears to worsen the prognosis significantly and is often associated with alterations in reactivity to challenge with dinitrochlorobenzene (DNCB), as described by Master et al. (1970). Successful therapy of bone lesions requires more

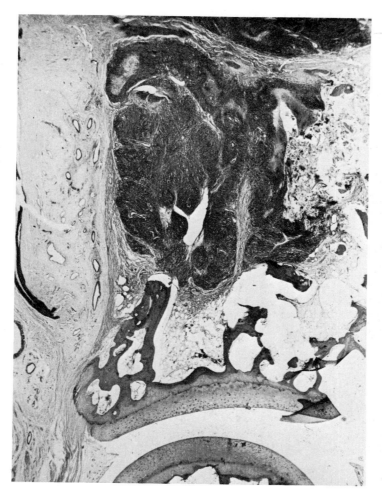

Figure 52–14 Terminal phalanx of a finger, showing tumor in the medulla.

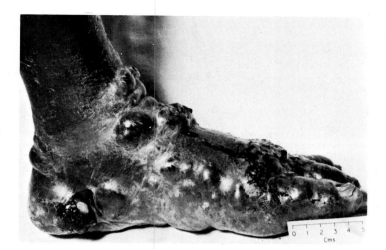

Figure 52–15 Aggressive lobulated tumor of the foot. (Courtesy of Dr. John Taylor.)

prolonged drug administration than is necessary for cutaneous lesions.

Lymph Node Involvement. Enlargement of lymph nodes occurs very frequently in Kaposi's sarcoma. In the majority of cases the enlarged node shows reactive changes. Reaction is also seen throughout the reticuloendothelial system, and changes have been noted in the spleen, nodes, and bone marrow (Stats, 1946; Tedeschi, 1958). More rarely the lymph node may be involved by

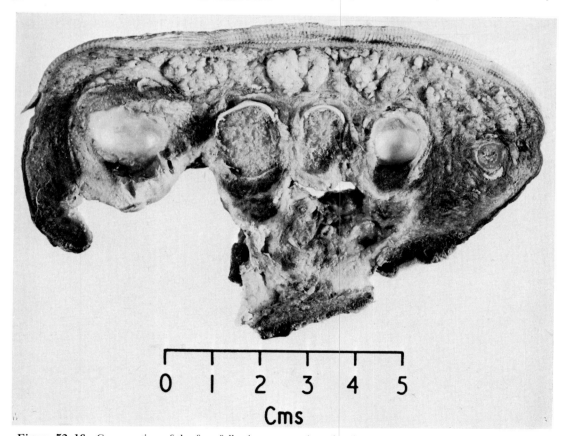

Figure 52–16 Cross-section of the foot following amputation, showing tumor surrounding the metatarsals.

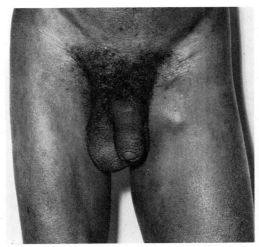

Figure 52–17 Enlargement of femoral nodes in the same patient due to tumor involvement.

tumor. Such involvement occurs in one of four disease patterns (Bhana et al., 1970):

1. Generalized nodal involvement
   (a) without significant cutaneous disease (Fig. 52–7)
   (b) with extensive visceral and cutaneous involvement

2. Localized nodal involvement
   (a) with cutaneous disease (Figs. 52–15 to 52–17)
   (b) without local cutaneous lesions

Patients with nodular disease only rarely show involvement of lymph nodes, but it occurs more frequently in other patterns.

Formation of Bullae and Hyperkeratosis. Large bullae may develop over the surface of the nodules, particularly on the feet and legs. This may create difficulties in diagnosis, and it is for this reason that reports of the concurrence of bullous eruptions and Kaposi's sarcoma should be treated with caution. In the majority of cases those bullae are the result of ectasia of subcutaneous lymph channels which appear to have been obstructed by tumor growth. Such areas are often covered by a thick hyperkeratotic layer (Fig. 52–18).

Development of Aggressive Lesions. Patients with nodular disease may develop aggressive lesions. This occurs much more frequently in African patients, though it also occurs in whites (Reynolds et al., 1965). Such lesions may develop from a preexisting nodule in the dermis or more frequently from one more deeply placed.

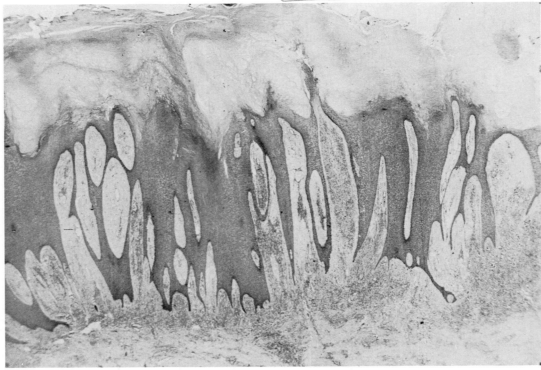

Figure 52–18 Edema and hyperkeratosis overlying a plaque of tumor.

AGGRESSIVE DISEASE

Such lesions are usually solitary (Fig. 52–5) and often have a lobulated appearance (Fig. 52–15). They are found most frequently on the feet and legs, but the upper limb or trunk and viscera may be affected. Tumors may develop de novo or more commonly from preexisting nodular disease, particularly nodules more deeply placed in the limb. These tumors correspond to the "true sarcomas" of other authors (Reynolds et al., 1965). The term "locally aggressive disease" is preferred for two reasons. First, nodular nonaggressive disease is probably also a true sarcoma; second, the aggressive lesions seem to possess a lower metastatic potential than other "true sarcomas" of connective tissue.

Clinically the lesion is usually a fungating mass with the surface composed of granulation tissue, unless covered by a necrotic slough. The color varies from pink to black, depending upon the amount of bleeding which has occurred into the site. The tumor may have a narrow pedicle and expand in a cauliflower shape. It is more often lobulated and appears to be an amalgam of numerous nodules growing in a plateau which may be of enormous dimensions. Less frequently the tumor shows a rather different growth pattern, which has been called the infiltrative type (Fig. 52–19) (Taylor et al., 1971b). The skin is often not ulcerated, but tumor tissue is found deep in the feet, and bones are usually involved. The separation of this pattern of growth is important, because the differential diagnosis from maduromycosis may be difficult in African patients. Histologically such tumors often show extensive sclerosis, and response to therapy appears to be less rapid (Reynolds et al., 1965; Vogel et al., 1971).

Spread of tumor by local invasion is usually slow but inexorable. Metastasis to the draining nodes is found from time to time (Bhana et al., 1970) (Fig. 52–17), but hematogenous spread seems to be unusual, in contrast to the behavior of many other types of sarcoma. Nevertheless, the prognosis in these cases seems to be poorer than in patients with nonaggres-

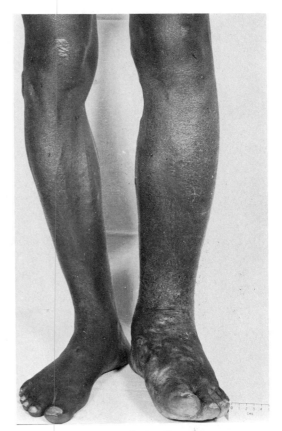

Figure 52–19 Lower limb affected by an aggressive lesion of the infiltrative type. (Courtesy of Dr. John Taylor.)

sive disease (Kyalwazi, 1969), and a vigorous therapeutic approach is justified.

More rarely the aggressive lesion grows extremely rapidly, and extensive necrosis is seen in the tumor mass. These cases are distinguishable histologically in that there is a much greater cellular pleomorphism than in other aggressive lesions (Taylor et al., 1971b). The response to cytotoxic therapy is less satisfactory than in other fungating lesions (Vogel et al., 1971). The proportion of such cases in Africa is fairly high, but they have been recognized elsewhere (e.g., Reynolds et al., 1965, Case No. 7).

Another feature of aggressive disease is the widespread occurrence of woody edema in the involved limb (Fig. 52–20). This is a result of widespread subcutaneous tumor growth, often at the level of the junction of dermis with subcutaneous fat. This involvement renders the limb

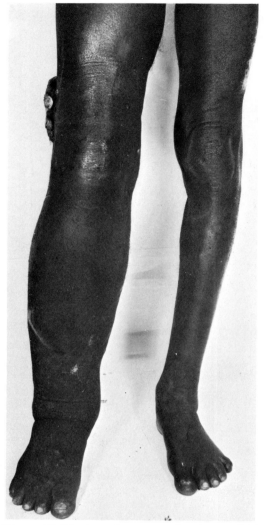

Figure 52-20 Agressive tumor in the poplitial fossa on a limb which is grossly edematous. (Courtesy of Dr. John Taylor.)

painful and also creates considerable difficulty if curative surgery is contemplated. Patients with locally aggressive lesions frequently do not respond to challenge with clinitrochlorobenzene (DNCB) (Master et al., 1970). This indicates that the thymic-dependent system is depressed and may explain why the tumor is able to erode local structures. Conversely, it implies that in nodular disease this system is important in maintaining the nodular structure of the tumor and perhaps its relatively good prognosis. Lymphocyte transformation is depressed in patients with locally aggressive lesions (Taylor et al., 1971a).

GENERALIZED DISEASE

The speed of development of generalized lesions varies markedly. For example, Reynolds et al. (1965) recorded a patient (Case No. 5) who died with visceral involvement 32 years after developing skin nodules, contrasting with their Case No. 6, who died of generalized disease within two years. Experience in Uganda has led to the conclusion that there are two fairly distinct clinical patterns.

Nodular Disease Progressing to Generalized Involvement

This usually occurs in males over the age of 50 years. The progress of the disease is slow and may be measured in years. After a period of relative quiescence, the tempo of the disease seems to accelerate, and new nodules appear at a rapid rate. Edema often becomes marked, and lesions in the mouth and pharynx may appear. The lymph nodes are less frequently involved than in the other type of generalized disease, but the distribution of lesions is otherwise similar. Such cases with necropsy data are recorded by Dillard and Weidman, 1925; Becker and Thatcher, 1938; Symmers, 1941 (Case No. 8); Stats, 1946; Epstein, 1957; Rothman, 1962; Jackson and Madoff, 1963; and Reynolds et al., 1965 (Case No. 5).

Generalized Disease at Presentation

This form occurs at a much younger age than the preceding clinical pattern. The sex ratio shows a smaller male excess, and widespread involvement of lymph nodes is frequently seen. This group of cases may be further subdivided into two types:

Nodal Predominance (Fig. 52-7). This form occurs in African children and is very rare in non-Africans (Dutz and Stout, 1960; Davies and Lothe, 1962; Sla-

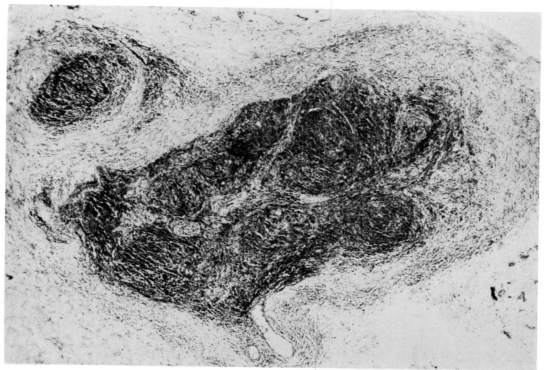

Figure 52–26   A regressing nodule surrounded by a zone of fibrous tissue and inflammatory cells, mainly lymphocytes.

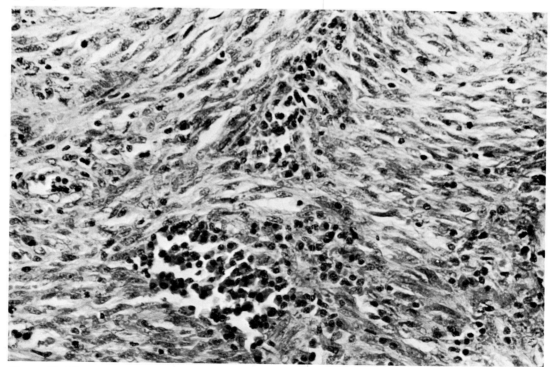

Figure 52–27   An aggressive lesion composed of spindle cells without a vascular component containing clumps of plasma cells.

be found within histiocytes or endothelial cells or, more rarely, extracellularly. Minimal proliferation of fibroblastic cells may be visible. The positive diagnosis of Kaposi's sarcoma by histologic means alone is difficult at this stage and is more likely to be made in retrospect.

The next change to be noted is a vascular response, with increasing tortuosity of vessels and thickening of the walls due to proliferation of the endothelium and other cells surrounding the vessel. Histiocytes are found more frequently at this stage, and proliferation of spindle cells may be seen. Other inflammatory cells appear less numerous, and iron pigment is rather less obvious. This is referred to as the *granulomatous phase*.

Angiomatous changes occur when the vascular proliferation has reached such proportions as to dominate the picture. The vessels appear to be a mixture of hematogenous and lymphatic type. Interspersed between the vessels are numerous large, pale cells with a macrophage function. Many of these cells contain iron, and some appear to have ingested red cells which may be seen in large vacuoles. The proportion of spindle cells gradually increases as the nodule forms and passes to the stage of *angiosarcoma*.

There are two basic patterns of growth at this phase of development, *nodules* and *plaques*. The nodule lies in the dermis and appears partially encapsulated. As it grows, collagen accumulates around it, and the epidermis becomes gradually flattened and often appears to grip the nodule (Fig. 52–28). There is usually a narrow band of fibrous tissue between the nodule and the epidermis, and this zone usually contains many dilated lymphatic vessels. These vessels may become very large indeed, and reactive epithelial hyperplasia may occur. The plaque grows in a loose sheet, spreading along the level of the skin accessories, often showing some accentuation around those structures (Fig. 52–29). The same basic ingredients are found as in the nodule, but the very diffuse nature of the change often makes it difficult to diagnose. Transitions between

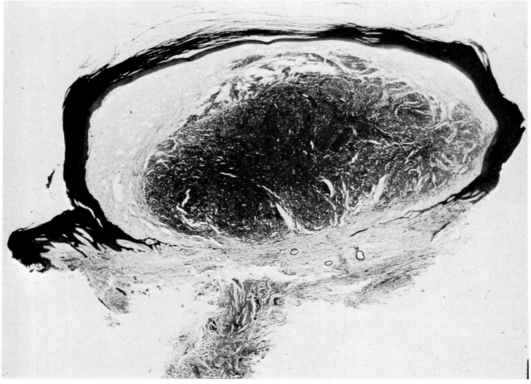

Figure 52–28   Cutaneous nodule showing an undermining of tumor tissue by ingrowth of a collarette of epidermis.

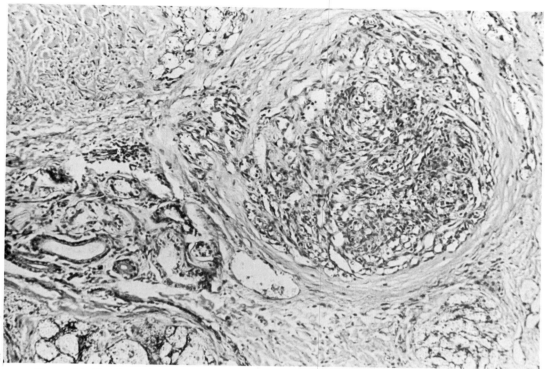

Figure 52–29 Photomicrograph of a plaque lesion, showing tumor at the level of a sweat gland.

these forms may occur, as, for example, when a nodule develops within a plaque.

The vascular component of nodules represents an amalgam of many different origins. Blood vessels are present in the periphery of the nodule and may give rise to the tiny vascular slits present throughout the tumor tissue. Lymphatic vessels also appear in the periphery and probably contribute to the tumor itself. That lymph and arterial blood are carried into the nodule may be proved by lymphangiography or arteriography, both of which delineate nodules well. Material injected directly into a nodule passes both to veins and lymphatics, whereas hemangiomas drain only to the veins (Palmer, 1962). This proves that connections are established with both vascular systems and suggests the possibility that Kaposi's sarcoma is derived from a cell capable of manufacturing both types of vessel.

A characteristic finding in tumor nodules is the presence of globules of hyaline eosinophilic material (Fig. 52–30). These are found extracellularly or in vacuoles in the spindle or macrophage cells. Such globules are found in the majority of cases, particularly if the tumor was stained with phloxine-tartrazine (Lendrum). The appearance and staining characteristics of this material are very similar to those of Russell bodies. They appear as laminated rounded bodies on electron microscopic examination and are commonly referred to as myelin figures. Their origin is obscure, but they may be products of lysosomal degeneration or effete red cells. In some cases when the differential diagnosis from granuloma pyogenicum is difficult to make, the finding of these globules is helpful in confirming the diagnosis of Kaposi's sarcoma (Lee, 1968).

The histologic appearance of nodular lesions is very similar in any part of the body and in a wide variety of clinical situations. Murray and Lothe (1962) commented on the remarkable homogeneity of appearance in their series of 497 cases and on the large measure of agreement between published descriptions from different parts of the world. Thus it is difficult to distinguish a nodule of tumor from the node of a child who will die

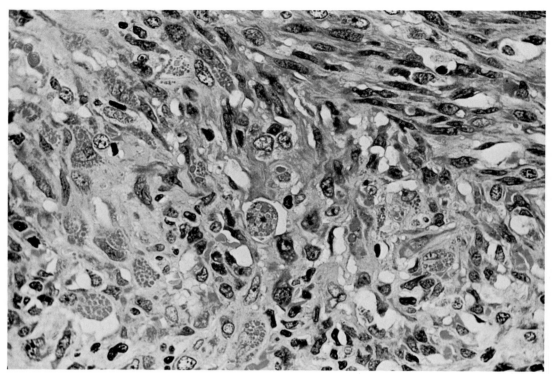

Figure 52–30   Eosinophilic inclusions in Kaposi's sarcoma. This section was processed in plastic and cut at 1μ. The amount of globular material seen is much greater when this technique is used. (Courtesy of Dr. Dennis H. Wright.)

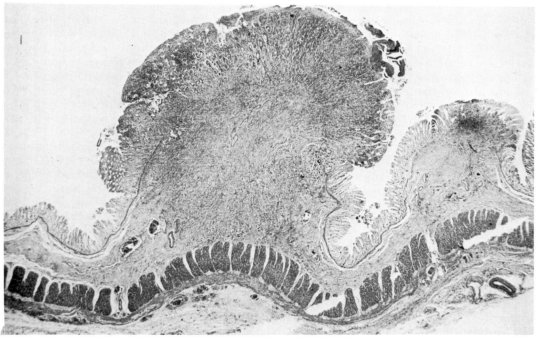

Figure 52–31   A nodule in the small intestine situated in the mucosa and submucosa, interrupting the muscularis mucosae but not invading the circular layer.

frequently—probably in about 2 percent of cases, but in others progression is rapid and inexorable. A patient presenting with generalized disease is likely to die within two years. Aggressive lesions are also sometimes lethal, even though widespread tumor metastasis is unusual. Nodular disease is compatible with very long survival. Reynolds et al. (1965) recorded one patient who was still alive 50 years after initial diagnosis. The average survival is in the region of 8 to 10 years (Cox and Helwig, 1959), and many of these patients die of intercurrent disease rather than Kaposi s sarcoma.

Available treatment may be summarized as follows:

1. Surgery—diagnostic, cosmetic, symptomatic, palliative, or curative.

2. X-ray therapy—conventional or mega voltage, implants.

3. Cytotoxic agents—administered locally or systemically.

4. Immunotherapy—with BCG or vaccinia virus or other nonspecific stimuli.

5. Supportive measures—antibiotics, blood transfusion, and so forth.

6. Arsenic—now largely abandoned, though claimed to be effective.

7. Symptomatic—elastic stockings, analgesics, reassurance, and so forth.

The contribution of each mode of treatment will be different in each case, but the majority of patients fall into a limited number of clinically and histologically defined groups.

Patients With Nodular Disease

In the majority of cases the lesions will be restricted to the limbs, and the natural history of the disease is usually that of slow progression.

At postmortem examination the majority of patients show visceral lesions, but clinical methods reveal lesions in a very small proportion. The true frequency of such involvement is unknown. If lesions occur in a large proportion of cases, as seems likely, it is perhaps illogical to treat the limb only, and there would be theoretic reasons for giving systemic drugs in every case. Controlled trials of these methods are urgently required but will not produce results for some years because of the slow progress of the disease.

Examination of the patient should include careful assessment of the mouth and pharynx, sigmoidoscopy, and x-ray of long bones and feet. It is probably worthwhile testing such patients with DNCB challenge (Master et al., 1970), since this may give some indication of the likelihood of visceral lesions. If any lesions are present in the viscera, more vigorous therapy on the lines of that advocated for generalized disease is probably justified. Treatment of the skin nodules may be by surgery if they are solitary or localized, but in most cases x-ray therapy or cytotoxic drugs will be required. Excision of solitary nodules is often curative; a large proportion of patients suffer no recurrence and may have no disease elsewhere many years later (Pack and Davis, 1954). The treatment of lesions by radiotherapy is well discussed by Cohen et al. (1962), who recommended fractionated doses at 100 k. for superficial nodules, 2500 rads at 25 k. for subcutaneous disease, and megavolt doses in cases in which the whole limb is involved. Great care is required at the periphery of edematous limbs to avoid damage to the skin. Hansson (1940) used radium implants with some success, but few authorities use this method. In the majority of cases such treatment is swift, effective, and obviously the treatment of choice; for example, in a series reported by Reynolds et al. (1965), 40 of 49 patients had excellent initial response to x-ray therapy. Radiotherapy is much more successful when the lesions are of recent onset (McCarthy and Pack, 1950) than it is on the older plaquelike lesions. Following superficial radiotherapy, most patients retain good function of the limb and require little further therapy other than an elastic stocking to reduce the accumulation of edema.

Relapse of the disease requires caution in therapy, since the skin is more sensitive and the tumor less sensitive to therapy. When radiotherapy is not available (most often in those areas where the tumor is most common) or in relapse following radiotherapy, drug treatment should be used. Monaco and Austen (1959) recommended extracorporeal perfusion on the basis of experience with two patients, both of whom responded. Cook (1962) recommended intra-arterial nitrogen mustard; although this is effective, the rate of late complications, such as contracture, is unacceptably high for a nonlethal condition, and its use has been abandoned in Uganda. Kyalwazi (1968 and 1969) has obtained very favorable results using Trenimon (Bayer 3231), an oral cytotoxic agent given in a weekly dose. This enables treatment to be carried out on an outpatient basis, though frequent hematologic investigation is needed. The rate of complications, such as leukopenia or thrombocytopenia, is low. Other drugs which have been found to be effective include cyclophosphamide (Spencer, 1966), vinca-leukoblastine (Scott and Voight, 1966), spiramycin (Back et al., 1964), and actinomycin (Kyalwazi et al., 1971; Vogel et al., 1971). By contrast, Kyalwazi (1969) found cyclophosphamide, methotrexate, orthomelphalan, and vinblastine largely ineffective. The average survival with therapy is in excess of ten years (Reynolds et al., 1965), and a significant proportion of patients will die of intercurrent disease rather than of Kaposi's sarcoma. It is difficult to predict which patients are likely to show visceral extension of the disease except that, in general, the younger the age of onset the more likely is generalized disease to occur (Hansson, 1940).

Arsenicals are sometimes claimed to be effective but are seldom used in the present day. It has also been suggested that penicillin is effective in the treatment of superficial lesions. This is doubtful, and the drug probably acts by reducing secondary infection rather than affecting the tumor itself. Because of the gross excess of males suffering from this disease, estrogen therapy has been used but was only found to be effective in one case (Hurlbut and Lincoln, 1949). Other authors have found no effect clinically, and added hormone has no effect upon growth of cells in tissue culture.

Aggressive Lesions

Radiotherapy for such tumors requires higher voltage and higher doseage, e.g., 5000 rads at 2 mv. Treatment is not nearly as successful as with nodular disease (Reynolds et al., 1965) and may be virtually without effect, particularly in those patients with atypical histology. Treatment with cytotoxic drugs is often successful. Vogel et al. (1971), in a controlled, randomized clinical trial, found a good response with actinomycin in high doses, whereas cyclophosphamide was relatively ineffective. Other drugs are at present under trial. Local perfusions by intra-arterial injection will often result in improvement (Cook, 1962), but once again the rate of complications appears higher than with systemic therapy without commensurately better results. Surgery may be used in such cases to reduce tumor bulk or to prevent hemorrhage or sepsis, but in many patients this would necessitate amputation in order to achieve sufficient margin around the tumor. Surgery is therefore usually reserved for those lesions which do not respond to conservative measures. If the histologic appearances are those of an anaplastic variant, it is likely that radiotherapy or cytotoxic drugs will be ineffective (Reynolds et al., 1965; Vogel et al., 1971). In such cases amputation may be the only effective remedy, and survival after amputation may be prolonged. The prognosis after amputation depends upon the nature and extent of disease elsewhere in the body. For example, many patients have nonaggressive lesions on other limbs, in which case after amputation the treatment and prognosis become those of nodular disease. Such patients are probably more likely to develop a second aggressive lesion than are patients with nodular disease. Because of the relative infrequency of metastatic spread, amputation even in advanced cases is justified and effective. In many cases, however, there is woody induration of the whole limb, which would require heroic surgery to circumvent. In these latter cases, symptomatic treatment is probably all that can be offered, particularly as many of these patients are old and doubtful surgical risks.

Some patients die quite early in the course of the disease, but survival may be prolonged. Experience with Ugandan cases indicates that the cause of death in such patients is usually one of the complications of the disease or of the therapy rather than generalized tumor metastases. For example, patients may die of pulmonary emboli, cerebral hemorrhage or pulmonary tuberculosis (Templeton, 1972).

Generalized Disease

This form of the disease is rapidly fatal, and the only feasible treatment is chemotherapy. Actinomycin has been successful in some cases (Taylor et al., 1971b), but long-term results are not as yet available. In the untreated cases, the mortality is virtually 100 percent within three years of onset.

REFERENCES

Ackerman, L. V., and Murray, J. F.: Symposium on Kaposi's Sarcoma. Basel, S. Karger, 1962.

Aegerter, E. E., and Peale, A. R.: Kaposi's sarcoma. A critical survey. Arch. Pathol., 34:413, 1942.

Alexander, M.: Kaposi's sarcoma with ocular manifestations. Am. J. Ophthal., 55:625, 1963.

de Amicis, T.: Dermopolimelano-sarcoma idiopathico. Quoted by Ronchese, 1958.

André, R., Duperrat, B., and David, V.: Association of Kaposi's disease with Waldenstrom's disease. Bull. Soc. Fr. Dermatol., 73:469, 1966.

Anthony, C. W., and Koneman, E. W.: Visceral Kaposi's sarcoma. Arch. Pathol., 70:740, 1960.

El Arini, A. F.: Idiopathic multiple haemorrhagic sarcoma of Kaposi (with report of a case associated with lymphosarcoma). Alexandria Med. J., 4:35, 1958.

Attygalle, D., Ratnaike, V. T., and Suntharalingam, M.: A case of Kaposi's sarcoma. Ceylon Med. J., 14:196, 1969.

Austregesilo, A.: Un cas d'angiokératome semblable au Pied de Madura. Arch. Schiffs. Trop. Hyg., 16:622, 1912.

Ayer, J. P., Paul, O., and Capps, R. B.: Clinicopathologic Conference. Am. Heart J., 63:566, 1962.

Babini, G.: A case of Kaposi's disease associated with chronic lymphatic leukaemia. Arch. Ital. Dermatol. Venereol., 34:450, 1966.

Bacaloglu, C., Iliescu, C., and Raileanu, C.: Les thrombus myxoides du coeur. Presse Med., 41:2074, 1933.

Back, N., Ambrus, J. L., Klein, E., Milgrom, H., Velasco, H., Ausman, R. K., Stutzman, L., and Sokal, J. E.: Systemic and local anti-tumor effect of the antibiotic spiromycin, a pharmacologic and clinical study. Acta Un. Int. Cancr., 20:300, 1964.

Basset, A., and Payet, M.: Caractères cliniques de la maladie de Kaposi dans l'Ouest Africain. Différences avec le Kaposi Européen. Acta Un. Int. Cancr., 18:376, 1962.

Becker, B. J. P.: The histogenesis of Kaposi's sarcoma. Acta Un. Int. Cancr., 18:477, 1962.

Becker, S. W., and Thatcher, H. W.: Multiple idiopathic haemorrhagic sarcoma of Kaposi. Historical review. Nomenclature and theories relative to the nature of the disease and experimental studies of 2 cases. J. Invest. Dermatol., 1:379, 1938.

Belloni, M. L.: Maladie de Kaposi à l'evolution lymphosarcomateuse (contribution à l'étude des mesenchymopathies hyperplasticoneoplasiques). Ann. Dermatol. Syphiligr. (Paris), 86:45, 1949.

Berg, J. W.: The incidence of multiple primary cancers. 1. Development of further cancers in patients with lymphomas, leukaemias and myeloma. J. Natl. Cancer Inst., 38:41, 1967.

Bertacinni, G.: Sopra un case di sarcoma idiopathico di Kaposi (angioendothelioma cutaneo). Ital. Mal. Vener., 61:589, 1920.

Bhana, D., Templeton, A. C., Master, S. P., and Kyalwazi, S. K.: Kaposi's sarcoma of lymph nodes. Br. J. Cancer, 24:464, 1970.

Bhana, D., Hillier, K., and Karim, S. M. N.: Vasoactive substances in Kaposi's sarcoma. Cancer, 27:233, 1971.

Biggs, B., Cooke, R. A., and McGovern, V. J.: Kaposi's sarcoma. Report of a case from New Guinea. Aust. J. Dermatol., 7:131, 1964.

Birch, N. H.: A case of Kaposi's sarcoma of the small intestine. E. Afr. Med. J., 44:343, 1967.

Bluefarb, S. M.: Kaposi's Sarcoma. A.M.A. Arch. Dermatol. Syph., 73:603, 1956.

Bluefarb, S. M.: Kaposi's Sarcoma. Springfield, Ill., Charles C Thomas, Publisher, 1957.

Bluefarb, S. M., and Adams, L. A.: Arteriovenous malformation with angiodermatitis. Stasis dermatitis simulating Kaposi's disease. Arch. Dermatol., 96:176, 1967.

Browne, S. G.: The hemorrhagic type of regression in Kaposi's sarcoma. Arch. Dermatol., 94:328, 1966.

Camain, R.: Aperçus sur le cancer en A.O.F. Bull. Soc. Pathol. Exot., 47:614, 1954.

Camain, R., and Quenum, A.: Histopathologie et histogenèse de la maladie de Kaposi. Acta Un. Int. Cancr., 18:453, 1962.

Chaboeuf, M.: Notes sur le cancer chez les Indigènes du Sud Caméroun. Rev. Soc. Méd. Pharm. Vétér. l'Afr. Fr. Libre, 2:379, 1945.

Chadli, A., and Philippe, E.: La physionomie du cancer en Tunisie. Arch. Inst. Pasteur Tunis., 37:397, 1960.

Choisser, R. M., and Ramsey, E. M.: Angioreticuloendothelioma (Kaposi's disease) of the heart. Am. J. Pathol., 15:155, 1939.

Choisser, R. M., and Ramsey, E. M.: Etiology of Kaposi's disease. Preliminary report of investigations. South. Med. J., 33:392, 1940.

Chopra, S., and Templeton, A. C.: Cancer in East African Indians. Int. J. Cancer, 8:176, 1971.

van Cleve, J. V., and Hellwig, C. A.: Case of idiopathic hemorrhagic sarcoma (Kaposi) with autopsy findings. Urol. Cutan. Rev., 39:246, 1935.

Coetzee, T., and LeRoux, C. G.: Kaposi's sarcoma, presentation with intestinal obstruction. S. Afr. Med. J., 41:442, 1967.

Cohen, F. B., Kannerstein, M., and Klosk, E.: Kaposi's sarcoma and macroglobulenaemia. J. Newark Beth Israel Hosp., 16:30, 1965.

Cohen, L., Palmer, P. E. S., and Nickson, J. J.: Treatment of Kaposi's sarcoma by radiation. Acta Un. Int. Cancr., 18:502, 1962.

Collins, M. D., and Fisher, H.: A case of generalised haemangiosarcomatosis erroneously considered as generalised tuberculosis. Am. Rev. Tuberc., 61:257, 1950.

Contreras, F.: Angiosarcoma de Kaposi primario del corazan, revision de la litteratura y descripcion del sexto case. Arch. Inst. Cardiol. Mex., 27:763, 1957.

Cook, J.: The treatment of Kaposi's sarcoma with nitrogen mustard. Acta Un. Int. Cancr., 18:494, 1962.

Cox, F. X., and Helwig, E. B.: Kaposi's sarcoma. Cancer, 12:289, 1959.

da Cuhna Motta, L.: Hemangio reticulo-endotelioma. An. Fac. Med. Univ. São Paulo, 17:627, 1941.

Dalla Favera, G. B.: Über das sog. Sarcoma idiopathicum multiplex haemorrhagicum (Kaposi). Klinische und histologische Beitrage. Arch. Dermatol. Syph. (Berl.) 109:387, 1911.

Dallinger, M. R., and Faye, L. V., Jr.: Kaposi's sarcoma and coexistent giant follicular lymphoblastoma. Yale J. Biol. Med., 38:449, 1966.

Davies, A. G. M.: Bone changes in Kaposi's sarcoma. An analysis of 15 cases occurring in Bantu Africans. J. Fac. Radiol., 8:32, 1956.

Davies, J. N. P., and Lothe, F.: Kaposi's sarcoma in African children. Acta Un. Int. Cancr., 18:394, 1962.

Davies, J. N. P., Knowelden, J., and Wilson, B. A.: Incidence rates of cancer in Kyadondo County, Uganda, 1954–1960. J. Natl. Canc. Inst., 35:789, 1965.

Dayan, A. D., and Lewis, P. D.: Origin of Kaposi's sarcoma from the reticuloendothelial system. Nature (Lond.), 213:889, 1967.

Dillard, G. J., and Weidman, F. D.: Multiple hemorrhagic sarcoma of Kaposi. Histologic studies of 2 cases, one disclosing intestinal lesions at necropsy. Arch. Dermatol. Syph. 11:203, 1925.

Dörffel, J.: Histiogenesis of multiple idiopathic haemorrhagic sarcoma of Kaposi. Arch. Dermatol. Syph., 26:608, 1932.

Dorfman, R. F.: Kaposi's sarcoma. The contribution of enzyme histochemistry to the identification of cell types. Acta Un. Int. Cancr., 18:464, 1962a.

Dorfman, R. F.: Enzyme histochemistry and fluorescence microscopy of Kaposi's sarcoma, malignant haemangio-endothelioma and post-mastectomy lymphangiosarcoma. S. Afr. Med. J., 36:989, 1962b.

Dorn, H. F., and Cutler, S. J.: Morbidity from cancer in the United States. Part 1. Variation in incidence by age, sex, marital status, and geographic region. Washington, D.C., Public Health Monograph No. 29, 1955, p. 121.

Dupont, A.: L'angioreticulomatose cutanée. Sarcomatose multiple idiopathique pigmentaire de Kaposi. Rev. Belge. Pathol. Exp., 20:375, 1951.

Dutz, W., and Stout, A. P.: Kaposi's sarcoma in infants and children. Cancer, 13:684, 1960.

Ecklund, R. E., and Valaitis, J.: Kaposi's sarcoma of lymph nodes. Arch. Pathol., 74:224, 1962.

Edington, G. H.: Malignant disease in the Gold Coast. Br. J. Cancer, 10:595, 1956.

Ehrenberg, L.: Zwei falle von tumor im herzen. Arch. Klin. Med., 103:293, 1911.

Ellis, F. A.: Multiple idiopathic hemorrhagic sarcoma of Kaposi. Report of a case in an American Negro. Arch. Dermatol. Syph., 30:706, 1934.

Epstein, E.: A case for diagnosis. ? Kaposi's sarcoma. Arch. Dermatol. Syph., 43:409, 1941.

Epstein, E.: Extracutaneous manifestations of Kaposi's sarcoma. A systemic lymphoblastoma. Calif. Med., 87:98, 1957.

Ewing, J.: Neoplastic Diseases. Ed. 3. Philadelphia, W. B. Saunders, 1928, p. 270.

de Foria, J. L.: Multiple reticulo histiocytosarcoma with a principal localisation in the heart; its relationship to Kaposi's disease. Folia Clin. Biol., 17:59, 1951.

Gelfand, M.: Kaposi's haemangiosarcoma of the heart. Br. Heart J., 19:290, 1957.

Gellin, G. A.: Kaposi's sarcoma. 3 cases of which two have unusual findings in association. Arch. Dermatol., 94:92, 1966.

Gilbert, T. T., Evjy, J. T., and Edelstein, L.: Hodgkins disease associated with Kaposi's sarcoma and malignant melanoma. Cancer, 28:293, 1971.

Giraldo, G., Beth, E., and Hpsuenac, F.: Herpes type virus particles in tissue culture of Kaposi's sarcoma from different geographic regions. I. Natl. Cancer Inst., 49:1509, 1972.

Gonzalez Crussi, F., Mossanen, A., and Robertson, D. M.: Neurological involvement in Kaposi's sarcoma. Can. Med. Assoc. J., 100:481, 1969.

Gordon, J. A.: Kaposi's sarcoma, a review of 136 Rhodesian African cases. Postgrad. Med. J., 43:513, 1967.

Greco, N. V., Bigatti, A., Ponce de Leon, S., Gunche, F. F., and Capurro, J.: Un segundo caso familiar de enfermedad (sarcomatosis) de Kaposi, con el hongo patogeno especifico el cryptococcus haematicon. Sem. Med., 45:989, 1938.

Grossman, A., and Williams, M. J.: Kaposi's sarcoma simulating renal carcinoma. J. Urol., 88:473, 1962.

Grupper, C.: Hereditary Kaposi's sarcoma (father and son). Bull. Soc. Fr. Dermatol. Syphiligr., 75:768, 1968.

Hadida, E., Bourdonnesques, J., and Sayag, J.: Kaposi's disease with cranial location and neurologic disorders. Therapeutic results. Bull. Soc. Fr. Dermatol. Syphiligr., 77:55, 1970.

Haim, S.: Kaposi's sarcoma developing in association with immunosuppressive therapy. Israel J. Med. Sci., 8:1993, 1972.

Hallenberger, O.: Multiple angiosarkome der Haut bei einem Kamerunneger. Arch. Schiffs. Trop. Hyg., 18:647, 1914.

Hansson, C. J.: Kaposi's sarcoma. Clinical and radiotherapeutic studies on 23 patients. Acta Radiol. (Stockh.), 21:457, 1940.

Hare, P. J.: Stasis syndrome mimicking Kaposi's sarcoma. Proc. R. Soc. Med., 53:381, 1960.

Hasegawa, K.: A case of Kaposi's sarcoma. Jap. J. Dermatol., 72:379, 1962.

Hashimoto, K., and Lever, W. F.: Kaposi's sarcoma. Histochemical and electron microscopic studies. J. Invest. Dermatol., 43:539, 1964.

Hazen, H. H., and Freeman, C. W.: Skin cancer in the American Negro. Arch. Dermatol. Syph., 62:622, 1950.

Hennessey, R. S. F.: A note on endotheliomatous tumors encountered in Uganda. E. Afr. Med. J., 19:236, 1942.

Hewer, T. F., and Kemp, R. P.: Malignant haemangioendothelioma of the heart, report of a case. J. Pathol. Bacteria, 43:511, 1936.

Higginson, J., and Oettlé, A. G.: Cancer incidence in the Bantu and Cape Coloured races of South Africa. Report of a cancer survey in the Transvaal, 1953–1955. J. Natl. Cancer Inst., 24:589, 1960.

Hogeman, O.: Hyperhemolysis of nonsplenic origin. Acta Med. Scand., 144:247, 1953.

Howland, W. J., Ambrecht, E. C., and Miller, J. A.: Oral manifestations of multiple idiopathic haemorrhagic sarcoma of Kaposi. A report of two cases. J. Oral. Surg., 24:445, 1966.

Huriez, C., Desmans, F., Agache, P., Benoit, P., and Bombart-Thoreux, M., Aspect clinique de maladie de Kaposi au cours d'une leucose lymphoide. Bull. Soc. Fr. Dermatol. Syphiligr., 68:463, 1961.

Húrlbut, W. B., and Lincoln, C. S., Jr.: Multiple haemorrhagic sarcoma and diabetes mellitus. A review of a series with report of 2 cases. Arch. Intern. Med., 84:738, 1949.

Jackson, D. R., and Madoff, I. M.: Kaposi's sarcoma. Report of a unique case with visceral metastases presenting as an idiopathic chylothorax. Boston Med. Quarterly, 14:57, 1963.

Johnstone, G.: Kaposi's sarcoma in Tanganyika. J. Trop. Med. Hyg., 68:1, 1965.

Justus, J.: Sarcoma idiopathicum Kaposi. Arch. Dermatolol. Syph. (Berl.), 151:436, 1926.

Kalomkarian, A. A., and Sych, L. I.: A case of coexistence of mycosis fungoides and Kaposi's sarcoma. Vestn. Dermatol. Venerol. 42:12, 1968.

Kaminer, B., and Murray, J. F.: Sarcoma idiopathicum multiplex haemorrhagicum of Kaposi, with special reference to its incidence in the South African Negro and two case reports. S. Afr. J. Clin. Sci., 1:1, 1950.

Kaposi, M.: Idiopathisches multiples Pigmentsarkom der Haut. Arch. Dermatol. Syph. (Berl.), 4:265, 1872.

Kaposi, M.: Pathologie und Therapie der Hautkrankheiten. Urban & Schwarzenberg, Wien and Leipzig, 1887.

Kaposi, M.: Zur nomenclatur des idiopathischen Pigmentsarkom Kaposi. Arch. Dermatol. Syph. (Berl.), 29:164, 1894.

Kingsley, H. J.: Kaposi's sarcoma associated with lymphoma. Central Afr. J. Med., 2:264, 1965.

Kocsard, E.: Kaposi's sarcoma in a Chinese boy (aged 16) with localisation on the left lower extremity and on the right caruncula lacrimalis. Dermatologica, 99:43, 1949.

Kren, O.: Sarcoma idiopathicum Hemorrhagicum (Kaposi). In Jadassohn, J.: Handbuch der Haut- und Geschlechtskrankheiten. Vol. 12. 1933, Springer-Verlag, Berlin, p. 841.

Kusnezow, W. N.: A case of sarcoma multiplex idiopathicum (Kaposi) with fatal outcome. Urol. Cutan. Rev., 37:230, 1933.

Kyalwazi, S. K.: Chemotherapy of Kaposi's sarcoma, experience with trenimon. E. Afr. Med. J., 45:17, 1968.

Kyalwazi, S. K.: Kaposi's sarcoma (one or two diseases). E. Afr. Med. J., 46:459, 1969.

Kyalwazi, S. K., Bhana, D., and Master, S. P.: Actinomycin D in malignant Kaposi's sarcoma. E. Afr. Med. J., 48:16, 1971.

Lee, F. D.: A comparative study of Kaposi's sarcoma and granuloma pyogenicum in Uganda. J. Clin. Pathol., 21:119, 1968.

Linsell, C. A., and Martyn, R.: Personal communication, 1963, quoted by Davey, W. W., *In* Companion to Surgery in Africa, Edinburgh, Livingstone, 1968, p. 349.

Loring, W. E., and Wolman, S. R.: Idiopathic multiple haemorrhagic sarcoma of the lung (Kaposi's sarcoma). N.Y. J. Med., 65:668, 1965.

Lothe, F.: Kaposi's sarcoma in Uganda Africans. Acta Pathol. Microbiol. Scand., Suppl. 161, 1:1, 1963.

Lothe, F., and Murray, J. F.: Kaposi's sarcoma. Autopsy findings in the African. Acta Un. Int. Cancr., 18:429, 1962.

Mallory, T. B.: Clinico-Pathologic Conference. Case 22491. Primary sarcoma (probably fibrosarcoma) of right auricle. Case records of Massachusetts General Hospital. New Engl. J. Med., 215:1082, 1936.

Maberry, J. D., and Stone, O. J.: Kaposi's sarcoma with thymoma. Arch. Dermatol., 95:210, 1967.

McCarthy, W. D., and Pack, G. T.: Malignant blood vessel tumours. A report of 56 cases of angiosarcoma and Kaposi's sarcoma. Surg. Gynecol. Obstet., 91:465, 1950.

McGinn, J. T., Ricca, J. J., and Currin, J. F.: Kaposi's sarcoma following allergic angiitis. Ann. Intern. Med., 42:921, 1955.

McKinney, B.: Kaposi's sarcoma and Burkitt's lymphoma. E. Afr. Med. J., 44:417, 1967.

McLaren, D. S.: Kaposi's sarcoma of the eyelids of an African child A.M.A. Arch. Ophthalmol., 63:859, 1960.

MacLean, C.M.U.: Kaposi's sarcoma in Nigeria. Br. J. Cancer, 17:195, 1963.

Marshall, A. H. E.: An outline of the cytology and pathology of the reticular tissue. Edinburgh, Oliver and Boyd, 1956.

Martensson, J., and Henrikson, H.: Immuno-hemolytic anemia in Kaposi's sarcoma with visceral involvement only. Acta Med. Scand., 150:175, 1954.

Martinotti, L.: Arch. Ital. Dermatol., 14:367, 1938. Quoted by Dupont, A. (1951).

Master, S. P., Taylor, J. F., Kyalwazi, S. K., and Ziegler, J. L.: Immunological studies on Kaposi's sarcoma in Uganda. Br. Med. J., 1:600, 1970.

Mazzaferri, E. L., and Penn, G. M.: Kaposi's sarcoma associated with multiple myeloma. Report of a patient and review of the literature. Arch. Intern. Med., 122:521, 1968.

Moe, N.: Hodgkin's disease and Kaposi's sarcoma. Report of a case. Acta Pathol. Microbiol. Scand., 68:189, 1966.

Moertel, C. G.: Multiple Primary Malignant Neoplasms. Vol. 7. Recent Results in Cancer Research. Berlin, Springer-Verlag, 1966.

Moertel, C. G., and Hagedorn, A. B.: Leukaemia or lymphoma and coexistent primary malignant lesions. A review of the literature and a study of 120 cases. Blood, 12:788, 1957.

Monaco, A. P., and Austen, W. G.: Treatment of Kaposi's sarcoma of the lower extremity by extracorporeal perfusion with chemotherapeutic agents. New Engl. J. Med., 261:1045, 1959.

Mortada, A.: Conjunctival regressing Kaposi's sarcoma. Br. J. Ophthalmol., 51:275, 1967.

Murray, J. F., and Lothe, F.: The histopathology of Kaposi's sarcoma. Acta Un. Int. Cancr., 18:413, 1962.

Mussini-Montpellier, J.: Angioreticuloendotheliosarcomatose de Kaposi en Afrique du Nord. Acta Un. Int. Cancr., 9:353, 1953.

Mustakallio, K. K.: Levenen, E., and Raekallio, J.: Histochemistry of Kaposi's sarcoma. 1. Hydrolases and phosphorylase. Exp. Mol. Pathol., 2:303, 1963.

Myers, B. D., Kessler, E., Levi, J., Rich, A., Rosenfeld, J. R., and Tikvah, P.: Kaposi's sarcoma in kidney transplant recipients. Arch. Intern. Med., 133:307, 1974.

Mysterious sarcoma. Lancet, 2:1290, 1967.

Nesbitt, S., Mark, P. F., and Zimmermann, H. M.: Disseminated visceral idiopathic hemorrhagic sarcoma (Kaposi's disease). Report of a case with necropsy findings. Ann. Intern. Med., 22:601, 1945.

Niemi, M., and Mustakallio, K. K.: The fine structure of the spindle cell in Kaposi's sarcoma. Acta Pathol. Microbiol. Scand., 63:567, 1965.

Niemi, M., Raekallio, J., Levonen, E., and Mustakellio, K. K.: Histochemistry of Kaposi's sarcoma. II. Cholinesterases, monoamine oxidase, adenosine triphosphatase. Exp. Mol. Pathol., 3:648, 1964.

O'Brien, P. H., and Brasfield, R.: Kaposi's sarcoma. Cancer, 19:1497, 1966.

Oettlé, A. G.: Geographical and racial differences in the frequency of Kaposi's sarcoma as evidence of environmental or genetic causes. Acta Un. Int. Cancr., 18:330, 1962.

Osborne, E. D., Jordan, J. W., Hoak, F. C., and Pschierer, F. J.: Nitrogen mustard therapy in cutaneous blastomatous disease. J.A.M.A., 135:1123, 1947.

Pack, G. T., and Ariel, I. M.: Tumors of the Soft Somatic Tissues. New York, Harper & Row, 1958.

Pack, G. T., and Davis, J.: Concomitant occurrence of Kaposi's sarcoma and lymphoblastoma. A. M.A. Arch. Dermatol. Syph., 69:604, 1954.

Palmer, D. E. S.: The radiological changes of Kaposi's sarcoma. Acta Un. Int. Cancr., 18:400, 1962.

Palmer, P. E. S.; Angiopathy and lymphography in Kaposi's sarcoma. *In* Shivas, A. A. (Ed.): Racial and Geographical Factors in Tumour Incidence. Edinburgh, University Press, 1967.

Paolini, R.: Sul sarcoma molteplice promitivo di Kaposi con speciale riguardo alle localizzazioni viscerali. Studio clinico anatomo-isto-pathologico e bacteriologico. Z. Haut. Geschlechtskr., 26:816, 1928.

Pardo-Castello, V.: Sarcoma hemorragico de Kaposi. Relacion de un case en un individuo de la raza de color. Bol Soc. Cubana Dermatol., 2:100, 1931. Quoted by Persky and Lisa, 1944.

Pautrier, L. M., and Diss, A.: Kaposi's idiopathic sarcoma is not a genuine sarcoma but a neurovascular dysgenesis. Br. J. Dermatol. Syph., 41:93, 1929.

Pelissier, A.: La maladie de Kaposi en Afrique Noire (angioreticuloendotheliofibrosarcomatose). A propos de 18 cas. Bull. Soc. Pathol. Exot., 46:832, 1953.

Penn, I.: Malignant tumors in organ transplant recipients. Recent Results in Cancer Research. Vol. 35. Berlin, Springer-Verlag, 1970.

Pepler, W. J., and Theron, J. J.: An electron microscope study of Kaposi's haemangiosarcoma. J. Pathol. Bacteriol., 83:521, 1962.

Persky, B. P., and Lisa, J. R.: Multiple idiopathic hemorrhagic sarcoma of Kaposi in a full-blooded Negro. Arch. Dermatol. Syph., 49:270, 1944.

Phillipson, L.: Ueber das Sarcoma Idiopathicum cutis Kaposi. Ein Beitrag zun Sarcom Uhre. Virchows Arch., 167:58, 1902.

Pick, W.: Zur kenntris des senilen angioms und seiner beziekungen zum endothelium. Arch. Dermatol. Syph. (Berl.), 99:109, 1910.

Prates, M. D.: Malignant neoplasms in Mozambique. A frequency ratio study from 1944–1957 and a comparison with other parts of Africa. Br. J. Cancer, 12:177, 1958.

Quenum, A., and Camain, R.: Los aspects africains de la maladie de Kaposi, reticulopathie maligne systématisée. Ann. Anat. Pathol. (Paris), 3:337, 1958.

Radaeli, F.: Sul proceso anatoma-patologica del sarcoma idiopatico di Kaposi (angio-endotelioma cutaneo di Kaposi). Ital. Dermatol. Sif., 71:1501, 1930. Quoted by Dupont, A., 1951, and Bluefarb, S. M., 1957.

Rajan, R. K., Goodman, S., and Floch, M. H.: Gastroscopic findings in Kaposi's sarcoma. Gastrointest. Endosc., 16:104, 1969.

Rajka, G.: Kaposi's sarcoma associated with Hodgkin's disease. Acta Derm. Venereol. (Stockh.), 45:40, 1965.

Reynolds, W. A., Winkelmann, R. K., and Soule, E. H.: Kaposi's sarcoma. Medicine, 44:419, 1965.

Ringertz, N., Sjöström, A., Ericsson, J., and Olinder, B.: Cancer incidence in Sweden, 1958. Stockholm, The Swedish Cancer Registry, National Board of Health, 1960, p. 85.

Robb Smith, A. M. T.: The reticular tissue and the skin. Br. J. Dermatol., 56:151, 1944.

Ronchese, F.: Kaposi's sarcoma. An overlooked essay of 1882. A.M.A. Arch. Dermatol., 77:542, 1958.

Ross, C. M. D.: Personal communications, quoted by Gordon, J. A., 1967.

Rothman, S.: Remarks on sex, age and racial distribution of Kaposi's sarcoma and on possible pathogenetic factors. Acta Un. Int. Cancr., 18:322, 1962.

Rouhani, A.: Kaposi's sarcoma. The first case observed in Afganistan. Lyon Med., 216:194, 1966.

Rywlin, A. M., Recher, L., and Hoffman, E. P.: Lymphoma-like presentation of Kaposi's sarcoma. Three cases without characteristic skin lesions. Arch. Dermatol. Syph., 93:554, 1966.

Schirren, C. G., and Burkhardt, L.: Kaposi's sarcoma with metastasis to the brain. Arch. Klin. Exp. Dermatol., 201:99, 1955.

Schonland, M., and Bradshaw, E.: Cancer in the Natal African and Indian, 1964–1966. Int. J. Cancer, 3:304, 1968.

Scott, W. D., and Voight, J. A.: Kaposi's sarcoma. Management with vincaleucoblastine. Cancer, 19:557, 1966.

Seagrave, K. H.: Kaposi's disease, report of a case with unusual visceral manifestations. Radiology, 51:248, 1948.

Serafino, X., Testu, J., and Diop, A.: Maladie de Kaposi à début viscéral. Bull. Soc. Med. Afr. Noire Lang. Fr., 9:302, 1964.

Shelburne, S. A.: Primary tumors of the heart. Ann. Int. Med., 9:340, 1935.

Shklar, G., and Meyer, I.: Vascular tumours of the mouth and jaws. Oral Surg., 19:335, 1965.

Siegal, J. H., Janis, R., Alper, J. C., Schutte, H., Robbins, L., and Blaufox, M. D.: Disseminated visceral Kaposi's sarcoma. Appearance after human renal homograft operation. J.A.M.A. 207:1493, 1969.

Silverberg, S. G., Kay, S., and Koss, L. G.: Post-mastectomy lymphangiosarcoma. Ultra-structural observations. Cancer, 27:100, 1971.

Sipos, J., Feher, L., and Sellyei, M.: Simultaneous occurrence of Kaposi's sarcoma, myeloid leukaemia and lung cancer. Orv. Hetil., 104:413, 1963.

Slavin, G., Cameron, H. M., and Singh, H.: Kaposi's sarcoma in mainland Tanzania. A report of 117 cases. Br. J. Cancer, 23:349, 1969.

Slavin, G., Cameron, H. M., Forbes, C., and Morton Mitchell, R.: Kaposi's sarcoma in East African children. A report of 51 cases. J. Pathol., 100:187, 1970.

Smith, D. S.: Neoplastic involvement of the heart. J.A.M.A., 109:1192, 1937.

Smith, E. C., and Elmes, B.G.T.: Malignant disease in the natives of Nigeria. An analysis of 500 tumours. Ann. Trop. Med. Parasitol., 28:461, 1934.

Smith, R., and Wolfe, L. G.: Kaposi's sarcoma: Electron microscopic and tissue culture studies. Abstract No. 85, Am. Assoc. Pathologists and Bacteriologists, 67th Annual Meeting, St. Louis, Mo., March 7–10, 1970. Quoted by Silverberg, 1971.

Spencer, M. C.: Cytoxan treatment of Kaposi's idiopathic haemorrhagic sarcoma. Illinois Med. J., 129:252, 1966.

Stats, D.: The visceral manifestations of Kaposi's sarcoma. J. Mount Sinai Hosp., 12:971, 1945.

Steiner, P. E.: Cancer, Race and Geography. Some etiological, environmental, ethnological, epidemiological and statistical aspects in Caucasoids, Mongoloids, Negroids and Mexicans. Baltimore, Williams & Wilkins, 1954.

Sternberg, C.: Ueber das sarcoma multiplex haemorrhagicum (Kaposi). Arch. Dermatol. Syph. (Berl.), 111:331, 1912.

Stewart, F. W., and Treves, N.: Lymphangiosarcoma in post-mastectomy lymphedema. Report of 6 cases in elephantiasis chirugica. Cancer 1:64, 1948.

Symmers, D.: Kaposi's sarcoma. Arch. Pathol., 32:764, 1941.

Taylor, J. F., Junge, U., Wolfe, L., Dienhardt, F., and Kyalwazi, S. K.: Lymphocyte transformation in patients with Kaposi's sarcoma. Int. J. Cancer, 8:468, 1971a.

Taylor, J. F., Templeton, A. C., Vogel, C. L., Ziegler, J. C., and Kyalwazi, S. K.: Kaposi's sarcoma in Uganda. A clinicopathological study. Int. J. Cancer, 8:122, 1971b.

Tedeschi, C. G.: Some considerations concerning the nature of the so-called sarcoma of Kaposi. Arch. Pathol., 66:656, 1958.

Tedeschi, C. G., Folsom, H. F., and Carnicelli, T. J.: Visceral Kaposi's disease. Arch. Pathol., 43:335, 1947.

Templeton, A. C.: Studies in Kaposi's sarcoma: I. Postmortem findings. II. Disease patterns in women. Cancer, 30:854, 1972.

Templeton, A. C., and Viegas, O. A. C.: Racial variations in tumour incidence in Uganda. Trop. Geogr. Med., 22:431, 1970.

Thijs, A.: L'angiosarcomatose de Kaposi au Congo Belge at au Ruanda Urundi. Ann. Soc. Belg. Méd. Trop., 37:295, 1957.

Tye, M. J.: Bullous pemphigoid and Kaposi's sarcoma. Arch. Dermatol. 101:690, 1970.

Uys, C. J., and Bennett, M. B.: Kaposi's sarcoma occurring in a coloured male. S. Afr. Med. J., 32:577, 1958.

Vogel, C. L., Templeton, C. J., Templeton, A. C., Taylor, J. F., and Kyalwazi, S. K.: Treatment of Kaposi's sarcoma with actinomycin D and cyclophosphamide. Results of a randomised clinical trial. Int. J. Cancer, 8:136, 1971.

Weller, G. L., Jr.: The clinical aspects of cardiac involvement (right auricular tumour) in idiopathic haemorrhagic sarcoma (Kaposi's disease). Ann. Intern. Med., 14:314, 1940.

White, J. A., and King, M. H.: Kaposi's sarcoma presenting with abdominal symptoms. Gastroenterology, 46:197, 1964.

Wigley, J. E., Rees, D. L., and Symmers, W. S.: Kaposi's idiopathic haemorrhagic sarcoma. Proc. R. Soc. Med., 48:449, 1955.

Williams, E. H., and Williams, P. H.: A note on an apparent similarity in distribution of onchocerciasis, femoral hernia and Kaposi's sarcoma in the West Nile District of Uganda. E. Afr. Med. J., 43:208, 1966.

Willis, R. A.: Pathology of tumors. St. Louis, Mo., C. V. Mosby Company, 1948, p. 780.

Willius, F. A.: Clinic on refractory right heart failure of relatively short duration; comments; post mortem findings (primary fibrosarcoma of right auricle). Proc. Staff Meetings Mayo Clin., 13:331, 1938.

Wise, F.: Idiopathic hemorrhagic multiple sarcoma of the skin (Kaposi) with special reference to early diagnosis. Med. Record, 88:513, 1915.

Yesudian, P.: A case of Kaposi's sarcoma. Indian J. Derm., 14:121, 1969.

Zak, F. G., Solomon, A., and Fellner, N. J.: Viscerocutaneous angiomatosis with dysproteinaemic phagocytosis, its relation to Kaposi's sarcoma and lymphoproliferative disorders. J. Pathol. Bacterol., 92:594, 1966.

Zeligman, I.: Kaposi's sarcoma in a father and son. Bull. John Hopkins Hosp., 107:208, 1960.

Zemek, L., Strom, L., Gordon, G., and Elguezabel, A.: Haemolytic anaemia with Kaposi's sarcoma. Report of a case. J.A.M.A., 187:232, 1964.

53

Lymphomas and Leukemias of the Skin

Samuel M. Bluefarb, M.D., and William A. Caro, M.D.

LYMPHOMAS OF THE SKIN

Malignant lymphomas may be defined as malignant neoplasms of the lymphoreticular tissue. As such these lesions have a diversity of cellular patterns and sites of origin reflecting the complexity and widespread distribution of the parent tissue. Lymphoreticular tissue also gives rise to benign proliferative lesions, which have been called reactive lymphoid hyperplasias or pseudolymphomas and which may closely simulate malignant lymphomas morphologically.

The reticular tissue has been defined as ". . . a tissue composed of fixed cells (primitive reticular cells) supporting a framework of fibrils and including all cells in the body derived from this tissue" (Marshall, 1956). Reticular tissue may be found in such fixed structures as lymph nodes, thymus, spleen, and bone marrow.

The pioneering work of Maximow showed that primitive reticular (primitive mesenchymal) cells are widely distributed throughout the body and have the capacity of differentiating toward blood cells or toward the various cellular components of connective tissue (Maximow, 1924). Cells of the histiocytic series (reticulum cells) and of the lymphoid series are the fundamental cells involved in lymphoreticular neoplasms, whether benign or malignant. Robb-Smith extended the observations of Maximow by discussing the skin as a site of reticular tissue and thus a site for lymphoreticular hyperplasia and neoplasia (Robb-Smith, 1944).

Of the various malignant neoplasms of man, malignant lymphomas constitute approximately 2 to 4 percent (Thorson and Brown, 1955; World Health Organization, 1961). Skin lesions occur in approximately 20 to 30 percent of patients with malignant lymphoma (Epstein and MacEachern, 1937; Gall and Mallory, 1942; Rosenberg et al., 1961), although the incidence in Hodgkin's disease may be as high as 50 percent (Epstein and MacEachern, 1937).

The skin lesions of malignant lymphoma fall into two general categories, specific and nonspecific (Bluefarb, 1959). Specific lesions represent actual lymphomatous infiltrates in the skin and may arise through several mechanisms (Altman and Winkelmann, 1960). A cutaneous lymphomatous lesion may arise ei-

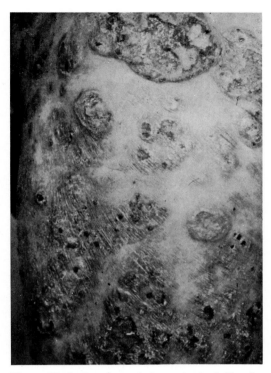

Figure 53–4 Papules and plaques in the infiltrative stage.

not marked, in the ability to form circulating antibodies.

Treatment involves superficial roentgen ray therapy in suberythema doses. Topical corticosteroid lotions or creams are useful because of their antipruritic effect. Cyclophosphamide (Cytoxan) in daily doses of 100 mg. until remission is obtained, then in weekly doses of 500 mg., has shown considerable promise. However, if one can still stimulate the immune mechanism of the host, then a more rational approach to therapy is obtained. The sensitization with nitrogen mustard or other primary irritants needs further study, for I believe the treatment of the future will be along these lines.

The prognosis is poor to fair.

Stage 3 — Tumor Stage

This stage develops gradually through the appearance of tumors only in infiltrated lesions. The tumor usually appears first at the border of an old plaque of infiltration and rarely occurs in a recent area of infiltration. Should the lesions appear suddenly on normal skin, this would be the true "d'emblée" type.

On palpation of an infiltrated lesion which will develop into a tumor, the sensation is that of a subcutaneous nodule. Nodular tumors often merge into larger, lobulated, deeply furrowed tumors which are of a dull red color, soft, and hemispherical and have nodular surfaces. These nodules have a broad base and may become fungating from constriction of the base. The face, back, and proximal parts of the extremities are common sites of localization, while involvement of the scalp is rare. The intact tumors are not painful, but the ulcerated ones are extremely painful.

The tumors are discrete and localized at the onset but increase rapidly in size and number; each tumor is round or oval in shape. The center is sometimes depressed, suggesting lobulation, and, more rarely, it becomes pedunculated. When

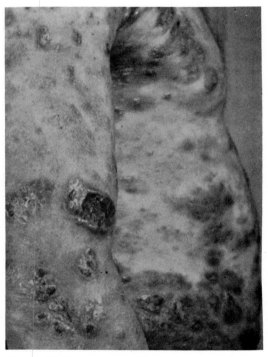

Figure 53–5 Plaques and beginning tumor formation. (*From* Bluefarb: Cutaneous lymphomas and leukemia cutis. *In* Pack and Ariel (Eds.): Treatment of Cancer and Allied Diseases. Vol. 9. Lymphomas and Related Diseases. 2nd ed. New York, Hoeber-Harper, 1964, p. 195.)

confluence takes place, the appearance is described as "more hideous than that of any other vegetating growth of the skin."

The tumors are soft and semi-fluid in consistency with a vinous coloration; interstitial hemorrhage may result in a dark color suggesting melanotic carcinoma. The tumors may regress and disappear in any stage of development. Usually no evidence of their presence remains, and scar tissue occurs only when the tumors ulcerate. They may, however, leave brownish pigmented macules, and there is alopecia of the hairy surfaces.

In the last stage the tumors may disintegrate, diminish in size, and disappear, with a pigmented atrophic scar remaining. The tumors may also clear in the center and progress peripherally, forming rings and circles. The majority, however, become excoriated and secondarily infected. These may be large round ulcers with a sloughing base which are invaded by progenic organisms and which cause severe toxemia, which results in the exhaustion preceding death.

Trauma and friction are common causes of ulceration and result in superficial erosions. The nodules often soften in the center, fluctuate, and finally ulcerate, leaving crater-shaped ulcers with ragged margins covered with shreds of tissue. The ulcers usually extend only to the subcutaneous tissue, rarely to the bone. The general health of the patient declines during the period, and there is usually diarrhea, cachexia, and fever.

Although the premycotic lesions are highly pruritic, the tumors are not pruritic. Pruritus is present as long as there is a defense reaction of the skin (lymphocytes) against the deposition of foreign cells. The pruritus subsides after the infiltrating tumor has become established and started unlimited growth.

The final stage of the disease is the ulceration of the tumors, which indicates that death is imminent. The skin over the tumor becomes tender and the center becomes ulcerated. At first the base consists of clear, bright red granulation tissue, but it soon develops into a purulent cavity as a result of secondary infection. The ulcer extends only to the subcutaneous tissue.

In this stage in which ulcerated tumors are the usual course, immunity is lost. The patient is unable to react to skin test antigens. It is difficult to sensitize these patients to nitrogen mustard.

At this stage, treatment is palliative. There is no drug or agent that will cure mycosis fungoides at this point. Roentgen therapy, electron beam therapy, and cytotoxic drugs may be tried. The only result from increasing the duration of remission is the comfort of the patient.

The appearance of ulcerated tumors is indicative of a poor prognosis.

Summary of Mycosis Fungoides (Alibert's Disease)

Stage 1

Clinical Features
> Pruritus
> Polymorphous eruption
> Persistent patches, usually crescentic or discoid, are frequently pathognomonic

Immunity
> Immunity usually intact
> Normal response to skin test antigens and DNCB sensitization
> Rejection of normally allogenic skin grafts

Pathology
> Lymphocytic predominance over histiocytes
> Many cell types
> Pautrier abscesses

Prognosis
> Fair to good

Treatment
> Topical steroid therapy
> Ultraviolet light
> Grenz ray therapy
> Nitrogen mustard plaster

Stage 2

Clinical Features
> Variegated eruptions of Stage 1 gradually subside
> Plaques develop—infiltrated lesions
> Lesions persistent

Immunity
> Varying degrees of impairment, al-

though not usually marked, in ability to form circulating antibodies

Pathology
    Mixed cellularity—lymphocytes and histiocytes about equal in number
    Dissolution of basement membrane
    Pautrier abscesses

Prognosis
    Poor to fair

Treatment
    Topical nitrogen mustard
    Superficial x-ray therapy
    Cytoxan (cyclophosphamide)

Stage 3

Clinical Features
    Tumors appear in infiltrated patches
    Tumors may merge
    Ulceration of tumors
    Pruritus absent

Immunity
    Immunity usually lost

Pathology
    Lymphocytic depletion
    Histiocyte is dominant cell, almost assuming a monomorphous pattern
    Nests of mycotic cells evident

Prognosis
    Poor

Treatment
    Irradiation
    Cytotoxic agents

The "Erythroderma" Form

This condition is sometimes described as the *"l'homme rouge"* or *"femme rouge"* stage of mycosis fungoides. This so-called "erythroderma" or diffuse form of mycosis fungoides was first described by Hallopeau and Besnier. The symptoms, entirely different from those of classic mycosis fungoides, consist of an uncharacteristic, universal, exfoliative dermatitis occurring as the only manifestation of the disease. This eruption is frequently preceded by pruritus; it develops rapidly on previously normal skin and eventuates in tumor formation. However, we believe that histopathologically these cases are either lymphocytic leukemia, Hodgkin's disease, reticulum cell lymphosarcoma, Sézary

syndrome, or some other form of malignancy rather than mycosis fungoides.

The erythema is associated with peeling of the skin and varies from branlike scales to large lamellar flakes. There is usually severe pruritus and thickening of the skin, causing formation of large folds resulting from diffuse cutaneous infiltration, which is particularly marked on the trunk (cutis laxa). Because of the intense pruritus and underlying systemic pathology, lymphadenopathy is frequent and the course rapidly fatal.

Trophic changes, such as alopecia of the affected areas and nail involvement, may occur when cutaneous edema and lymphadenopathy are present. Superficial ulcers and "white patches" may occasionally involve the lips and buccal mucosa. Nodules and tumors subsequently develop, but the characteristic tumors have not always appeared at the time of death.

Tumor "d'Emblée" Type

This form of the disease, which we believe to be lymphosarcoma rather than mycosis fungoides, was first described by Vidal and Brocq. The sites of involvement, in order of frequency, appear to be the extremities, head, back, and trunk. Some degree of trauma has frequently been described as a participating factor in the d'emblée type.

The characteristic clinical features of the "d'emblée" form were described by Vidal and Brocq in 1885. They stated:

The lesions are much more circumscribed, do not have the characteristics of the preceding types, never are generalized if they are multiple, form sometimes one or more tumors which are well defined and of a fixed character. One does not observe the premycotic or infiltrative stage. This form is a much more grave type and cases end fatally rapidly.

As early as 1900 Brocq stated that this "d'emblée" type was closely related to lymphosarcoma of the skin.

Eosinophilia is usually present in this form of the disease, which has no premonitory signs or symptoms. However, since these cases described as mycosis fungoides "d'emblée" are actually a localized form of lymphosarcoma, they should be so designated and not be included with mycosis fungoides.

Internal organ involvement may occur in this form of lymphosarcoma, as well as in the erythroderma form. Internal organ involvement is not common in the classic type (Alibert) of mycosis fungoides.

Dermatoses Believed to be Precursors of Mycosis Fungoides

The various dermatoses which have been reported to be precursors of mycosis fungoides include (1) psoriasis, (2) parapsoriasis, (3) poikiloderma atrophicans vasculare, and (4) congenital icthyosiform erythroderma. A detailed account of this subject can be found in Bluefarb (1955c).

Pathology of Mycosis Fungoides

The histopathologic picture of mycosis fungoides varies considerably with the stage of the disease, and in patients with this clinical diagnosis, the spectrum ranges from a banal, nonspecific inflam-

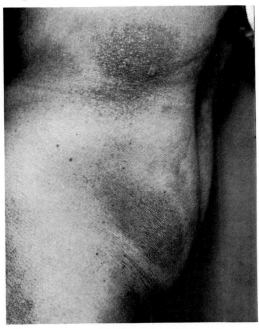

Figure 53–6 Poikiloderma vasculare atrophicans. (*From* Bluefarb: Cutaneous manifestations of the leukemia-lymphoma group. Postgrad. Med., 41:476, 1967.)

matory reaction to frank lymphomatous involvement. The skin is the site of origin of mycosis fungoides, although a variable proportion of patients develop extracutaneous disease.

In the eczematous or premycotic stage the histopathologic features are those of a chronic dermatitis. The epidermis is covered by a variable parakeratotic scale, and one usually sees mild acanthosis. Mild spongiosis may be present, and at this stage there may be some migration of normal lymphocytes into the lower epidermis. Within the dermis one sees an inflammatory infiltrate of lymphocytes and variable numbers of normal-appearing histiocytes. Occasional eosinophils and plasma cells may be encountered. The infiltrate usually has a loose perivascular configuration, although it may be more diffuse. As in simple dermatitis, the inflammatory infiltrate tends to be located superficially.

As the disease progresses to the plaque or infiltrated stage, a number of changes take place, leading to the diagnostic histopathologic picture of mycosis fungoides. The point in this progression at which a specific diagnosis can be made is not precise, and transitional pictures often present diagnostic problems.

In the infiltrated stage the histiocytes play the crucial role. These cells exhibit considerable pleomorphism, ranging from normal to bizarre forms which may resemble Sternberg-Reed cells or the cells of reticulum cell lymphoma. Mitotic figures may be frequent.

A characteristic histiocytic alteration results in the "mycosis fungoides" cell. Under light microscopy this is a large abnormal-appearing cell with an irregular hyperchromatic nucleus. Electron microscopic studies (Brownlee and Murad, 1970; Lutzner et al., 1971) reveal a large nucleus with infolding cleft formation and lobulation. The nucleus is heterochromatic with dense aggregates throughout the nucleus. The nucleolus is prominent. The cytoplasm has no distinguishing characteristics. These cells have the same basic appearance as the abnormal cells in peripheral blood, skin, and lymph nodes of Sézary syndrome (Lutzner and Jordan, 1968), but in Sézary syndrome these

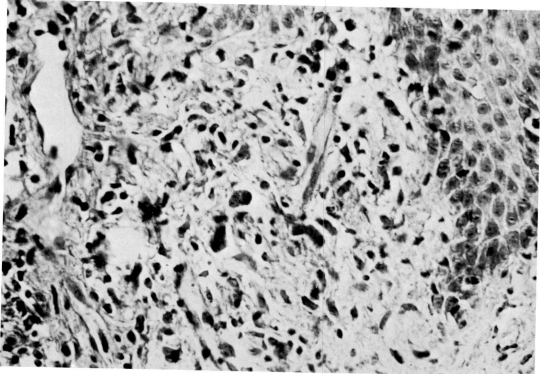

Figure 53–7   Lymphocytes predominating and few histiocytes are present.

changes are more pronounced (Lutzner et al., 1971).

The role of this cell in mycosis fungoides and in Sézary syndrome is subject to debate, because morphologically identical cells have been identified in unrelated conditions, including lichen planus (Lutzner et al., 1971; Flaxman et al., 1971), discoid lupus erythematosus, cutaneous vasculitis, psoriasis, actinic keratoses, and basal cell carcinoma (Flaxman et al., 1971).

In addition to the abnormal histiocytic cells, infiltrated plaques also show a polymorphous infiltrate of the usual inflammatory cells: lymphocytes, eosinophils, and plasma cells. The inflammatory infiltrate usually is of greater density than that found in ordinary dermatitis and often extends into the deeper levels of the dermis.

The epidermis in the infiltrative stage shows important features. Most characteristic is the Pautrier microabscess. This microabscess results from the migration of cells of the dermal infiltrate into the dermis and appears as a small, round,

cell-filled space, usually in the lower epidermis. These abscesses are differentiated from spongiotic vesicles and from spongiform pustules by the lack of associated spongiosis and by the presence of abnormal histiocytic cells. Pautrier microabscesses also occur in reticulum cell lymphoma (Kim et al., 1963).

Less commonly one finds a more diffuse migration of abnormal cells into the lower epidermis, and in these cases the basal layer appears disrupted and suggests liquefaction degeneration. The presence of these abnormal cells in the epidermis, whether as microabscesses or diffusely, makes the histopathologic diagnosis of mycosis fungoides considerably easier.

In the tumor stage the infiltrate is dense and extensive, occupying the entire thickness of the dermis and often extending into the subcutaneous fat. Extensive epidermal invasion results in ulceration. In the tumor stage one sees a high proportion of abnormal histiocytic cells, although the inflammatory component usually remains until late in the disease.

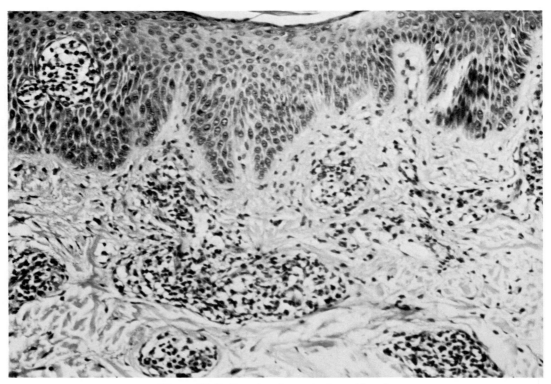

Figure 53–8 Pautrier abscess in the epidermis.

The abnormal cells often have a more bizarre pattern than in the infiltrative stage, and the picture may be indistinguishable from that of Hodgkin's disease or of reticulum cell lymphoma (Lever, 1967).

The incidence of internal involvement varies widely in published studies, and this variance in data is due, in part, to the differing criteria for the diagnosis of mycosis fungoides. Of 67 autopsied cases of mycosis fungoides from selected series, 58 or 86.6 percent had evidence of visceral involvement (Gates, 1938; Berman, 1940; Cawley et al., 1951; Rauschkolb, 1961; Block et al., 1963). Many of these cases, however, did not fit the strict criteria for mycosis fungoides and represented cutaneous expressions of other malignant lymphomas, such as Hodgkin's disease and reticulum cell lymphoma. In contrast, Allen believed the incidence of visceral involvement to be approximately 15 percent when strict histopathologic criteria were employed (Allen, 1967).

After the skin, the lymph nodes are most frequently involved (Cawley et al., 1951; Block et al., 1963), and here one encounters a spectrum ranging from reactive hyperplasia to frank involvement with malignant lymphoma. In many cases the cellular infiltrate in the lymph nodes appears identical to that in the skin. In other cases the lymph node diagnosis is Hodgkin's disease, reticulum cell lymphoma, lymphocytic lymphoma, or plasmacytosis (Block et al., 1963). Other significant organ involvement includes the spleen, liver, kidneys, lungs, heart, and gastrointestinal tract (Cawley et al., 1951; Block et al., 1963; Cyr et al., 1966).

SÉZARY SYNDROME

It has been convenient to divide leukemic reticuloendotheliosis into three hematologic types: a primitive cell variety, a monocytic (Schilling), and a lymphocytic type. In some cases of the lymphocytic type of leukemic reticuloendotheliosis, a chronic course indicates the benign nature of the proliferation (Sézary and Bouvrain, 1938). The chronic form may

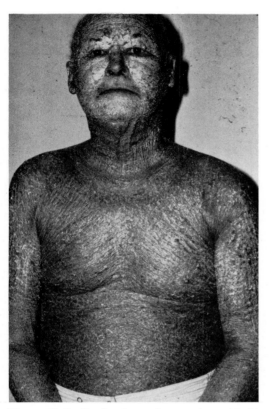

Figure 53–9 Erythroderma in a patient with Sézary syndrome. (See also Color Plate VIII-E.)

persist for 10 years or more, and among its manifestations is erythroderma. Some of these erythrodermic cases are now recognized as the Sézary form of erythrodermic reticulemia. A constellation of clinical findings—erythroderma, edema, alopecia, hyperpigmentation, hypopigmentation, and hyperkeratosis of the palms and soles—seems to point toward the diagnosis of the Sézary syndrome. Skin biopsy, dermal touch smears, and the peripheral blood smears confirm the diagnosis. The bone marrow is normal, and the results of the general physical examination are usually unremarkable.

In 1938 Sézary and Bouvrain described a general exfoliative dermatitis characterized by an intense pruritus and a cutaneous infiltrate primarily composed of atypical mononuclear cells which were also found in the marrow, liver, and spleen. They interpreted the changes as secondary to a malignant reticulosis involving the skin and lymph nodes, accompanied by monocytic leukemia. The following year, Baccareddo (1939) reported a similar clinical entity but interpreted the findings as representing a benign hyperplasia of the reticulohistiocytic system of the skin without involving the internal organs.

Fleischmajer and Eisenberg (1964) 25 years later reviewed the reported cases of Sézary syndrome. At that time 23 patients had been reported; of these 16 were dead. Only in two of these was the clinical course suggestive of progressive systemic malignant lymphoma. They suggested that Sézary's reticulosis may represent a distinct malignant hyperplasia of the reticuloendothelial system not related to the leukemias or lymphomas; furthermore, they suggested that it may be a reticulosis of the skin and superficial lymph nodes, sparing the bone marrow and internal organs. It was their belief that the leukemic component results from the release of the reticular cells from the skin into the blood stream. They pointed out that some evidence seems to suggest that Sézary reticulosis is a syndrome that may precede by many years the establishment of definitive malignant neoplastic process of the lymphoreticular system.

Taswell and Winkelmann (1961) reviewed the diagnostic features of the syndrome. They included the following: exfoliative erythroderma with intense pruritus, edema, pigmentation, superficial lymphadenopathy, hepatomegaly, leonine facies, alopecia, dystrophic nails, and hyperkeratosis of the palms and soles. A cutaneous infiltrate of atypical mononuclear cells is present and is associated with an increased leukocyte count and an abundance of atypical cells in the peripheral blood. This atypical cell is characterized by a large convoluted nucleus, with a narrow rim of cytoplasm frequently containing numerous vacuoles in a necklace type of arrangement around the nucleus. Within these vacuoles is an intensely PAS-positive mucopolysaccharide. Patients with this disease remain in good condition for long periods of time. There is no evidence of distant metastatic lesions or involvement of other organs. Treatment with superficial irradiation, steroids, and cytotoxic agents yields only temporary relief. Death occurs from unrelated causes approximately five years after the first symptoms.

The identification of the Sézary cell—a mature monocytoid lymphocyte with or without vacuoles—is the key to the diagnosis. Vacuolated lymphocytes are usually found in small numbers and are associated with specific nuclear or cytoplasmic changes in the cell, as in lymphoblastic lymphoma or infectious mononucleosis. It must be emphasized that the Sézary cell is not a malignant lymphocytic cell. The detection of polysaccharide in the cytoplasmic vacuoles of the lymphocyte is interesting and requires further investigation. Periodic acid–Schiff granules have been found in the lymphocyte on many occasions. In most cases these have proved to be diastase-digestible, and they are said to be composed of glycogen. Such granules are found in immature and neoplastic lymphocytes. The Sézary cell may be characterized by PAS-positive, diastase-resistant granules, which are assumed to be made up of neutral mucopolysaccharide. This picture has not been recognized as a useful feature in the diagnosis of any lymphocytic disease heretofore, and continued study of the lymphocytic form of leukemic reticuloendotheliosis by this means may establish the source of these polysaccharide granules and the extent of their usefulness in diagnosis.

As the disease progresses, the Sézary cell increases in number in the peripheral blood until the count may be 30,000 to 60,000 cells per cubic millimeter of blood. What is the source of these cells? The marrow is normal, the lymphatic tissue is not hyperplastic, and the patient is in good general health. It seems an inescapable conclusion that the skin is forming these cells as an extramedullary site of hyperplastic reticulosis.

Because of the cutaneous lesions, this condition has been diagnosed as mycosis fungoides. Because of the atypical lymphocytes in the peripheral smear, it has been diagnosed as chronic lymphatic leukemia. Erythrodermic mycosis fungoides is the condition most frequently confused with the Sézary syndrome. Such cases are recognized as unusual on both clinical and histologic grounds. It is our contention (Bluefarb, 1955c) that "erythroderma" and "d'emblée" types of mycosis fungoids cannot be accepted as representing classic mycosis fungoides. The entity of Sézary syndrome gives us one answer to the question of the nature of some of these confusing borderline cases. It should be emphasized that the early lesions of Sézary syndrome may be serpiginous or annular plaques, which may be confused with similar lesions of mycosis fungoides. The histologic pictures of mycosis fungoides and the Sézary syndrome are characterized by an infiltrate of mononuclear cells limited to the upper portion of the dermis. In such cases, recognition of the Sézary cell in the peripheral smear and in the skin is of great importance in making the correct diagnosis (Taswell and Winkelmann, 1961). The erythrodermic form of lymphocytic leukemic reticuloendotheliosis (Sézary syndrome) may thus be a primary cutaneous expression of a proliferative reticulosis.

Pathology of Sézary Syndrome

The major pathologic features of Sézary syndrome include changes in the skin, peripheral blood, and lymph nodes. The skin in Sézary syndrome shows a variable histopathologic picture, but most cases have the features of mycosis fungoides (Taswell and Winkelmann, 1961; Fleischmajer and Eisenberg, 1964; Clendenning et al., 1964). Within the upper dermis one finds an infiltrate of abnormal-appearing histiocytic cells, usually associated with Pautrier abscesses. As in mycosis fungoides, there is a variable proportion of chronic inflammatory cells, although in Sézary syndrome the appearance may more closely resemble reticulum cell lymphoma (Taswell and Winkelmann, 1961; Tedeschi and Lasinger, 1965).

The Sézary cell, present in skin, peripheral blood, and lymph nodes, is slightly larger than a neutrophil but has a nucleus which occupies at least 80 percent of the cell (Taswell and Winkelmann, 1961). With light microscopy the nucleus is round to markedly irregular, and the cytoplasm usually appears amorphous and contains vacuoles which have been variously described as PAS-positive,

alopecia, and nail changes, are frequently present in Hodgkin's disease.

The onset of icthyosis vulgaris in an adult with no personal or family history of this disease is unusual. The simultaneous occurrence of Hodgkin's disease and icthyosis, therefore, should arouse suspicion of a cause and effect relationship.

J. R. Webster and Bluefarb (1952) presented a 22 year old Negro who had icthyosis associated with Hodgkin's disease. He first developed a small "knot" in the left axilla 11 months previously, which gradually enlarged to the size of a small "grapefruit" and became painful. He had lost 23 pounds in weight, and dryness of the skin had begun at the time the lymphadenopathy appeared. There were occasional mild pruritus of the arms and slight scaling of the lower extremities, as well as a moderate follicular keratosis. The liver and spleen were palpable. The lymphadenopathy decreased slightly following triethylenemelamine therapy.

Another case of icthyosis associated with Hodgkin's disease was presented by Bluefarb and Goldberg (1953). This patient, a 58 year old woman, had cervical, axillary, and inguinal lymphadenopathy for five years before the development of fever, night sweats, fatigue, and anorexia.

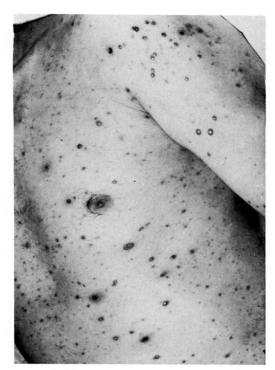

Figure 53–13 Generalized zoster associated with Hodgkin's disease.

She had received intensive roentgenotherapy and nitrogen mustard therapy during this period. The skin had become red and scaly one year after the lymphadenopathy appeared and had slowly increased in severity. The skin, particularly that of the face and extremities, appeared erythematous with a generalized exfoliation. There was hyperkeratosis of the palms and soles, and the hair of the scalp was sparse and coarse while the axillary and eyebrow hair was absent. There were a few palpable inguinal lymph nodes.

Herpes Zoster. Herpes zoster is more frequently present in Hodgkin's disease and lymphosarcoma (4 to 7 percent) than in lymphocytic leukemia (1 percent). Although there are few reports of herpes zoster associated with Hodgkin's disease, undoubtedly many cases are observed and not reported, since this association is not rare and occurs more frequently than is generally recognized.

In Hodgkin's disease, the specific virus of zoster is stimulated by the compression of the granuloma along the nerve or ganglion. The severity of zoster associated

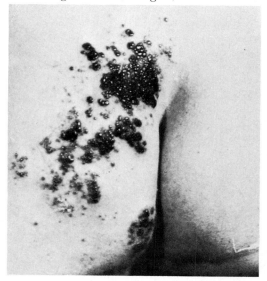

Figure 53–12 Herpes zoster associated with Hodgkin's disease. (*From* Bluefarb and Schwartz: Scientific exhibits; cutaneous manifestations of leukemia-lymphoma group. A.M.A. Arch. Dermatol., 73:189, 1956.)

with Hodgkin's disease is often emphasized, since the hemorrhagic or gangrenous type is frequent, and severe scarring often results. Deep gangrenous
sloughing ulceration has also been described.

Purpura.   Although the occurrence of
purpura has been observed in Hodgkin's
disease, it is more frequent in the leukemias. The hemorrhagic tendencies are
usually a terminal manifestation in Hodgkin's disease but may be an initial symptom in leukemia. When the purpuric lesions occasionally show a specific rather
than a nonspecific infiltrate histologically,
they are classified with the lymphogranulomatids.

Poikiloderma.   The cutaneous features of this sign are discussed under
mycosis fungoides. Cases have been reported of poikiloderma of the skin associated with Hodgkin's disease.

SPECIFIC CUTANEOUS LESIONS

The specific cutaneous lesions occurring in Hodgkin's disease may be classified as: (1) papules, (2) infiltrates or
plaques, (3) nodules or tumors, (4) ulcerated lesions, (5) mixed or combinations
of these, and (6) erythroderma. Specific
cutaneous lesions, associated with nonspecific or toxic lesions, may also be present.

Papular Lesions.   The papular lesion
appears as small, brownish red, flattened
papules of a rather firm consistency.

Infiltrates and Plaques.   The cutaneous infiltrations in Hodgkin's disease,
when situated deeply, are frequently discernible only on palpation. They are
usually diffuse and appear to be most
frequent in the breast.

Nodules and Tumors.   A further sub-
division of specific cutaneous Hodgkin's
disease is the primary or initial lymphogranulomatous cutaneous lesion, which
develops in the skin proper and is not
merely an extension from a deeper lesion
of a contiguous lymph node. The primary
lesion may be a nodule, infiltrate, or specific ulcer. French investigators have designated this lesion "*le chancre lymphogran-
ulomateux.*" Thus Hodgkin's disease would
have a primary lesion such as occurs in
tuberculosis, syphilis, sporotrichosis, and

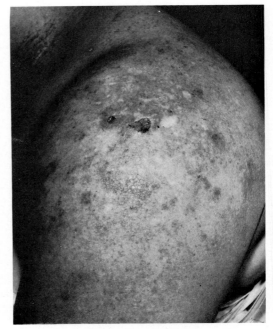

Figure 53–14 Ulcerated nodules in Hodgkin's disease. (*From* Bluefarb: Cutaneous manifestations of
the leukemia-lymphoma group. Postgrad. Med.,
41:476, 1967.

other conditions. The similarity of these
lesions to those of mycosis fungoides
"d'emblée" is one of the many reasons for
the confusion regarding the "d'emblée"
form of mycosis fungoides.

The scalp appears to be a frequent site
of the initial lesion in cutaneous Hodgkin's disease.

Ulcerative Lesions.   Ulcerative cutaneous lesions are as infrequent but important form of specific involvement in
Hodgkin's disease. In a comparative review of this subject, Senear and Caro
(1937) described three initial forms which
occur in this type. In the first, the ulceration is limited in extent and develops a
few cutaneous nodules, with the necrosis
usually starting at the top of the nodule
and gradually extending until the surface
of the nodule is almost completely covered. In the second type, cutaneous involvement results from lymphogranulomatous
changes in the underlying structures. The
involved lymph nodes or underlying
structures, such as bone or other tissues,
gradually become inflamed and then form
fistulae, leading to ulceration. The third

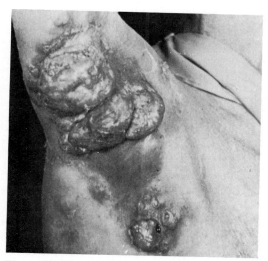

Figure 53–15 Tumors associated with Hodgkin's disease. (*From* Bluefarb and Schwartz: Scientific exhibits; cutaneous manifestations of leukemia-lymphoma group. A.M.A. Arch. Dermatol., 73:189, 1956.)

type represents extensive ulceration developing in large cutaneous infiltrations without involvement of the underlying structure. This type has been confused with mycosis fungoides "d'emblée," since the cutaneous lesions may precede the lymphadenopathy by a period of months to many years.

Erythroderma Form. Erythroderma may be specific or nonspecific in Hodgkin's disease. Although the specific form is not common, such cases have been described.

LYMPHOGRANULOMATIDS

At times, there is no definite distinction between toxic or nonspecific cutaneous lesions and true tumors or specific lesions of Hodgkin's disease or leukemia. The unity of these two conditions, which frequently cannot be separated clinically or pathologically, is often evidenced by cases described in the literature. The merging of these conditions may be almost imperceptible. The connecting link between these two disease groups are the "ids": lymphogranulomatids when associated with Hodgkin's disease, and leukemids when associated with leukemia. Clinically they resemble nonspecific or toxic lesions, but histologically they resemble

specific or true cutaneous infiltration by either Hodgkin's disease or leukemia.

Treatment

Aggressive radiotherapy is still the treatment of choice in the early stages of the disease. A combination of four potent chemotherapeutic drugs is used in the late stages of Hodgkin's disease.

Treatment consists of the administration of 40 mg. of prednisone daily on days zero to 14 inclusive; 100 mg. per sq. meter of procarbazine daily on days zero to 14; 10 mg. of vinblastine intravenously on days zero, seven, and 14; and 6.0 mg. per sq. meter of mustine hydrochloride on days zero and seven. This two-week course of treatment is repeated for six courses, with a four-week rest between treatments. Further treatment consists of a course every one to four months, depending on the clinical condition.

Pathology

The pathologic changes of Hodgkin's disease are more complex than those of the monomorphous lymphomas because of the interrelationship of neoplastic and inflammatory features. The predominant pathologic feature in early Hodgkin's disease is an inflammatory response, and in these stages the bulk of the lesion may be due almost entirely to a proliferation of inflammatory cells (Rappaport, 1966). As the disease progresses the inflammatory response is gradually replaced by a neoplastic picture, and in late stages the entire picture may be neoplastic. This progression is widely felt to represent the initially adequate but gradually deteriorating ability of the host to resist the neoplastic assault of the disease (Lukes et al., 1966a).

During the evolution of Hodgkin's disease, five basic pathologic tissue responses may be encountered (Higgins, 1968): (1) lymphocytic proliferation, (2) alteration in histiocytic cells, (3) polymorphous infiltrate of leukocytes, (4) necrosis, and (5) fibrosis. The currently employed classification of Hodgkin's disease is based on these alterations.

The early stages of Hodgkin's disease are characterized by a proliferation of mature small lymphocytes, often with concomitant proliferation of histiocytes. This is a relative change and is in no way specific for the disease.

During the course of the disease the histiocytes undergo a number of progressive changes. Histiocytes in early cases are of a reactive type, although with progression these cells become larger and more abnormal appearing with the development of the Sternberg-Reed cell so characteristic of Hodgkin's disease. In certain cases the histiocytes appear more anaplastic and simulate the cells of reticulum cell lymphoma.

A mixed infiltrate of inflammatory cells is another characteristic feature of Hodgkin's disease, and one frequently encounters neutrophils, eosinophils, and plasma cells.

In later stages necrosis may be a significant feature and usually is of a caseous type. Calcification may occur within the necrotic areas.

Fibrosis occurs in localized nodular forms and also occurs extensively late in the disease when it may accompany the proliferation of Sternberg-Reed cells or may be associated with cellular depletion.

The original widely used classification of Hodgkin's disease into paragranuloma, granuloma, and sarcoma (Jackson and Parker, 1947) finds less use today because of the relatively few cases of paragranuloma and sarcoma (8 percent and 1 percent, respectively) and the high incidence of granuloma (91 percent) (Lukes, 1963). The granuloma group was found to be heterogeneous, and the designation provided no help as to prognosis (Lukes et al., 1966a).

The newer classification of Lukes (Table 53–2) (Lukes et al., 1966a and 1966b) correlates more closely with the clinical spectrum of the disease and also correlates well with prognosis (Lukes et al., 1966a; Keller et al., 1968; Kadin et al., 1971). We should note that the pathologic

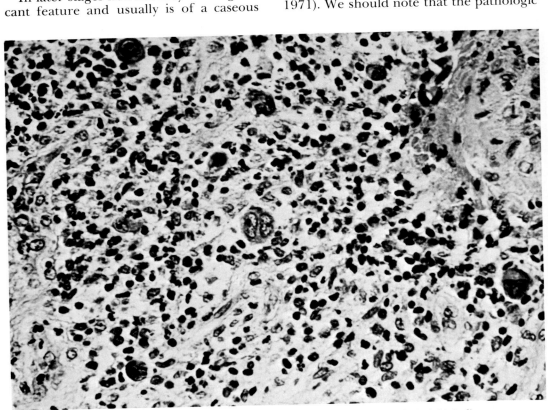

Figure 53–16   Mixed cellularity and Sternberg-Reed cells from a nodule of Hodgkin's disease.

TABLE 53-2

Jackson and Parker (1947)	Lukes et al. (1966a and 1966b)
Paragranuloma	Lymphocytic predominance
	a. Nodular
	b. Diffuse
	Nodular sclerosis
Granuloma	Mixed cellularity
	Lymphocytic depletion
	a. Diffuse fibrosis
Sarcoma	b. Reticular type

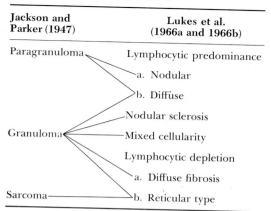

classification of Hodgkin's disease depends upon examination of lymph nodes. The histopathologic responses of the skin are more limited.

The picture of lymphocytic predominance usually occurs early in the course of Hodgkin's disease and generally is associated with a good prognosis. Mature lymphocytes and histiocytes are present in variable proportions, and other inflammatory cells and abnormal cells are absent or present in minimal numbers. Such cases usually fall into the old paragranuloma group.

Nodular sclerosis, a frequently encountered pattern, also has a good prognosis and is characterized by interconnecting bands of connective tissue and by atypical histiocytic cells and Sternberg-Reed cells lying in lacunae. Hodgkin's disease with nodular sclerosis stands somewhat apart from other forms of the disease, with a predilection for females and a high incidence of mediastinal involvement. These cases are included in Hodgkin's granuloma.

Hodgkin's disease with mixed cellularity represents a transitional form between lymphocytic predominance and lymphocytic depletion. The number of lymphocytes varies, but neutrophils, eosinophils, and plasma cells become prominent. In addition, one sees many Sternberg-Reed cells, as well as some irregular fibrosis and foci of necrosis. Such lesions lie within the spectrum of Hodgkin's granuloma, and the prognosis is less favorable than in lymphocytic predominance or nodular sclerosis.

Lymphocytic depletion includes lesions with greatly decreased or absent lymphocytes and is associated with the poorest prognosis. Two types are recognized. In diffuse fibrosis ones sees extensive disorderly fibrosis, which contrasts sharply with the well-organized pattern of nodular sclerosis. Lymphocytes and other inflammatory cellular components are suppressed, and variable foci of necrosis occur within the fibrotic masses. Such cases are included in Hodgkin's granuloma. The reticular type of lymphocytic depletion includes lesions with a predominance of atypical histiocytic cells. In some cases these cells are of the Sternberg-Reed type, while in other cases the pattern simulates reticulum cell lymphoma. The reticular pattern has been included in Hodgkin's granuloma and in Hodgkin's sarcoma.

The skin in Hodgkin's disease, although it may be the site of specific lesions, seldom shows a histopathologic pattern diagnostic of the disease. Diagnostic Sternberg-Reed cells rarely appear in skin lesions, although they may be present in abundance in involved lymph nodes. The most common histopathologic pattern of specific skin lesions reveals a polymorphous infiltrate of inflammatory cells, including lymphocytes, neutrophils, eosinophils, and plasma cells. In addition, abnormal cells of the histiocytic series usually are present, and these may have the appearance of the cells of stem cell or reticulum cell lymphoma. Infrequent lesions have Sternberg-Reed cells. These cells are large, 12 to 40 micra in diameter, and have large prominent nuclei. The nuclei may be single or multiple, and a characteristic feature is a double bean-shaped nucleus with a mirror image appearance. The nuclear chromatin is coarse and tends to concentrate near the nuclear membrane. Each nucleus usually contains a large, homogeneous-appearing nucleus which often is eosinophilic and which resembles an inclusion body (Lukes et al., 1966a). Mitotic figures may be frequent among the abnormal histiocytic cells. Skin lesions also may show foci of necrosis and ultimately considerable fibrosis. These lesions fall into the broad category of Hodgkin's granuloma.

In certain cases the dermal infiltrate contains few inflammatory cells and consists almost entirely of stem cells, reticulum cells, and Sternberg-Reed cells. Such cases show lymph node features of the reticular type of lymphocytic depletion (Hodgkin's sarcoma).

The diagnosis of Hodgkin's disease cannot be made with certainty from the skin lesions unless Sternberg-Reed cells are present. The polymorphous cellular picture may simulate mycosis fungoides, but Hodgkin's disease lacks Pautrier microabscesses, and mycosis fungoides cells do not resemble Sternberg-Reed cells. Reticular Hodgkin's disease may be indistinguishable from malignant lymphoma of the stem cell or reticulum cell type, although this form of Hodgkin's disease is uncommon in the skin.

LYMPHOSARCOMA

Lymphosarcoma is a malignant neoplastic disease involving the lymphoid tissue. It is capable of arising in any lymphoid aggregate and may occur primarily or secondarily in the skin. The course of the disease may be acute or chronic. The lesions are nearly always radiosensitive.

Lymphosarcoma, like Hodgkin's disease, appears to begin as a localized disease. Its onset is usually in one of three regions: the nasopharyngeal ring of lymphoid tissue, the mediastinal lymph nodes or thymus, and the abdomen, most likely from the gastrointestinal nodes or perhaps the lymphoid tissue of the alimentary canal. Rarely, it may be primary in the skin, but usually it is secondary to lymphosarcoma elsewhere.

Clinical Features

Systemic symptoms (chills, fever, lassitude, increased sweating, weight loss) are conspicuously absent early in lymphosarcoma, rarely appearing until the disease is far advanced, in contrast to the case in Hodgkin's disease.

Mikulicz's syndrome may be associated with lymphosarcoma. Mikulicz's disease is a symptom complex characterized by symmetrical lymphadenopathy of the lacrimal, orbital, and salivary glands due to infiltration of small round cells. The predominant clinical signs and symptoms are caused by pressure from the lymph nodes and dryness of the mouth and throat; exophthalmos and impaired hearing and vision may occur.

Cutaneous Lesions

NONSPECIFIC CUTANEOUS LESIONS

The nonspecific cutaneous manifestations of Hodgkin's disease and lymphosarcoma show a close parallelism.

Pruritus. Pruritus occurs somewhat more frequently in Hodgkin's disease than in lymphosarcoma.

Prurigo-like Papules. Prurigo-like papules (prurigo lymphadenique) occur with lymphosarcoma, just as in leukemia and Hodgkin's disease. Occasionally the intensely pruritic prurigo-like papules resemble dermatitis herpetiformis.

Erythema Multiforme. Erythema multiforme is noted, especially after roentgen ray therapy.

Herpes Zoster. When associated with lymphosarcoma, the mechanism of herpes zoster is due, as in Hodgkin's disease, to compression by the new growth, which results in a stimulation of the virus and the development of zoster along the distribution of the affected nerve.

Exfoliative Dermatitis. Exfoliative dermatitis may occur in association with chronic lymphocytic leukemia and Hodgkin's disease, as well as in lymphosarcoma. Clinically, the erythrodermatous type is indistinguishable from that present in leukemia or Hodgkin's disease.

Purpura. Purpura occasionally occurs in association with lymphosarcoma and has the same mechanism and significance as purpura associated with Hodgkin's disease.

Pigmentation. The mechanism for pigmentation in lymphosarcoma is similar to that in Hodgkin's disease.

Trophic Changes. Icthyosiform atrophy of the skin in lymphosarcoma has been reported.

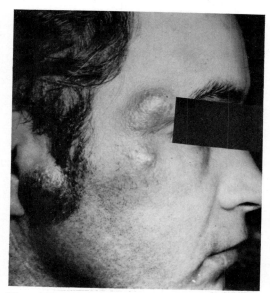

Figure 53–17 Nodules of lymphocytic lymphosarcoma.

Oral Lesions. There are reports of lymphosarcomatous involvement of the tonsil, tongue, and hard palate.

SPECIFIC CUTANEOUS LESIONS

The specific nodular cutaneous lesions of lymphosarcoma are one or several, "pea to hazel nut" in size, firm, round or oval, bluish red, elastic tumors at the onset. They are not painful on palpation, are freely movable over the underlying structures, and appear to arise in the subcutaneous tissue of the skin. The tumors increase reapidly in size to that of an "egg" or an "apple" and increase in number. The color varies from bright red to deep blue, depending upon their depth. Ulceration of the nodules, although not common, has been observed.

Pathology of the Monomorphous Lymphomas

The histopathologic features of the cutaneous lesions of stem cell, reticulum cell, and lymphocytic lymphomas are similar, and differentiation is based on identification of the proliferating cell. All these lesions have certain features in common (Caro, 1971). The epidermis usually is not involved except for thinning and infrequently ulceration, resulting from the underlying infiltrate. The migration into the epidermis of cells of the dermal infiltrate as seen in mycosis fungoides does not occur in these lymphomas, and in many cases a zone of uninfiltrated dermis separates the epidermis from the underlying dermal infiltrate (grenz zone). The dermal infiltrate is diffuse or patchy in nature, and these patches tend to be randomly distributed throughout the dermis and frequently in the subcutis.

True lymphoid follicles are rare in malignant lymphomas. While lymphoid follicles have peripheral lymphocytes and germinal centers composed primarily of reticulum cells, the follicle-like structures seen in malignant lymphomas are monomorphous, with the central areas showing a lesser density of the parent tumor cell.

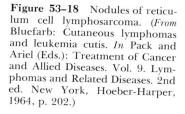

Figure 53–18 Nodules of reticulum cell lymphosarcoma. (*From* Bluefarb: Cutaneous lymphomas and leukemia cutis. *In* Pack and Ariel (Eds.): Treatment of Cancer and Allied Diseases. Vol. 9. Lymphomas and Related Diseases. 2nd ed. New York, Hoeber-Harper, 1964, p. 202.)

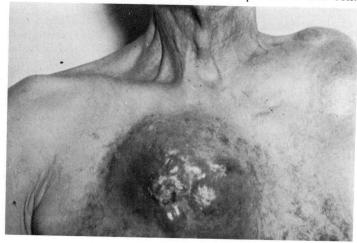

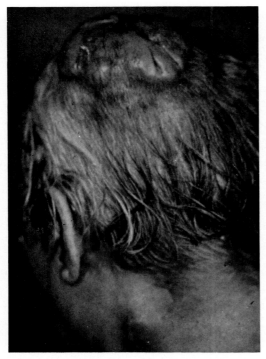

Figure 53–19 Tumors of reticulum cell lympho-sarcoma. (*From* Bluefarb and Schwartz: Scientific exhibits; cutaneous manifestations of leukemia-lymphoma group. A.M.A. Arch. Dermatol., 73:189, 1956.)

These areas do not represent germinal centers. Any type of malignant lymphoma may produce such a pseudofollicular or nodular pattern, usually early in the course of the disease, and such a picture does not represent a separate type of malignant lymphoma (Rappaport et al., 1956).

Although in well-differentiated lymphocytic lymphoma the infiltrate tends to be patchy, in poorly differentiated lymphocytic lymphoma and in reticulum cell lymphoma the infiltrate tends to be more diffuse.

In stem cell lymphoma (Gall and Mallory, 1942; Rappaport, 1966), the neoplastic elements represent primitive lymphoreticular cells without differentiation along lymphocytic or histiocytic lines. The stem cell is large, 15 to 35 micra in diameter, and has abundant pale-staining cytoplasm. These cells often lie in a syncytial arrangement so that cell boundaries are not distinct. The nucleus is large and round to oval, with a delicate, irregularly distributed chromatin pattern. Mitotic figures are usually numerous. A single vesicular nucleolus can be identified. Because of the primitive nature of these cells, no reticulum is produced.

The definition of reticulum cell lymphoma has not been precise because of the varying characterization of the reticulum cell (Gall, 1955 and 1958). We have not attempted to subclassify reticulum cell lymphoma but rather consider it simply a neoplasm of cells differentiating along histiocytic lines. Because of wide variations in degree of differentiation, reticulum production, and phagocytic function, the morphology of reticulum cell lymphoma will show considerable variability (Kim et al., 1963; Rappaport, 1966).

The reticulum cells participating in this tumor lie between stem cells and mature histiocytes in size and have indistinct to sharply defined borders, depending upon the degree of differentiation. Nuclei range from round or oval to deeply lobulated or reniform. The chromatin pattern is coarser than in stem cell lymphoma, and the nucleoli are usually larger (Rappaport, 1966). The cytoplasm varies in amount and staining quality, depending on the degree of differentiation, and poorly differentiated lesions have a larger proportion of eosinophilic staining cytoplasm. Mitotic figures vary in number but usually are frequent.

In well differentiated lesions fibrile formation is evident, and some lesions show evidence of phagocytic function. Although reticulum cell lymphoma is classified as monomorphous, it is not unusual to find variable numbers of poorly differentiated and well differentiated lymphocytes within the lesion (Director and Kern, 1963; Kim et al., 1963; Caro, 1971).

Lymphocytic lymphoma (lymphosarcoma) presents a histopathologic spectrum ranging from lesions with poorly differentiated cells to lesions with cells indistinguishable from normal-appearing small lymphocytes. In poorly differentiated lymphocytic lymphoma (Gall and Mallory, 1942; Rappaport, 1966), the cells range from 10 to 20 micra in diameter and are larger than well differentiated lymphocytes. The nucleus is large, round, or indented to irregular and has relative-

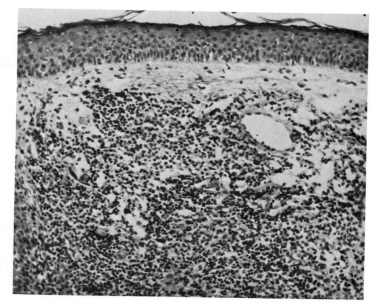

Figure 53–20 Lymphocytic lymphosarcoma.

ly course, evenly distributed chromatin which is not clumped. About the nucleus one sees a narrow rim of basophilic cytoplasm. Mitotic figures are usually numerous. No reticulum is produced.

Many of these cells have an admixture of stem cells and reticulum cells, usually in small numbers, and some lesions have well differentiated lymphocytes (Gall and Mallory, 1942; Rappaport, 1966).

Well differentiated lymphocytic lymphoma is characterized by cells which are

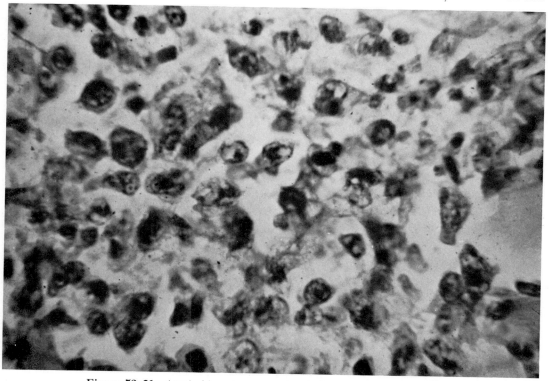

Figure 53–21 Atypical lymphocytes and reticulum cells in lymphosarcoma.

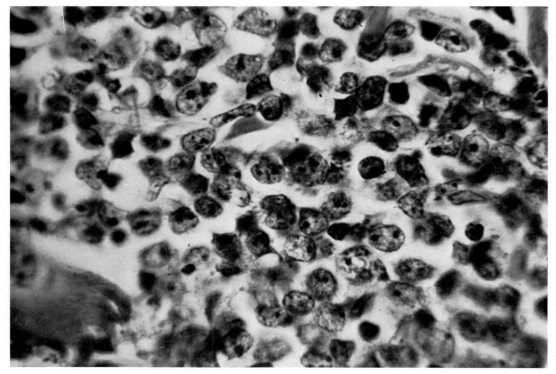

Figure 53–22   Atypical lymphocytes and reticulum cells in lymphosarcoma.

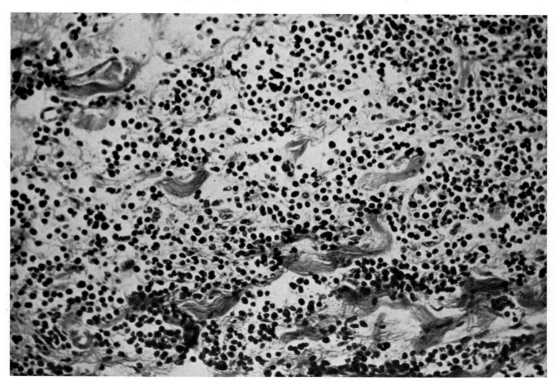

Figure 53–23   Lymphocytic lymphosarcoma.

indistinguishable from normal lymphocytes (Gall and Mallory, 1942; Rappaport, 1966). The cellular pattern usually is uniform, and mitotic figures are infrequent. Although the infiltrate in stem cell, reticulum cell, and poorly differentiated lymphocytic lymphomas often is diffuse and massive, in well differentiated lymphocytic lymphoma there is a common tendency for the infiltrate to be segregated into discrete patches. One also will find single rows of lymphocytes infiltrating between collagen fibers from the cellular patches ("Indian-file sign").

These skin lesions cannot be differentiated histopathologically from the specific lesion of chronic lymphocytic leukemia; the microscopic picture is the same.

LEUKEMIA

Leukemia is usually classified according to the duration of the process and the type of cell that predominates in the peripheral blood or bone marrow. In the acute forms, the cells are often so immature that it is impossible to identify their origin, whether from granulocytic, lymphocytic, or monocytic cells. The most immature type of cell is the so-called stem or blast cell. Cases of acute leukemia in which these cells predominate are designated "stem cell" or "blast cell" leukemia.

Acute Leukemia

In acute leukemia, physical examination usually reveals marked pallor and generalized lymphadenopathy, while splenomegaly may or may not be present, and the skin may show hemorrhagic manifestations or true leukemic infiltrations. Anemia is invariably present in acute leukemia and may be extremely severe. Thrombocytopenia is also a characteristic finding.

Onset of acute leukemia, regardless of cell type, is usually rapid, although occasionally the prodromal phases are insidious. Initial signs are usually related to bone marrow replacement, such as overwhelming infection incident to a decrease in the leukocytic precursors or thrombo-

cytopenia with hemorrhage. Anemia secondary to marrow erythrocytic cell replacement is often severe at the time of diagnosis. The profound debility of some patients with acute leukemia is frequently out of proportion to the severity of the clinical signs.

CUTANEOUS LESIONS

The cutaneous manifestations of acute leukemia may be divided into nonspecific or toxic lesions and specific lesions.

Nonspecific Cutaneous Lesions

PALLOR. Pallor is a marked feature of the acute leukemic state and is probably due to the rapidly developing anemia.

HEMORRHAGIC PHENOMENA. Acute leukemia is usually accompanied by spontaneous hemorrhages. In the acute forms this hemorrhagic state is probably dependent, to a great extent, upon the paucity of blood platelets. The petechial lesions may be generalized or may be limited to one area of the body. Frequently they occur in the form of successive crops which appear for no apparent reason. The most frequent site of predilection of ecchymoses is in the region of the sacrum. In the great majority of cases, there is hemorrhage from the gums, manifested by the persistent oozing of blood.

Bleeding of the gingivae appears to be associated with stomatitis as an early manifestation of acute granulocytic leukemia and consequently occurs more frequently in adults.

ORAL LESIONS. The intraoral lesions occurring in acute leukemia are numerous and varied. Pathologic processes affecting the mucous membranes are chiefly hemorrhage, necrosis, and hypertrophy of the gingivae. Leukemic manifestations of the mouth are mainly confined to the gingival tissues and mucous membranes. The most common lesion is bleeding from the gums, which is probably due in part to infiltration of the bone marrow by leukemic cells, which crowd out or inhibit megakaryocytes with the resulting blood platelet deficiency. In some cases the bleeding gums are pale and of normal contour. In others, the gums are hypertrophic and edematous

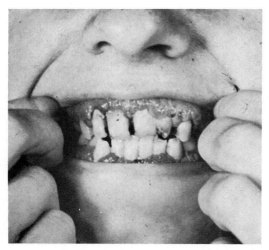

Figure 53–24 Hypertrophic gums associated with leukemia. (*From* Bluefarb and Schwartz: Scientific exhibits; cutaneous manifestations of leukemia-lymphoma group. A.M.A. Arch. Dermatol., 73:189, 1956.)

and resemble the appearance of gums in scurvy or acute stomatitis. As the leukemia progresses, the epithelial and submucous layers of the gums undergo exudative and necrotic changes, so that there is sloughing of irregular areas of the lining membrane.

Infiltration of the gums by leukemia cells occurs in acute leukemia and results in swollen gums, which are painful and bleed easily on slight trauma. At times this swelling is so extreme that the gums cover the teeth.

The next most frequent oral manifestation consists of areas of necrosis which may appear on the buccal surfaces of the cheeks, on the labial surfaces of the lips, on the gums, on the hard or soft palate, or on two or more of these areas.

Pyoderma. Pyoderma occurs frequently in acute leukemia as a result of the reduction in the number of mature granulocytes. Viral infections are common because of a deficiency in the immune mechanism.

Specific Cutaneous Lesions. Specific infiltrative cutaneous lesions are rare in acute lymphocytic and acute granulocytic leukemia but are characteristic in acute monocytic leukemia. When these lesions do occur in acute lymphocytic leukemia, they resemble the specific cutaneous lesions present in chronic lymphocytic leukemia, being nodular or papular, small in size, and of "plum" color.

Lymphocytic Leukemia

The symptoms of chronic leukemia are generally referable to (1) a local accumulation of cells which causes symptoms by mechanical means, such as marked splenomegaly, cervical and axillary lymphadenopathy, and cutaneous tumors; and (2) a diminution of formed elements of the blood caused by the myelophthisic replacement of the normal cell elements with the leukemic cell. The various syndromes associated with anemia, such as granulocytopenia, manifested by lessened resistance to infection, and thrombocytopenia, manifested by a hemorrhagic tendency, are all characteristic of the second group. General symptoms may include tachycardia, increased sweating, loss of weight, "nervousness," and easy fatigability.

Cutaneous lesions

The majority of specific cutaneous lesions occur more frequently in chronic lymphocytic leukemia than in other types of leukemia. However, there is a much higher incidence of cutaneous involvement in monocytic leukemia, although the total number of cases is much lower.

A diagnosis of primary leukemia cutis is made only when there are no changes in the peripheral blood, lymph nodes, or internal organs and the only symptoms are in the skin. A diagnosis is possible only by histologic examination of the cutaneous lesions and this diagnosis is later verified by the clinical course of the disease. The conception of infiltrating cutaneous tumors resulting from lymphocytic and granulocytic migrations is no longer considered to be correct, whereas the theory of autochthonous development has been accepted and is supported by Ribbert's theory on the ubiquitous presence of the lymphatic tissue. The foci of lymphocytic cells usually occur in minute numbers and begin to proliferate as the result of the leukemic toxin.

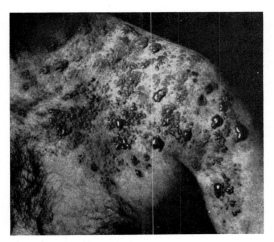

Figure 53–25 Severe herpes zoster in leukemia. (*From* Bluefarb: Cutaneous manifestations of the leukemia-lymphoma group. Postgrad. Med., 41:476, 1967.)

Leukemic infiltrations develop locally from the undifferentiated mesenchyma which is distributed widely throughout the body, particularly around the smaller blood vessels. This undifferentiated mesenchyma can normally develop to free histiocytes and probably to lymphocytes and plasmacytes when irritated. However, in leukemia a fundamental change occurs in the reactivity of the mesenchyma in that a slight, physiologic stimulation will induce an abundant proliferation of perivascular cells, which may differentiate into lymphocytic and granulocytic tissue. Therefore, the leukemic tissue develops locally and not by metastasis from a primary focus.

Specific Cutaneous Lesions. The various specific cutaneous lesions which may be associated with chronic lymphocytic leukemia are (1) nodules, (2) infiltrations or plaques, (3) ulcerative lesions, and (4) exfoliative erythroderma. The characteristic papules or nodules are blue or red in color. The infiltrations may result in thickening or wrinkling of the skin, and when the face, especially the cheeks and forehead, are involved, the large folds and grooves produce an appearance described as "resembling the convolutions of the brain." Not infrequently, deep cutaneous ulcerations resembling a gumma occur.

NODULES. As a rule, the cutaneous nodules are well defined, slightly elevated, smooth, and semiglobular, and they vary markedly in size. They may be 1 mm. in size or as large as 10 cm., and the large tumors frequently become lobulated from coalescence of the smaller nodules. Ringed, festooned lesions, resulting from central involution, spreading of a single patch, or juxtaposition of individual smaller patches, are an unusual occurrence in lymphocytic leukemia, although they frequently occur in mycosis fungoides. The cutaneous tumors are usually persistent, but occasionally they following roentgenotherapy. If a concurrent hemorrhagic diathesis occurs, the nodules may be hemorrhagic and simulate a melanoma. When the nodules are localized, only in the deep portion of the cutis or in the subcutaneous tissue, the surface of the lesions may appear normal or have only a slight bluish tinge. The typical nodules are yellowish brown or yellowish red to reddish blue or purple in

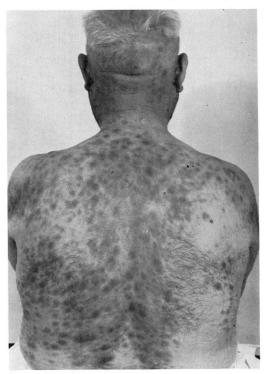

Figure 53–26 Specific nodules of lymphocytic leukemia. (*From* Bluefarb: Cutaneous manifestations of the leukemia-lymphoma group. Postgrad. Med., 41:476, 1967.)

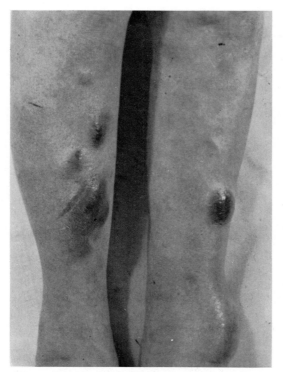

Figure 53–27 Specific nodules of lymphocytic leukemia. (*From* Bluefarb: Leukemia Cutis. Springfield, Ill., Charles C Thomas, Publisher, 1960.)

color and often appear translucent on pressure. These nodules may develop slowly and rarely become ulcerated. In cases having ulceration, it is found to be due to trauma or sepsis or both. The nodules are usually soft or firm, elastic, and edematous; they invariably remain localized to the skin or the subcutaneous tissues, and the deeper structures are not involved. The cutaneous nodules may grow rapidly in size for a time and then remain stationary for years, or they may regress following therapy without scar formation. These nodules usually do not ulcerate and rarely become necrotic. The surrounding skin is usually atrophic, glossy, and transversed by telangiectases. Cutaneous atrophy also occurs in areas not involved by tumors, thereby simulating acrodermatitis chronica atrophicans, while in other instances it may resemble scleroderma or dermatomyositis. The subjective symptoms usually consist of a "burning" sensation and slight pain or discomfort on pressure. Pruritus is not a prominent feature.

The appearance of cutaneous nodules is usually considered to be a grave prognostic sign, although many patients have had such nodules one to several years before death.

INFILTRATIONS AND PLAQUES. Infiltrated or plaquelike lesions are not a frequent specific cutaneous manifestation of lymphocytic leukemia. As in the nodular form, the face appears to be the site of predilection for these lesions.

ULCERATED LESIONS. The cutaneous nodules which are associated with leukemia seldom become ulcerated. The ulceration is usually the result of infection or trauma. The majority of reports of ulcerated lesions appear to indicate that the extremities are the sites of predilection.

Another uncommon manifestation is cutaneous ulceration of the genitalia with a clinical picture simulating that of primary syphilis or other venereal diseases. Three patients having this involvement were reported by Bluefarb and Webster (1953).

ERYTHRODERMA. When generalized

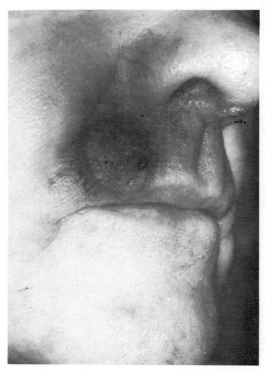

Figure 53–28 Infiltrated plaques of lymphocytic leukemia. (*From* Bluefarb: Leukemia Cutis. Springfield, Ill., Charles C Thomas, Publisher, 1960.)

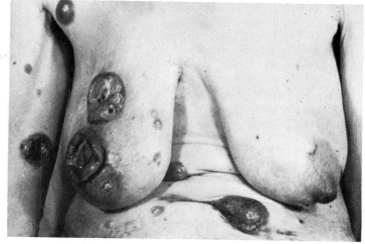

Figure 53–29 Ulcerated tumors of lymphocytic leukemia. (*From* Bluefarb and Schwartz: Scientific exhibits; cutaneous manifestations of leukemia-lymphoma group. A.M.A. Arch. Dermatol., 73:189, 1956.)

erythroderma is present, the skin is dry, scaling, reddened, thickened, and pruritic.

Granulocytic Leukemia

Leukocyte counts in chronic granulocytic leukemia are among the highest of any disease and usually exceed 100,000 per mm.³ in untreated patients. Liver and spleen are diffusely infiltrated; the spleen may be massively enlarged and weigh several thousand grams. Lymph nodes are inconspicuous and, if involved, are diffusely infiltrated; the architecture, in-

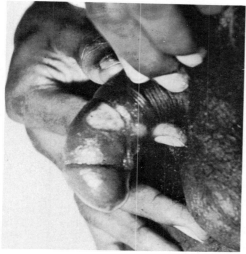

Figure 53–30 Ulcerated lesions of penis on lymphocytic leukemia. (*From* Bluefarb: Leukemia Cutis. Springfield, Ill., Charles C Thomas, Publisher, 1960.)

cluding the follicles, is characteristically preserved.

The only consistent chromosomal anomaly that has been demonstrated in a hematopoietic neoplasm is the Philadelphia chromosome (Ph¹) that has been observed in the blood cells of 90 percent of patients with chronic granulocytic leukemia. This anomalous formation of a single chromosome is observed only in the cells of blood and bone marrow, not other cells, and is acquired rather than inherited. There is evidence that patients with chronic granulocytic leukemia who do not have the pH¹ chromosome have a poorer prognosis than those in whom it is present. Young children did not have the Ph¹ chromosome in one series.

Survival of patients with chronic granulocytic leukemia is ordinarily less than two or three years following diagnosis. As in acute forms of leukemia, death occurs as a result of hemorrhage or infection incident to the replacement of the bone marrow elements.

Cutaneous lesions

Specific cutaneous lesions may occur in the course of granulocytic leukemia or its "aleukemic" form. The typical nodular lesions associated with granulocytic leukemia result from infiltration of granulocytic cells into the cutis, subcutis, and cutaneous appendages. These nodules are described as varying from "pinhead" to "cherry" size, and their color ranges from that of normal skin to deep purple. The cutaneous nodules associated with lymphocytic leukemia have a predilection for the face, while the nodules occurring with granulocytic leukemia primarily involve the trunk. The face, scalp, and extremities are rarely affected, and local symptoms usually do not occur. Cutaneous lesions do not occur as frequently in granulocytic leukemia as in lymphocytic leukemia. The cutaneous lesions do not usually ulcerate, but there is a tendency toward ulceration when the mucous membranes are involved.

Monocytic Leukemia

CUTANEOUS LESIONS

The cutaneous manifestations of monocytic leukemia usually consist of nonspecific lesions, such as ulcerative gingivitis, petechiae, and subcutaneous hemorrhages. The two types of specific cutaneous lesions which are commonly present

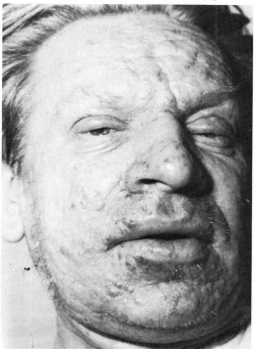

Figure 53-31 Nodules associated with monocytic leukemia giving leonine appearance. (*From* Bluefarb: Cutaneous lymphomas and leukemia cutis. *In* Pack and Ariel (Eds.): Treatment of Cancer and Allied Diseases, Vol. 9. Lymphomas and Related Diseases. 2nd ed. New York, Hoeber-Harper, 1964, p. 204.)

are (1) red or brown macules or papules which usually later become blue in color, and (2) pale, shotty papules which lie deeper in the skin and may develop into larger nodules. The nodules may either disappear or break down to form ulcers; bullae sometimes occur. One or more cutaneous lesions are usually present during some stage of monocytic leukemia and more often in monocytic leukemia than in other types of leukemia. The cutaneous lesions resemble those present in secondary syphilis.

Macules and Papules. These cutaneous lesions, which are usually generalized, have an asymmetric distribution. The typical roseolar maculopapular eruption, resembling early secondary syphilis, changes from day to day and may be of a cyclic nature. These are often minute red dots and fine bluish lines in these lesions. Following subsidence of the erythema, a slightly indurated, slate-blue area may remain. When involution occurs, the eruption often leaves faint gray areas which result in a mottled appearance. The lesions are sometimes tender to pressure, but pain and pruritus are rarely present.

Nodules and Plaques. These "shot-like," pale cutaneous lesions are usually more readily palpable than visible and are situated deeper in the cutis than the macules or papules. Occasionally, the center of the lesion softens and sloughs, leaving an irregular crateriform ulcer having an indurated base and raised, infiltrated edges. Usually some degree of secondary infiltration occurs. All stages of transition between macules and papules and nodules and plaques may occur.

Nonspecific Cutaneous Lesions Associated With the Leukemias

When nonspecific cutaneous lesions are associated with leukemia, they may precede the internal organ involvement or the specific cutaneous lesions by a period of weeks or years. However, they occasionally do not appear until late in the course of the disease. The character or duration of these lesions is not constant in any one type of leukemia or in any one individual. They may be protean and evanes-

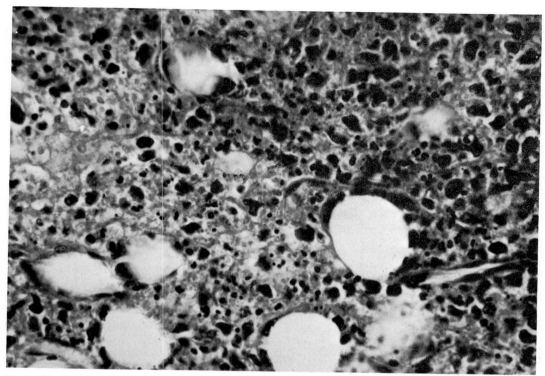

Figure 53–32 Atypical monocytes associated with monocytic leukemia. (*From* Abele and Griffin: Histiocytic medullary reticulosis. Arch. Dermatol., 106:319, 1972.)

cent and may disappear and recur spontaneously, without any obvious relation to the underlying disease process. Specific cutaneous lesions may sometimes develop from these nonspecific lesions. The head of the body appears to be more frequently involved with nonspecific lesions than it is with specific cutaneous lesions.

The most frequent nonspecific cutaneous lesions associated with lymphocytic leukemia are the prurigo-like papules, bullae, purpura, herpes zoster, and exfoliative dermatitis, while urticaria, pigmentation, herpes simplex, eczematoid lesions, pyoderma, and trophic changes occur less frequently. Priapism is sometimes present.

Nonspecific cutaneous lesions do not occur as frequently in granulocytic leukemia as in lymphocytic leukemia. There have been occasional reports of prurigo-like papules or hemorrhagic lesions such as purpura, while herpes zoster and urticaria are rarely described.

Nonspecific cutaneous lesions associated with monocytic leukemia usually involve the oral mucosa and consist of soreness, bleeding from the gingivae, and swelling and necrosis of the mucous membranes which may extend to the tonsil or soft palate. There may be purpuric lesions and widespread *Staphylococcus* infections, including furuncles, carbuncles, and abscesses, as well as exfoliative dermatitis.

Cutaneous manifestations appear to be more frequent in lymphocytic than in other forms of leukemia, although the highest incidence of cutaneous involvement occurs in monocytic leukemia.

Prurigo-like Papules. The term "prurigo-like papules" would seem to be preferable to "prurigo lymphatica," since morphologically this same type of lesion occurs in Hodgkin's disease, lymphosarcoma, tuberculosis, dermatitis herpetiformis, and occasionally malaria. In some cases it is impossible to determine the cause of this nonspecific cutaneous lesion without peripheral blood studies, sternal bone marrow examinations, histologic examination of a lymph node, and a roentgenogram of the chest.

Purpura. Hemorrhage is a frequent

clinical manifestation of all types of leukemia. These hemorrhages may occur in the skin and mucous membranes or in any organ of the body and may appear as isolated or multiple, diffusely distributed, purpuric lesions. The hemorrhages may develop spontaneously or may result from trauma and may sometimes occur in association with a blood platelet deficiency. However, the number of blood platelets may be normal or increased. In some cases a tissue factor which causes fragility of the blood vessels may be present, and in others an added factor, not manifest in the peripheral blood, causes direct damage to the smaller blood vessels or even rupture of these vessels. There may also be a combination of all three of these factors. Leukemic infiltrations are not of primary importance in the production of bleeding. Abnormal bleeding usually occurs as petechiae, particularly in acute leukemia. Purpura in the form of petechiae and ecchymoses are more frequent, more extensive, and of longer duration in chronic lymphocytic leukemia than in chronic granulocytic leukemia.

The hemorrhagic diathesis is particularly distressing in acute leukemia and in the acute exacerbations of chronic leukemia. It has been suggested that an important factor in bleeding associated with leukemia is damage to the integrity of the blood vessel walls.

Purpura, in the form of petechiae and ecchymoses, is the most frequent cutaneous manifestation of chronic granulocytic leukemia, despite the fact that thrombocytopenia rarely occurs in this type of leukemia.

Herpes Zoster. The occurrence of herpes zoster appears to be frequently associated with lymphocytic leukemia and appears to represent a definite relationship rather than a mere coincidence (see Fig. 53–25).

From a study of the reported cases, herpes zoster appears to be frequently associated with lymphocytic leukemia, rarely with granulocytic leukemia, and has been reported only once in association with monocytic leukemia.

Exfoliative Erythroderma. Exfoliative dermatitis is defined as a universal or extremely extensive exfoliation of the skin associated with inflammatory redness, which varies from bright red to dull red, to a dusky violaceous hue, or even to a yellowish tint. There may be associated pruritus, secondary pyoderma with exudation, or fissuring accompanied by systemic manifestations of dehydration, toxemia, or hypoproteinemia. The patient becomes extremely sensitive to external temperature changes, especially cold, and to pressure and friction. The skin becomes dry and loses its normal elasticity. There may be loss of nails and hair, and when the disturbance is unusually severe, atrophy of the skin may occur.

The subjective symptoms of exfoliative dermatitis are varied. Frequently there are no subjective symptoms, as in some cases of exfoliative psoriasis or pityriasis rubra pilaris. More frequently, however, pruritus is a prominent symptom in the majority of patients having cutaneous exfoliation from any cause. The most frequent complaint is general "tenderness" of the skin associated with pruritus, and paresthesias may be present. Temperature changes exaggerate the discomfort, and cool or moving air is not tolerated because of the excessive loss of body heat through radiation from dilated superficial blood vessels. There is often a sensation of chilliness due to a rapid loss of heat from the erythematous and inflamed skin.

There may also be various general symptoms, such as diarrhea, fever, headache, malaise, or lassitude, depending on the cause of the condition and the severity of the process. The skin often has a "musty" odor.

The skin has a dull red hue, is frequently lichenified, and presents varying degrees of scaling. The type of scaling is usually not characteristic but is sometimes suggestive, as in the case of pemphigus foliaceus. The skin is usually dry but may become moist, especially in the body folds and on the sides of the trunk. Eventually the skin becomes markedly infiltrated and the normal markings exaggerated.

The cutaneous appendages are involved early in the disease. There may be temporary loss of hair, and the nails frequently become opaque, lusterless, brittle, furrowed, and soft, lose their attachments, and are gradually shed. Infiltrations of the skin around the eyes may result in ectropion. The palms and soles may remain normal but are frequently thickened, fissured, and painful. There is usually generalized lymphadenopathy, and the mucous membranes may show an inflammatory reaction.

Erythema Multiforme (Including Bullous Lesions). There are few reports of bullous lesions associated with leukemia. In the majority of cases, pruritus is usually present.

Polymorphous bullous lesions precipitated by high voltage roentgenotherapy are believed to occur in predisposed persons as a result of absorption of products of cellular degeneration, probably proteins present in both the irradiated lesions and healthy tissue.

Pyoderma. The increased tendency toward the development of infection in all types of leukemia is well recognized, since normal resistance to infections is very low when there is an absence of normal defense cells. The most frequent sites of involvement for infection appear to be around the teeth and gums and in the tonsils and rectum. Infection occurs most often in acute leukemia, since leukopenia is frequent and the number of polymorphonuclear leukocytes in the peripheral blood and tissues is reduced. However, such infections may also occur in chronic leukemia when fever is usually present.

Pigmentation. Pigmentation is not frequently associated with chronic leukemia. The cutaneous pigmentation is grayish brown in color, resembling that of Banti's disease, in chronic granulocytic leukemia, but a hemorrhagic diathesis may occur in acute granulocytic leukemia.

Trophic Cutaneous Changes. Trophic changes associated with leukemia usually occur with exfoliative dermatitis. Patients who had trophic changes of the nails, skin, and hair are described under Exfoliative Dermatitis.

HISTIOCYTIC MEDULLARY RETICULOSIS

The terms "histocytosis" and "reticuloendotheliosis" have been used for clinical and pathologic features of the systemic proliferative diseases in which histiocytes in varying maturation predominate. Three groups of histiocytoses can be distinguished (Rappaport, 1966):

1. The reactive histiocytic proliferations that occur in response to known infectious agents or as the result of metabolic disturbances.

2. The systemic proliferations of differential histiocytes that are characteristic of Letterer-Siwe disease and Hand-Schüller-Christian disease, although these differentiated histiocytes lack the cytologic abnormalities of neoplastic cellular proliferations; they are invasive, progressive, and of unknown etiology.

3. The systemic proliferations of neoplastic, morphologically malignant histiocytes.

Histiocytic medullary reticulosis would be classified in the third group as a malignant histiocytosis. The entity seems not to have gained general acceptance, for it is not yet included in most standard textbooks of medicine and pathology. It appears likely that similar cases have been and are being classified as atypical Hodgkin's disease, reticulum cell sarcoma, or reticulohistiocytosis.

Scott and Robb-Smith (1939) presented four patients of their own and six from the literature who they felt presented a unique disorder of the reticuloendothelial system with a "clear-cut clinical and pathological picture." The typical clinical course was characterized by "fever, wasting and generalized lymphadenopathy associated with splenic and hepatic enlargement; in the final stages jaundice and purpura with profound leukopenia may occur." Postmortem examination revealed a "systematized hyperplasia of histiocytes actively engaged in phagocytosis of erythrocytes." They proposed the term "histiocytic medullary reticulosis" for this syndrome.

Histiocytic medullary reticulosis is a rapidly fatal disease, characterized by pyrexia, weight loss, hepatosplenomegaly, generalized lymphadenopathy, anemia, and frequently leukopenia, thrombocytopenia, and jaundice. Postmortem examination of all these patients demonstrated a systematized proliferation of histiocytes with active erythrophagocytosis.

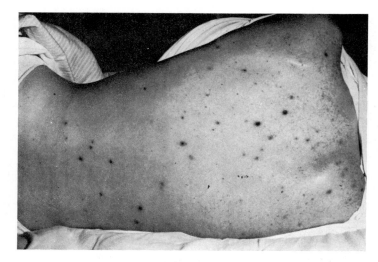

Figure 53–33 Specific nodules of histiocytic medullary reticulosis. (*From* Abele and Griffin: Histiocytic medullary reticulosis. Arch. Dermatol., 106:319, 1972.)

In spite of the uniform clinical and histologic picture, the diagnosis has not usually been made until the postmortem examination. All previous diagnoses ante mortem have been made by finding numerous phagocytic histiocytes in the bone marrow. Skin lesions other than purpura or jaundice have been uncommon. Specific purplish nodules have been reported by Anderson (1944), Israels (1953), Civin et al. (1954), Friedman and Steigbegel (1965), and DeVilliers (1969). Abele and Griffin (1970) reported two cases in which the cutaneous lesions were the initial presenting complaint, and both cases were diagnosed ante mortem by cutaneous biopsy.

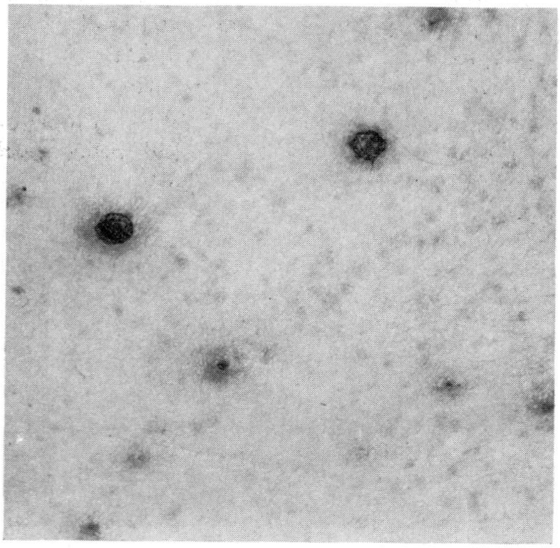

The differential diagnosis mainly must exclude atypical Hodgkin's disease, "adult" Letterer-Siwe disease, and reticulum cell lymphosarcoma. Giant cells seen in histiocytic medullary reticulosis are identical with those seen in Hodgkin's disease. This explains why cases of histiocytic medullary reticulosis have been misdiagnosed as "atypical" Hodgkin's disease. However, eosinophilis, plasma cells, and fibrosis are invariably absent in histiocytic medullary reticulosis. In addition, patients with Hodgkin's disease usually exhibit a more protracted course and ordinarily respond, at least temporarily, to treatment.

The histologic picture of histiocytic medullary reticulosis is characterized by multifocal proliferations of histiocytes and their precursors, predominantly in the skin, spleen, liver, lymph nodes, and bone marrow. In some cases cytologic abnormalities of the histiocytes may be so slight that the disease cannot be distinguished from benign reactive histiocytosis. In other cases the histologic features may be difficult to distinguish from those of malignant lymphoma of the histiocytic or reticulum cell type. The neoplastic histiocytes show nuclear variations, mitoses, and large nucleoli which suggest the malignant nature of the proliferation. They may contain phagocytized material, including pyknotic nuclei, hemosiderin, and

Figure 53–34 Specific nodules of histiocytic medullary reticulosis. (*From* Abele and Griffin: Histiocytic medullary reticulosis. Arch. Dermatol., 106:319, 1972.)

lor is the outstanding clinical sign of this anemia. Glossitis and koilonychia may be associated with iron deficiency anemia. One patient in Snapper's series (1953) had koilonychia.

In the presence of leukopenia, numerous cases will show pyoderma. When the bone marrow is replaced with plasma cells, a granulocytopenia results; an agranulocytopenic membrane may be present in the gums. This occurred in two of our cases.

About one-third of these patients show an increased tendency to bleeding, particularly from the nose (epistaxis) and gums. The clotting factor is usually not defective, but many patients evidence thrombocytopenia.

Purpura and petechiae of the skin may also occur. The purpura usually results from infiltration of the blood vessel walls with amyloid, resulting in damage to the vessel walls, but this is not a complete explanation of the purpura since amyloid is not always demonstrable in the blood vessel walls. Snapper et al. (1953) called attention to the fact that these patients with a hemorrhagic tendency demonstrate a higher incidence of elevated serum globulins than the average patient with no bleeding tendency.

Three possible causes of purpura occurring in myeloma are advanced by Esser (1950): (1) damage to the bone marrow with secondary thrombocytopenia, (2) liver damage with secondary derangement of the clotting mechanism, and (3) vascular amyloidosis in the skin. The reticuloendothelial system, particularly the liver, is more frequently involved as an extramedullary lesion. Logically this would lead to the speculation by Limarzi (1951) that hypothrombinemia may contribute to the cause of bleeding in myeloma. Another mechanism frequently mentioned is the uremia resulting from extensive renal impairment in myeloma. The mechanism of bleeding here is due to toxic damage to the endothelium of the smaller vessels in addition to further toxic depression of thrombocytopoiesis.

TOXIC CUTANEOUS LESIONS

Many toxic cutaneous lesions, such as alopecia, are usually associated with amy-loidosis. This subject is well covered by Goltz (1952). However, so-called "toxic" cutaneous lesions not associated with amyloidosis may be present.

Spiethoff (1911) described a 58 year old man who had redness and pruritus of the face and hands and an indurated, localized erythroderma. A 39 year old man reported by Heidenström and Tottie (1943) had polyarthritis and an exanthem of follicular craters on the extremities and buttocks. A diagnosis of multiple myelomatosis was suggested by the finding of cryoglobulinemia in the patient described by Blades (1931). This patient also had xeroderma. Three patients in our series presented associated icthyosiform atrophy of the skin.

Seborrheic Dermatitis. The incidence of seborrheic dermatitis of the face appeared to be more than average in our series of cases. The dermatitis was of the oily, greasy type and predominated in the nasolabial folds. This characteristic seborrhea frequently led our hematologists to suspect the presence of multiple myeloma.

Plasma Cell Leukemia

The general concept is that plasma cell leukemia is merely a variant of multiple myeloma in which large numbers of plasma cells reach the peripheral blood stream.

Patek and Castle (1934) described a 60 year old woman having plasma cell leukemia. She presented various sized ecchymotic areas of the skin of the left hand and wrist, thighs, left groin, and both pectoral regions. The paient reported by Ghon and Roman (1913) was a 49 year old man with plasma cell leukemia who had bleeding from the gums and petechiae of the neck and upper chest.

Treatment

Lee et al. (1971) stated:

... patients who respond to melphalan and cyclophosphamide currently appear to be living longer than non-responders. Other alkylating agents may be just as effective, but to date these two drugs are the agents of choice in the therapy of myeloma, and a good drug response suggests a better than average prognosis. Cross-resistance does appear to exist. No patient who has had a well-documented melphalan failure has been reported to respond to cyclophosphamide, or vice versa.

PSEUDOLYMPHOMATOUS REACTIONS OF THE SKIN

Studies of cutaneous lymphoreticular infiltrates have revealed a large group of lesions which may mimic malignant lymphomas histopathologically but which are clinically benign (Caro and Helwig, 1969). These lesions comprise a heterogeneous group, ranging from reactions to insect bites to tumors arising apparently de novo. The histopathologic picture varies widely and includes some lesions with masses of lymphocytes or reticulum cells, suggesting one of the monomorphous lymphomas, and other lesions with a multiplicity of cell types, suggesting Hodgkin's disease or an atypical granulomatous process. Most investigators believe that these benign lymphoreticular lesions represent hyperplasias of preexisting cutaneous lymphoid tissue and are not true neoplasms (Hirsch and Lukes, 1965; Mach and Wilgram, 1966a and 1966b).

In this discussion we shall consider lymphocytoma cutis (lymphadenosis benigna cutis), arthropod bite granuloma, lymphomatoid papulosis, actinic reticuloid, and pseudolymphomatous reactions to anticonvulsant drugs.

Lymphocytoma Cutis

This term (Kaufmann-Wolf, 1921) is widely employed by dermatologists in this country to describe benign nodular and plaque lesions which have heavy lymphocytic dermal infiltrates. A diagnosis of lymphocytoma is ambiguous to the pathologist, however, as this term also has been employed for the lesions of malignant lymphoma. Lymphadenosis benigna cutis (Bäfverstedt, 1943, 1960), cutaneous lymphoplasia (Mach, 1965; Mach and Wilgram, 1966a and 1966b), and cutaneous

lymphoid hyperplasia (Caro and Helwig, 1969) are terms more descriptive of this benign hyperplastic process.

The terms Spiegler-Fendt sarcoid (Lewis, 1935) and pseudolymphoma of Spiegler-Fendt (Lever, 1967) have been employed for this lesion, but these designations are ambiguous and are best avoided. Of Spiegler's original six cases (Spiegler, 1894), one had evidence of malignant lymphoma with gastrointestinal involvement, and Spiegler viewed the condition with a guarded prognosis because of the likelihood of systemic involvement. Fendt's single case (Fendt, 1900), a 16 year old boy, had cutaneous lesions which pursued a benign course and which would fall into today's classification of lymphocytoma cutis.

Bäfverstedt's extensive studies (1943, 1960) have helped to delineate the nature and spectrum of this condition. His designation of lymphadenosis benigna cutis has not found favor in this country, although it is widely employed in Europe. Lymphocytoma cutis occurs in all age groups from childhood through senescence and is two to three times more frequent in women than in men (Bluefarb, 1960b). Although the etiology is unknown, insect bites, trauma, sun, and wind (Bluefarb, 1960b) and malignant tumors (Bäfverstedt, 1953) have been cited as inciting stimuli.

Two clinical forms have been recognized, a localized form and disseminated form (Bäfverstedt, 1943, 1960). Patients with the localized form develop one or more lesions in an area such as the face, ear lobes, and nose, and exposed areas are favored. Grouped lesions also occur on the nipple, scrotum, and elsewhere. Localized lesions may develop in any age group, and the process tends to be chronic, although some lesions regress spontaneously.

The disseminated form is much less common and occurs in adults. These patients develop multiple lesions over the body without any localization in any particular area. This form has great chronicity, and new lesions may continue to develop over the course of many years.

Individual lesions of lymphocytoma cutis are usually firm and dome-shaped with a dusky erythematous to bluish or

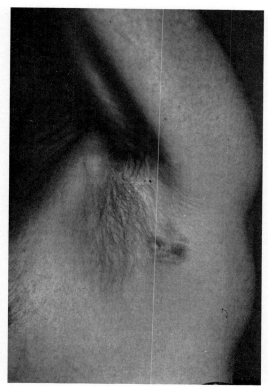

Figure 53–36 Nodular lesions of lymphocytoma cutis. (See also Color Plate VIII-F.)

brownish hue. The surface is often smooth with a waxy appearance, although some lesions have an irregular surface. The size ranges from small superficial papules to large plaques and nodules, and the larger lesions may be subcutaneous in location.

Although the clinical findings in lymphocytoma cutis are limited to the skin, there is evidence that other lymphoid tissue participates. A significant number of patients have had lymphadenopathy and peripheral lymphocytosis (Caro and Helwig, 1969), and bone marrow examinations in other patients have revealed a small increase in mature lymphocytes and reticulum cells (Mach and Wilgram, 1966a).

The clinical appearance is at best suggestive of the diagnosis, and microscopic examination is necessary for accurate diagnosis. Lymphocytoma cutis must be differentiated clinically from malignant lymphoma, sarcoidosis, granuloma faciale, dermatofibroma, urticaria pigmentosa,

polymorphous light eruption, lymphocytic infiltration of Jessner-Kanoff, facial angiofibromas, and trichoepitheliomas.

The histopathologic picture of lymphocytoma cutis varies from lesion to lesion, but all lesions show a benign proliferation of lymphoreticular tissue (Mach and Wilgram, 1966a; Caro and Helwig, 1969). The epidermis appears normal but may be thinned by a heavy underlying cellular infiltrate. Occasionally one encounters acanthosis. Frequently the epidermis is separated from the dermal infiltrate by a band of uninvolved collagen, a grenz zone similar to that seen in malignant lymphomas.

Within the dermis one sees a dense infiltrate of well differentiated lymphocytes and histiocytes. The proportion of these cells varies in different lesions. The infiltrate is patchy in nature, and many lesions may show well developed lymphoid follicles with germinal centers. In these structures the histiocytes lie centrally, whereas in areas without lymphoid follicles there is a diffuse admixture of lymphocytes and histiocytes. Occasional lesions have eosinophils or plasma cells in the infiltrate. All lymphocytomas have an infiltrate of at least two cell types, and this polymorphous nature helps to distinguish these lesions from malignant lymphomas (Caro and Helwig, 1969).

These lesions also show stromal alterations, including fibrosis, fibrocellular proliferation, and compression of the stroma by the infiltrate. Many lesions also show vascular changes, such as endothelial swelling and proliferation (Caro and Helwig, 1969).

The important histopathologic differential diagnosis is cutaneous malignant lymphoma. Features favoring a benign diagnosis include a polymorphous infiltrate of well differentiated cells, lymphoid follicles, and stromal and vascular changes.

Lymphocytoma cutis is a highly radiosensitive lesion which regresses rapidly using low dosages of fractionated superficial x-ray. Penicillin injection has been reported to be of benefit in the past (Bäfverstedt, 1960; Mach and Wilgram, 1966b). This mode of treatment is not unequivocally successful, and improvement

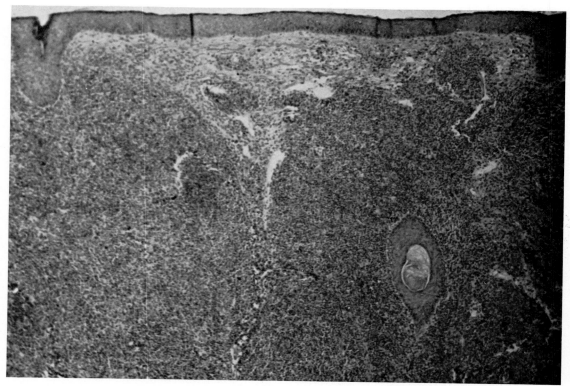

Figure 53–37   Dense infiltrate of lymphocytes and histiocytes. (*From* Caro and Helwig: Cutaneous lymphoid hyperplasia. Cancer, 24:487, 1969.)

with penicillin administration must be weighed against the natural history of the disease in which spontaneous regression does occur.

More recently satisfactory results have been achieved using intralesional injections of corticosteroid suspensions, such as triamcinolone acetonide (Self et al., 1969).

The prognosis for both localized and disseminated forms of lymphocytoma cutis is excellent, and the lesions almost always regress with treatment. Although in the disseminate form of the disease new lesions may appear over several decades, the benign nature of the disease is maintained (Bäfverstedt, 1960). In rare cases lymphocytoma cutis has been associated with malignant lymphomas of the skin (Herzberg, 1952; Gertler, 1955; Caro and Helwig, 1969). In these cases lymphocytoma may have arisen as a lymphoid hyperplastic response to the underlying disease, as has been reported with other malignant tumors (Bäfverstedt, 1953),

while in exceptional cases transformation of lymphocytoma to malignant lymphoma has been reported (Herzberg, 1952; Gertler, 1955).

Arthropod Bite Granuloma

The bite of a number of arthropods may produce lesions with a histopathologic appearance closely simulating malignant lymphomas (Allen, 1948), and the underlying mechanism also appears to be a reactive proliferation of cutaneous lymphoreticular tissue with an inflammatory component. These lesions occur in all age groups, may be single, or multiple, and favor exposed areas. Clinically they have no distinguishing features but usually present as erythematous to brownish papules or nodules, often with a central crusted area. Arthropod bites undergo an evolutionary process, and removal early in their course will reveal acute inflammation (Winer and Strakosh, 1941). Chronic

Schulze's case (1971), although the case of Wyse (1969) did respond to chlorambucil. We have not seen an evaluation of systemic antibiotics or corticosteroids in these patients.

Lymphomatoid papulosis has been delineated too recently to allow an authoritative statement on prognosis. Although the process appears to be chronic and benign, one such case diagnosed as Mucha-Habermann's disease ultimately died of malignant lymphoma (Wilson Jones, 1969).

Actinic Reticuloid

Actinic reticuloid is a recently described disorder characterized by a chronic photosensitivity of unknown etiology and a histopathologic picture suggesting malignant lymphoma (Ive et al., 1969). In the original series and in subsequent reports (Jensen and Sneddon, 1970; Mitchell, 1970), all patients have been male and 10 of the 12 have been older than 60 years. The process begins as an erythematous scaling to eczematous eruption on exposure sites such as the head, neck, and dorsa of the hands, with gradual spread to covered areas as well. Continuing spread results in a generalized erythroderma with increasing lichenification. In the fully developed state the clinical appearance suggests a malignant lymphoma such as Sézary syndrome. Patients have no previous history of photosensitivity and often do not recognize the eruption as being photosensitive in nature because of the ultimate spread to covered areas and the lack of seasonal fluctuation.

The photosensitive nature of the disease is clearly recognized with phototesting, which reveals a broad spectrum of reacting wavelengths extending from ultraviolet to 500 to 600 mm. in the visible spectrum. Clinical confirmation of this photosensitivity state may be seen with the marked improvement which occurs when the patient is confined to a darkened room.

Microscopic examination reveals a variable picture. Within the dermis one sees an extensive, dense cellular infiltrate, usually of mononuclear cells. These cells may show considerable atypia, and epidermal invasion with microabscesses re-sembling Pautrier microabscesses also may be seen. Other inflammatory cells, such as lymphocytes, eosinophils, and plasma cells are present in variable numbers. The histopathologic picture may resemble mycosis fungoides, other malignant lymphomas, or an atypical granulomatous response. In differential diagnosis actinic reticuloid may be distinguished from other forms of photosensitivity by the broad spectrum of exciting wavelengths and by the histopathologic picture. The differentiation from true cutaneous malignant lymphomas is more difficult. Lymphomatous erythroderma, Sézary syndrome, and mycosis fungoides ordinarily are not associated with sensitivity, although it may be possible to rule out a malignant lymphoma in individual cases.

Treatment of actinic reticuloid has been difficult, and the process generally has been resistant to topical corticosteroids, sun screens, and antimalarials. Methotrexate and systemic corticosteroids have been given equivocal results. The most favorable response has occurred by confining the patient to a darkened room, and in this circumstance topical and systemic steroids have hastened resolution.

Our knowledge of actinic reticuloid is as yet too young to permit unequivocal statements on prognosis. Affected patients have had a prolonged course, and one reported patient ultimately developed a malignant lymphoma nine years after the onset of actinic reticuloid (Jensen and Sneddon, 1970).

Pseudolymphomatous Reactions to Anticonvulsant Drugs

Patients receiving certain anticonvulsant drugs may develop a reactive hyperplasia of the reticuloendothelial system mimicking the features of a malignant lymphoma (Saltzstein and Ackerman, 1959; Rosenfeld et al., 1961; Schreiber and McGregor, 1968). Diphenylhydantoin (Dilantin) and mephenytoin (Mesantoin) have been the usual offenders, although most hydantoin derivatives have been implicated. Exposure to the drug may range from a week to two years (Schreiber and McGregor, 1968).

Affected patients develop malaise,

fever, generalized lymphadenopathy, hepatosplenomegaly, and often arthralgia. The patient may develop a polymorphous skin eruption with maculopapular and vesicular lesions. Lymph node biopsy closely simulates one of the malignant lymphomas, such as Hodgkin's disease or lymphocytic lymphoma (Saltzstein and Ackerman, 1959; Rosenfeld et al., 1961). Biopsy of affected skin may suggest mycosis fungoides or may be normal (Schreiber and McGregor, 1968). Treatment depends upon recognizing the hydantoin drug responsible and discontinuing the medication. Improvement usually begins rapidly with complete clearing. Re-exposure to the drug may be anticipated to reproduce the syndrome.

REFERENCES

Abele, D. C., and Griffin, T. B.: Paper Read at the Am. Dermatol. Assoc. Meeting, March, 1970.

Allen, A. C.: Persistent "insect bites" (dermal eosinophilic granulomas simulating lymphoblastomas, histiocytoses, and squamous cell carcinomas. Am. J. Pathol., 24:367, 1948.

Allen, A. C.: The Skin. A Clinicopathologic Treatise. Ed. 2. New York, Grune & Stratton, 1967, p. 1131.

Altman, J., and Winkelmann, R. K.: Lymphosarcoma of skin and testes. Arch. Dermatol., 82:943, 1960.

Anderson, R. G.: Histiocytic medullary reticulosis with transient skin lesions. Br. Med. J., 1:220, 1944.

Baccareddo, A.: Reticulohistiocytosis cutanea hyperplastica benigno cum melanodermis. Arch. Dermatol. Syph., 179:209, 1939.

Bäfverstedt, B.: Über Lymphadenosis Benigna Cutis. Ein klinische und pathologisch-anatomitche Studie. Acta Derm. Venereol. (Stockh.), Suppl. 24, 11:1, 1943.

Bäfverstedt, B.: Lymphadenosis benigna cutis as a symptom of malignant tumours. Acta Derm. Venereol. (Stockh.), 33:171, 1953.

Bäfverstedt, B.: Lymphadenosis benigna cutis (LABC): Its nature, course and prognosis. Acta Derm. Venereol. (Stockh.), 40:10, 1960.

Berman, L.: Pathologic nature of mycosis fungoides. Arch. Pathol., 29:530, 1940.

Blades, A. N.: Cryoglobulinemia in multiple myelomatosis. Br. Med. J., 1:169, 1931.

Blaylock, W. K., et al.: Normal immunologic reactivity in patients with the lymphoma mycosis fungoides. Cancer, 19:233, 1966.

Block, J. B., Edgecomb, J., Eisen, A., and Van Scott, E. J.: Mycosis fungoides. Natural history and aspects of its relationship to other malignant lymphomas. Am. J. Med., 34:228, 1963.

Bluefarb, S. M.: Cutaneous manifestations of multiple myeloma. (review). Arch. Dermatol., 72:506, 1955a.

Bluefarb, S. M.: Exfoliative dermatitis. Quart. Bull. Northwestern University Med. School, 29:304, 1955b.

Bluefarb, S. M.: Is mycosis fungoides an entity? Arch. Dermatol., 71:293, 1955c.

Bluefarb, S. M.: Cutaneous Manifestations of the Malignant Lymphomas. Springfield, Ill., Charles C Thomas, Publisher, 1959.

Bluefarb, S. M.: Leukemia Cutis (review). Springfield, Ill., Charles C Thomas, Publishers, 1960a.

Bluefarb, S. M.: Lymphocytoma cutis. In Cutaneous Manifestations of the Benign Inflammatory Reticuloses. Springfield, Ill., Charles C Thomas, Publisher, 1960b, pp. 131–199.

Bluefarb, S. M.: The staging of mycosis fungoides. Cutis, 7:393, 1971.

Bluefarb, S. M., and Goldberg, A.: Hodgkin's Disease with Trophic Changes. Chicago Dermatol. Soc. Meetings, January, 1953.

Bluefarb, S. M., and Wbster, J. M.: Leukemia cutis simulating venereal disease. Quart. Bull. Northwestern Univ. Med. School, 27:18, 1953.

Borrie, P. F.: Lymphomatoid papulosis. Proc. R. Soc. Med., 62:159, 1969.

Brownlee, T. R., and Murad, T. M.: Ultrastructure of mycosis fungoides. Cancer, 26:686, 1970.

Brunsting, L. A., and MacDonald, I. D.: Primary systematized amyloidosis with macroglossia: A syndrome related to Bence-Jones proteinuria and myeloma. J. Invest. Dermatol., 8:145, 1947.

Caro, W. A.: Benign lymphoid hyperplasia and malignant lymphoma of the skin. In Helwig, E. B., and Mostoli, F. K., (Eds.): The Skin. International Academy of Pathology Monograph. Baltimore, The Williams & Wilkins Company, 1971, pp. 558–577.

Caro, W. A., and Helwig, E. B.: Cutaneous lymphoid hyperplasia. Cancer, 24:487, 1969.

Cawley, E. P., Curtis, A. C., and Leach, J. E. K.: Is mycosis fungoides a reticuloendothelial neoplastic entity? Arch. Dermatol. Syph., 64:225, 1951.

Christian, H. A.: Multiple myeloma: A histological comparison of six cases. J. Exp. Med., 9:325, 1907.

Civin, H., Gotschalk, H. C., and Okazaki, K.: Histiocytic medullary reticulosis: Report of two cases. Arch. Intern. Med., 94:375, 1954.

Clendenning, W. E., and Van Scott, E. J.: Skin autografts and homografts in patients with the lymphoma mycosis fungoides. Cancer Res., 25:1844, 1965.

Clendenning, W. E., Brecher, G., and Van Scott, E. J.: Mycosis fungoides. Relationship to malignant cutaneous reticulosis and Sézary syndrome. Arch. Dermatol., 89:785, 1964.

Custer, R. P., and Bernhard, W. G.: Interrelationship of Hodgkin's disease and other lymphatic tumors. Am. J. Med. Sci., 216:625, 1948.

Cyr, D. P., Geokos, M. C., and Worsley, G. H.: Mycosis fungoides. Hematologic findings and terminal causes. Arch. Dermatol., 94:558, 1966.

DeVilliers, D. M.: Histiocytic medullary reticulosis. S. Afr. Med. J., 43:756, 1969.

Director, W., and Kern, A. B.: Reticulum cell sarcoma. Arch. Dermatol. and Syph., 62:69, 1963.

Dupont, A.: Langsam verlaufende und klinisch gutarige Retikulopathie mit höchst Maligner histologische Struktur. Hautarzt, 16:284, 1965.

Duvoir, M., Pollet, L., Dechaune, M., and Gaultier, M.: Myelomes multiples avec tumeurs cutanées. Bull. Mem. Soc. Hôp. Paris, 54:687, 1938.

Epstein, E., and MacEachern, K.: Dermatologic manifestations of the lymphoblastoma-leukemia group. Arch. Intern. Med., 60:867, 1937.

Esser, H.: Über seltene Befunde beim Plasmocytom (Beitag zur Purpura hyperglobulinaemia). Z. Klin. Med., 146:535, 1950.

Fendt, H.: Beiträage zur Kenntnis·der sogenannten sarcoiden Geschwülste der Haut. Arch. Dermatol. Syph. (Berl.), 53:213, 1900.

Feuerman, E. J., and Sandbeck, M.: Lymphomatoid papulosis. An additional case of a new disease. Arch. Dermatol., 105:233, 1972.

Fine, R. M., and Meltzer, H. D.: Lymphomatoid papulosis. J. Med. Assoc. Georgia, 58:453, 1969.

Flaxman, B. A., Zelazny, G., and Van Scott, E. J.: Nonspecificity of characteristic cells in mycosis fungoides. Arch. Dermatol., 104:141, 1971.

Fleischmajer, R., and Eisenberg, S.: Sézary reticulosis. Arch. Dermatol., 80:9, 1964.

Friedman, R. M., and Steigbegel, N. H.: Histiocytic medullary reticulosis. Am. J. Med., 38:130, 1965.

Gall, E. A.: Enigmas in lymphoma. Reticulum cell sarcoma and mycosis fungoides. Minn. Med., 38:674, 1955.

Gall, E. A., The cytological identity and interrelationship of mesenchymal cells in connective tissue. Ann. N.Y. Acad. Sci., 73:120, 1958.

Gall, E. A., and Mallory, T. B.: Malignant lymphoma. A clinico-pathologic survey of 618 cases. Am. J. Pathol., 18:381, 1942.

Gall, E. A., Morrison, H. R., and Scott, A. T.: The follicular types of malignant lymphoma: A survey of 63 Cases. Ann. Intern. Med., 14:2073, 1941.

Gates, D.: Cutaneous tumors in leukemia and lymphoma. Arch. Dermatol. Syph., 37:1015, 1938.

Gertler, W.: Retikulosarkomatöse Umwandlung tumorartiger Lymphocytome. Dermatol. Wochenschr., 132:1035, 1955.

Ghon, A., and Roman, B.: Über pseudoleukämische und leukämische Plasmazellen-hyperplasie. Folia haematol., 15:72, 1913.

Goldman, L., Rockwell, E. M., and Richfield, D. F.: Histopathological studies on cutaneous reactions to the bites of various arthropods. Am. J. Trop. Med., 1:514, 1952.

Goltz, R. W.: Systematized amyloidosis. Medicine, 31:381, 1952.

Hedinger, E.: Zur Frange des Plasmocytomes Granulationsplasmocytom in Kombination mit einem krebsig umgewandelten Schweissdrusenadenom des behaarten Kopfes. Z. Pathol., 7:343, 1911.

Heidenström, N., and Tottie, M.: Haut- und Gelenkveränderungen bei multiplen Myelom. Acta Derma. Venereol. (Stockh.), 24:192, 1943.

Hellwig, C. A.: Extramedullary plasma cell tumors as observed in various locations. Arch. Pathol., 36:95, 1943.

Herzberg, J.: Retikulosarkomatöse Umwandlung subkutaner Lymphocytome bei acrodermatitis chronica atrophicans. Dermatol. Wochenschr., 125:422, 1952.

Higgins, G. K.: Pathologic anatomy in Hodgkin's disease. *In* Molander, D. W., and Pack, G. T. (Eds.): Hodgkin's Diseases. Springfield, Ill., Charles C Thomas, Publisher, 1968, pp. 20–63.

Hirsch, P., and Lukes, R.: Reactive pseudolymphoma, nodular type. Arch. Dermatol., 91:408, 1965.

Hurst, D. W., and Meyer, O. O.: Giant follicular lymphoblastoma. Cancer, 14:753, 1961.

Israels, M. C. G.: The reticuloses: A clinicopathologic study. Lancet, 265:525, 1953.

Ive, F. A., Magnus, I. A., Warin, R. P., and Wilson Jones, E.: "Actinic reticuloid"; a chronic dermatosis associated with severe photosensitivity and the histological resemblance to lymphoma. Br. J. Dermatol., 81:469, 1969.

Jackson, H., Jr., and Parker, Jr.: Hodgkin's Disease and Allied Disorders. Oxford, Oxford University Press, 1947, pp. 17–34.

Jensen, N. E., and Sneddon, I. B.: Actinic reticuloid with lymphoma. Br. J. Dermatol., 82:287, 1970.

Kadin, M. E., Glatstein, E., and Dorfman, R. F.: Clinicopathologic study of 117 untreated patients subjected to laparotomy for the staging of Hodgkin's disease. Cancer, 27:1277, 1971.

Kaplan, H. S.: On the Natural History, Treatment and Prognosis of Hodgkin's Disease. *In* The Harvey Lectures, 1968–1969. New York, Academic Press, 1970, pp. 215–259.

Kaufman-Wolf, M.: Uber gutarige lymphocytare Neubilgungen der Scrotalhaut des Kindes. Arch. Dermatol. Syph. (Berl.), 130:425, 1921.

Keder, A. R., Kaplan, H. S., Lukes, R. J., and Rappaport, H.: Correlation of histopathology with other prognostic indicators in Hodgkin's disease. Cancer, 22:487, 1968.

Kim, R., Winkelmann, R. K., and Dockerty, M.: Reticulum sarcoma of the skin. Cancer, 16:646, 1963.

Kin, S. S.: Beitag zur Kenntnis der Kahlerschen Krankheit mit Mycosis fungoides, besonders über die Genese der Geschwulstzellen. Arch. Jap. Chir., 16:79, 1939.

Kobro, M.: Further observations of zoster and spinal diseases. Acta Med. Scand., 104:1, 1940.

Lee, B. J., Pinsky, C., and Miller, D. F.: The management of plasma cell neoplasm. Med. Clin. North Am., 55:703, 1971.

Lerner, A. B., and Watson, C. J.: Studies of cryoglobulin. I. Unusual purpura associated with the presence of a high concentration of cryoglobulin (cold precipitable serum globulin). Am. J. Med. Sci., 214:410, 1947.

Lever, W. F.: Histopathology of the Skin. Ed. 4. Philadelphia, J. B. Lippincott Company, 1967.

Lewis, G. M.: Is Spiegler-Fendt sarcoid a clinical or histological entity? Arch. Dermatol. Syph., 31:67, 1935.

Limarzi, L. R.: Diagnostic and therapeutic aspects of multiple myeloma. Med. Clin. North Am., 35:189, 1951.

Lubarsch, O.: Zur Kenntis ungewohnlicher Amyloisablagerungen. Arch. Pathol. Anat., 271:867, 1929.

Lukes, R. J.: Relationship of histologic features to clinical stages in Hodgkin's disease. Am. J. Roentgenol., 90:944–955, 1963.

Lukes, R. J.: The pathologic picture of the malignant lymphomas. *In* Zarafoneti's, C. J. D. (Ed.): Proceedings of the International Conference on Leukemia-Lymphoma. Philadelphia, Lea and Febiger, 1968, pp. 333–354.

Lukes, R. J., Butler, J. J., and Hicks, E. B.: Natural

history of Hodgkin's disease as related to its pathologic picture. Cancer, 19:317, 1966a.

Lukes, R. J., Craver, L. F., Hull, T. C., Rappaport, H., and Ruben, P.: Report of the Nomenclature Committee. Cancer Res., 26:1311, 1966b.

Lutzner, M. A., and Jordan, H. W.: The ultrastructure of an abnormal cell in Sézary syndrome. Blood, 31:719, 1968.

Lutzner, M. A., Hobbs, J. W., and Horvath, P.: Ultrastructure of abnormal cells in Sézary's syndrome, mycosis fungoides and parapsoriasis en plaque. Arch. Dermatol., 103:375, 1971.

Macaulay, W. L.: Lymphomatous papulosis. A continuing self-healing eruption clinically benign—histologically malignant. Arch. Dermatol., 97:23, 1968.

Mach, K. W., and Wilgram, G. F.: Characteristic histopathology of cutaneous lymphoplasia (lymphocytoma). Arch. Dermatol., 94:26, 1966a.

Mach, K. W., and Wilgram, G. F.: Cutaneous lymphoplasia with giant follicles. A report of eight cases. Arch. Dermatol., 94:749, 1966b.

Marshall, A. H. E.: An Outline of the Cytology and Pathology of the Reticular Tissue. Edinburgh, Oliver and Boyd, 1956.

Maximow, A. A.: Relation of blood cells to connective tissues and endothelium. Physiol. Rev., 4:533, 1924.

Mitchell, D.: Actinic reticuloid. Br. J. Dermatol., 83:706, 1970.

Mitus, W. J., Bergna, L. J., Mednicoff, I. B., and Dameschek, W.: Cytochemical studies of glycogen content of lymphocytes in lymphocytic proliferations. Blood, 13:748, 1958.

Montgomery, H.: Mycosis fungoides, lymphoblastoma of the skin and allied conditions as general diseases, Oxford Med., 4:44, 1920.

Muller, S. A., and Schulze, M.: Mucha-Habermann Disease mistaken for reticulum cell lymphoma. Arch. Dermatol., 103:423, 1971.

Patek, A. J., Jr., and Castle, W. B.: Plasma cell leukemia. Folia Haematol., 52:369, 1934.

Plenck, A., and Pretl, K.: Peripheres endobronchiales Plasmocytom der Lunge mit Osteopathica hypertrophicans. Wien. Med. Wochenschr. 103:450, 1953.

Rappaport, H.: The histological aspects of malignant lymphoreticular neoplasms. The lymphoreticular tumors in Africa. 174:210, 1963.

Rappaport, H.: Tumors of the Hematopoietic System. Atlas of Tumor Pathology, Section III, Fascicle 8. Washington, D.C., Armed Forces Institute of Pathology, 1966.

Rappaport, H., Winter, W. J., and Hicks, E. B.: Follicular lymphoma. A re-evaluation of its position in the scheme of malignant lymphoma. Based on a study of 253 cases. Cancer, 9:782, 1956.

Rauschkolb, R. B.: Mycosis fungoides. Discussions and clinical experiences at Cleveland Metropolitan General Hospital. Arch. Dermatol., 83:217, 1961.

Rigdon, R. H.: Diffuse amyloidosis of the skin accompanying primary systemic amyloidosis. Am. Pract., 2:423, 1948.

River, G. L., and Schorr, W. F.: Multiple skin tumors in multiple myeloma. Arch. Dermatol., 93:432, 1966.

Robb-Smith, A. H. T.: The reticular tissue and the skin. Br. J. Dermatol., 56:151, 1944.

Rosenberg, S. A., Diamond, H. D., Jaslowitz, B., and

Craver, L. F.: Lymphosarcoma: A review of 1269 cases. Medicine, 40:31, 1961.

Rosenfeld, S., Swiller, A. I., Shanroy, M. V., and Morrison, A. N.: Syndrome simulating lymphosarcoma induced by diphenylhydantoin sodium. J.A.M.A., 176:491, 1961.

Schreiber, M. M., and McGregor, J. G.: Pseudolymphoma syndrome. A sensitivity to anticonvulsant drugs. Arch. Dermatol., 97:297, 1968.

Scott, R. B., and Robb-Smith, A. H. T.: Histiocytic medullary reticulosis. Lancet, 2:194, 1939.

Self, S. J., Carter, V. H., and Noojin, R. O.: Disseminated lymphocytoma cutis. Case reports of miliarial and nodular types. Arch. Dermatol., 100:459, 1969.

Senear, F. E., and Caro, M. R.: Ulcerative Hodgkin's disease of the skin. Arch. Dermatol. Syph., 35:114, 1937.

Sézary, A., and Bouvrain, Y.: Erythrodermie avec Présence de Cellules Monstrueuses dans Dermie et Sang Circulant. Bull. Soc. Fr. Dermatol. Syphiligr., 45:254, 1938.

Shelley, W. B., and Lehman, J. M.: Generalized anhidrosis associated with multiple myeloma. Arch. Dermatol. 83:903, 1961.

Snapper, I., Turner, L. B., and Muscovitz, H. L.: Multiple Myeloma. New York, Grune & Stratton, 1953.

Spiegler, E.: Uber die sogenannte Sarkomatosis Cutis. Arch. Dermatol. Syph. (Berl.), 27:163, 1894.

Spiethoff, cited by Hazen, H. H.: Skin changes in the leukemias and allied conditions. J. Cutan. Dis., 29:521, 1911.

Saltzstein, S. L., and Ackerman, L. V.: Lymphadenopathy induced by anticonvulsant drugs and mimicking clinically and pathologically malignant lymphomas. Cancer, 12:164, 1959.

Taswell, H. F., and Winkelmann, R. K.: Sézary syndrome—A malignant reticulemic erythroderma. J.A.M.A., 177:465, 1961.

Tedeschi, L. G., and Lasinger, D. T.: Sézary syndrome. A malignant leukemic reticuloendotheliosis. Arch. Dermatol., 92:257, 1965.

Thorson, T. A., and Brown, D. V.: A study of the lymphomas. 1. Distribution and incidence. A.M.A. Arch. Pathol., 60:353, 1955.

Van Scott, E. J.: Paper read at the Am. Dermatol. Assoc. Meeting, March, 1970.

Verallo, V. M.: Lymphomatoid papulosis. Arch. Dermatol., 104:435, 1971.

Verallo, V. M., and Haserick, J. R.: Mucha-Habermann's disease simulating lymphoma cutis. Report of two cases. Arch. Dermatol., 94:295, 1966.

Webster, J. R., and Bluefarb, S. M.: Icthyosis associated with Hodgkin's disease. Arch. Dermatol. Syph., 65:368, 1952.

Webster, J. R., and Bluefarb, S. M.: Prurigo-like papular eruption of the extremities—Hodgkin's disease. Arch. Dermatol., 67:424, 1953.

Wilson Jones, E.: In Borrie, P. F.: Lymphomatoid papulosis. Proc. R. Soc. Med., 62:159, 1969.

Winer, L. H., and Strakosh, E. A.: Tick bites—*Dermacenter variabilis* (Say). J. Invest. Dermatol., 4:249, 1941.

World Health Organization: Morbidity statistics; Malignant neoplasms for certain countries. Epidemiology. Vital Statistics Rep., 14:429, 1961.

Wyse, C. W.: Atypical mycosis fungoides or lymphomatoid papulosis. Cutis, 5:1227, 1969.

54

Neoplasms Metastatic to the Skin

Amir H. Mehregan, M.D.

DEFINITION

This chapter examines secondary involvement of the skin by malignant neoplasms originating within the underlying tissues or internal organs.

MODE OF SPREAD

Cutaneous metastasis may occur in one of the following ways.
1. Direct invasion of the skin from underlying growth.
2. Continuous extension of the tumor cells through lymphatics.
3. Lymphatic emboli.
4. Hemic emboli.
5. Accidental implantation of the tumor cells through the surgeon's glove or instruments.

INCIDENCE

Cutaneous involvement from internal malignancies is rare in comparison with metastases to other organs of the body.

Gates (1937) found this evidence in only 2.7 percent of cases. Abrams et al. (1950), in a survey of 1000 autopsied cases with malignant neoplasms of epithelial origin, found cutaneous metastases occurring only in 44 cases, and Leu (1964) reported 34 instances of cutaneous metastasis among 1367 autopsies with malignant neoplasia. Certain malignant tumors show a tendency for cutaneous metastasis. In women, breast carcinoma is the best example of this type. Warren and Witham (1933) found 61 instances of cutaneous metastasis in a series of 162 cases with breast carcinoma. In a study by Brownstein and Helwig (1970), breast carcinoma was found to be the primary site of cutaneous metastasis in 67 percent of cases in their female series. In their evaluation, the pattern of frequency for men was found to be strikingly different, and the most common primary lesions in order of prevalence were bronchogenic carcinoma, adenocarcinoma of the digestive tract, malignant melanoma, and squamous cell carcinoma of the oral cavity. Gechman (1946) stated that rarity of cutaneous metastasis is probably due to the fact that this occurs only when the body has lost its quality of defense.

AGE AND RACE

The greatest incidence of cutaneous metastasis is between the fourth and sixth decades of life. As certain malignancies occur earlier in life, their cutaneous metastases are also observed in younger individuals. Such is the case with malignant melanoma and neuroblastoma of childhood (Shown and Durfee, 1970). The race factor also contributes to some statistical differences; for example, malignant melanoma is extremely rare in Negroes.

LOCATION

Localization of cutaneous metastases depends upon the mode of spread of the primary lesion. Certain regions appear to be sites of predilection for cutaneous metastasis. Frequency of scalp involvement has been well recognized. In Gates' (1937) report, 12 out of 33 cutaneous metastases from breast carcinoma, as well as 20 percent from other sources, were located on the scalp. The scalp as the only site of metastasis of hypernephroma has been mentioned by Halstead (1907), Smyth (1939), Gates (1937), Cohen (1960), and Winer and Wright (1960). In the series studied by Connor et al. (1963), of 52 cutaneous metastases observed in 40 cases with renal cell carcinoma (hypernephroma), 26 lesions were located on the scalp. Involvement of the anterior abdominal wall, especially the periumbilical region, from malignancies of the digestive tract and urinary system has been pointed out by Poinso et al. (1953). Involvement of the operation scar occurred in 16 instances in a series of 69 cases with hypernephroma studied by Rosenthal and Lever (1957). A similar incidence occurred in 11 cases in the series reported by Connor et al. (1963). Metastatic malignant tumors of the eyelids have been studied by Riley (1970). In his series of 15 cases, six originated from carcinoma of the breast, six were metastatic malignant melanoma, two were adenocarcinoma of the stomach, and

one was secondary to a squamous cell carcinoma of the lung.

CLINICAL PICTURE

Carcinomas metastatic to the skin may appear in any one or a combination of the following morphologic forms.

Carcinoma en Cuirasse

This name was proposed by Velpeau in 1838 (cited by Willis, 1952) for an advanced stage of cutaneous invasion by malignant cells. Early lesions consist of scattered, lenticular, hard papules or small, dermal nodules seated over a red or reddish blue smooth surface. Eventually the papulonodular lesions coalesce to form hard and sclerotic plaques. In this process, the inflammatory signs are minimal or may be completely absent.

Carcinoma en cuirasse is most commonly secondary to breast carcinoma, and only occasionally may other types of malignant tumors produce this form of cutaneous involvement. Such rare instances have been reported by Harvey and Cochrane (1950) from carcinoma of the stomach and by Leu (1964) from carcinoma of the prostate, uterus, and pancreas. A localized variety of carcinoma en cuirasse, most commonly secondary to breast malignancy, occurs on the scalp of

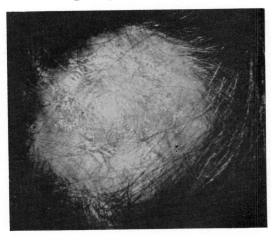

Figure 54–1   Breast carcinoma metastatic to scalp, resembling a patch of chronic discoid lupus erythematosus. (Courtesy of Dr. W. Schorr.)

women in the form of singular or multiple well-defined areas of alopecia (Delacrétaz and Chapuis, 1958). In these areas, the skin appears atrophic and is bound down to the underlying tissue, resembling clinically a scarring alopecia (Baran, 1969), patches of discoid lupus erythematosus (Mehregan, 1961), or alopecia areata (Schorr et al., 1970). Examples of this form have been described under the term "alopecia neoplastica" by Cohen et al. (1961) (Fig. 54–1).

Inflammatory Carcinoma (Carcinoma Erysipelatoïdes)

This form of carcinoma metastatic to the skin was first described by Hutchinson in 1886 (cited by Ingram, 1958) as cancer erythema. Lee and Tannebaum (1924) reported a series of 28 cases under the term "inflammatory carcinoma." Küttner

(1924), Rasch (1931), and later Dawson and Shaw (1937) proposed the name "carcinoma erysipelatoïdes." In this form, involvement of the skin occurs in rapid fashion (Taylor and Meltzer, 1938; Leavell and Tillotson, 1951). Inflammatory signs, such as erythema, edema, and pain, are present. The skin is red, warm, and slightly brawny with well-demarcated borders resembling erysipelas (Fig. 54–2). Purplish papules and hemorrhagic pseudovesicles may be present on the surface of the lesion (Freeman and Lynch, 1937). Mild fever and signs of toxicity may complicate the picture. A variety of carcinoma erysipelatoïdes, characterized by the presence of dilated capillaries and pin-point telangiectases, has been described by Weber (1933) as "carcinoma telangiectaticum."

Nodular Metastatic Carcinoma

This is by far the most common form of cutaneous involvement from internal malignancies (Suzuki, 1918). Metastatic nodular lesions may be singular or multiple and intradermal or subcutaneous in location (Figs. 54–3 and 54–4). Intradermal lesions may show superficial erosion or ulceration and closely resemble a benign or a primary malignant cutaneous neoplasia (Fig. 54–5). Cutaneous metastasis of bronchial carcinoma resembling keratoacanthoma has been described by Hunziker et al. (1969). Large and multilobulated growth

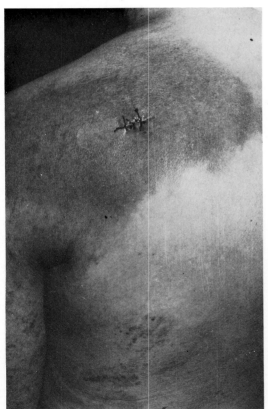

Figure 54–2 Inflammatory (erysipelatous) carcinoma of breast involving the chest wall and shoulder. (Courtesy of Dr. L. Shapiro.)

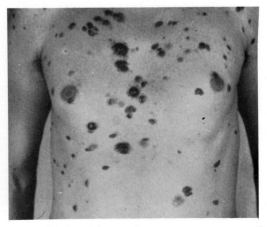

Figure 54–3 Widespread cutaneous metastases of malignant melanoma.

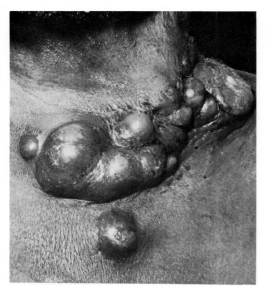

Figure 54–4   Large, nodular metastases of a bronchogenic carcinoma in the skin and subcutaneous tissue of clavicular area. (Courtesy of Dr. M. Mir.)

of scalp, resembling turban tumor, originating from a carcinoma of the prostate, has been reported by Ronchese (1940). Cauliflower-like lesions of the lower abdomen secondary to carcinoma of the uterus have been described by Bade (1939). Nodular cutaneous metastases of renal cell carcinoma may be highly vascular, resem-

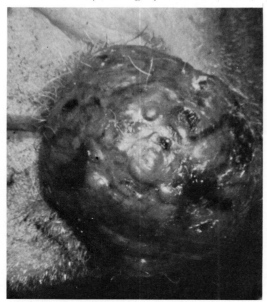

Figure 54–5   Oat cell carcinoma of lung metastatic to the skin, clinically resembling a primary malignant tumor of cheek. (Courtesy of Dr. L. Shapiro.)

bling a hemangioma. Selmanowitz (1968) has included cutaneous metastases of renal cell carcinoma and thyroid carcinoma in the group of pulsating tumors of the skin. Nodular metastatic lesions located deep in the skin or within the subcutaneous tissue are usually covered by normal skin. Deep lesions may resemble an epithelial cyst or lipoma. Newborns with deep-seated cutaneous metastatic lesions of neuroblastoma have been described as blueberry muffin babies (Shown and Durfee, 1970). Involvement of the subcutaneous fat tissue by pancreatic carcinoma simulating cellulitis has been reported by Edelstein (1950). The nodular cutaneous metastases are usually asymptomatic. Metastatic carcinoid, however, may be sensitive to palpation.

Dermatitis-like Metastatic Carcinoma

In this relatively rare form, crusted, patchy lesions occur which resemble an eczematous dermatitis. Examples of this type include Paget's disease of the nipple and extramammary Paget's disease secondary to underlying sweat gland carcinoma or malignancies of the lower intestinal tract.

HISTOPATHOLOGY

The histopathologic pattern of metastatic tumors may fall into two categories. In one group the growth consists of completely undifferentiated cells, and the primary site cannot be recognized histologically. In the second group, the histopathologic pattern of the metastatic lesion is so characteristic that the source of origin can be easily identified (Fig. 54–6). Histopathologic findings of some of the most common carcinomas metastatic to the skin are described below.

Metastatic Breast Carcinoma

In the sclerotic form or carcinoma en cuirasse, diffuse invasion of the corium occurs by numerous small nests and thin

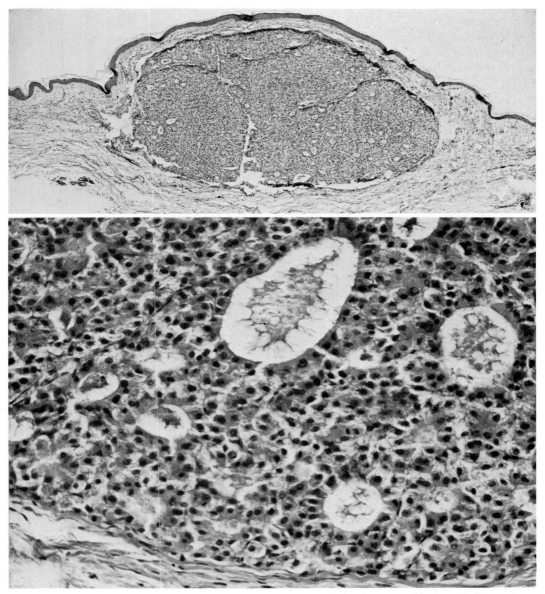

Figure 54–6 Hepatocellular carcinoma metastatic to the skin. Lobulated masses of hepatocellular carcinoma show numerous bile-containing canaliculi. *H & E, ×45 and ×225.* (*From* Kahn et al.: Arch. Dermatol., 104:299, 1971.)

cords of tumor cells. Individual cells may line up in between the collagen bundles and show "Indians in a file" arrangement (Fig. 54–7). This form of breast carcinoma is characterized by production of fibrous tissue (desmoplasia), and the anaplastic tumor cells are surrounded by a scarlike fibrous stroma. Isolated tumor cells embedded in dense stroma may resemble atypical fibroblasts. Invasion of the overlying epidermis may lead to formation of junctional or intraepidermal nests of anaplastic cells (Bálus et al., 1968). In the inflammatory form of breast carcinoma metastatic to the skin, the superficial dermal capillary blood vessels and lymphatics are dilated and are filled with clusters of tumor cells (Fig. 54–8). The tumor nests consist of cells with atypically large and hyperchromatic nuclei, which also

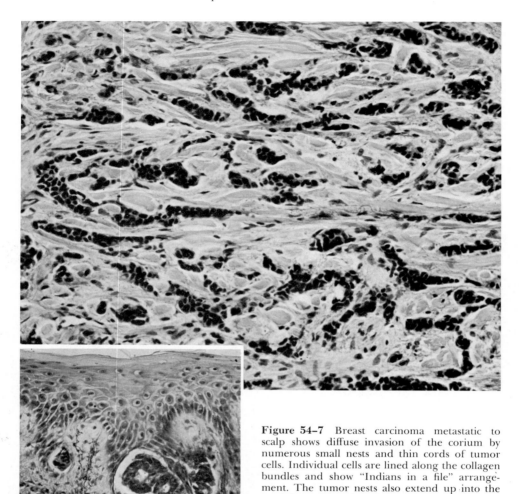

Figure 54–7 Breast carcinoma metastatic to scalp shows diffuse invasion of the corium by numerous small nests and thin cords of tumor cells. Individual cells are lined along the collagen bundles and show "Indians in a file" arrangement. The tumor nests also extend up into the overlying epidermis and show pagetoid phenomenon. *H & E, ×180.*

show mitotic figures. Mild dermal edema and perivascular inflammatory cell infiltrate are present. In carcinoma telangiectaticum, in addition to the tumor emboli, some of the superficial capillary blood vessels are markedly dilated and are engorged with erythrocytes (Fig. 54–9).

Metastatic Renal Cell Carcinoma (Hypernephroma)

The histopathology of the cutaneous metastatic lesions of renal cell carcinoma is characteristic. The findings are similar to those of the primary tumor and in some instances have led to the discovery of a silent primary lesion. Intradermal or subcutaneous tumor masses consist of large polyhedral cells forming tubular or glandular structures (Fig. 54–10). The tumor cells show round or ovoid central nuclei and abundant clear and finely granular cytoplasm which contains both glycogen and lipid. The tumor stroma is richly vascular and often shows extensive extravasation of erythrocytes into the tubular structures, lending the growth an angiomatous appearance. In histopathologic differential diagnosis of metastatic cutaneous renal cell carcinoma, sebaceous carcinoma and clear cell hidradenoma should be taken into consideration.

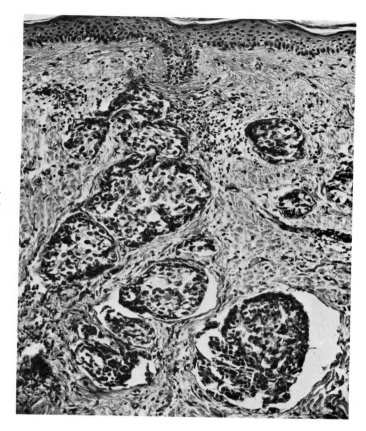

Figure 54–8 Inflammatory metastatic carcinoma of breast shows extensive involvement of dermal capillaries and lymph spaces by anaplastic tumor masses. *H&E, ×135.*

Metastatic Carcinoma of Gastrointestinal Tract

Metastatic tumors originating from malignancies of the digestive tract are characterized by formation of acid mucopolysaccharide by the anaplastic cells (Winer and Wright, 1960). The mucin-producing anaplastic cells may form numerous tubular or glandular structures or invade the corium in the form of irregular sheets of signet-ring cells (Figs. 54–11 and 54–12).

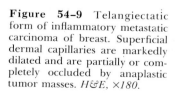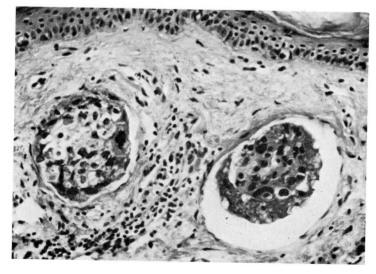

Figure 54–9 Telangiectatic form of inflammatory metastatic carcinoma of breast. Superficial dermal capillaries are markedly dilated and are partially or completely occluded by anaplastic tumor masses. *H&E, ×180.*

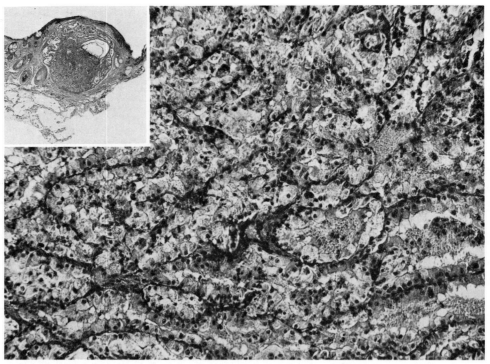

Figure 54–10   Renal cell carcinoma metastatic to the skin. The tumor masses consist of large, polyhedral cells forming tubular structures. There is also extensive extravasation of erythrocytes. *H&E, ×180.*

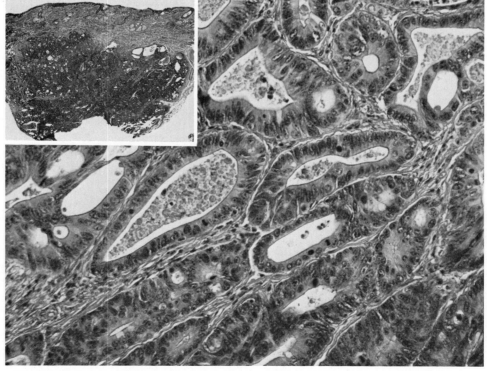

Figure 54–11   Carcinoma of colon metastatic to the skin shows numerous tubular and glandular structures. *H&E, ×180.*

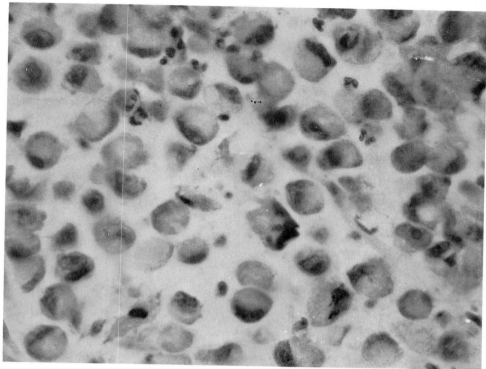

Figure 54–12 Carcinoma of colon metastatic to the skin. In this lesion the corium is invaded by masses of mucin-containing signet-ring cells. *H&E, ×225.*

The mucinous material is PAS-positive and diastase-resistant. It is also Alcian blue– and aldehyde fuchsin–reactive and shows color reaction similar to sialomucin. Mucin production is not exclusive to metastatic carcinoma of the digestive tract and can also be demonstrated in metastatic lesions from other sources, such as in carcinoma of the prostate or breast (Foster and Levine, 1963; Cawley et al., 1964). Metastatic lesions originating from the gastrointestinal tract with tubular or glandular structures should be histologically differentiated from primary benign or malignant tumors of the sweat glands (Montgomery and Kierland, 1940; Reingold, 1966).

Metastatic Bronchogenic Carcinoma

Cutaneous metastasis of bronchogenic carcinoma is often in the form of poorly keratinizing squamous cell carcinoma (Fig. 54–13). Diffuse invasion of the corium, dermal capillary blood vessels, and lymphatics occurs by numerous solid masses and nests of anaplastic cells. Paucity of dermal reaction and normal appearance of the overlying epidermis are helpful in differentiating the metastatic lesion from a primary epidermoid carcinoma.

Metastatic Malignant Melanoma

A nodular lesion of metastatic malignant melanoma in which the tumor cells show melanogenesis can be easily identified. The absence of junctional activity and epidermal invasion and lack of dermal inflammatory cell reaction differentiate the metastatic growth from a primary lesion (Fig. 54–14). Epidermal invasion, however, may occur in some metastatic lesions in rare instances. In a completely amelanotic lesion, the identification of the metastatic tumor may be difficult and may require special histochemical stains, such as Masson-Fontana's

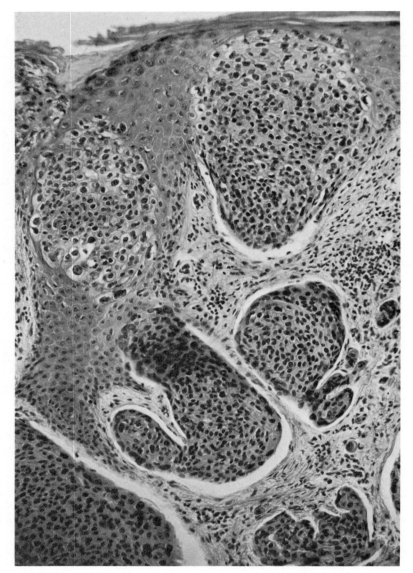

Figure 54-13   Bronchogenic carcinoma metastatic to the skin. There is extension of the tumor masses from the superficial dermal lymphatics into the overlying epidermis (Paget phenomenon). *H&E, ×180.*

ammoniacal silver nitrate method, or demonstration of tyrosinase activity.

Metastatic Carcinoid

In cutaneous metastases of carcinoid, invasion of dermis and subcutis occurs by irregular sheets of cells with small and hyperchromatic nuclei (Rudner et al., 1965). Argentaffin granules may be demonstrated in carcinoid tumors originating from the intestinal tract and are rarely ob-

served in carcinoid tumors of other organs.

TREATMENT

Treatment of carcinomas metastatic to the skin is palliative. Small and localized lesions should be surgically excised. Larger lesions may be treated by radiation. Systemic anticancer medications may be used for patients with extensive and disseminated lesions.

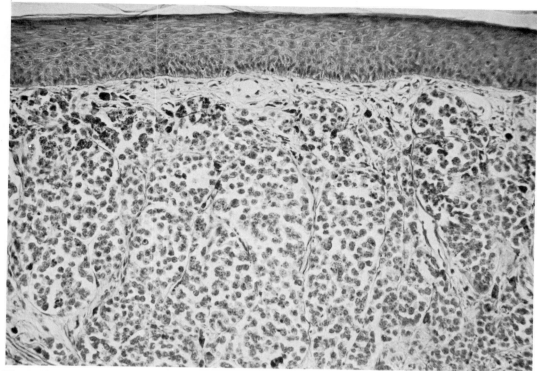

Figure 54–14 Malignant melanoma metastatic to the skin. The corium is solidly replaced by the anaplastic melanoma cells. There is no evidence of epidermal involvement or junctional activity. *H&E, ×180.*

PROGNOSIS

In a small percentage of cases, cutaneous metastases appear early as the first sign of internal malignancy (Leu, 1964). Cutaneous involvement has also occurred as late as 12 to 14 years after the surgical removal of the malignant tumor. In general, involvement of the skin is considered as a late occurrence in the phenomenon of metastasis of malignant tumors to various organs of the body. The prognosis is poor, and death usually occurs within a period of a few weeks to several months (Suzuki, 1918). Regressive changes of cutaneous metastases have been reported in a few cases following dissemination of malignant melanoma.

REFERENCES

Abrams, H. L., Spiro, R., and Goldstein, N.: Metastases in carcinoma. Analysis of 1000 autopsied cases. Cancer, 3:74, 1950.

Bade, W.: Das Metastatische Carcinom der Haut in Anschluss an Carcinom innerer Organe. Arch. Dermatol. Syph. (Berl.), 179:257, 1939.

Bálus, L., Harap, E., and Gogonea, L.: Über die intraepidermale metastasierung. Arch. Klin. Exp. Dermatol., 231:371, 1968.

Baran, R.: Les métastases alopéciantes scléro-atrophiques des cancers mammaires (Revue générale sur 18 cas). Dermatologica, 138:169, 1969.

Brownstein, M. H., and Helwig, E. B.: Patterns of Cutaneous Metastasis. Arch. Dermatol., 105:862, 1972.

Cawley, E. P., Hsu, Y. T., and Weary, P. E.: The evaluation of neoplastic metastases to the skin. Arch. Dermatol., 90:262, 1964.

Cohen, D. M.: Hypernephroma metastases to skin and bones. Arch. Dermatol., 81:622, 1960.

Cohen, I., Levy, E., and Schreiber, H.: Alopecia neoplastica due to breast carcinoma. Arch. Dermatol., 84:490, 1961.

Connor, D. H., Taylor, H. B., and Helwig, E. B.: Cutaneous metastasis of renal cell carcinoma. Arch. Pathol., 76:339, 1963.

Dawson, E. K., and Shaw, J. J.: Mammary cancer with generalized telangiectatic carcinoma (carcinoma erysipelatoides). Br. J. Surg., 25:100, 1937.

Delacrétaz, J., and Chapuis, H.: Métastases cutanées alopéciantes. Dermatologica, 116:372, 1958.

Edelstein, J. M.: Pancreatic carcinoma with unusual metastasis to the skin and subcutaneous tissue simulating cellulitis. New Engl. J. Med., 242:779, 1950.

Foster, E. A., and Levine, A. J.: Mucin production in metastatic carcinomas. Cancer, 16:506, 1963.

Freeman, C. D., and Lynch, F. W.: Carcinoma of the breast with peculiar cutaneous metastases. Report of a case. Arch. Dermatol., 35:643, 1937.

Gates, O.: Cutaneous metastases of malignant disease. Am. J. Cancer, 30:718, 1937.

Gechman, E.: Ueber metastatische hautkarzinom. Wien. Klin. Wochenschr., 58:748, 1946.

Halstead, A. E.: Case of hypernephroma. Surg. Gynecol. Obstet., 4:654, 1907.

Harvey, G., and Cochrane, T.: Carcinoma en cuirasse. Primary lesion in stomach. Arch. Dermatol., 62:651, 1950.

Hunziker, N., Djalali, A., and Laugier, P.: Métastase cutanée de cancer bronchique simulant le keratoacanthome. Bull. Soc. Fr. Dermatol. Syphiligr., 76:552, 1969.

Ingram, J. T.: Carcinoma erysipelatodes and carcinoma telangiectaticum. Arch. Dermatol., 77:227, 1958.

Kahn, J. A., Sinhamohapatra, S. B., and Schneider, A. F.: Hepatoma presenting as a skin metastasis. Arch. Dermatol., 104:299, 1971.

Küttner, H.: Beiträge zur pathologie des mammacarcinoms. Beitr. Z. Klin. Chir., 131:1, 1924.

Leavell, U. W., Jr., and Tillotson, F. W.: Metastatic cutaneous carcinoma from the breast. Arch. Dermatol., 64:774, 1951.

Lee, B. J., and Tannebaum, N. E.: Inflammatory carcinoma of the breast. Surg. Gynecol. Obstet., 39:580, 1924.

Leu, F.: Les metastases cutanees des cancers visceraux. These, presentee á la Faculte de Medicine de l'Universite de Lausanne pour l'obtention du grade de docteur en medecine. Lausanne, 1964.

Mehregan, A. H.: Metastatic carcinoma to the skin. Dermatologica, 123:311, 1961.

Montgomery, H., and Kierland, R. R.: Metastasis of carcinoma to the scalp. Distinction from cylindroma and from carcinoma of the dermal appendages. Arch. Surg., 11:672, 1940.

Poinso, R., Callas, E., and Sauve, M.: Les metastases cutanées et sous-cutanées des cancers de l'estomac. Presse Med., 61:1188, 1953.

Rasch, C.: Carcinoma erysipelatodes. Br. J. Dermatol., 43:351, 1931.

Reingold, I. M.: Cutaneous metastases from internal carcinoma (review). Cancer, 19:162, 1966.

Riley, F. C.: Metastatic tumors of the eyelids. Am. J. Ophthalmol., 69:259, 1970.

Ronchese, R.: Metastases of the scalp simulating turban tumors. Arch. Dermatol., 41:639, 1940.

Rosenthal, A. L., and Lever, W. F.: Involvement of the skin in renal carcinoma. Arch. Dermatol., 76:96, 1957.

Rudner, E. J., Lentz, C., and Brown, J.: Bronchial carcinoid tumor with skin metastases. Arch. Dermatol., 92:73, 1965.

Schorr, W. F., Swanson, P. M., Gomez, F., and Reyes, C. N.: Alopecia neoplastica. Hair loss resembling alopecia areata caused by metastatic breast cancer. J.A.M.A., 213:1335, 1970.

Selmanowitz, V. J.: Diagnosis of pulsatile tumors of the skin. Cutis, 4:949, 1968.

Shown, T. E., and Durfee, M. F.: Blueberry muffin baby: Neonatal neuroblastoma with subcutaneous metastases. J. Urol., 104:193, 1970.

Smyth, M. J.: Silent hypernephromata. Br. J. Surg., 27:266, 1939.

Suzuki, N.: Multiple skin metastases from cancer of internal organs. J. Cancer Res., 2:357, 1918.

Taylor, G. W., and Meltzer, A.: "Inflammatory carcinoma" of the breast. Am. J. Cancer, 33:33, 1938.

Warren, S., and Witham, E. M.: Studies on tumor metastasis. The distribution of metastases in cancer of the breast. Surg. Gynecol. Obstet., 57:81, 1933.

Weber, P. F.: Bilateral thoracic zosteroid spreading marginate telangiectasis probably a variety of "carcinoma erysipelatodes" (C. Rasch)—Associated with unilateral mammary carcinoma and better termed "carcinoma telangiectaticum." Br. J. Dermatol., 45:418, 1933.

Willis, R. A.: The Spread of Tumors in the Human Body. St. Louis, Mo., C. V. Mosby Company, 1952.

Winer, L. H., and Wright, E. T.: Über den sekundären (metastatischen) hautkrebs: klinische und pathologische untersuchungen. Hautarzt, 11:23, 1960.

55

Dermatoses That May Be Accompanied By Carcinoma

Erich Landes, M.D., Adolf Kúta, M.D.,
and Burkhard Metz, M.D.

PSORIASIS

The first report on the simultaneous occurrence of carcinoma and psoriasis was made early (Pozzi, 1874; White, 1885). At that time Hutchinson (1887) drew attention to the development of carcinoma in psoriatics treated with arsenic. Autochthonous growth of carcinoma in psoriasis has been the subject of numerous investigations. In 1921, Alexander compiled the cases known until then. Of 18 cases, 11 were malignant degenerations of arsenical keratoses, while in 7 a so-called autochthonous psoriasis carcinoma was assumed. Psoriasis carcinoma meant that the tumor growth was a psoriatic lesion. It was said that no arsenic had been administered, and that neither radiotherapy nor long-term tar treatment had been applied before. It was also said that manipulations of a different nature did not lead to irritations. The patient, whom Alexander assumed to have a primary psoriasis carcinoma, had been given arsenicals; to this he did not attach any importance, because

treatment dated five years back. Burgener (1939) compiled another 18 cases of psoriasis with carcinoma. He came to the conclusion that there are no autochthonous psoriasis carcinomas. Biltz (1953), who reinvestigated the cases reported after Burgener's publication, agreed with this conclusion. In the ninth case, one of his own, he considered the possibility of a psoriasis carcinoma; but here, too, arsenicals had been administered 20 years previously. Unna, Memmesheimer, and Herzberg (1963) described four more cases of carcinoma with psoriasis, in which all patients had been treated with carcinogens (arsenic, thorium X, x-rays, tar). In none of the cases were the criteria of a psoriasis carcinoma met. The report speaks not only of different types of carcinoma (squamous cell carcinomas, basal cell epitheliomas, bowenoid carcinomas), but also of simultaneous occurrence of squamous cell carcinoma, bowenoid carcinoma, and arsenical keratosis, as well as seborrheic keratosis. In one case a melanoma was described (Unna et al., 1963),

1291

but the fact that this might be a coincidence must be considered.

The majority of squamous cell carcinomas in psoriasis have grown on arsenical keratoses. In the description by Kleine-Natrop (1959), an ulcerating squamous-cell carcinoma on one finger and a bowenoid carcinoma on the back developed 40 years after the onset of psoriasis and 20 years after the beginning of arsenic therapy. Arsenic as the cause of carcinoma is excluded by a number of authors, because the arsenic treatment had been given a very long time before (Kromeyer, 1938; Arsenic treatment 22 years previously). Frequently x-ray therapy of a psoriatic lesion has been observed to be carcinogenic (Goodman and Brice, 1930; Nexmand, 1961; Fuss, 1932; carcinoma after 30 to 40 x-ray treatments of a psoriatic lesion).

Upon perusal of the relevant literature it becomes apparent that there is no case of autochthonous psoriasis carcinoma. In all cases a multitude of carcinogens (arsenic, ultraviolet light, x-rays, tar) had been applied (Goodman et al., 1954). In the few cases in which arsenic was not mentioned in the anamnesis, one must take into account that patients frequently do not recall the therapy applied before. The simultaneous occurrence of internal carcinomas in cases of negative arsenic anamnesis is a significant indication of arsenic administration. The combination of squamous cell carcinoma, Bowen's disease, basal cell epithelioma, and benign neoformations may be indicative of arsenical origin.

According to Sommer and McManus (1953), the latency period of arsenical cancer varies from 3 to 50 years. Knoth (1966) was able to demonstrate in young mice that, if transplacental or lactogenic arsenic is administered, carcinomas may develop; thus he proved the oncogenic effect of arsenic. Fierz (1966) pointed out that the formation of carcinoma in psoriatics increases after arsenical treatment. The reason for this is that psoriasis patients on the average have taken larger doses of arsenic than is usual in other diseases. Obviously the type of carcinoma is dependent on the dose of arsenic applied, not on the latency period. Basal cell

epitheliomas in the skin of the trunk may occur after a total quantity of only 70 ml. of arsenic, whereas squamous cell carcinomas occur mostly after the intake of 500 ml. or more.

Considering the incidence of psoriasis (0.27 to 2.48 percent, according to Grüneberg, 1958), it seems quite possible to find the accidental occurrence of carcinoma in a psoriatic. This is why Unna et al. (1963) spoke of a triad: psoriasis-carcinoma-arsenic; however, it is still under discussion whether the epithelial irritation, characteristic of psoriasis, is the precondition for the neoformation. Changes existing for years might be conducive to the cancerization process, as for instance in the patient observed by Bild (1961), who had had psoriatic lesions existing for years on both elbows, where later squamous cell carcinoma appeared. Here, too, however, treatment with arsenic was the case. Upon critical consideration of cases reported in the literature, and taking into account the frequency of the clinical picture, one must say that there is no psoriasis carcinoma in the true sense: it is always a secondary carcinomatosis caused by carcinogens (arsenic, x-rays, thorium X, tar, ultraviolet light) (Figs. 55–1 and 55–2).

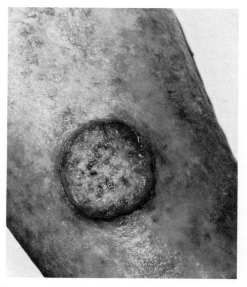

Figure 55–1 Squamous cell carcinoma in a psoriatic lesion. (Courtesy of Prof. H. Grimmer, Wiesbaden.)

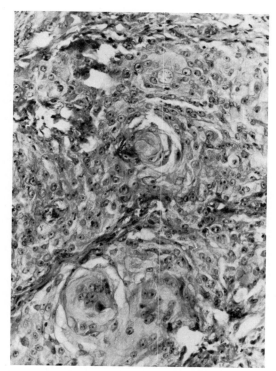

Figure 55–2 Biopsy of squamous cell carcinoma in psoriatic lesion seen in Figure 55–1. (Courtesy of Prof. H. Grimmer, Wiesbaden.)

ECZEMA

Hillström and Swanbeck (1969, 1970a, and 1970b), in their study of the localization of 548 squamous cell carcinomas which had been registered in Sweden from 1958 to 1965, demonstrated that in 9 cases psoriasis and in 16 cases eczema had been in the location of the carcinoma. The incidence of both diseases on the trunk and in the face was the same; on the arms and hands the eczema dominated (7:1); the same was true for the lower extremities (6:5). In contrast to psoriasis, an "eczema carcinoma" has never been mentioned. No histogenetic explanation for the formation of carcinoma on eczema can be found, so the sum of therapeutic measures (arsenic, x-rays, tar, and actinic factors) must be considered as the cause.

LICHEN PLANUS

Steigleder (1963), in his classification of precancerous stages, places lichen planus

of the mucous membrane among the precancerous stages in a broader sense. Greither (1966) has also placed lichen planus of the mucous membrane among the group of symptomatic leukoplakias, characterizing it as a facultative precancerous stage. Malignant degeneration of lichen planus of the skin is rare. Degenerations of banal lichen planus lesions are rarely described (Hampel, 1940; squamous cell carcinoma with lichen planus on the dorsum of the hand after arsenic and x-rays; Rohde, 1966; squamous cell carcinoma with lichen planus on the chest among a group of 558 patients with lichen planus). Neoplasia of lichen planus of the skin develops mainly with verrucous lichen planus or lichen corneus (Brennan and Teplitz, 1958; Kronenberg et al., 1971); it develops as well with atrophic and ulcerating forms (Jansen and Groothuis, 1960) and with sclerobullous lichen planus (Midana and Depaoli, 1967; after arsenic therapy dated four years previously).

The rare neoplasias on lichen planus of the skin occur predominantly on the lower leg (see also Hillström and Swanbeck, 1969; Hansen, 1955). Particularly impressive is the observation by Kronenberg et al. (1971). In a 39 year old male patient with lichen planus, the authors could observe, over a period of five years, the growth of squamous cell carcinomas developing from hyperkeratotic changes in the verrucous plaques on the lower leg. Histologically the squamous cell carcinoma was located in a region of extensive pseudoepitheliomatous hyperplasia. In addition, there was anhidrosis with compensatory hyperhidrosis in the head and neck.

The reported observations of malignant degeneration of lichen planus of the skin permit the conclusion that special factors, such as atrophy, pseudoepitheliomatous hyperplasia, and chronically relapsing inflammation, rather than therapeutic measures, such as arsenic and x-rays, lead to malignant degeneration. Midana and Depaoli, 1967; Hampel, 1940). Thus there is a pathomechanism for carcinogenesis similar to that for carcinoma on ulcer cruris.

In the literature of the past 60 years, more than 50 well-documented publications on malignant degeneration of lichen planus were issued. During the Symposium of the American Dermatological Association in 1919, the first statistical investigation of the connection of lichen planus and carcinoma was carried out.

In 1966, Muissus was able to compile 57 cases from the world literature. In the meantime, further reports were published by Bureau et al., 1970; Grinspan et al., 1966; and Opperbeck, 1971. The carcinoma predominates in the oral mucosa, and is less frequently found on the tongue (Fig. 55–3) and on the lip. Carcinoma with lichen planus has been described on the genitals too (Jänner et al., 1967; a keratinizing squamous cell carcinoma in the clitoris region). Here a relation to lichen sclerosus et atrophicus must be assumed. Carcinomas with lichen planus of the mucous membrane, as well as the rare cases occurring on the skin, are exclusively squamous cell carcinomas.

According to Rohde's (1966) compilation of 47 case reports, 25 lesions occurred on the oral mucosa, 10 on the tongue, and 3 on the vermilion border. The remaining 9 patients had carcinoma on the lips and the skin. Jänner (1971) was able to make a follow-up examination of 150 out of 585 lichen planus patients. In eight cases a carcinoma was diagnosed; only in one case had arsenical treatment been applied. Schürmann (1958) did not look upon previous arsenical treatment or radiotherapy as the cause for the majority of carcinomas in lichen planus. Essentially, the cause of cancerization is to be found in chronic inflammatory processes, degenerative changes, and local irritation, in which a decisive role is attributed mainly to the atrophic mesenchymal changes (Gottron, 1954; Jänner, 1971). Atrophy of the tongue with its reduction of the papillary structures particularly seems to favor the development of neoplasms (Greither and Hornstein, 1966). Because of the frequently difficult diagnosis of lichen planus of the mucous membrane, histologic examination is essential. The clinically convincing lichen planus of the mucous membrane may as well be a true precancerous leukoplakia, and even Bowen's disease may present as a lichen planus (Steigleder, 1963). Malignant neoformations in other variants of lichen planus, the lichen planopilaris (Graham-Little-Lassueur syndrome), are not described. With lichen nitidus, malignant neoformations were not observed either.

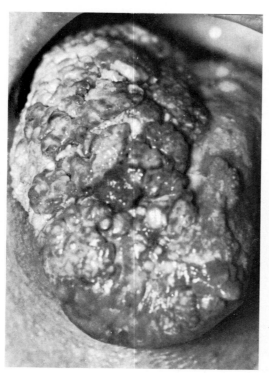

Figure 55–3 Squamous cell carcinoma of the tongue in lichen planus. (Courtesy of Prof. T. Nasemann, Frankfurt.)

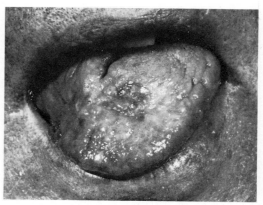

Figure 55–4 Squamous cell carcinoma in glossitis granulomatosa of the tongue. (Courtesy of Prof. O. Hornstein, Erlangen.)

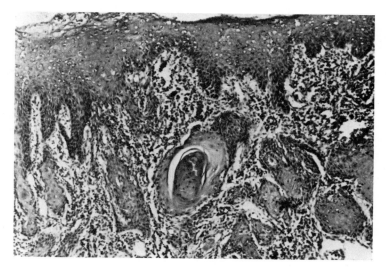

Figure 55–5 Biopsy of squamous cell carcinoma seen in Figure 55–4. (Courtesy of Prof. O. Hornstein, Erlangen.)

GLOSSITIS GRANULOMATOSA

According to Hornstein (1965), squamous cell carcinoma on glossitis granulomatosa (Schürmann-Miescher) is rare (Figs. 55–4 and 55–5). Similar to carcinomas in lupus or carcinomas on lichen planus, the interaction of proliferative inflammatory conditions with permanently cicatricial transformation processes and therapeutic aggression—in the present case, radiotherapy—is assumed to be the cause.

CANDIDIASIS OF THE ORAL MUCOSA

The occurrence of carcinoma in candidiasis of the oral mucosa may be considered a rare observation. Degos et al. (1970) observed a squamous cell carcinoma in candidiasis of the oral mucosa, mainly in the region of the left corner of the mouth. In the course of nearly nine years, biopsies were made repeatedly. In 1960, the diagnosis was made: papillomatous and keratotic moniliasis. However, in 1967 a metastasizing squamous cell carcinoma could be found histologically, from which the patient died. It is important that the patient reacted anergically to *Candida* antibodies, because this anergic reaction might be responsible for the occurrence of the carcinoma. Williamson (1969), too, was able

to observe the growth of a squamous cell carcinoma in hyperplastic moniliasis of the angle of the mouth.

LUPUS ERYTHEMATOSUS

Chronic discoid lupus erythematosus (CDLE) belongs to the chronically inflammatory dermatoses, which show a considerable amount of malignant degeneration. As early as 1886, Curie mentioned the degeneration of a CDLE lesion. In 1904, Jadassohn had compiled 13 such cases from the literature. In 1948, Grana was already able to mention 130 carcinomas in CDLE terrain. Based on information reported in the literature, Kappesser (1952) concluded that one out of every 50 CDLE's degenerates into a malignant tumor. Several other observations of this kind followed, all dealing with problems of pathogenetic connections of malignant degeneration of the chronic CDLE lesions. Grana (1956) stated that the period from the onset of CDLE to the formation of the neoplasm is seldom only a few years; it may even take 30 to 40 years. He presented a case of his own, in which, in a CDLE localized on the dorsum of the nose, a basosquamous epithelioma developed four months after an injury. Malignant degeneration of a CDLE lesion usually occurs as solitary squamous cell carcinoma. Grana could find in the literature only five basal cell epitheliomas in CDLE terrain. Other observations confirmed and documented these data (Vilanova, 1957; Landi and Nardi, 1961; Storck et al., 1961).

Without doubt, not only the external factors but also the internal ones must be assumed to be a cause of malignant degeneration of a CDLE lesion. Of the external carcinogenic factors, all the carcinogens known for the skin must be considered, especially ultraviolet light and x-rays. Seen in the light of clinical experience, rather indifferent factors (chronically repeated mechanical irritation, maceration, and chemical irritation by various external therapeutic agents) must be taken into account, which do not show carcinogenic effects on the healthy skin.

This information clearly speaks for the fact that the immediate carcinogenic impulses are coming from the primary subepidermal changes and are of a more or less biologic nature; only their summation and torpid effect within a limited area are not physiologic. With reference to the poorly vascularized cicatricial structures in the CDLE lesions, it seems to be absolutely justified to assume that the epidermal cell system is suffering from a permanent hypoxidosis. Thus the epidermal cells actually are continuously "suffocated," and their physiologic degeneration is accelerated, i.e., the keratinization is increased (hyperkeratosis). Finally, there is malignant degeneration in this terrain because, in the end, cell elements or cell generations are formed to which the hypoxidosis of this terrain is congenial.

Their further proliferation determines the entire character of the new pathologic process—the character of the malignant autonomous tumor growth, which, even under the poor conditions of permanent hypoxidosis, can develop· optimally. It seems to be quite logical and natural that exogenous carcinogens or cocarcinogens are able to assist this degeneration even further (Kúta, 1967).

Based on the literature mentioned above, and the facts or pathophysiologic connections quoted, one might range chronic discoid lupus erythematosus among the facultative or precancerous lesions in a broader sense (Steigleder, (1963). This should be kept in mind

when starting therapy, and any irritating local treatment should be avoided, including x-rays, especially because epitheliomas in this terrain are extraordinarily resistant to x-rays (Landi and Nardi, 1961).

POROKERATOSIS MIBELLI

Observations of carcinomatous degeneration of porokeratosis Mibelli (PM) are found more and more in the literature, especially in recent years.

In 1931 Moncorps, in his elaborate monograph on PM, was able to mention only one single case of this type, which Lombardo had described in 1907: a squamous cell carcinoma of the skin in an area of porokeratosis on the extensor surface of the right wrist of a patient aged 56.

Observations to follow only several years later were made by Vigne (1942), Lovel and Puchol (1947), Smith (1950), Gandola (1951), Savage and Lederer (1951), Rodin (1953), Johnston (1958), Beurey et al. (1961), Bazex et al. (1965), Kúta (1965), Ciaula (1966), Bazex and Dupré (1968), Oberste-Lehn and Moll (1968), Degos et al. (1970), and Ehlers and Rothe (1971).

In view of the rather infrequent occurrence of PM, these observations cannot be considered merely accidental. In addition, carcinomatous degeneration of this dermatosis is mainly possible because of the nature of the underlying pathologic process. In order to clarify the pathogenetic situation, we shall discuss the essential features of PM, which by now are quite well known.

The cutaneous lesions in PM occur mostly on the extremities, particularly on the exposed extensor surfaces. Rather frequently, however, head and genitals are affected too. Involvement of the mucous membranes is less frequent, and involvement of the cornea is exceptional (Kiessling, 1952).

Detailed histomorphologic analysis of these initial lesions, on the basis of biopsies taken from the periphery of the flat, widespread plaques, established that the pathologic cellular changes at this stage of the process are practically always located in the hair follicles, and that the changes occur in the walls of the hair follicles, and only exceptionally in the sweat pores (Kúta, 1965).

Even in the initial intrafollicular manifestations, the development of the disease reveals all the characteristics of a primary epidermal hyper-regenerative to proliferative process (see also Pinkus), accompanied by a peculiar impairment of keratinization, characteristic of PM: the so-called cornoid lamella (Fig. 55–6). Subsequently, the epidermis becomes involved, and through simultaneous central regression and atrophy the characteristic changes of PM are produced.

To clarify the pathogenetic connections (PM and carcinoma), the following may be said here: microscopically two significant pathologic features stand out: acanthosis and hyperkeratosis with a marked focal dyskeratinization. The same features—though in a different presentation—are also found in the cellular structures of

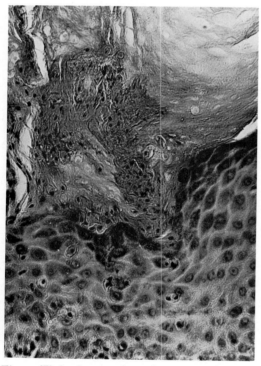

Figure 55–6 Cross-section of cornoid lamella in porokeratosis Mibelli. The compact cornoid body emerges from the stratum spinosum. The granular layer is partially defective. In the stratum spinosum are signs of dyskeratosis (grains).

dermatoses known as obligatory precanceroses of the skin (Melczer, 1961) or primary epidermal precancerous stages (Kúta, 1960 and 1965) (keratosis senilis and the other actinic keratoses, arsenic keratoses, tar keratoses, and epidermodysplasia verruciformis). With these two histologic features alone, PM is very close to the precanceroses of the skin. This should be reason enough to consider the possibility of malignant degeneration in this process (see also Moncorps, 1931).

The two histopathologic features of the obligatory precancerous lesions of the skin (progressive acanthosis, degenerative dyskeratosis) may be explained by the chronic effect of some carcinogenic factors: ultraviolet light and x-rays, arsenic, tar and its components, and viruses (e.g., epidermodysplasia verruciformis of Lewandowsky-Lutz) (see Chapter 24). This effect partly causes irritation (acanthosis) and partly damage to the more sensitive cells (dyskeratosis). With the continuous effect of a carcinogen in this terrain, or with an additional different or banal factor, the hyperregenerative process, so far still reversible, may enter a new stage, i.e., autonomous malignant tumor growth. This happens gradually and is at first histomorphologically unnoticeable, until finally there are clear signs of a malignant proliferation: distinct cellular polymorphism and marked atypical mitoses.

The obligatory presence of atrophy in the porokeratosis foci and the degenerative changes in the upper corium, although the latter are secondary, are important for the process of cancerization in PM (Ehlers and Rothe, 1971). These superficial intradermal changes may even favor the process of cancerization.

The clinical features of PM reveal striking analogies with proliferative epithelial processes of viral etiology (Kúta, 1960 and 1965). In this connection the epidermodysplasia verruciformis should be mentioned. More recently, the viral etiology of this disease has been demonstrated (Ruiter and van Mullen, 1966; Baker, 1968; Jablonska et al., 1968). In epidermodysplasia verruciformis, malignant degeneration of the verrucous changes of the skin is practically obligatory, especially in sun-exposed areas, where squamous cell carcinomas appear. Doubtless the epitheliomatous structures of epidermodysplasia represent a sensitive terrain, in which ultraviolet light can have a carcinogenic effect. The same etiopathogenetic explanation of malignant degeneration may be assumed for PM in sun-exposed areas.

Lately the so-called "disseminated superficial actinic porokeratosis" has been mentioned as a peculiar, actinically provoked, and highly light-sensitive form of this disease (e.g., Chernosky and Freeman, 1967). According to our own observations, in this form the differential diagnosis of scattered arsenical keratoses has to be considered (Kúta, 1960 and 1965).

Most of the observations made so far on malignant degeneration in PM can be explained by the carcinogenic effect or the associated effect of ultraviolet rays. The known biologic activity of x-rays should always be taken into account in porokera-

tosis lesions treated previously with irradiation. Other factors (chronic chemical and mechanical irritation, maceration), however, may doubtless stimulate the malignant degeneration of porokeratosis, as mentioned in some of the observations described above.

In practically all cases of malignant degeneration of porokeratosis published so far, a squamous cell carcinoma developed in this terrain. Fully developed invasive squamous cell carcinomas with nuclear pleomorphism (e.g., Ehlers and Rothe, 1971; Figs. 55–7 to 55–9), as well as bowenoid carcinomas which are still intraepidermal but with regard to the cells unequivocal, were described (Kúta, 1960 and 1965; Bazex and Dupré, 1968), this would be in accordance with the carcinogenesis of porokeratosis mentioned above. The occurrence of basal cell epitheliomas in porokeratosis is mentioned as an exception (Bazex and Dupré, 1968).

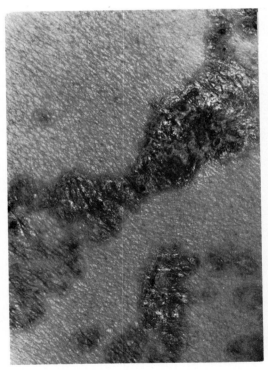

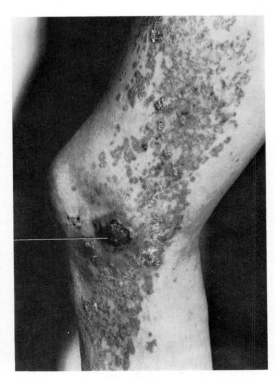

Fig. 55–7   Fig. 55–8

Figure 55–7   Porokeratosis Mibelli with malignant transformation. In central part of atrophic area there is bowenoid senile keratosis. (Courtesy of Prof. G. Ehlers, Munich.)

Figure 55–8   Porokeratosis Mibelli with squamous cell carcinoma. Malignant epithelial tumor in the porokeratosis Mibelli zoniformis. Biopsy revealed squamous cell carcinomas (see Fig. 55–9). (Courtesy of Prof. G. Ehlers, Munich.)

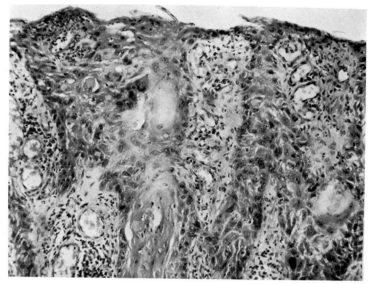

Figure 55–9 Squamous cell carcinoma in porokeratosis Mibelli. Biopsy of epithelial tumor from Fig. 55–8. Neoplastic proliferation of the prickle cells of the rete mucosum with numerous mitotic figures and abnormalities in size and shape of the cells; monocellular keratinization. (Courtesy of Prof. G. Ehlers, Munich.)

In our own observation of a basal cell epithelioma in the skin of the trunk in the sacral region of a female patient with disseminated, superficial actinic PM, which was treated with arsenic according to the anamnesis, there seems to have been a combination or coincidence of two processes—PM and arsenic–basal cell epithelioma—rather than a true degeneration of the porokeratosis (Figs. 55–10 and 55–11).

The above mentioned malignant degeneration and all other characteristics of the disease would make PM a precancerosis in the broader sense (according to the classification by Steigleder-Miescher).

ACRODERMATITIS CHRONICA ATROPHICANS HERXHEIMER

It is known that, in the terrain of acrodermatitis chronica atrophicans Herxheimer, intradermal, i.e., mesenchymal, hyper-regenerative changes (fibrous nodes, scleroderma-like lesions or band-like collagenous hyperplasia) and truly be-

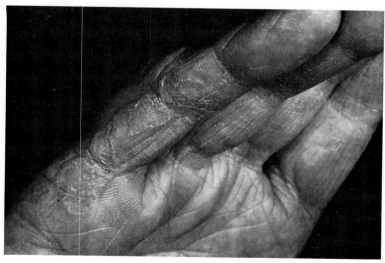

Figure 55–10   Porokeratosis Mibelli. A characteristic lesion on the right hand. (Courtesy of Prof. G. K. Steigleder, Köln.)

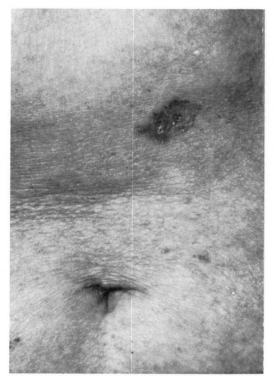

Figure 55–11   Basal cell carcinoma in a patient with porokeratosis Mibelli (see Fig. 55–10). (Courtesy of Prof. G. K. Steigleder, Köln.)

nign (fibromas, lymphocytomas) as well as malignant tumors (sarcomas, lymphosarcomas, and reticulosarcomas) can occur (Gans and Steigleder, 1955; Helle, 1959; Herzberg, 1952).

It is only in recent years that observations of carcinomas have been reported (Swanbeck and Hillström, 1970; Lagerholm et al., 1970). In their statistical review of incidence and localization of the carcinomas, Swanbeck and Hillström found eight squamous cell carcinomas in this terrain. Seven of these were localized on the lower legs, and only one squamous cell carcinoma was found on the hand. In this connection we may mention our own observation of a grade I squamous cell carcinoma on a massive hyperkeratosis in the region of the inner malleolus (Fig. 55–12). According to our knowledge, only one single observation of a basal cell epithelioma is mentioned in the literature (Lagerholm et al., 1970): a superficial basal cell epithelioma on the left

thigh. Even though until now observations of this kind in the literature have been rather infrequent, the carcinomatous degeneration of Herxheimer's acrodermatitis chronica atrophicans is not unusual. Particularly since the underlying conditions mentioned in the section on chronic discoid lupus erythematosus are valid also for acrodermatitis chronica atrophicans (atrophy, hypoxidosis), the possibility of cancerization must be taken into account.

The study by Swanbeck and Hillström (1970) of the localization of carcinomas on the lower extremities mentions that 7 out of 157 patients had acrodermatitis chronica atrophicans. The authors therefore believe that, at least in Sweden, Herxheimer's acrodermatitis chronica atrophicans is the dermatosis which most favors the development of squamous cell carcinomas. It would be followed by stasis ulcers of the leg (see below).

The same authors found a squamous cell carcinoma in one case of scleroderma on the lower leg. No other reference to the occurrence of carcinoma with scleroderma could be found in the literature.

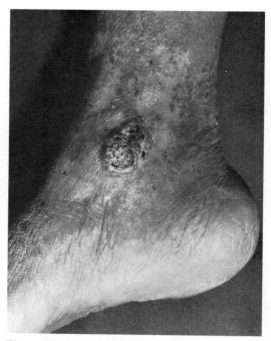

Figure 55–12   Squamous cell carcinoma (in situ) on the ground of keratoma in terrain of acrodermatitis chronica atrophicans Herxheimer. (Skin Clinic, Darmstadt.)

LICHEN SCLEROSUS ET ATROPHICUS

No carcinomas have been described in lichen sclerosus et atrophicus of the skin, in contrast to that of the mucous membranes or the transitional mucous membrane. Lichen sclerosus et atrophicus of the male genitals which has also been described as balanitis xerotica obliterans of Stühmer and as kraurosis penis et praeputii Del Banco, and which since has been found to be identical with lichen sclerosus et atrophicus, may lead to the development of squamous cell carcinomas, particularly in case of noncircumcision (Hauser, 1958; Stühmer, 1958; Frühwald, 1931 and 1935; Grütz, 1937). The possibility of this degeneration is increased if in lichen sclerosus of the genital region there are proliferative epithelial changes like those seen in leukoplakia or leukokeratosis (leukoplakia-kraurosis). In this context it is interesting that Marchionini (1953) did not find lichen sclerosus of the male genitalia in circumcised patients in Turkey.

As for the female genitals, the identity of lichen sclerosus et atrophicus with kraurosis vulvae has been confirmed by numerous authors (Laymon and Freeman, 1944; Pillsbury et al., 1961; Steigleder and Raab, 1961; Grimmer, 1967a, 1967b, and 1967c). Grimmer believed that a carcinoma on a lichen sclerosus of the vulva occurs only through hyperplastic epithelial changes, as in leukoplakia. In this process cocarcinogenic factors, such as those discussed in lichen planus of the oral mucosa (chronic irritation, inflammation, candidiasis, and radiotherapy), play a cumulative role. It is doubtful that the relation of the vulva to the hormonal system plays a part in the tendency toward malignancy, as is assumed by Wallace and Whimster (1951), because carcinomas in lichen sclerosus are also observed in menopausal women. We have observed a basal cell epithelioma in a kraurosis vulvae in a female patient aged 76. The peculiarity of this observation is the fact that this was a basal cell epithelioma and not a squamous cell carcinoma, as is usually the case.

Over a follow-up period of five years, Grimmer observed one squamous cell car-

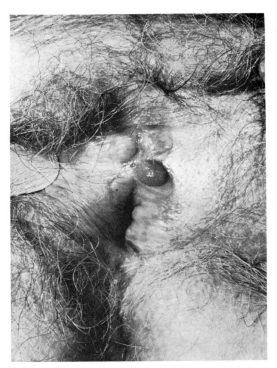

Figure 55–13 Squamous cell carcinoma in lichen sclerosus et atrophicus of the vulva. (Courtesy of Prof. H. Grimmer, Wiesbaden.)

cinoma in lichen sclerosus of the vulva (Figs. 55–13 and 55–14) and one case of Bowen's disease in 57 female patients with lichen sclerosus et atrophicus of the genital region. According to a survey by Suurmond (1964), which Grimmer supplemented in 1967, the incidence of carcinoma in 962 cases of lichen sclerosus et atrophicus was 16 percent. In spite of this, Grimmer hesitates to regard lichen sclerosus et atrophicus of the genitalia as a precancerosis unless there are leukoplakia-like or leukokeratotic changes present. Steigleder (1963), however, is ranging lichen sclerosus et atrophicus among the precanceroses in a broader sense (see Chapter 26).

ULCUS CRURIS

If one considers the extraordinary frequency of the varicose and post-thrombotic symptoms, the incidence of carcinomatous degeneration of ulcus cruris is rare. According to Sigg (1958 and 1967),

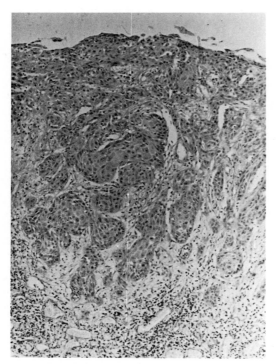

Figure 55–14   Biopsy of squamous cell carcinoma seen in Fig. 55–13. (Courtesy of Prof. H. Grimmer, Wiesbaden.)

about 15 percent of the population is suffering from varicose veins and 0.5 percent from leg ulcers. Fischer (1961) and Sigg stated that the percentage of carcinomas in ulcus cruris is less than 0.1 percent. Until 1928, Muchra and Mras had compiled about 80 cases of carcinomas in ulcus cruris. Fischer reported 113 cases until 1961. In 200 ulcers of the leg, Nobl (1928) could observe only one carcinoma, and Sigg only one carcinoma in 6500 ulcers. Maerz (1957), too, could remember only one or two malignant degenerations among thousands of ulcera cruris. Van der Molen and Lukkes put the percentage of "malignant ulcers of the leg" at nearly 0.06 percent, as compared with all other carcinomas.

The uncertainty in the catamnestic recording of carcinomas in ulcus cruris and the varying results may be due to the lack of a distinct definition of the ulcers. Thus, statistics of carcinoma in ulcus cruris also include frostbite ulcers, osteomyelitis, burns, lupus, and syphilis (Fischer, 1961).

Varicose symptoms or the post-thrombosis syndrome are not mentioned in this context. This becomes obvious in the study by Swanbeck and Hillström (1969), who are concerned, however, only with the incidence of squamous cell carcinomas on the lower leg. In 143 patients with squamous cell carcinoma on the lower extremity, the so-called hypostatic ulcers could not be separated with certainty and therefore were ranged among the group of nonspecific ulcers.

The above authors found 68 ulcers with carcinomas on the lower extremity, 19 in male and 49 in female patients. Proceeding on the assumption that the sex incidence of the varicose ulcer is 4:1 (female:male), according to Fischer (1961), this nearly coincides with the ratio established by the authors. The time required from the onset of the ulcer to the growth of carcinoma also gives a certain lead to the pathogenesis. Malignant degeneration seems to occur earlier after burns, mechanical trauma, and osteomyelitis than it does in hypostatic ulcers of the lower leg (Swanbeck and Hillström, 1969). According to van der Molen (1962), the danger of malignant degeneration is present if the varicose ulcers have been present for more than 10 years (see also Schneider and Fischer, 1969). Fischer found an ulcer of less than five years' duration only in two cases. Swanbeck and Hillström were able to demonstrate that the incidence of carcinomas on the lower leg markedly increases with age; the peak is reached in the age group between 70 and 80 years, while in the case of carcinomas developing in other diseases, the peak is reached earlier. According to Fischer, the highest percentage of 61.8 percent is reached in the age group of 60 to 70 years. Obviously the ulcus cruris has a predisposition for malignant growths of various types. The simultaneous occurrence of squamous cell carcinoma and fibrous sarcoma is reported by Knoth and Lanz (1955). Schulz and Schüller (1969) found a carcinoma simultaneously with a fibrosarcoma which, starting from the periosteum of the tibia, probably triggered the degeneration of the ulcus, while the squamous cell carcinoma developed multilocularly on the margin of the ulcus. Black (1962) found a fibrosarcoma and an osteosarcoma. Similar evidence was produced by van der Molen (1962) (metastasizing sarcoma on an ulcer after thrombosis) and Rodermund (1964) (reticulum cell sarcoma on a varicose ulcer). In a survey Fischer found 94 percent carcinomas and 6 percent sarcomas. However, fibroepithelioma (Ebner and Niebauer, 1967) and one cylindroma (Hübschmann and Jedlicka, 1940) have also been found on an ulcus cruris. Most of the observations refer to squamous cell carcinomas (Albertazzi et al., 1967; Fischer, 1961; Nödl, 1953) (Figs. 55–15 to 55–17). Metastases with bone involvement are possible and are responsible for a mortality rate of about 10 percent, while for the rest the prognosis is relatively favorable (Fischer, 1961). Frequently the malignant tumor growth starts on the papillomatous-verrucous hyperplasia, as observed by van der Molen and Lukkes (1962), who report a benign papillomatous tumor developing on a varicose ulcer which had been recurring for 10 years; the tumor developed into a squamous cell carcinoma. Kuske

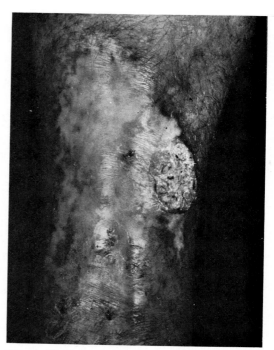

Figure 55–16 Squamous cell carcinoma in an atrophic lesion in ulcus cruris. (Courtesy of Prof. T. Nasemann, Frankfurt/M.)

and Soltermann (1957) found on an ulcer of 23 years' duration a nonspecific cauliflower-like granulation tissue. This was thought to be a pseudoepitheliomatous epidermal proliferation. The defect was excised and covered with a graft; immediately after that a squamous cell carcinoma developed. Pages et al. (1964) observed a malignant melanoma on a post-traumatic ulcer. Van der Molen and Lukkes (1962), too, reported a melanoma on an ulcus cruris. We saw a malignant melanoma developing two years after onset of an ulcus cruris in a woman aged 76. Multiple cauliflower-like metastases on the lower leg and inguinal lymph node metastases were present. Observation over a period of one year did not reveal further progression to this day.

The development of carcinomas in ulcus cruris is progressive from normal proliferative processes on the margins of the ulcers to atypical epithelial proliferation to pseudocarcinomatous changes and finally to carcinoma. The starting point is the margin of the ulcer. Gans and Steigleder (1957) emphasized the difficulty of histologic differentiation between

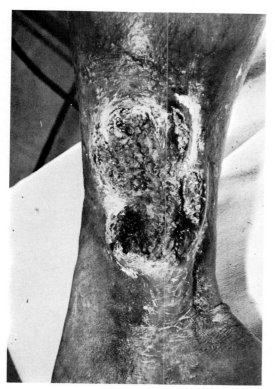

Figure 55–15 Squamous cell carcinoma in ulcus cruris. (Courtesy of Prof. T. Nasemann, Frankfurt/M.)

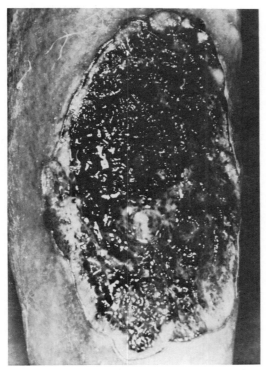

Figure 55–17 Squamous cell carcinoma in ulcus cruris. (Courtesy of Prof. F. Nödl, Homburg/Saar.)

atypical epithelial proliferation and carcinomatous changes. In the epithelial proliferation, the deep portions of the varicose ulcer corresponding to the collagen bundles remain mostly unaffected. The cancerous proliferation is limited to the upper dermis.

The chronic inflammation and the sclero-atrophic-hypoxemic environment of the ulcer are of decisive significance, the marked atrophy representing one of the essential preconditions for malignant degeneration. The rare carcinomas forming in the center of the ulcer develop from pseudoepitheliomatous, cauliflower-like proliferations (Black, 1962; Nödl, 1953). It is certainly justified to count the varicose or post-thrombotic ulcer as well as other ulcerations of the lower leg of the post-traumatic type and ulcers formed through chronic inflammatory changes (osteomyelitis) among the facultative precanceroses.

LEPROSY

Occurrence of carcinomas in syphilis and tuberculosis is known. It is therefore not too surprising that malignant tumors also not infrequently occur in leprosy. Klingmüller (1970) cited the incidence of carcinoma in leprosy as 1.72 percent (see also Terencio de las Aguas, 1970). Michalany (1967) cited the rate at 1 percent. Until 1966, this author had observed 94 carcinomas and identified 539 cases from a vast histologic material. This list included internal carcinomas, however. Until 1965, Keil observed 85 cases of carcinoma in leprosy. The author made the interesting observation that the incidence of squamous cell carcinoma as compared to basal cell epithelioma is nearly equal. Less frequently Bowen's disease, melanoma, and sarcoma are observed. The frequency of malignant neoplasms and the type of tumor seem to be coincidental, as is borne out by single observations; for example, Tarabini et al. (1960) reported an ulcus rodens in a female leprosy patient aged 63, who had had basal cell epitheliomas before contracting leprosy. The mucous membrane, too, can be affected (Asano, 1959; basal cell epithelioma on the tongue). Michalany (1967) pointed out that intense sun exposure might play a role, because most of the lepra patients with carcinoma are white farm laborers in a leprosary and the epitheliomas predominantly occur on the exposed parts of the body (Fig. 55–18).

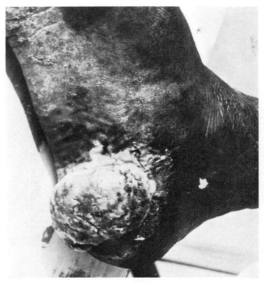

Figure 55–18 Melanoma in leprosy. (Courtesy of Prof. G. Klingmüller, Bonn.)

Job and Riedel (1970) and Riedel (1967) described six cases of squamous cell carcinoma on plantar ulcers in the anesthetic region in lepra patients. All ulcers were of more than five years' duration. According to Klingmüller (1970), the chronic irritation provokes the formation of malignant tumors. It is interesting that the carcinomas show a preference for lepromatous leprosy. In the compilation by Keil (1965), carcinoma occurred in lepromatous leprosy in 45 cases, while there were only 18 cases each in indeterminate and tuberculoid leprosy. This author is of the opinion that the better immunity in tuberculoid leprosy might give some protection, while nonspecific immunologic insufficiency in hypoergic and anergic lepromatous leprosy also favors the growth of carcinomas. Michalany (1967) and Terencio de las Aguas (1970)—the latter in 95 percent of the cases—confirmed the greater incidence in lepromatous leprosy. Histologically (Tarabini et al., 1960) the carcinomas (squamous cell carcinomas and basal cell epitheliomas) invade the lepromatous tissue, while the Virchow's cells do not participate in the process.

A violent stroma reaction is always present; the tumor cells and Virchow's cells are disposed at random. In some cases the Virchow's cell is surrounded by the tumor cells.

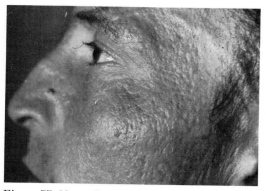

Figure 55–20   Follicular atrophodermia of the face. (Courtesy of Prof. A. Dupré, Toulouse.)

FOLLICULAR ATROPHODERMIA, WITH BASAL CELL EPITHELIOMAS AND HYPOTRICHOSIS

In 1966, Bazex and Dupré observed a peculiar clinical picture, occurring in six members of one family. The major symptom of the disease was hypotrichosis in all of the affected persons, with main localization in the region of the first cervical vertebra and the auriculotemporal regions. The eyebrows were missing, and the eyelashes were rudimentary. An essential second symptom was a follicular atrophodermia, especially of the dorsum of the hand and foot and of the face, here mainly on the cheeks (Figs. 55–19 and 55–20). These were dotlike depressions in the center of the sebaceous glands. The third symptom was basal cell epitheliomas on the face, predominantly in the region

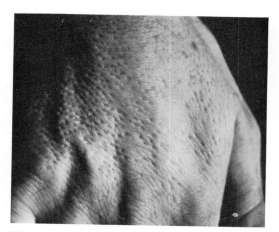

Figure 55–19   Follicular atrophodermia of the hand. (Courtesy of Prof. A. Dupré, Toulouse.)

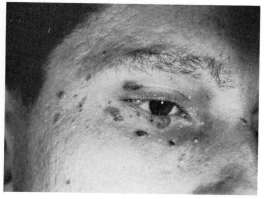

Figure 55–21   Basal cell epitheliomas in the region of the eyelids. (Courtesy of Prof. A. Dupré, Toulouse.)

of the upper and lower eyelids (Fig. 55–21) but also on the forearms and on the dorsa of the hands. A fourth symptom was a hypo- or anhidrosis of the face. With the help of the genealogic tree, the authors were able to establish a dominant hereditary line with preference to the male sex. Obviously this was a phakomatosis, in which, beside the symptoms of ectodermal dysplasia (hypotrichosis, atrophodermia, anhidrosis), a special proneness to basal cell epitheliomas was present.

REFERENCES

Psoriasis

Alexander, A.: Arch. Dermatol. Syph. (Berl.), 129:5, 1921.
Bild: Cited by Melczer (1961).
Biltz, G.: Dermatol. Wochenschr., 128:667, 1953.
Burgener, J.: Dermatologica, 80:86, 1939.
Fierz, U.: Arch. Klin. Exp. Dermatol., 227:286, 1966.
Fuss, S.: Z. Haut. Geschlechtskr., 41:550, 1932.
Goodman, H., and Brice, C.: Arch. Phys. Ther. (Omaha), 11:209, 1930.
Goodman, H., Alexander, O. B., and Macrosson, K. J.: Br. Med. J., 4896:1089, 1954.
Grüneberg, T.: Psoriasis vulg. *In* Gottron, H. A., and Schönfeld, W.: Dermatologie und Venerologie. Bd. 21. Stuttgart, Thieme Verlag, 1958.
Hutchinson, J.: Br. Med. J., 11:1280, 1887.
Kleine-Natrop, H. E.: Hautarzt, 10:224, 1959.
Knoth, W.: Arch. Klin. u. Exp. Dermatol., 227:228, 1966.
Kromeyer, E.: Z. Haut. Geschlechtskr., 62:612, 1938.
Lagerholm, B., and Skog, E.: Acta Derm. Venereol. (Stockh.), 48:128, 1968.
Melczer, N.: Praecancerosen und primäre Krebse der Haut. Budapest, Verlag der Ungarischen Akademie der Wissenschaften, 1961.
Nexmand, P. H.: Cited by Melczer (1961).
Pozzi: Cited by Unna, Memmesheimer, and Herzberg, (1963).
Sommer, S. C., and McManus, R. G.: Cancer, 6:347, 1953.
Unna, P. J., Memmesheimer, A., Jr., and Herzberg, J. J.: Das Carcinom bei Psoriasis vulgaris—post hoc oder propter hoc? Mit 4 Kasuistischen Beiträgen. Arch. Klin. Exp. Dermatol., 217:321, 1963.
White, E.: Cited by Melczer (1961).

Eczema

Hillström, L., and Swanbeck, G.: Acta Derm. Venereol. (Stockh.), 49:427, 1969.
Hillström, L., and Swanbeck, G.: Acta Derm. Venereol. (Stockh.), 50:129, 1970a.
Hillström, L., and Swanbeck, G.: Acta Derm. Venereol. (Stockh.), 50:350, 1970b.

Lichen Planus

Brennan, B. B., and Teplitz, R.: Arch. Dermatol., 77:332, 1958.

Bureau, Y., Barrière, H., Litoux, P., and Bureau, B.: Bull. Fr. Dermatol. Syphiligr., 77:128, 1970.
Depaoli, M.: Minerva Dermatol., 38:311, 1963.
Gottron, E.: Dermatol. Wochenschr., 129:462, 1954.
Greither, A.: Arch. Klin. u. Exp. Dermatol., 227:798, 1966.
Greither, A., and Hornstein, O.: Krankheiten der Mundschleimhaut und der Lippen. (H. Schürmann 3. Aufl. München-Berlin, Urban u. Schwarzenberg, 1966.
Hampel, E.: Z. Haut. Geschlechtskr., 65:132, 1940.
Hansen, A.: Acta Derm. Venereol. (Stockh.), 35:225, 1955.
Jänner, M.: Hautarzt, 22:267, 1971.
Jänner, M., Muissus, E., and Rohde, B.: Dermatol. Wochenschr., 153:515, 1967.
Jansen, L. H., and Groothuis, F. B. G.: Ann. Dermatol. Syphiligr. (Paris), 87:371, 1960.
Kronenberg, K., Fretzin, D., and Potter, B.: Arch. Dermatol., 104:304, 1971.
Midana, A., and Depaoli, M.: Minerva Dermatol., 42:447, 1967.
Muissus, E.: Inauguraldissertation, Hamburg, 1966.
Opperbeck, J.: Z. Laryngol. Rhinol. Otol., 50:442, 1971.
Rohde, B.: Arch. Klin. Exp. Dermatol., 227:815, 1966.
Schürmann, H.: Krankheiten der Mundschleimhaut und der Lippen. München-Berlin, Urban u. Schwarzenberg, 1958.

Glossitis Granulomatosa

Hornstein, O.: Hautarzt, 16:90, 1965.

Candida Mycosis of the Oral Mucosa

Degos, R., Touraine, R., Escande, J. P., and Delizant, O.: Ann. Dermatol. Syphiligr. (Paris), 97:361, 1970.
Williamson, D. M.: Br. J. Dermatol., 81:125, 1969.

Lupus Erythematosus

De Feo, C. P.: Arch. Dermatol., 96:474, 1967.
Grana, A.: G. Ital. Dermatol. Sif., 88:416, 1947.
Grana, A.: Rass. Dermatol., 9:435, 1956.
Jadassohn, J.: Mracek Hbch. III, 1904.
Kappesser, W.: Z. Haut. Geschlechtskr., 12:495, 1952.
Kúta, A.: *In* Polak, E., and Kol, A.: Chirurgische Praecancerosen. Prague, SZN, 1967.
Landi, G., and Nardi, S.: Dermatologia (Napoli), 12:215, 1961.
Storck, H., Schnyder, U. W., and Schwarz, K.: Dermatologica, 122:315, 1961.
Vilanova, and Oller Corominas, F.: Act. Dermosifiliogr. (Madr.), 48:352, 1957.

Porokeratosis Mibelli

Baker, H.: Proc. R. Soc. Med., 61:589, 1968.
Bazex, A., and Dupré, A.: Ann. Dermatol. Syphiligr. (Paris), 95:361, 1968.
Bazex, A., Salvador, R., Dupré, A., and Christol, B.: Bull. Soc. Fr. Dermatol. Syphiligr., 72:182, 1965.
Beurey, J., Rousselot, R., and Wolfowicz, G.: Bull. Soc. Fr. Dermatol. Syphiligr., 68:653, 1961.
Chernosky, M., and Freemann, R.: Arch. Dermatol., 96:611, 1967.
Ciaula, U.: Minerva Dermatol., 41:354, 1966.
Degos, R., Delort, J., Duterge, M., and Schnitzler, R.: Bull. Soc. Fr. Dermatol. Syphiligr., 77:24, 1970.

Ehlers, C., and Rothe, A.: Hautarzt, 22:68, 1971.

Gandola, M.: Boll. Soc. Med. Chir. Pavia, 64:273, 1951. (Ref. Z. Haut. Geschlechtskr., 80:370, 1952.)

Jablonska, S., Biczysko, W., Jakubowicz, J., and Dabrowski, J.: Dermatologica, 137:113, 1968.

Johnston, E.: Br. J. Dermatol., 70:381, 1958.

Kiessling, W.: Dermatol. Wochenschr., 126:1168, 1952.

Kúta, A.: Porokeratosis Mibelli Respighi. Prague, Publ. House of the Czechosl. Academy of Sciences, 1965.

Kúta, A.: Acta Univ. Carol. [Med.] (Praha), Suppl. 10:200, 1960.

Lombardo, G.: G. Ital. Mal. Vener., 48:699, 1907. Cited by Moncorps (1931).

Lovel, A., and Puchol, J.: Act. Dermo-sifiliogr. (Madr.), 38:929, 1947.

Melczer, J.: Praekancerosen und primäre Krebse der Haut. Budapest, Verlag der ungarischen Akademie der Wissenschaften, 1961.

Miescher, Q.: Arch. Dermatol. Syph. (Berl.), 181:532, 1941.

Moncorps, C.: *In* Handbuch der Haut- und Geschlechtskrankheiten. VIII, 2:463, Berlin, Springer-Verlag, 1931.

Oberste-Lehn, H., and Moll, B.: Hautarzt, 19:399, 1968.

Pinkus, H.: Cited by Ehlers and Rothe (1971).

Rodin, H.: Arch. Dermatol., 67:526, 1953.

Ruiter, M., and van Mullem, P. J.: J. Invest. Dermatol., 47:247, 1966.

Savage, J., and Lederer, H.: Br. J. Dermatol., 63:187, 1951.

Smith, P.: Cited in Bazex and Dupré (1968).

Vigne, P.: Ann. Dermatol., 8:5, 1942.

Acrodermatitis Chronica Atrophicans Herxheimer

Gans, O., and Steigleder, G. K.: Histologie der Hautkrankheiten. Berlin, Springer-Verlag, 1955.

Helle, J.: Acta Derm. Venereol. (Stockh.), 39:58, 1959.

Herzberg, J. J.: Dermatol. Wochenschr., 125:422, 1952.

Lagerholm, B., Molin, L., and Gip, L.: Acta Derm. Venereol. (Stockh.), 50:218, 1970.

Swanbeck, G., and Hillström, L.: Acta Derm. Venereol. (Stockh.), 50:350, 1970.

Lichen Sclerosus et Atrophicus

Frühwald, R.: Z. Haut. Geschlechtskr., 35:605, 1931.

Frühwald, R.: Z. Haut. Geschlechtskr., 50:98, 1935.

Grimmer, H.: Z. Haut. Geschlechtskr., 42:19, 1967a.

Grimmer, H.: Z. Haut. Geschlechtskr., 42:113, 1967b.

Grimmer, H.: Z. Haut. Geschlechtskr., 42:121, 1967c.

Grütz, O.: Dermatol. Wochenschr., 105:1206, 1937.

Hauser, W.: Atrophien: Dermatologie und Venerologie, Gottron-Schönfeld, Band 2, Teil 2, Stuttgart, Thieme Verlag, 1958.

Laymon, C. W., and Freeman, C.: Arch. Dermatol., 49:57, 1944.

Marchionini, A.: Hautarzt, 4:409, 1953.

Montgomery, H., and Hill, W. R.: Arch. Dermatol., 42:755, 1940.

Pillsbury, D. M., Shelley, W. B., and Kligman, A. M.: Manual of Cutaneous Medicine. Philadelphia, W. B. Saunders Company, 1961.

Steigleder, G. K.: Hautarzt, 14:87, 1963.

Steigleder, G. K., and Raab, W. B.: Arch. Dermatol. Syph., 84:219, 1961.

Stühmer, A.: Cited by Hauser (1958).

Suurmond, D.: Arch. Dermatol., 90:143, 1964.

Wallace, H. J., and Whimster, J. W.: Br. J. Dermatol., 63:241, 1951.

Ulcus Cruris

Albertazzi, F., Leigheb, G., and Visetti, M.: Minerva Dermatol., 42:213, 1967.

Black, W.: Br. J. Cancer, 6:120, 1962.

Ebner, H., and Niebauer, G.: Z. Haut. Geschlechtskr., 42:417, 1967.

Fischer, H.: Hautarzt, 12:548, 1961.

Gans, O., and Steigleder, G. K.: Histologie der Hautkrankheiten. Bd. II, 2. Aufl. 393. Berlin, Springer-Verlag, 1957.

Hübschmann, K., and Jedlicka, V.: Acta Derm. Venereol. (Stockh.), 21:239, 1940.

Knoth, W., and Lanz, W.: Dermatol. Wochenschr., 131:569, 1955.

Kuske, H., and Soltermann, W.: Dermatologica, 115:758, 1957.

Maerz, F. R.: Die ambulante Behandlung des varikösen Symptomenkomplexes. Stuttgart, Gustav Fischer Verlag, 1957.

Muchra, V., and Mras, F.: *In* Jadassohn's Handbuch der Haut- und Geschlechtskrankheiten. VI, 2:441, Berlin, Springer-Verlag, 1928.

Nobl, G.: Cited by Muchra and Mras (1928).

Nödl, F.: Z. Haut. Geschlechtskr., 15:256, 1953.

Pages, F., Lapeyre, J., Many, P., and Misson, R.: Bull. Soc. Fr. Dermatol. Syphiligr., 716:701, 1964.

Rodermund, O. E.: Z. Haut. Geschlechtskr., 36:1, 1964.

Schneider, W., and Fischer, H.: Die chronisch venöse Insuffizienz. Stuttgart, Ferdinand Enke Verlag, 1969, p. 128.

Schulz, H., and Schüller, W.: Chirurg, 40:138, 1969.

Sigg, K.: Varizen, Ulcus cruris und Thrombose. Berlin, Springer-Verlag, 1958.

Sigg, K.: Beinleiden, Entstehung und Behandlung. Berlin, Springer-Verlag, 1967.

Swanbeck, G., and Hillström, L.: Acta Derm. Venereol. (Stockh.), 49:427, 1969.

van der Molen, H. R., and Lukkes, J.: Zentralb. Phlebol., 1:139, 1962.

Leprosy

Asano, M.: Z. Haut. Geschlechtskr., 103:69, 1959.

Job, C. K., and Riedel, R. G.: Cited by Klingmüller (1970).

Keil, E.: Krebsarzt, 20:269, 1965.

Klingmüller, G.: *In* Jadassohn's Handbuch der Haut- und Geschlechtskrankheiten. VI, 1B:330, Berlin, Springer-Verlag, 1970.

Michalany, J.: Ref. Z. Haut. Geschlechtskr., 122:557, 1967.

Riedel, R. G.: Ref. Z. Haut. Geschlechtskr., 122:557, 1967.

Tarabini, G., Sotelo, C., and Contreras, F.: Ref. Z. Haut. Geschlechtskr., 106:124, 1960.

Terencio de las Aguas: Cited by Klingmüller (1970).

Follicular Atrophodermia, With Basal Cell Epitheliomas and Hypotrichosis

Bazex, A., Dupré, A., and Christol, B.: Ann. Dermatol. Syphiligr. (Paris), 93:241, 1966.

56

Skin Lesions and Internal Carcinoma

Helen Ollendorff Curth, M.D.

In the discussion of benign (Table 56–1), premalignant (Table 56–2), or malignant cutaneous lesions associated with internal carcinoma, we shall disregard cutaneous metastases of malignant internal tumors.

Since the time that I began in the course of studies on acanthosis nigricans

to investigate the relationship between benign dermatoses and malignant internal tumors, an increasing number of dermatologic conditions related to malignant internal tumors has been reported. Part of this increase is real and based on greater knowledge of dermatoses and the associated tumors; another part, however, is spurious. The great enthusiasm which comes from having discovered yet another association of a benign dermatosis with a malignant tumor sometimes masks the possibility that certain associations have occurred by chance.

A causal relationship between a dermatosis and a malignant internal disease exists when the following criteria are fulfilled:

1. Both conditions start at about the same time (i.e., dermatomyositis).

TABLE 56–1 BENIGN DERMATOSES ASSOCIATED WITH INTERNAL CARCINOMA

"Malignant" acanthosis nigricans
Dermatomyositis
Malignant down
Flushing
Tylosis palmaris et plantaris
Punctate palmar keratoses
Alopecia mucinosa
Acquired ichthyosis
Erythema gyratum repens and Erythema annulare centrifugum
Acquired pachydermoperiostosis
Reticulohistiocytoma
Gardner's syndrome
The Peutz-Jeghers-Touraine syndrome
Arsenical keratoses
Herpes zoster
Dermatitis herpetiformis
Pemphigoid

TABLE 56–2 PREMALIGNANT DERMATOSES ASSOCIATED WITH INTERNAL CARCINOMA

Bowen's disease
Extramammary Paget's disease
Psoriasiform acrokeratosis (Bazex)

2. Both conditions follow a parallel course (i.e., malignant acanthosis nigricans).

3. In certain syndromes neither the course nor the onset of one of the two manifestations is dependent on those of the other manifestation, because the two conditions are part of a genetic syndrome and are therefore coordinated with each other (i.e., Gardner's syndrome).

4. It is a specific tumor (i.e., adenocarcinoma in malignant acanthosis nigricans) which occurs in connection with a certain dermatosis.

5. The dermatosis is usually not common (i.e., erythema gyratum repens).

6. A high percentage of the association of the two conditions is noted (i.e., reticulohistiocytoma).

Such a syndrome will, if one searches further, either fulfill criteria 1, 2, 4, or 5 or show a genetic basis as postulated in criterion 3.

Attempts at classification of the conditions to be dealt with have been unsuccessful because of a lack of knowledge of the mechanism which produces the tumor or the dermatosis. Which factor comes first? If it is the tumor, we would have to conclude that, for example, in cases of malignant acanthosis nigricans which may precede the cancer by about 15 years, the tumor has been present in some form in order to induce the cutaneous manifestation. Is a special genetic make-up of the cancerous patient necessary so that the dermatosis will "take"? Or is this cancer a special one and different from the cancer in those other instances in which no dermatosis is associated with it, such as the internal adenocarcinoma without malignant acanthosis nigricans? Are perhaps both needed—the genetic make-up and a special cancer—for the syndrome of malignant acanthosis nigricans and cancer? Could it be the cutaneous manifestation that induces the cancer? A few dermatoses result from the secretion of the tumor; for example, flushing and its sequelae are due to a malignant carcinoid. In certain syndromes the primary internal manifestation is benign but may become malignant; this occurs rarely in the Peutz-Jeghers syndrome but regularly in Gardner's syndrome.

"MALIGNANT" ACANTHOSIS NIGRICANS

Pollitzer (1890) and Janovsky (1890) described acanthosis nigricans in the same issue of the International Atlas of Rare Skin Diseases. Each author's patient also had a malignant internal tumor and suffered, therefore, from malignant acanthosis nigricans. Not all cases of acanthosis nigricans, however, are associated with a malignant internal tumor. For this reason the disorder has been divided into two types—the malignant form (with tumor) and the benign form (without tumor)—but both were considered variants of one disease. In 1952, Curth concluded that each type constituted a separate disease entity. In 1943, she had shown that the cancer associated with acanthosis nigricans is an adenocarcinoma.

Only the "malignant" type of acanthosis nigricans, one of the four types of acanthosis nigricans (Fig. 56–1), is associated with a malignant internal disorder. The other three types are all benign in the wide sense of the word because they are not associated with a malignant tumor. One distinguishes (1) "benign" acanthosis nigricans, (2) pseudo-acanthosis nigricans, and (3) acanthosis nigricans as part of a syndrome (Curth, 1968).

The presence of a malignant tumor in one of these three types would have to be considered coincidental to acanthosis nigricans.

The axillae and most of the other body folds show hyperpigmented, verrucous, elevated, and confluent ridges (Fig. 56–2). The nipples and the umbilicus are hyperkeratotic and hyperpigmented. The oral mucous membranes show papillomatous, nonpigmented changes. Brown and Winkelmann (1968) reported on edema and inflammation, a velvety hypertrophic quality or diffuse pigmentation of the oral mucous membranes. The palms and soles become keratotic. The skin of the entire body can become affected. The eruption may be accompanied by itching.

The histology of all four types is identical. It shows acanthosis, hyperkeratosis, and hyperpigmentation.

How, then, can one differentiate "malignant" acanthosis nigricans, the poten-

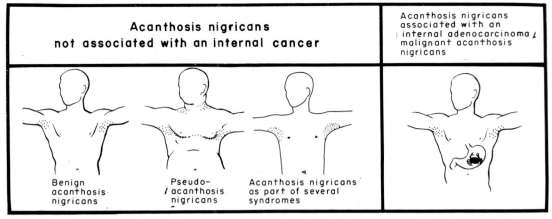

Figure 56–1 The four types of acanthosis nigricans. (*From* Curth: Cutaneous manifestations associated with malignant internal disease. *In* Dermatology in General Medicine. Copyright 1971 by McGraw-Hill, Inc. Used by permission of McGraw-Hill Book Company.)

tially most serious type, from the three other types? This may be done by answering the following questions:

1. *What was the age of the patient at the onset of the dermatosis?* Patients suffering from "malignant" acanthosis nigricans are usually beyond puberty. They are young, middle-aged, or old adults. (It must be added, however, that in a few

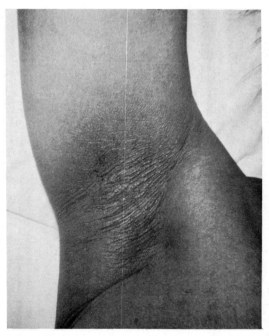

Figure 56–2 Acanthosis nigricans. Axilla of 62 year old black woman suffering from gastric cancer. (See also Color Plate IX–A.)

cases of "malignant" acanthosis nigricans the dermatosis had its onset in childhood.) "Benign" acanthosis nigricans is usually present at birth or starts in childhood. It may begin or have its climax at puberty. Pseudo—acanthosis nigricans can start at any age when marked obesity develops (Curth, 1951). When acanthosis nigricans is part of a syndrome, the other signs are usually easily recognizable and the dermatosis begins as a rule in childhood or at puberty (Curth, 1962).

2. *Is the patient obese?* Patients suffering from "malignant" acanthosis nigricans are usually nonobese, or if they are obese at the onset of the dermatosis, they will soon lose their excess weight in the presence of a growing tumor. Obese persons showing signs of acanthosis nigricans are usually suffering from pseudo–acanthosis nigricans (Curth, 1951).

3. *Is the dermatosis progressive?* In patients suffering from "malignant" acanthosis nigricans, the dermatosis usually progresses, whereas in "benign" acanthosis nigricans the dermatosis has either disappeared or become stationary after puberty. When acanthosis nigricans is part of a syndrome, it is usually nonprogressive. Pseudo–acanthosis nigricans will progress with a gain in weight and regress when the patient reduces considerably.

If the answers to these questions indicate that the patient has "malignant" acanthosis nigricans, this diagnosis must be made, even in the apparent absence of

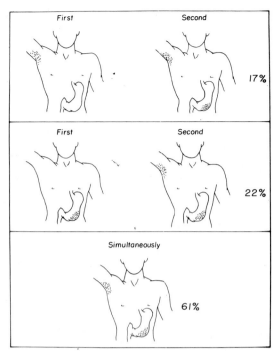

Figure 56-3 Sequence of events in malignant acanthosis nigricans. (*From* Curth: A.M.A. Arch. Dermatol. Syph., 71:95, 1955. Copyright 1955, American Medical Association.)

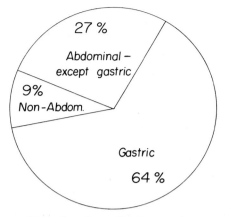

Figure 56-4 Location of adenocarcinoma associated with malignant acanthosis nigricans. (*From* Curth: A.M.A. Arch. Dermatol. Syph., 71:95, 1955. Copyright 1955, American Medical Association.)

a malignant tumor*. All efforts from now on should be made to locate this tumor.

In most cases (61 percent) of malignant acanthosis nigricans, both signs, the cancer and the dermatosis, appear at about the same time (Fig. 56-3). In 17 percent of cases, however, the dermatosis appears first. The interval between the manifestation of the dermatosis and that of the tumor may take up to 16 years. In the remaining 22 percent, the dermatosis appears after the cancer—not too much later, however, since the high degree of malignancy of the tumor does not leave much time. However, the interval between the removal of a mammary cancer and the onset of metastases and acanthosis nigricans amounted to 4½ years in Engel's (1969) case.

The cancers associated with "malignant" acanthosis nigricans (Fig. 56-4) occur (Curth, 1962 and 1970) in the stomach (64 percent) (Fig. 56-5), esophagus, colon, rectum, liver, pancreas, hepatic ducts, cystic duct, uterus, ovaries, lungs, mammary gland, prostate gland, and testis* (Braun and Schlang, 1970).

The belief that the cancer associated with "malignant" acanthosis nigricans is always fatal has fortunately been shattered. In a case of my own (Curth, 1970) the adenocarcinoma of the colon was discovered and removed before it caused any symptoms. It had been looked for because the patient showed a slight increase in papillary hypertrophy of lesions of the lower lip. He survived the operation by 6½ years and died at the age of 90 of a heart attack. "Malignant" acanthosis nigricans completely disappeared after the removal of the colonic cancer. After the onset of acanthosis nigricans—10 years before his death—without any effect on the dermatosis, this same patient had undergone removal of a squamous cell cancer of the urinary bladder, and of a

---

*It has been found recently that acanthosis nigricans may be caused by prolonged use of birth control pills.

---

*Pigmentation with hyperkeratosis of the face and arms occurred in a 39 year old male patient with a malignant testicular dysembryoma. The authors (Thivolet and Perrot, 1971) ruled out malignant acanthosis nigricans because of the unreported association of testicular carcinoma with malignant acanthosis nigricans. Such an association was recently described however, (Braun and Schlang, 1970).

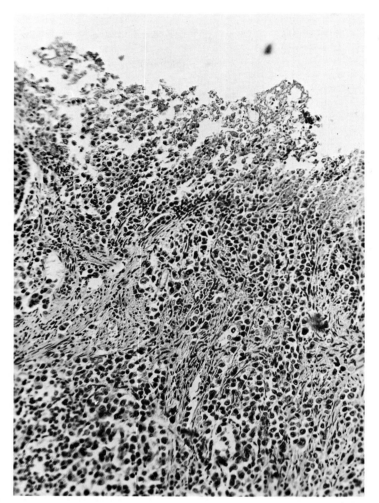

Figure 56–5 Gastric adenocarcinoma in 46 year old man with acanthosis nigricans. Histology. (*From* Curth: A.M.A. Arch. Dermatol. Syph., 71:45, 1955. Copyright 1955, American Medical Association.)

transitional cell carcinoma of the left kidney and subtotal gastrectomy for leiomyoma of the stomach. The other case (Brown and Winkelmann, 1968) of survival concerns a 34 year old woman who survived an operation for adenocarcinoma (Grade 2) of the sigmoid colon by 14 years, with complete regression of the dermatosis after the operation. It is interesting to note that in both instances of survival the tumor was an adenocarcinoma of the sigmoid colon.

With the exception of these two cases, the duration from the onset of the dermatosis to death was 11.9 months (Curth, 1952), or 22.7 months in 12 cases reported by Brown and Winkelmann (1968).

Curth et al. (1962) had Dr. H. L. Stewart and A. W. Hilberg of the National Cancer Institute examine 46 cases of tumors associated with acanthosis nigricans. Adenocarcinoma was found in 36 specimens, in two of which it was highly anaplastic. Another specimen was interpreted as showing anaplastic carcinoma in a lymph node. The diagnosis of "cancer" was made in six cases in which the material submitted was inadequate to permit a definite classification of the tumor. In one section, the slide submitted was inadequate for histologic diagnosis, but an adenocarcinoma was found at autopsy. One specimen came from a patient with squamous cell cervical cancer. We mentioned in our report (1962) that this cancer probably represented a coincidental cancer unrelated to the dermatosis. The patient is the only one of the group still alive – 14 years after the onset of the dermatosis.* Brown and Winkelmann (1968) cited this case with squamous cell cancer as proof that not all cancers associated with malignant acanthosis nigricans are adenocarcinomas. They further assumed that one of the cases "most probably was a reticulum cell sarcoma," although in the original paper reasons were brought forward why Stewart, Hilberg, Stout, Lattes, and Frantz, who studied the slides, believed that the evidence spoke against a reticulum cell sarcoma. The clinical picture also disproved it.

In several other instances the diagnosis quoted by Brown and Winkelmann as not being adenocarcinoma had already been refuted in my 1962 paper. In some cases the association with a nonadenocarcinomatous tumor seemed fortuitous; in others the dermatosis was not characteristic of acanthosis nigricans (Summons, 1960; Graham and Helwig, 1959; and Schlammadinger, 1934). Another patient (Miller and Davis, 1954) had a squamous cell carcinoma of the hypopharynx 5½ years before onset of acanthosis nigricans and died a year after the onset of the dermatosis. No autopsy was performed. A survival of 6½ years is unusual for a patient with a tumor associated with acanthosis nigricans. One single case of lymphosarcoma associated with acanthosis nigricans quoted by Brown and Winkelmann was mentioned by Rosenberg et al. (1961), in a report on 1269 cases of lymphosarcoma. This case was reported with no history or data on the duration of the dermatosis, so that this may not have been malignant acanthosis nigricans at all but one of the other types. There are, however, two cases reported of squamous cell cancer of the lung associated with acanthosis nigricans (Hadida et al., 1970) and

one case of a squamous cell cancer of the esophagus (Hamidou et al., 1968). The slides of these cases have not yet been reviewed by Stewart and Hilberg. In Ive's (1963) case of squamous cell cervical cancer the patient also suffered from pemphigoid, and radiologic and clinical pictures suggested a lung tumor. There are no data on operation, biopsy, or autopsy. Sanderson's (1962) patient had Hodgkin's disease, but the histologic picture of ₋acanthosis nigricans was atypical.

In their own series, Brown and Winkelmann found that all tumors were adenocarcinomas except for one squamous cell cancer of the uterine cervix and three lymphomas; lymph node biopsies of two of these showed Hodgkin's disease. In these four cases, no data on duration of the dermatosis, follow-up of the patients, results of operations, or autopsies were given, so that the possibility of types other than malignant acanthosis nigricans or of future development of adenocarcinoma exists.

Lerner's (1969) hypothesis of a peptide hormone from malignant visceral tumors playing a role in malignant acanthosis nigricans is interesting, but such a hormone has as yet not been found in a single case of malignant acanthosis nigricans. There were no increased amounts of melanin stimulating hormone (MSH) found in several of my patients with malignant acanthosis nigricans, and Lerner did not find any darkening agent in the tissue of the adenocarcinoma of the sigmoid colon of one of my patients.

Gordon (1970) found growth hormone disturbance in a case of acanthosis nigricans associated with lipodystrophy but did not find it in another case of acanthosis nigricans associated with dermatomyositis, calcinosis cutis, and exogenous hypercortisonism. Winkelmann (1970) found growth hormone disturbance in a case of malignant acanthosis nigricans with lung cancer. Theoretically, as Winkelmann pointed out, the hormone should not be purely pituitary, since, if adrenal hormones are responsible for acanthosis nigricans, they would suppress the pituitary hormones.

Criteria 1, 2, 4, 5, and 6 are fulfilled, so that malignant acanthosis nigricans ap-

---

*This patient was represented before the Metropolitan Dermatological Society of Los Angeles by Dornbush in 1956. Having now followed this patient for 15 years, I believe that she may have been erroneously placed among cases of malignant acanthosis nigricans. I did not observe her dermatosis, which began before a uterine squamous cell carcinoma was found. She is now 64 years old and has for many years been free of the dermatosis. Her weight during these years ranged from 144 to 197 lbs. She should perhaps have been classified as a case of pseudo–acanthosis nigricans.

pears as the classic association of a benign dermatosis with a malignant internal tumor.

DERMATOMYOSITIS

In 1916 an observation of a man suffering from polymyositis and gastric cancer was published by Stertz. It was Bezecny in 1935, however, who first referred to the relationship between dermatomyositis and internal cancer. He observed ovarian cancers in two patients and a mammary cancer in another patient with dermatomyositis.

Whereas polymyositis, with its principal clinical feature of muscular weakness, may occur with or without accompanying skin lesions, *dermato*myositis always shows cutaneous and muscular changes. Carcinoma is more common with dermatomyositis than with pure polymyositis (Braverman, 1970). The percentage of patients with dermatomyositis and cancer varies in the various statistics from 13 percent (Schuermann, 1952), 15.3 percent (Williams, 1959), 17.7 percent (Curth, 1971), and "less than 20 percent" (Pearson, 1966) to 36 percent (Midana and Leone, 1963). Since with very few exceptions (Braverman, 1970) cancer does not occur in children with dermatomyositis (Muller et al., 1959; Sneddon, 1968), statistics for the association of dermatomyositis are meaningful only if they are restricted to adults with dermatomyositis. In one study (Bureau and Barrière, 1963) that dealt with patients over the age of 30 with dermatomyositis, cancer occurred in 40 percent; in another (Arundell et al., 1961) that dealt with patients over 40 years old with dermatomyositis, cancer occurred in 52.2 percent.

Dermatomyositis is characterized by bluish red discoloration around the eyes (Fig. 56–6) and part of the entire face, neck, chest, and extremities. Facial, especially periorbital, edema is prominent. There is erythema of the nail folds and fingers. The mucous membranes of the buccal and pharyngeal surfaces are only rarely affected. When they are, they show red, atrophic, and occasionally ulcerated surfaces (Pearson, 1966). Calcinosis of

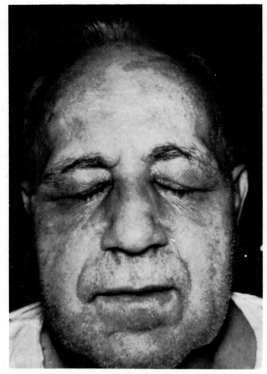

Figure 56–6   Male patient suffering from dermatomyositis and also from a carcinoma of the nasopharynx.

muscles and skin has been observed in long-standing cases of dermatomyositis in adults but occurs in 74 percent of cases in children.

The pelvic girdle, thighs, shoulder girdle, arms, neck, and sometimes esophagus show muscular weakness. Dysphagia, however, is more commonly caused by weakness of the striated musculature in the posterior pharynx (Pearson, 1966).

Pearson sets up rules about the behavior of skin and muscles in those cases of dermatomyositis that are associated with malignant internal tumors: "The muscular disorder takes the form of a florid dermatomyositis, which is easily recognized. In a few persons the skin changes are only minor; muscular weakness is characteristically proximal in distribution and dysphagia may be a particularly prominent complication." Whether these differences between dermatomyositis with and dermatomyositis without cancer are distinct enough to differentiate between the two

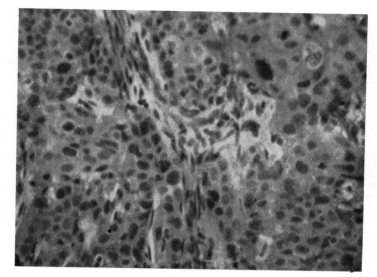

Figure 56–7 Squamous cell cancer of cervix in a woman with dermatomyositis. Histology. (*From* Curth: A.M.A. Arch. Dermatol. Syph., 71:101, 1955. Copyright 1955, American Medical Association.)
(See also Color Plate IX–B.)

forms of dermatomyositis seems questionable. It is always necessary to look for an internal tumor in adult patients with dermatomyositis.

Values of enzymatic tests for CPK, SGOT, and SGPT are usually elevated but may—at least at later stages of the disease—be normal (Schorr, 1970).

Patients with dermatomyositis may show skin hypersensitivity to extracts of their own tumors (Curtis et al., 1952). This, however, does not prove that dermatomyositis can be explained as a phenomenon of autosensitivity (Grace and Dao, 1959), because certain tumors show circulating antibodies, even in the absence of dermatomyositis.

The tumor associated with dermatomyositis does not fulfill criterion 4, since it is extremely variable: some tumors are squamous cell tumors (Fig. 56–7), some are adenocarcinomas. However, all may perhaps contain a certain—still unknown—principle capable of provoking the characteristic dermatosis. Moreover, a certain (genetic) disposition of the patient, which predisposes him to the characteristic cutaneous changes in the presence of various kinds of tumors, may have to be present. Some bilateral tumors of the breasts and ovaries were noted (Curth, 1971). Bureau and Barrière (1963) found in 162 observations of cases of their own of dermatomyositis the following tumors: 71 in breast and genitals (mostly in women), 37 in stomach or rectum, 24 in the respiratory tract (mostly in men), 22 with diverse locations, some being sarcomas, some occurring in the kidney, and 8 cases of reticuloendothelioses, of which 5 were diagnosed as Hodgkin's disease.

Usually dermatomyositis precedes the cancer, but the tumor may acutally have been present although not recognized. Dermatomyositis may be overt and the malignancy symptomatically minor or unrecognized, even up until the time of death (Pearson, 1966). In rare cases, dermatomyositis develops late, 6 and even 12 months after the cancer (Bureau and Barrière, 1963). The dermatosis regresses after the elimination of the tumor or its metastases but does not always exacerbate following renewed activity of the tumor (Curth, 1971) (see a similar situation in pemphigoid, p. 1331); a remarkable parallelism between tumor and dermatosis is quite evident in malignant acanthosis nigricans. Holzmann (1971) concluded that the diagnosis of dermatomyositis should initiate systematic search for a malignant tumor which might be curable.

Obviously, search for and elimination of the tumor is the logical treatment of cases of dermatomyositis that are associated with a malignant internal tumor. A cure of dermatomyositis can be achieved if the tumor can be completely resected. Howell (1963) observed a patient with dermatomyositis and mastectomy for cancer, who underwent hypophysectomy for metastasis 11 months after the first operation and showed regression of the dermatomyositis within five weeks. Another patient had three primary cancers: one in the rectum, one in the breast, and one in the transverse colon. After their removal, the dermatosis became stationary (Wilson et al., 1965).

Criteria 1 and 2, with certain reservations, since a recurrent tumor has not always been accompanied by an exacerbation of the dermatosis, or a recurrent dermatosis has not always been accompanied by a recurrent tumor, are fulfilled.

MALIGNANT DOWN (HYPERTRICHOSIS LANUGINOSA ACQUISITA)

In contrast to excessive lanugo hair present at birth, acquired excessive growth of lanugo-like hair (Figs. 56–8) over the body has been observed in association with bronchogenic carcinoma of un-

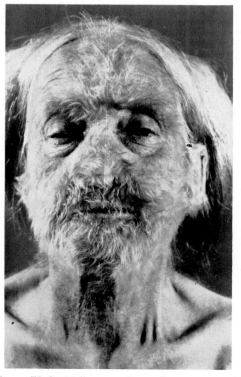

Figure 56–8 Malignant down in woman with adenocarcinoma, probably primary in rectum. (*From* Chadfield and Khan: Trans. St. John's Hosp. Dermatol. Soc., 56:30, 1970.)

differentiated cell type, carcinoma of the gallbladder with metastases, carcinoma of the urinary bladder with metastases, and rectal carcinoma. Hegedus and Schorr (1971) reported on two patients with cancers of the colon. Men and women are affected. Another report dealt with recurrent duodenal ulcerations.

The hair growth starts suddenly. In milder forms it is confined to the face; in pronounced cases it may involve the entire body except the palms and soles. Even bald areas of the scalp may become covered with hair. The hair may be longer than 10 to 15 cm. Interest has been focused on the prolongation of the anagen stage with synchronization of all follicular hair growth. Hegedus and Schorr (1971) reported a predominance of mantle hairs, some of which have lanugo follicles growing inferiorly almost parallel to the overlying epidermis. They also noted cherry-red tongue lesions. The tumor or its metastases become evident at about the same time the hair growth starts. In Chadfield and Khan's (1970) patient, a 78 year old woman, the rectal carcinoma developed eight months before the abnormal hair growth appeared. No endocrine disturbances seemed to be at fault. A case of hypertrichosis lanuginosa without cancer (Ormsby, 1930) does not seem to have been adequately investigated or followed. Fretzin's (1967) patient also showed numerous palmar punctate keratoses.

The tumor is not specific; the parallelism between time of onset and course of the two diseases, dermatosis and cancer, however, is noteworthy. The dermatosis is uncommon.

FLUSHING

Several reports concerning a new disorder called "the carcinoid syndrome" or the "functioning carcinoid" appeared in the early fifties in the Swedish, Swiss, and American literature. In the last decade reports of this association were published from many countries.

The tumors cause an acute reddish cutaneous flush, starting in the face and sometimes extending to the chest, arms, and legs. This lasts for seven to eight minutes (Olson and Gray, 1958). If the flushing persists, telangiectasia or permanent cyanosis results. In a number of patients pellagrous and sclerodermatous changes are associated with the flushing.

Carcinoids may be of the nonfunctioning type, but in all cases of flushing the carcinoid was of the functioning type and had metastasized to the liver (Olson and Gray, 1958). A common primary site of the tumor is the appendix. The neoplasm may originate elsewhere in the gastrointestinal tract, however, frequently in the ileum; it may also be present in the bronchi. Serotonin, identified as 5-hydroxytryptamine, can be extracted from the carcinoid tumor (Lembeck, 1953). This substance is chiefly destroyed in the liver, but in the presence of hepatic metastases it is produced there and escapes inactivation in this organ (Thorson et al., 1954; McKusick, 1956). The metabolite 5-hydroxy-3-idoleacetic acid is found in excess in the urine of patients with carcinoids. Serotonin is at least partially responsible for the flushing. An important role seems to be played also by bradykinin, which could either be the sole mediator of the symptoms of the carcinoid syndrome or act in conjunction with serotonin (Oates et al., 1964).

Single or multiple carcinoids usually progress slowly and then metastasize. Patients often give a history of asthma, diarrhea, and slow edema and show an enlarged liver. The tumors have been observed in patients aged 10 days to those aged 89 years (Ritchie, 1956). Surgery is recommended, even when metastasis is demostrated.

In patients with carcinoids, pellagra (Bridges et al., 1957) is explained by an altered tryptophan metabolism, and scleroderma is probably due to the cutaneous fibrous tissue proliferation, also observed in the heart and peritoneal cavity of patients suffering from carcinoids.

It is obvious that the tumor, which is of a distinctive type, is responsible for the cutaneous changes.

TYLOSIS PALMARIS ET PLANTARIS

The association of palmar and plantar keratoses with esophageal carcinoma was observed in familial and sporadic cases. Two families from Liverpool, England, who apparently were not related to each other, were reported by Clarke et al. (1957) and Howel-Evans et al. (1958). Most of the sporadic cases originated in the Middle West and were reported by Parnell and Johnson (1969) from Wisconsin.

In the familial cases diffuse palmar and plantar hyperkeratoses with hyperhidrosis began at the age of 14. In men doing manual labor, the keratoderma is more pronounced. Occasionally, only plantar keratosis is present.

Of 48 family members with keratosis palmoplantaris, 18 developed squamous cell cancer of the esophagus in later life. The tumor usually arose on the lower third of the esophagus, occasionally in the middle third, and rarely in the upper third. There was no evidence of esophageal hyperkeratosis preceding the tumor, and only once was leukoplakia observed. No family member without palmoplantar keratosis developed esophageal cancer. Parnell and Johnson said only one did. Clarke found two other patients with bronchial carcinoma and diffuse palmar and plantar keratosis. These two were unrelated to each other and to the members of the Liverpool families.

The presence of a bronchial carcinoma (instead of an esophageal carcinoma) associated with palmar and plantar tylosis is not surprising, since esophagus as well as bronchus is derived from the foregut (Parnell and Johnson, 1969). These authors observed such an association in a patient, and Everall reported another instance of bronchial carcinoma and palmar and plantar keratosis.

In a case reported from India (Patnaik and Krishneswamy, 1963), keratosis palmoplantaris had been present since childhood and esophageal cancer developed at the age of 70. In this instance the association of skin disease and internal cancer seemed fortuitous.

A pleiotropic autosomal dominant gene is most probably responsible for the association of palmar and plantar keratoses and bronchial or esophageal carcinomas in the familial cases. As in other genetic associations, time of onset and the course of each manifestation need not be and were not parallel.

Parnell and Johnson's patient was a 49 year old woman with bronchogenic carcinoma. They also reported on a 58 year old man with metastatic esophageal cancer, a 77 year old man with esophageal carcinoma, a 65 year old man with a grade II squamous cell carcinoma of the esophagus, and a 58 year old man with carcinoma of the mid-esophagus. The duration of the keratoses in their first, third, and fourth cases was not given, but apparently the keratoses of Case No. 2 were of recent origin. Other family members were not similarly affected.

Woscoff et al. (1970) also reported on acquired palmar and plantar keratoderma in a man who developed lung cancer. Following cobalt therapy of the tumor, the dermatosis improved. These instances of acquired keratoderma are suggestive of beginning malignant acanthosis nigricans, in which rough palms and soles may be the first cutaneous sign.

PUNCTATE PALMAR KERATOSES

In 1965 Dobson et al. found palmar keratoses—punctate, pearly, yellow or flesh-colored, translucent, hyperkeratotic papules surrounded by a collarette of scale—four to five times as frequently in persons with cancerous tumors as in control persons without cancer. In this connection it may be mentioned that Fretzin's (1967) patient suffering from an anaplastic bronchogenic cancer and malignant down had punctate keratoses of the palms and soles.

Various authors tried to confirm the findings of Dobson et al. (1965). This author examined in a New York hospital 42 men and women suffering from various kinds of internal cancer and cancers of the head and neck. Only in one man with a laryngeal cancer was a single keratotic lesion of the left palm found. Stolman et al. (1970) also were unable to confirm the statistical significance of the palmar keratoses in patients with systemic cancer. They examined in New York a group of cancer patients and a control group of noncancerous patients for the presence of palmar keratoses. Bean et al. (1965) from Minnesota also saw no increase in the frequency of palmar keratoses in patients with internal malignancies.

If it is the exposure to arsenic that explains palmar keratoses (and perhaps the internal cancer), then the different exposures to arsenic of dissimilar populations in the United States are perhaps responsible for the discrepancy in results. However, Bean et al. (1965), who could not confirm an association of internal cancer and palmar keratoses, point to a greater exposure to arsenic in Minnesota than in Oregon, the home of Dobson et al. (1965). Braverman (1970) sees no resemblance of palmar keratoses to lesions associated with arsenic.

ALOPECIA MUCINOSA (FOLLICULAR MUCINOSIS)

Pinkus (1957 and 1963) described alopecia mucinosa as an inflammatory dermatosis characterized clinically by infiltrated grouped folliculopapules with accompanying hair loss (alopecia), and histochemically by the accumulation of an acid mucopolysaccharide substance (mucin) in the outer root sheath of hair follicles and the secretory epithelium of associated sebaceous glands. There is a mild or more severe degree of inflammatory infiltrate about the affected follicles. The disorder occurs more frequently in men than women.

Lesions either clear spontaneously within a few months, then relapse but pursue a benign course over several years, or appear in about 15 (Felman et al., 1969) to 17 percent of patients (Emmerson, 1969) in association with lymphomas (Fig. 56–9) or mycosis fungoides. Of nine patients reported by Degos and Beuve-Mery (1966), six had reticulosis. The internal disease precedes the cutaneous changes or starts at the same time.

In patients without associated lymphomas, the cutaneous lesions are confined to the head and neck. There may, however, be associated reticulosis in patients whose lesions occur also on the trunk and extremities. In a case that came

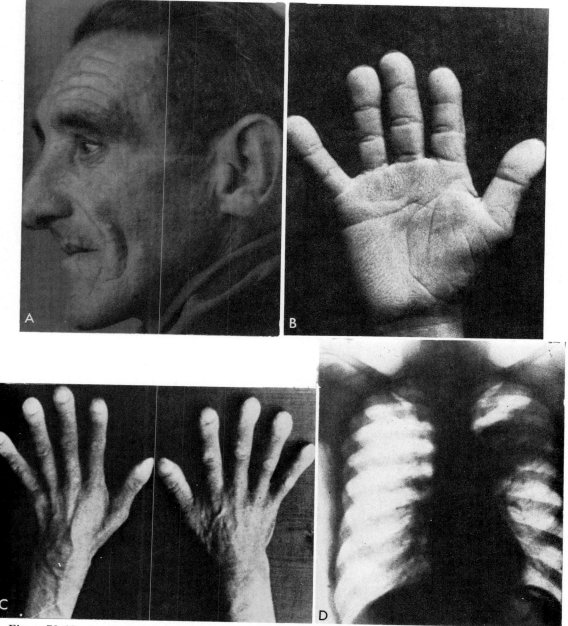

Figure 56–12 Acquired pachydermoperiostosis. *A*, Deep folds; *B*, rough palms; *C*, clubbed fingers; *D*, roentgenogram showing lung cancer in left upper lobe. (*From* Curth: A.M.A. Arch. Dermatol., 71:99, 1955. Copyright 1955, American Medical Association.)

toarthropathy. This type of the disorder occurs also in association with bronchiectasis, tuberculosis, empyema, lung abscess, mediastinal and congenital cardiac disease, sickle cell anemia, congenital syphilis, and hepatic disorders and is less often associated with cancer of the stomach, esophagus, and thymus (Rook et al., 1968).

The disease usually occurs in men aged 30 to 70 who are suffering from bronchogenic cancer. The first case described by Schiassi (1933), however, was that of a woman.

The association of two benign dermatoses, malignant acanthosis nigricans and pachydermoperiostosis, known to occur with internal carcinoma, was observed in two instances (Marmelzat, 1955; Stevanovic, 1966). This seemed to indicate, through the presence of malignant acanthosis nigricans, that the patient had an adenocarcinoma, which probably was located in the lung, as indicated by the presence of pachydermoperiostosis. Actually this could not be ascertained in either case. In Marmelzat's patient only one right hilar node could be examined at autopsy. It showed an anaplastic carcinoma. The second patient had a uterine cancer. At the time of the last report (1966), she was still alive and the lungs were free radiologically.

An increase in peripheral circulation during the active phase of the disorder explains the pathogenesis of many of the peripheral cutaneous and osseous changes (Vogl and Goldfischer, 1962; Rasmussen, 1952; Wyburn-Mason, 1948).

Acquired pachydermoperiostosis must be differentiated from the familial form of pachydermoperiostosis, which occurs predominantly in men and starts soon after puberty. This type of the disorder is also associated with arthropathy and clubbed fingers.

The cutaneous and osseous changes of the acquired type will regress if the tumor can be removed.

There is parallelism between the onset and the course of the two manifestations. The tumor is usually a bronchogenic carcinoma. Criteria 1, 2, and 4 are fulfilled.

RETICULOHISTIOCYTOMA (SYSTEMIC RETICULOHISTIOCYTOSIS, LIPOID DERMATOARTHRITIS)

In the first report on reticulohistiocytoma (Parkes Weber and Freudenthal, 1937), no associated tumor was noted. Recently, however, the following associated tumors were observed: axillary sarcoma, gastric adenocarcinoma, and bronchogenic carcinoma. These were observed respectively by Albert et al. (1960) (secondary carcinoma of the colon) and by Lyell and Carr (1959) (in another patient ma-

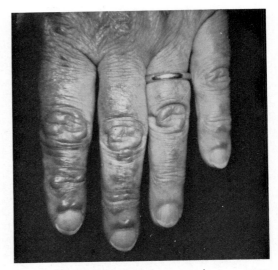

Figure 56-13 Reticulohistiocytoma in a woman who died of cancer of undetermined origin. (Courtesy of Dr. Lewis Shapiro.)

lignant involvement of the bronchial lymph nodes); by Labow and Shapiro (1965) (cancer of undetermined origin) (Fig. 56-13) and by Warin et al. (1957) (carcinoma suggestive of bronchial origin found at autopsy). Barrow and Holubar (1969) estimated that cancer occurred in 15 per cent of their 33 patients.

The generalized form of the disorder (to be distinguished from the localized form) affects the skin and the joints, which show destructive symmetric polyarthritis resembling rheumatoid arthritis. Rapid destruction of the joint and subarticular bone produces shortening of the fingers with redundant skin folds, the so-called telescopic or opera glass hand. The cutaneous changes affect the dorsa of the hands, the forearms, scalp, face, ears, trunk, and occasionally the mucosa of the lip (Warin et al., 1957). Firm red, brown, or yellow nodules and papules are observed. Xanthelasma is found in one-fourth of the patients (Jansen, 1967).

Histologically there is in the upper half of the corium a granulomatous reaction with giant cells. Scattered among these giant cells are smaller cells resembling histiocytes. The eruption fluctuates in severity and shows a protracted course. Elevation of total serum lipids may be present (Labow and Shapiro, 1965).

Affected by the disorder are women over 40 years of age. If the dermatosis is associated with a tumor, the two manifestations start at about the same time and run a parallel course. One autopsy (Warin et al., 1957) did not reveal a tumor. Some cases without a tumor do not seem to have been followed long enough. The disease is rare as well as unusual.

With regard to our criteria, course and time of onset of the two manifestations run about parallel. The tumor, however, is not specific.

GARDNER'S SYNDROME

Gardner's syndrome comprises multiple "soft" cutaneous tumors, osteomas, and polyposis of the large intestine. It is named after Gardner, who together with his co-workers investigated in the early fifties large Utah family groups with the disorder. The syndrome, however, is not confined to families from Utah (Weiner and Cooper, 1955) or the United States (Oldfield, 1953/54).

The cutaneous tumors are present at birth or in early childhood and consist of cystic lesions (Fig. 56–14*A*) and fibrous and fatty tumors. Epidermal inclusion cysts are more common than sebaceous cysts and occur mostly on the face and extremities. They gradually increase in size and number. We find among the fibrous tissue tumors simple fibromas, desmoid tumors, and fibrosarcomas.

Multiple polyps (Fig. 56–14*B*) occur in the colon and rectum and are as a rule not demonstrable before the second decade. Malignant degeneration (Fig. 56–14*C* and *D*) has been observed in young or middle-aged patients. It occurs in about 45 to 53 percent of adults, so that prophylactic colectomy and extirpation of large

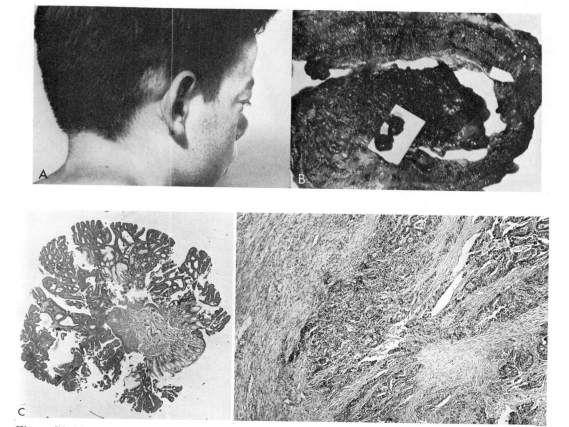

Figure 56–14 *A*, Cyst behind the right ear in a patient with Gardner's syndrome.(*From* Curth: A.M.A. Arch. Dermatol., 71:98, 1955. Copyright 1955, American Medical Association.) *B*, Intestinal polyps. *C*, Polyp with questionable transition to malignant tumor. *D*, Frank carcinoma of colon. (Courtesy of Dr. E. J. Eichwald.)

parts of the rectum (Leichtling, 1971) are warranted.

Lewis and Mitchell (1971) observed basal cell epitheliomas at the age of 44 in two brothers suffering from Gardner's syndrome. Actinic exposure probably served to induce the carcinomas, but the natural history of Gardner's syndrome may include basal cell epitheliomas.

The disorder is due to a dominant pleiotropic gene. The genetic basis of the components of the syndrome make the course of each component with regard to time and intensity independent of the other.

PEUTZ-JEGHERS-TOURAINE SYNDROME

Cases of the syndrome consisting of characteristically located pigmented spots on the skin and mucous membranes and polyps in the small intestines were reported from England (Conner, 1895; Hutchinson, 1896; Parkes Weber, 1919) before Peutz, a Dutch physician, in 1921, Jeghers, an American physician, in 1944, and Touraine, a French dermatologist, in 1945, studied affected families. Since that time additional reports have come from

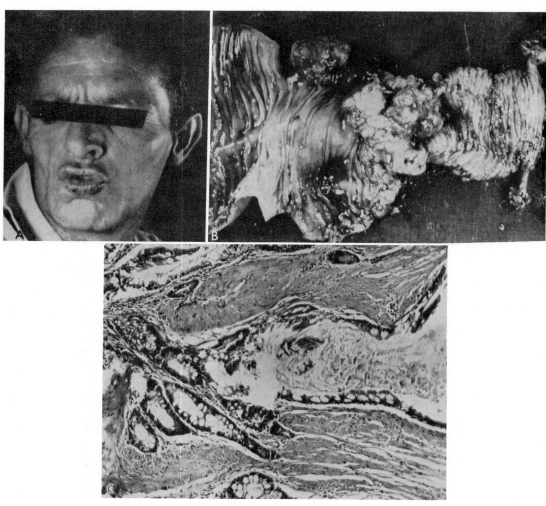

Figure 56–15   Peutz-Jeghers-Touraine syndrome. *A*, Melanin spots on lips, especially pronounced on lower lip. *B*, Constricting adenocarcinoma (center) of ileum and three adenomatous polyps (same patient). *C*. Adenocarcinoma invading the musculature from a section of the constricting tumor (preceding picture). (*From* Gastroenterology, 35:534, 1958.)

the United States and European countries.

Brown to black pigmented spots appear on the vermilion border, especially on the lower lip (Fig. 56–15*A*), in the oral cavity, periorally, perinasally, periorbitally, and on the fingers and toes. They may be present at birth or develop 6 to 12 months later; they usually disappear between puberty and the twenties.

The polyps, although already present, usually become manifest in the second decade of life, causing recurring bouts of abdominal pain, bleeding, anemia, and intussusception. The tumors are chiefly located in the small intestine, but some are occasionally found in the stomach, duodenum, colon, or rectum.

Although on the whole the general outlook for the patient is good, even if multiple operations may be required, as a report with a 30-year follow-up shows (McKittrick et al., 1971), some polyps undoubtedly degenerate into malignant tumors (Fig. 56–15*B* and *C*). Malignant transformation, however, rarely takes place in the polyp located in the small intestine. Associated rectal, duodenal (Gasser and Arquint, 1969), or gastric polyps are the ones that may undergo transformation into malignant tumors (Paglia et al., 1975).

Scully (1970) found a rare, distinctive ovarian sex cord tumor with annular tubules occurring in six women with the Peutz-Jeghers syndrome. Discovery of such a tumor associated with an abnormal menstrual pattern may be the first clue to the diagnosis of the Peutz-Jeghers syndrome. The tumor is perhaps better called a hamartoma. Other benign ovarian tumors have been observed in women with the Peutz-Jeghers syndrome. However, malignant tumors, such as the granulosa cell ovarian tumor (Berkowitz et al., 1955; Burdick et al., 1963; Dickson, 1944), have also occurred.

The syndrome is based on a single autosomal gene, which is fully penetrant and pleiotropic, causing the pigmentary disturbance and the intestinal polyposis. The disorder affects both sexes equally.

In case of bleeding and a sustained intussusception, the offending polyp must be removed. Genetic counseling is in order.

ARSENICAL KERATOSES

In 1959, 1963, and 1964 Graham and Helwig stated that arsenical keratoses are associated with cutaneous and internal cancer. They found arsenical keratoses on exposed and unexposed areas in 22 patients. Clinically and histologically, the arsenical keratoses were almost indistinguishable from Bowen's disease. Fifteen patients had a history of injections or contact with arsenic. Systemic cancer was found in three: one occurred in the ampulla of Vater, another in the breast, and a third represented a malignant carcinoid of the ileum and appendix with metastases. Graham and Helwig conclude that "because of the gross, microscopic, and chemical similarities of Bowen's disease and arsenical keratosis and their association with systemic cancer arsenic is probably a common etiologic factor."

No data were given by the authors for the time interval between the cutaneous and the internal lesions, so that no decision as to the parallelism between the onset and the course of the cutaneous and internal lesions (criteria 1 and 2 of our evaluation of a causal relationship between cutaneous and internal lesions) can be made.

HERPES ZOSTER

The first observation of the association of herpes zoster with malignant internal disease was published in 1895 by Carrière, who described herpes zoster along the left femoral nerve in a woman with uterine cancer.

In the unilateral eruption, grouped blisters or pustules are found in segmental distribution of posterior root ganglia of spinal nerves or of analogous ganglia of cranial nerves. The eruption frequently occurs in the segment corresponding to the location of the tumor or metastases. It was found in 20 out of 23 patients on the same side of the body (Huguenin et al., 1950). Whereas the unilateral eruption is associated with malignant disease in a relatively small number of cases (4 percent in women with breast cancer) (Huguenin et al., 1950), generalized herpes zoster is so associated in an unu-

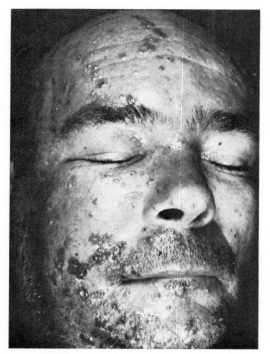

Figure 56–16 Herpes zoster in man suffering from Hodgkin's disease. (*From* Curth: A.M.A. Arch. Dermatol., 71:104, 1955. Copyright 1955, American Medical Association.)

sually high percentage (50 to 58 percent). Generalization (Fig. 56–16) is much less likely to occur in Hodgkin's disease than in chronic lymphatic leukemia, but the attack is likely to be severe, with pain and ulceration (Rook et al., 1968). In the study of Merselis et al. (1964), 11 of 17 patients with disseminated herpes zoster had serious underlying disease, primarily malignant disease of the hematopoietic system; nine of these patients had been treated with adrenocorticosteroids, x-ray, or radiomimetic drugs prior to dissemination of herpetic lesions. Four patients with an associated malignancy died during the course of disseminated herpes zoster.

The authors warn of the use of adrenocorticotropic hormone and systemic therapy with adrenocorticosteroids, x-ray, or radiomimetic drugs in patients with herpes zoster.

The malignant processes include lymphomas and myelomas—in women mammary, uterine, or ovarian carcinoma (also ovarian sarcoma); in men gastric cancer

and seminoma. Huguenin et al. (1950) found many cases of thoracic herpes zoster with thoracic cancers (five out of six men had tracheal or bronchial cancer, and all 17 women had mammary cancer).

The malignant disease preceded herpes zoster in all cases. In most instances irradiation of the tumor had taken place 4 to 40 months prior to the onset of the cutaneous lesions (Curth, 1955) (Fig. 56–17). The prognosis of the cancer does not seem to be influenced by the occurrence of herpes zoster, and Huguenin et al. (1950) reported survival times of several years after an attack of herpes zoster in patients with cancer.

Rogers and Tindall (1971) found among their pediatric patients with herpes zoster seven with malignancies, mostly lymphoproliferative disease. None had systemic herpes zoster, but two had surface dissemination.

By infiltration, pressure, or toxic influence on the reflex arc, the malignant process creates an ideal condition for the activation of the herpes virus.

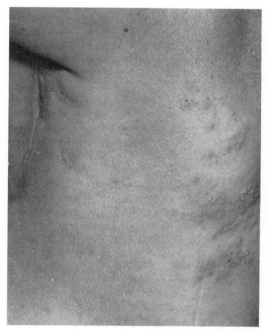

Figure 56–17 Herpes zoster of left side of back in 51 year old woman following radiation therapy for a questionable intraductal carcinoma of left mammary gland. (*From* Curth: A.M.A. Arch. Dermatol., 71:104, 1955. Copyright 1955, American Medical Association.)

The criterion regarding the time of onset of the two manifestations is fulfilled. Since herpes zoster is a self-limited disease, the course of the two conditions cannot run completely parallel. In cases of generalized herpes zoster, one must look for a malignant internal disease. But even in cases of unilateral herpes zoster, search may yield a malignant internal process.

BULLOUS DERMATOSES — DERMATITIS HERPETIFORMIS

Bogrow in 1909 was the first to observe the association of dermatitis herpetiformis with a cancer. This was not an internal carcinoma but a cancer of the labium. In 1931 Gougerot et al. described coexisting and subsequent eruptions of erythema annulare centrifugum and dermatitis herpetiformis in a patient with a malignant tumor of the larynx. Several reports of the association followed. Bureau and Barrière (1963) found 21 cases of their own of this association and believed that

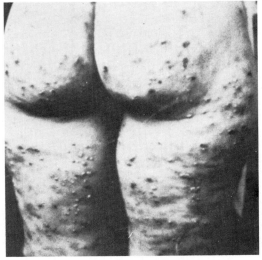

Figure 56–18 Dermatitis herpetiformis in patient suffering from papillary ovarian cancer with necrosis. (*From* Curth: A.M.A. Arch. Dermatol., 71:105, 1955. Copyright 1955, American Medical Association.)

the relationship between the cancer and the dermatosis was especially close.

Grouped papulovesicular lesions on an erythematous base are present on the

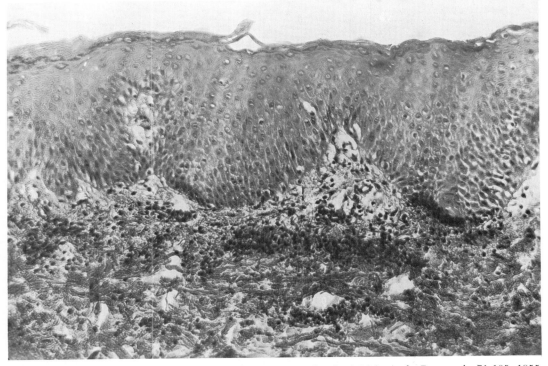

Figure 56–19 Histology of dermatitis herpetiformis. (*From* Curth: A.M.A. Arch. Dermatol., 71:105, 1955. Copyright 1955, American Medical Association.)

trunk (Fig. 56–18) and extremities with occasional involvement of the oral mucous membranes. Histologically dermatitis herpetiformis with cancer is not different from that without cancer (Fig. 56–19). It shows subepidermal bullae with eosinophils. Patients with dermatitis herpetiformis and internal carcinomas usually are middle-aged or older and in poor general health. In instances with malignant internal tumors, the cutaneous manifestations began between the ages of 44 and 83 years, according to Skog (1971). Patients suffering from dermatitis herpetiformis without cancer are usually below 40 years of age. The result of the treatment also permits a distinction between dermatitis herpetiformis with and without cancer: "idiopathic" dermatitis herpetiformis usually responds well to sulfapyridine or to sulfone drugs, but this therapy is valueless when cancer is present. Arrest of the carcinoma brings a prompt remission of the cutaneous disease (Cormia and Binford, 1967).

Structural changes of the intestinal mucosa resembling those of idiopathic steatorrhea are prevalent in dermatitis her-

petiformis. Gjone and Nördoy (1970) recently studied two middle-aged men with dermatitis herpetiformis of long duration and steatorrhea. One had an ulcerating jejunal tumor, probably originating from the reticuloendothelial system; the other had a large renal carcinoma.

Tumors other than the ones mentioned above in association with dermatitis herpetiformis are carcinoma of the uterus (Hartzell, 1918), chorionic carcinoma (Elliott, 1938), hydatidiform mole (Tillman, 1950), and papillary ovarian carcinoma (Tobias, 1951). Other cancers are carcinoma or sarcoma of the thyroid, gastric adenocarcinoma, and cancer of the cervix, pancreas, prostate (Grupper, 1961; Balabanov and Andreev, 1964), and bronchi (Duperrat, 1958). Other diseases are Hodgkin's disease, multiple myeloma, lymphatic leukemia (Coriciati, 1960), and a leukemoid reaction (Evan-Paz and Sagher, 1938). Necrosis is present in some tumors (Fig. 56–20) but absent in others.

The failure of dermatitis herpetiformis to recur when the tumor reappears is perhaps due to the absence of necrosis in the recurrent tumor. Balabanov and An-

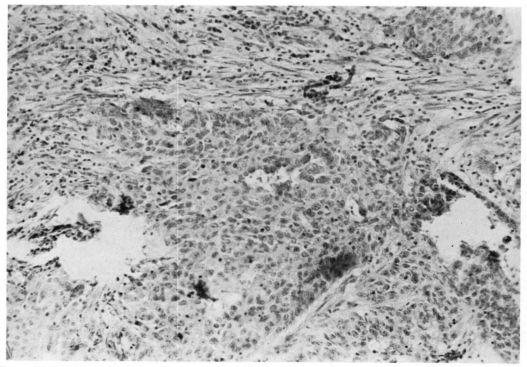

Figure 56–20 Dermatitis herpetiformis. Papillary ovarian cancer. (*From* Curth: A.M.A. Arch. Dermatol., 71:105, 1955. Copyright 1955, American Medical Association.)

dreev (1964) considered the presence of dermatitis herpetiformis in a patient with malignant disease an ominous sign, since all patients whose cases they reviewed died.

There exists a good correlation between the time of onset of both manifestations. The course of both may not run completely parallel, since in several patients the recurrent tumor was not accompanied by a reappearance of the dermatosis.

A generalized eruption resembling erythema multiforme rather than dermatitis herpetiformis has been observed 1 to 21 days after deep radiation for a malignant tumor. The tumors are cancers of the tongue, stomach, uterus, and breast; bronchogenic carcinoma; mediastinal lymphoblastoma; retroperitoneal lymphosarcoma; and myosarcomatosis (Curth, 1955), or cancer of the cervix (Sneddon, 1970). Shatin (1955) observed erythema multiforme following x-ray therapy. The

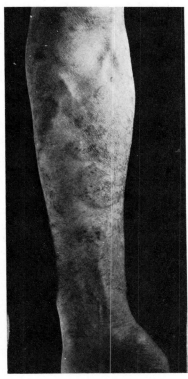

Figure 56–21 Erythema multiforme in man suffering from primary adenocarcinoma of adrenals with metastases. (*From* Curth: A.M.A. Arch. Dermatol., 71:102, 1955. Copyright 1955, American Medical Association.)

patient suffered from primary adenocarcinoma of the adrenals with metastases (Figs. 56–21 and 56–22). Arnold (1949) observed erythema multiforme following radiation therapy for abdominal metastases from a seminoma, an anaplastic urethral carcinoma, and a mammary carcinoma.

The cutaneous eruption results most probably from absorption of products of cellular degeneration, probably protein disintegration of tumor tissue and normal tissue as well.

PEMPHIGOID

In 1922 Davis described in two women with malignant uterine tumors a peculiar blisterous and bullous eruption, which suggested erythema annulare centrifugum or bullous pemphigoid. The dermatosis of one woman resolved after removal of the tumor.

Pemphigoid may resemble pemphigus vulgaris, but after rupture of the bullae the large denuded areas do not increase in size. In addition to covering wide areas of the trunk and extremities, pemphigoid associated with an internal tumor may affect the oral cavity (Lever, 1965; Rook and Waddington, 1953). The bullae are large, tense, and subepidermal.

Tumors associated with bullous pemphigoid are mammary (Wilson, 1961), pulmonary (Gold, 1961; two patients; Parsons and Savin, 1968), pancreatic (Kilby, 1965), and uterine (Davis, 1922; Parsons and Savin, 1968; one papillary adenocarcinoma, one squamous cell carcinoma); also associated are malignant melanoma (Marks, 1961; Parsons and Savin, 1968), a cancer of the gallbladder (Parsons and Savin, 1968), a lymphoblastic lymphosarcoma (Parsons and Savin, 1968), and a cystic adenoid basal cell carcinoma.

The presence of autoantibodies to the basement membrane zone of skin and mucous membrane in the sera of patients with bullous pemphigoid has been firmly established by immunofluorescent methods (Jordon et al., 1969). Thivolet et al. (1971) insisted that the presence of autoantibodies to the basement membrane occurs only in bullous pemphigoid and not in dermatitis herpetiformis, although

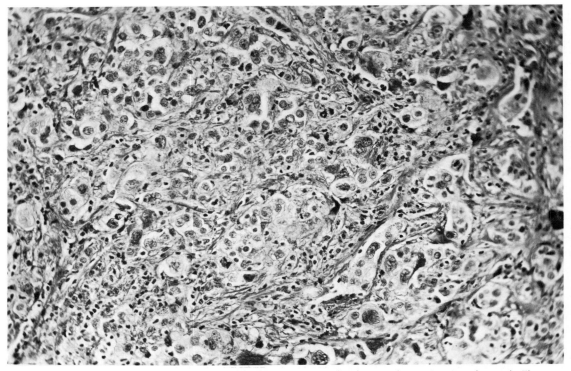

Figure 56–22   Left supraclavicular lymph node showing metastatic adenocarcinoma (same patient as in Figure 56–21). (*From* Curth: A.M.A. Arch. Dermatol., 71:102, 1955. Copyright 1955, American Medical Association.)

they found a report on a woman aged 78 with dermatitis herpetiformis, mammary adenocarcinoma, and elevated titers of antibodies. In their own patient, a man with pulmonary carcinoma and bullous pemphigoid, the authors were able to demonstrate antinuclear autoantibodies and those against the basement membrane.

Only a few instances of pemphigoid are associated with malignant tumors. In these the tumors were not uniform. The onset of the two manifestations occurred at about the same time. Parsons and Savin (1968) concluded that the association between dermatosis and neoplasms may be coincidental, although they could observe seven such associations in middle-aged or old persons. The course of the two was parallel in most of their cases; in others it was variable, i.e., the skin cleared up in two cases while the neoplasms continued to advance. A consistent relationship between the progression of the two disorders, however, was seen by other observers. The situation with regard to a parallel course may be somewhat comparable to that seen in dermatomyositis. After a time stimuli for the progression of the dermatosis other than the cancer may take over; on the other hand, the cancer may lose its capacity as a trigger with regard to the dermatosis.

BOWEN'S DISEASE

In 1959, 1961, and 1964 Graham and Helwig reported on the association of Bowen's disease of the skin with cutaneous and internal cancers.

The single or multiple lesions represent erythematous (nodular), scaly, and sometimes ulcerated plaques on all parts of the body (Fig. 56–23). Graham and Helwig (1959, 1961, 1964a, and 1964b) stated that, contrary to the general impression, the exposed areas are as frequently involved as the covered areas. Histologically cellular atypism in the form of multinucleated, vacuolated cells, mitotic figures, and a loss of normal architecture are seen (Fig. 56–24).

Fried, B. M.: Chronic pulmonary osteoarthropathy. Arch. Intern. Med., 72:565, 1943.

Marmelzat, W. L.: Pachydermoperiostosis associated with acanthosis nigricans–like syndrome. Arch. Dermatol., 72:90, 1955.

Rasmussen, H.: Peripheral vascular disease with hypertrophic osteoarthropathy as the first manifestation of bronchial carcinoma. Acta Med. Scand., Suppl. 266, 142:855, 1952.

Rook, A., Wilkinson, D. S., and Ebling, F. J. G.: Textbook of Dermatology. Vol. I. Oxford, Blackwell Scientific Publications, 1968, p. 71.

Schiassi, F.: Osteoartropatia ipertrofica pneuminica per metastasi ossee di cancero polmone. Radiol. Med., 20:753, 1933.

Stevanovic, D. V.: Personal communication, 1966.

Vogl, A., and Goldfischer, S.: Pachydermoperiostosis, primary or idiopathic hypertrophic osteoarthropathy. Am. J. Med., 33:166, 1962.

Wyburn-Mason, R.: Bronchial carcinoma presenting as polyneuritis. Lancet, 1:203, 1948.

Reticulohistiocytoma

Albert, J., Bruce, W., Allen, A. C., and Blank, H.: Lipoid dermato-arthritis. Reticulohistiocytoma of the skin and joints. Am. J. Med., 28:661, 1960.

Barrow, M. V., and Holubar, K.: Multicentric reticulohistiocytosis and review of 33 patients. Medicine, 48:287, 1969.

Jansen, G. T.: Skin lesions associated with systemic granulomas. *In* The Skin and Internal Disease. New York, McGraw-Hill Book Company, 1967, p. 32.

Labow, T. A., and Shapiro, L.: Giant cell reticulohistiocytoma associated with cancer. N.Y. State J. Med., 65:2941, 1965.

Lyell, A., and Carr, A. J.: Lipoid dermato-arthritis (reticulohistiocytosis). Br. J. Dermatol., 71:12, 1959.

Parkes Weber, F., and Freudenthal, W.: Nodular non-diabetic cutaneous xanthomatosis with hypercholesterolemia and atypical histological features. Proc. R. Soc. Med., Section on Dermatol., 30:552, 1937.

Warin, R. P., Evans, C. D., Hewitt, M., Taylor, A. L., Price, C. H. G., and Middlemiss, J. H.: Reticulohistiocytosis (lipoid dermato-arthritis). Br. Med. J., 1:1387, 1957.

Gardner's Syndrome

Gardner, E. J.: Genetic and clinical study of intestinal polyposis, predisposing factor for carcinoma of colon and rectum. A. J. Hum. Genet., 3:167, 1951.

Gardner, E. J., and Plenk, H. P.: Hereditary pattern for multiple osteomas in family group. Am. J. Hum. Genet., 4:31, 1951.

Gardner, E. J., and Richards, R. C.: Multiple cutaneous and subcutaneous lesions, occurring simultaneously with hereditary polyposis and osteomatosis. Am. J. Hum. Genet., 5:139, 1953.

Gardner, E. J., and Stephens, F. E.: Cancer of the lower digestive tract in one family group. Am. J. Hum. Genet., 2:41, 1950.

Lewis, R. J., and Mitchell, J. C.: Basal cell carcinoma in Gardner's syndrome. Acta Derm. Venereol. (Stockh.), 51:67, 1971.

Leichtling, J. J.: Gardner's syndrome: A report of four cases. Mt. Sinai J. Med., 38:311, 1971.

Oldfield, M. C.: The association of familial polyposis of the colon, with multiple sebaceous cysts. Br. J. Surg., 41:534, 1953/54.

Weiner, R. S., and Cooper, P.: Multiple polyposis of the colon, osteomatosis and soft tissue tumors. Report of a familial syndrome. New Engl. J. Med., 253:795, 1955.

Peutz-Jeghers-Touraine Syndrome

Berkowitz, S. B., Pearl, M. J., and Shapiro, H. H.: Syndrome of intestinal polyposis with melanosis of lips and buccal mucosa. Ann. Surg., 141:129, 1955.

Burdick, D., Prior, J. T., and Scanlon, D. T.: Peutz-Jeghers syndrome: A clinical-pathological study of a large family with a 10-year follow-up. Cancer, 16:854, 1963.

Conner, J. T.: Aesculapian Society of London. Lancet, II:1169, 1895.

Dickson, W. B.: Multiple adenomas of jejunum. Ann. Surg., 119:283, 1944.

Gasser, U., and Arquint, A.: Ein Fall von Peutz-Jeghers Syndrome mit maligner Entartung. Schweiz. Med. Wochenschr., 99:1894, 1969.

Hutchinson, J.: Pigmentations of the lips and mouth. Arch. Surg. (Lond.), 7:920, 1896.

Jeghers, H.: Pigmentation of skin. New Engl. J. Med., 231:88, 122, and 181, 1944.

McKittrick, J. B., Lewis, W. M., Doane, W. A., and Gerwig, W. H.: The Peutz-Jeghers syndrome, report of two cases, one with 30-year follow-up. Arch. Surg., 103:57, 1971.

Paglia, M. A., Ghosh, B., Sherlock, P., and Kurtz, R.: Peutz-Jeghers syndrome, N.Y. State J. Med., 75:402, 1975.

Parkes Weber, F.: Patches of deep pigmentation of the oral mucous membrane not connected with Addison's disease. Quart J. Med., 12:404, 1919.

Peutz, J. L. A.: Over een merkwaardige gecombineerde familiaire polyposis van de skijmvliezen van den tractus intestinalis met die van de neuskeelhote en gepaard met eigenardige pigmantatis van huid- en slijmvliezen. Ned. Tijdschr. Geneeskd., 10:134, 1921.

Scully, R. E.: Sex cord tumor with annular tubules, a distinctive ovarian tumor of the Peutz-Jeghers syndrome. Cancer, 25:1107, 1970.

Touraine, A., and Couder, F.: Syndrome de Peutz (lentigo-polypose digestive). Ann. Dermatol. Syphiligr. (Paris), Series 8:313, 1945.

Touraine, A., and Couder, F.: Lentiginose périorificielle et polypose viscérale. Presse Med., 54:405, 1946.

Arsenical Keratoses

Graham, J. H., and Helwig, E. B.: Bowen's disease and its relationship to systemic cancer. A.M.A. Arch. Dermatol., 80:133, 1959.

Graham, J. H., and Helwig, E. B.: Cutaneous precancerous conditions in man. *In* Conference on Biology of Cutaneous Cancer. Washington, D.C., National Cancer Institute Monograph No. 10, 1963, pp. 323–333.

Graham, J. H., and Helwig, E. B.: Pathology of precancerous dermatoses and precancerous skin lesions and systemic cancer. *In* Tumors of the Skin. Chicago, Year Book Medical Publishers, 1964, pp. 138 and 212.

Herpes Zoster

Carrière :Zona femoro-cutané dans un cas de cancer de l'uterus. Ann. Dermatol. Syphiligr. (Paris), Series 3, 6:892, 1895.

Huguenin, R., Fauvet, J., and Pierat, A.: Les zonas des cancereux. Bull. Mém. Soc. Méd. Hôp. Paris, 66:111, 1950.

Merselis, J. G., Jr., Kaye, D., and Hook, E. W.: Disseminated herpes zoster. A report of 17 cases. Arch. Intern. Med. 113:679, 1964.

Pendergrass, E. P., and Kirsh, D.: Role of irradiation in management of carcinoma of breast. Radiology, 51:767, 1948.

Rogers, R. S., III, and Tindall, J. P.: Pediatric herpes zoster. Paper read at the 120th A.M.A. Annual Convention, Atlantic City, June, 1971.

Rook, A., Williamson, D. S., and Ebling, F. J. G.: Textbook of Dermatology, Vols. I and II. Oxford, Blackwell, 1968.

Dermatitis Herpetiformis

Balabanov, A., and Andreev, V. F.: Dermatite erpetiforme di Duhring in a patient with carcinoma of the prostate. Dermatologica, 129:461, 1964.

Bogrow, B. L.: Zur Kasuistik der Dermatitis herpetiformis Duhring. Arch. Dermatol. Syph. (Berl.), 98:327, 1909.

Bureau, Y., and Barrière, H.: Dermatoses et cancers profonds. Laval Méd., 34:654, 1963.

Cormia, F. E., and Binford, R. T., Jr.: Vesiculobullous eruptions associated with internal disease. *In* The Skin and Internal Disease. New York, McGraw-Hill Book Company, 1967, p. 19.

Coriciati, L.: Dermatite erpetiforme di Duhring e leucemia linfatica cronica. Minerva Dermatol., 38:285, 1960.

Curth, H. O.: Dermatoses and malignant internal tumors. A.M.A. Arch. Dermatol., 71:106, 1955.

Duperrat, B., and Andrade, R.: Radiodermite et cancer; à propos de 52 observations de radiodermite dont 12 cancérisées. Presse Méd., 66(4):52, 1958.

Elliott, J. A.: Bullous dermatoses of toxic origin. Report of a case involving association with chorioncarcinoma. Arch. Dermatol., 37:219, 1938.

Even-Paz, Z., and Sagher, F.: High leucocytosis (leukamoid reactions) in dermatitis herpetiformis. Br. J. Dermatol., 71:325, 1938.

Gjone, E., and Nördoy, A.: Dermatitis herpetiformis, steatorrhea and malignancy. Br. Med. J., 1:610, 1970.

Gougerot, P., Blum, P., and Bralez, J.: Succession puis coexistence d'érythème annulaire centrifuge et de dermatite polymorphe douleureuse. Bull. Soc. Fr. Dermatol. Syphiligr., 38:616, 1931.

Grupper, G.: *In* discussion to Degos, R., Touraine, R., and Leclerc, A.: Maladia de Duhring et épithelioma vulvaire. Bull. Soc. Fr. Dermatol. Syphiligr., 68:864, 1961.

Hartzell, M. B.: Dermatitis herpetiformis: Its etiology and relationship in certain members of the bullous group of diseases. J. Cutan. Genitourinary Dis., 36:497, 1918.

Shatin, H.: Personal communication, 1955.

Skog, E.: Bläschen und blasenbilden-de Dermatosen als pareneoplastische Syndrome in Cutane paraneoplastische Syndrome. Stuttgart, Gustav Fischer Verlag, 1971, p. 35.

Sneddon, I. B.: Cutaneous manifestations of visceral malignancy. Postgrad. Med. J., 46:678, 1970.

Tillman, W. G.: Herpes gestationis with hydatidiform mole and chorion epithelioma. Br. Med. J., 1:1471, 1950.

Tobias, N.: Dermatitis herpetiformis associated with visceral malignancy. Urol. Cutan. Rev., 55:352, 1951.

Pemphigoid

Davis, H.: Two cases of exudative erythema associated with malignant disease of the uterus. Br. J. Dermatol., 34:12, 1922.

Gold, S. C.: Pemphigoid with malignant melanoma. Proc. R. Soc. Med., 54:226, 1961.

Jordon, R. E., Sams, W. M., Jr., and Beutner, E. H.: Complement immunofluorescent staining in bullous pemphigoid. J. Lab. Clin. Med., 74:548, 1969.

Kilby, P. E.: Carcinoma of the pancreas presenting with benign mucous membrane pemphigoid. Cancer, 18:847, 1965.

Lever, W. F.: Pemphigoid. In Jaddssohn's Handbuch der Haut- und Geschlechtskrankheiten. Ergänzungswerk II, 2:661, Berlin, Springer-Verlag, 1965.

Marks, J. M.: Pemphigoid with malignant melanoma. Proc. R. Soc. Med., 54:225, 1961.

Parsons, R. L., and Savin, J. A.: Pemphigoid and malignancy. Br. J. Cancer, 22:669, 1968.

Rook, A. J., and Waddington, E.: Pemphigus and pemphigoid. Br. J. Dermatol., 65:425, 1953.

Thivolet, J., Beyvin, A. J., and Perrot, H.: Maladie de Duhring-Brocq bulleuse paranéoplasique avec autoanticorps antimembrane basale et antinucleaires. Cutane paraneoplastische Syndrome. Stuttgart, Gustav Fischer Verlag, 1971, p. 39.

Wilson, H. T. H.: Discussions to Gold, 1961.

Bowen's Disease

Belisario, J. C.: Cutaneous manifestations associated with internal cancer. Cutis, I:513, 569, 1965, and II:34, 95, 1966.

Bowen, J. T.: Precancerous dermatoses: A sixth case of a type recently described. J. Cutan. Dis., 33:787, 1915.

Bureau, Y., and Barrière, H.: Dermatoses et cancers profonds. Laval Méd., 34:642, 1963.

Caro, M. R.: Discussion following Graham, J. H., Mazzanti, G. R., and Helwig, E. B.: Chemistry of Bowen's disease. Relationship to arsenic. J. Invest. Dermatol., 37:317, 1961.

Epstein, E.: Association of Bowen's disease with visceral cancer. Arch. Dermatol., 82:349, 1960.

Fraser, J. F.: Bowen's disease and Paget's disease of the nipples. Arch. Dermatol. Syph., 18:809, 1928.

Graham, J. H., and Helwig, E. B.: Bowen's disease and its relationship to systemic cancer. A. M. A. Arch. Dermatol. 80:133, 1959.

Graham, J. H., and Helwig, E. B.: Bowens disease and its relationship to systemic cancer. Arch. Dermatol., 83:738, 1961.

Graham, J. H., and Helwig, E. B.: Pathology of precancerous dermatoses. *In* Tumors of the Skin.

57

Cancer of the Lids and Ocular Adnexa

Paul Henkind, M.D., and Alan Friedman, M.D.

INTRODUCTION

This section deals with tumors of the eyelids and conjunctiva. In addition to the usual neoplasms which can involve any skin or mucosal area, there are a number of lesions unique to this region which present diagnostic or therapeutic problems. The regional anatomy will be briefly outlined, for knowledge of the local anatomy is essential in aiding in diagnosis and in planning therapy.

We believe that the ophthalmologist should be primarily responsible for managing lesions in and about the eye; however, this situation rarely prevails, even in large centers, because of the interests of dermatologists and plastic surgeons. However, certain general rules should apply to all who work in the anatomic area. First, when treating lesions which may affect the eye, a visual acuity should be obtained prior to any therapy. Poor or absent vision in the eye on the affected side can modify one's approach. Furthermore, diminished acuity may be claimed following treatment. Second, all lesions should be submitted for histopathologic examina-

tion. All too frequently specimens are discarded. As we shall point out, a large percentage of lid lesions, including malignancies, are misdiagnosed clinically. Third, an accurate history is necessary, and a complete examination of the lesion should be performed. The latter should include palpation of the lesion, palpation of regional lymph nodes, and transillumination whenever possible. Accurate drawings or photographs of lesions prove invaluable both as a teaching aid and for the clinical record.

ANATOMY

General Topography (Fig. 57–1)

The upper lid is limited superiorly by the eyebrow, which forms a definite boundary; the lower lid blends indefinably into the cheek. The medial portion of the lid lacks hair and has a smoother, shinier, and greasier skin than the temporal portion. The mucous membrane conjunctiva lines the inner surface of the

1345

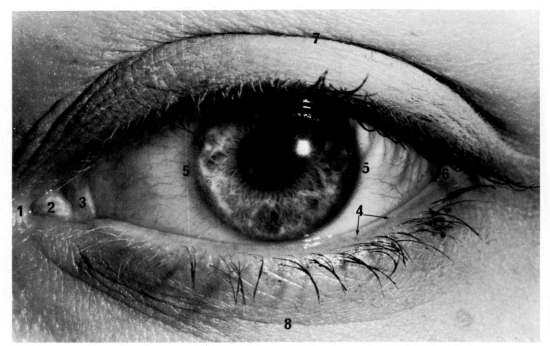

Figure 57–1   External photograph of the left eye. *1*, Medial canthus; *2*, caruncle; *3* plica semilunaris; *4*, gray line; *5*, limbus; *6*, lateral canthus; *7*, superior palpebral furrow; and *8*, inferior palpebral furrow.

lids and covers the anterior portion of the sclera.

Together, the lids and conjunctiva form a functional unit which protects the eyeball from injury, lubricates the globe, drains excess tears, aids the iris in modulating the amount of light entering the eye, and excludes light during sleep.

The Lids

Each upper and lower lid is composed of four distinct layers; skin, muscle, tarsus, and palpebral conjunctiva (Fig. 57–2). Lying between the external skin and internal palpebral conjunctiva are the orbicularis muscle and the more deeply placed tarsus. The lids may be surgically divided into an anterior skin-muscle lamina and a posterior tarsoconjunctival lamina. A convenient landmark to show the proper plane of separation of these layers is the sulcus called the "gray line," which extends the length of the eyelid behind the eyelashes and in front of the meibomian orifices (Fig. 57–2).

The skin of the eyelids, the thinnest in the body, is quite elastic and lacks fat. It is firmly attached to the tissue of the medial and lateral canthi and to the tarsus. Elsewhere, it is loosely attached to underlying tissues. The lid shows a microscopic organization similar to that of other areas of skin; however, papillae, hair follicles, and sebaceous and sweat glands are relatively inconspicuous except at the lid margin. Three rows of lashes grow from the anterior rounded portion of the lid. Holocrine sebaceous glands of Zeis, two to an eyelash, empty through a duct into the hair follicle. Apocrine sweat glands of Moll are unbranched spiral tubules which empty into the lash follicle.

Lying deep to the orbicularis muscle layer is the dense, collagenous tarsus which contains the sebaceous meibomian glands. Approximately 30 glands are present in the upper lid and 20 in the lower lid. The ducts of these holocrine glands open on the lid margin. The junction between skin and conjunctiva is located near the posterior edge of the lid margin just behind the openings of the meibomian glands.

1970a). Only one of our patients was Negro, this in spite of the fact that our hospital center served a large Negro and Oriental community. There seems little question that this neoplasm is uncommon in pigmented races (Payne et al., 1969).

Over 60 percent of our patients had their lid lesion for at least a year before seeking medical attention, and this is in line with other reports of BCE. In one series the mean duration of symptoms was well over five years (Aurora and Blodi, 1970a), while in another (Payne et al., 1969), 10 percent of cases had their lesion for at least 10 years. A number of our patients had previously treated "skin cancer," particularly of facial regions other than the lids. The symptoms of eyelid BCE are given in the following table:

There seems to be some disagreement as to the type of skin in which BCE develops. Some authors feel that the condition is most likely to occur in fair-skinned persons exposed to excessive amounts of sunlight or to chemical, mechanical, or thermal injury (Reeh, 1963). A positive relationship between light eye color and skin cancer, without specific reference to eyelid lesions, has been noted (Gellin et al., 1965). Reeh (1963) noted that chronic irritation of the lids, such as occurs in dermatitis, blepharitis, conjunctivitis, chronic ulcers, discharging sinuses, and irritation from spectacles, may be a predisposing factor in the production of basal cell epitheliomas. On the other hand, Boniuk (1962) felt that most cases develop in areas of normal skin, but that occasional tumors may occur in areas of senile keratosis and radiation dermatosis, as well as in patients with xeroderma pigmentosum.

TABLE 57–3 SYMPTOMS OF 173 PATIENTS WITH BASAL CELL EPITHELIOMAS OF THE EYELIDS*

	No. of Cases	%†
Mass of growth	66	38
Irritation	56	32
Ulceration	30	17
Bleeding	23	13
Cosmesis	15	9
Tearing	11	6
Trichiasis (inturned lashes)	3	2
Miscellaneous	10	6
Asymptomatic	39	23

*Modified from Payne et al.: Arch. Ophthalmol., 81:553, 1969. Copyright 1969, American Medical Association.

†Cases and % reflect more than one possible symptom.

We have not been impressed with any increased frequency of the neoplasm in patients with eyeglasses that press on the bridge or side of the nose.

The distribution of eyelid BCE is of interest. Most series indicate that the lower lid is the most common site, followed by the inner canthal area, the upper lid, and the outer canthal region (Table 57–4). In our series the upper lid was the second most frequent site of occurrence. According to Cobb et al. (1964), large and small lesions did not favor any particular region of the eyelids. Aurora and Blodi (1970a), found that circumscribed lesions were four times more frequent on the lower eyelid than on the inner canthus, whereas extensive lesions involved the inner canthus one and a half times more often than the lower eyelid.

Many cases of BCE of the eyelid present a typical appearance of an ulcerated nodule with telangiectatic vessels

TABLE 57–4 LOCATION OF BASAL CELL EPITHELIOMAS OF THE EYELIDS

Authors	Lower Lid	Inner Canthus	Upper Lid	Outer Canthus	Mixed
Martin (1939)	54.0%	28.0%	13.0%	5.0%	
Driver and Cole (1939)	50.0%	26.5%	9.3%	6.5%	7.7%
Hollander and Krugh (1944)	42.0%	38.0%	13.0%	7.0%	
Stetson and Schulz (1949)	48.2%	21.0%	14.6%	9.0%	7.2%
del Regato (1949)	40.9%	37.7%	10.7%	10.7%	
Barron (1962)	55.3%	18.8%	21.8%	4.1%	
Payne et al. (1969)	51.1%	24.2%	18.6%	6.1%	
Henkind and Friedman	67.0%	10.0%	20.0%	3.0%	

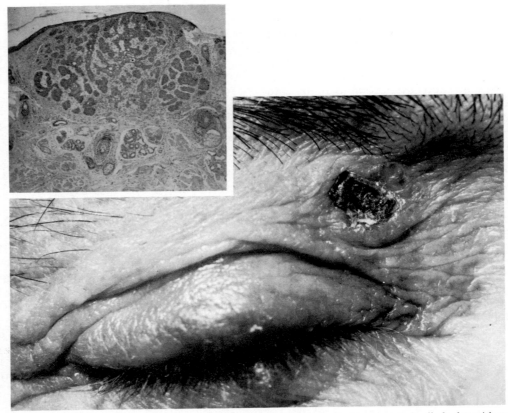

Figure 57–4 Basal cell epithelioma of the right upper lid. Note central ulceration and rolled edge with attendant telangiectatic vessels at border. Inset shows nests of tumor cells in the dermis with ulceration of overlying epithelium.

over its surface and rolled pearly edges (Figs. 57–4 and 57–5). There are, however, numerous instances of uncharacteristic lesions, and these range from small, solid nodules, "cysts," and long, linear ulcers to large, polypoid masses (Fig. 57–5). These can and do present diagnostic problems. In this regard Welch and Duke (1958) found that only 56 percent of the cases which they examined histopathologically had the correct clinical diagnosis. A later report from the same institution mentioned a correct clinical diagnosis in 60 percent of 273 cases (Payne et al., 1969). Papilloma, cyst, and nevus were the most frequent misdiagnoses.

A perhaps disquieting point noted in one more recent work (Einaugler and Henkind, 1969) was that only one-half of 40 eyelid BCE's submitted for histopathologic examination appeared to have been completely excised. Analysis of an additional 62 cases gives an incomplete excision rate of just under 50 percent (Henkind and Friedman, unpublished data). In this series there were numerous examples of tumor cords and nests beneath intact and otherwise normal appearing epithelium at the edge of the excised specimens (Fig. 57–6). Aurora and Blodi (1970a) reported that there was incomplete excision in 30 of their series of 129 primary cases of BCE of the eyelids. It seems that clinicians find it exceedingly difficult to determine the full extent of tumor involvement in many cases of this tumor. Another possibility is the reluctance of the surgeon (or radiotherapist) to excise or treat sufficient tissue for fear of involving the lacrimal drainage apparatus or of producing a poor cosmetic result. One must attack BCE of the eyelids boldly if one expects to eradicate the tumor; cosmesis should be a secondary concern. It is likely

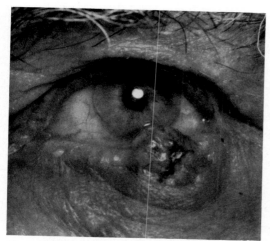

Figure 57–5 Large polypoid basal cell epithelioma located in the middle of the left lower lid. Central ulceration and prominent telangiectatic vessels are present.
(See also Color Plate X–A.)

that most cases of so-called recurrence of tumor involve incomplete excision (or incomplete radiation) of the primary lesion. The number of patients who will suffer "recurrence" after incomplete treatment is not known. The work of Gooding et al. (1965) suggested that only about one-third of lesions which show marginal extension will recur. Very few of their cases were from the eyelids.

If BCE of the eyelids is untreated or incompletely eradicated, it tends to pursue an unremitting, chronic course for many years, with spreading ulceration and invasion of soft tissue and ultimately of bone (Fig. 57–7). We have noted that the tarsus tends to prevent the tumor from invading the deeper lid structures until very late in the disease. Similarly, bony involvement seems to be uncommon except in previously treated lesions where natural boundaries have been disturbed by scalpel or x-ray. Those patients whom we have seen with the deepest involvement of the orbital structures, nasal passages, and even brain had generally been treated on multiple occasions. Patients may die from extension of eyelid BCE. Indeed, Birge (1938) reported an 11 percent mortality among a series of advanced cases of BCE.

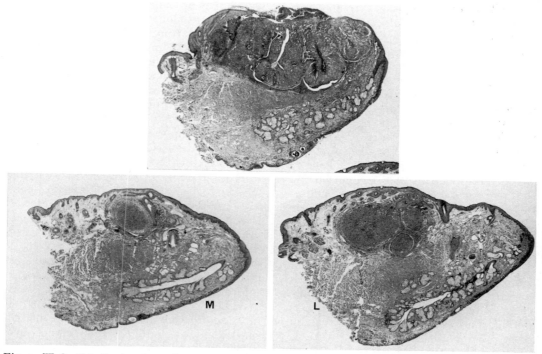

Figure 57–6 *Top,* Section through center of basal cell epithelioma of lid, showing large mass of tumor and ulceration of overlying epithelium. *Below, left* and *right,* medial *(M)* and lateral *(L)* edges of specimen, showing cords of tumor cells at the cut edges of the surgical excision. (*From* Einaugler and Henkind: Am. J. Ophthalmol., 67:413, 1969.)

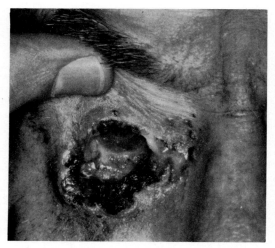

Figure 57–7 Far advanced basal cell epithelioma originating in the right lower lid. The tumor has destroyed the lid and invaded both medial and lateral canthi, the soft tissues of the orbit, and maxillary bone.
(See also Color Plate X–B.)

He felt that tumors involving the upper lid or inner canthus had a higher rate of mortality. Other authors have also noted a significant mortality due to extensive invasive BCE of the eyelids (Aurora and Blodi, 1970a; Payne et al., 1969). A striking finding reported by Payne and co-workers (1969) was that 25 percent of patients who underwent excision of an eyelid BCE were unaware of the diagnosis, apparently never having been told the potentially serious nature of their disease. In some cases patient follow-up was only desultory. We recommend periodic follow-up examinations for several years.

A variety of histologic classifications have been applied to BCE in general. We prefer to use Lever's (1967) classification. By far the most common tumor is the undifferentiated solid type (Fig. 57–8), composed of solid masses of uniform, dark-staining (basophilic) nuclei and scanty cytoplasm. There is characteristic palisading of the peripheral cells of the tumor cords. Not infrequently the tumor mass appears retracted from the surrounding tissue. In general, there is no inflammatory reaction around the neoplasm. Some BCE's are associated with marked melanin production and clinically can be confused with seborrheic keratosis or even malignant melanoma. Others have necrosis of the cells

in the center of the tumor lobule with "cyst" formation. The more differentiated adenoid type of BCE is the second most frequent histologic type (Einaugler and Henkind, 1969; Aurora and Blodi, 1970a). This type has been reported to occur more frequently in females than males (Aurora and Blodi, 1970a). In the past, the term "mixed basosquamous-type tumor" was reported with some frequency; Birge (1938) noted 14 percent in his series, and Driver and Cole (1939) 8.2 percent in their series. More recent authors do not utilize this classification but rather note that squamoid differentiation may be a prominent feature of certain lesions (Boniuk, 1964). Areas of pseudo-epitheliomatous hyperplasia in association with BCE's may also cause confusion.

How should one treat BCE's of the eyelids? Excision, curettage, cryosurgery, chemosurgery, chemical applications, and x-radiation have all been utilized. It is too tedious to recite the claims and counter-claims of proponents of the various modalities of treatment. Any method which will destroy the entire lesion while preserving, as much as possible, normal tissue will suffice. The problems in planning treatment are: (1) determining the extent of the lesion, and (2) preserving the structure and function of the lids and eyeball. Preservation of structure and function is meaningless if the tumor is not eradicated. Determining the extent of the lesion is a more difficult problem. Should one do multiple biopsies to delimit the borders of the lesion? This may be particularly worthwhile in very extensive lesions where radiation is considered to be the modality of choice, or if one is trying to preserve the lacrimal drainage apparatus. If the tumor is to be excised, at least 5 mm. of tissue, or one-half the diameter of the evident lesion, should be taken in excess at the borders, and care should be taken to mark the edges so the pathologist can report the location of free or involved margins. Very large lesions involving more than one half of the lids and medial canthal lesions, unless very small, are probably best handled by radiotherapy (Lederman, 1964a and 1964b). We are in agreement with other ophthalmic plastic surgeons (Fox, 1970; Smith and Cherubini,

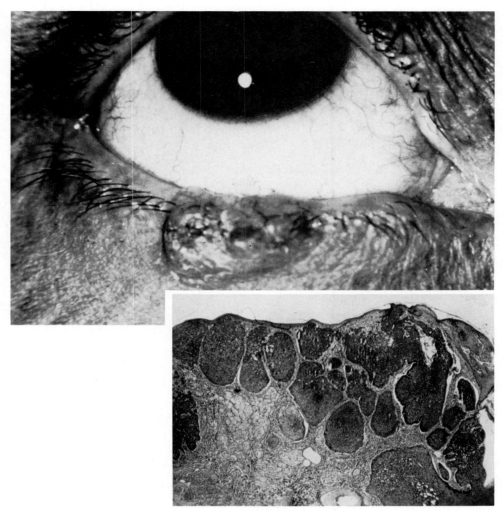

Figure 57–8 Solid basal cell epithelioma appearing on right lower lid. Inset shows nests of tumor cells infiltrating deeply within lid tissues.

1970) who have advocated surgical excision of large BCE's without plastic repair, for remarkably good cosmetic results have been effected; this is particularly so when dealing with lesions of the medial canthus (Fig. 57–9). For recurrent lesions, particularly those which have been treated on multiple occasions, we advocate Mohs' chemosurgery (Robbins et al., 1971). This modality of treatment may save otherwise "hopeless" cases.

Squamous Cell Carcinoma. Squamous cell carcinoma (SCC), the second most frequent malignancy involving the eyelids, is far less common than basal cell epithelioma. The ratio of occurrence appears to be at least 10:1 in favor of the

latter. Unfortunately, statistics from literature older than a decade cannot be relied upon with assurance, for the diagnosis of SCC often cannot be sustained in the light of modern scrutiny (Kwitko et al., 1963). For this reason we will consider eyelid SCC only in broad terms.

Squamous cell carcinoma tends to affect older individuals, particularly those with precancerous dermatoses, such as senile keratosis, radiation keratosis, and Bowen's disease. It also affects younger individuals afflicted with xeroderma pigmentosum. SCC affects the eyes of cattle, causing economic loss to ranchers (Russell et al., 1956). Occasional lesions may arise in otherwise normal skin. According to Bon-

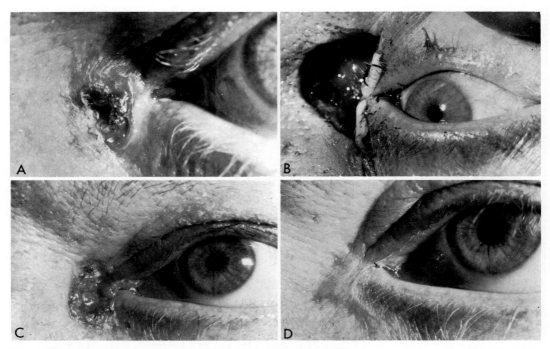

Figure 57-9 Basal cell epithelioma of the left medial canthus. The tumor was surgically excised and the wound allowed to heal by granulation only. *A,* Clinical picture of the tumor. *B,* Photograph taken in operating room just after excision of lesion. *C,* Three weeks postoperatively. *D,* Eight weeks postoperatively. The wound has healed by granulation with excellent cosmetic results.

iuk (1962), most such neoplasms are solitary on the lid, but the patient often has other skin tumors. While any part of the eyelid may be involved, the lower lid is the commonest site for SCC. This neoplasm has many guises, ranging from an ulcerated nodular lesion, resembling basal cell epithelioma, a warty lesion, or keratin horn, to the typical flat, crusty, ulcerated lesion (Fig. 57–10). In general the lesion grows relatively rapidly compared with BCE. Clinical differential diagnosis includes keratoacanthoma, keratin horn, senile keratosis, irritated seborrheic keratosis, inverted follicular keratosis, and basal cell epithelioma.

In all probability the mortality from SCC is higher than that reported with BCE, particularly since the former tumor has a predilection for metastasis to regional lymph nodes. Aurora and Blodi (1970b) were able to obtain follow-up data on 10 of 15 patients with this lesion examined at Iowa. Four patients had died of the tumor within two years of the diagnosis.

The management of SCC of the eyelids depends on the extent and location of the lesion. Surgical excision is recommended for small, noncanthal lesions, but radiation is the treatment of choice for large lesions and those involving the canthi, especially the median canthus. Mohs' chemosurgery should be reserved for recurrent or very extensive tumors.

Adenocarcinoma of the Sebaceous Glands. Sebaceous carcinoma is a rare tumor of the eyelid and adnexa accounting for less than 5 percent of malignant tumors in this area. We had no cases in our series of 557 lid lesions, but Aurora and Blodi (1970b) had 7 cases in 892 consecutive lid lesions (3.2 percent of their malignant lid tumors). Adenocarcinoma of the sebaceous glands of the eyelid and adnexa may arise in any of a number of locations: (1) the glands of Zeis; (2) the meibomian glands; (3) the sebaceous glands on the cutaneous surface of the eyelid; (4) the sebaceous glands of the eyebrow; and (5) the sebaceous glands located in the caruncle. Boniuk and Zim-

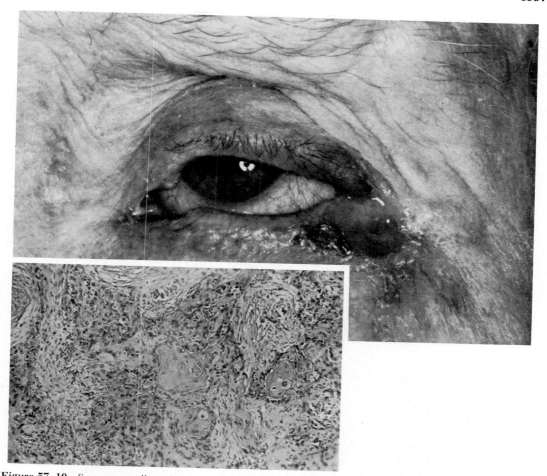

Figure 57–10 Squamous cell carcinoma of the left lateral canthus. Inset shows microscopic appearance of the tumor with well-developed horn pearls in the center of the field.

merman (1968) collected 88 cases of sebaceous carcinoma of the eyelid, eyebrow, and caruncle at the Armed Forces Institute of Pathology. In their series, the average age at time of diagnosis was 62 years, and females were involved in a 1.4:1 ratio to males. In most instances tumors developed in Caucasians. The site of origin is summarized in Table 57–5.

The lesions show a definite predilection for the upper lid: of the 78 cases arising in the eyelid, 47 arose in the upper lid, 21 in the lower lid, and 7 in both lids. In 24 instances, clinical presentation was on the conjunctival surface. Meibomian carcinoma often presents as an enlarging lid mass, usually with little evidence of ulceration of overlying skin. The clinical appearance may then simulate a chalazion,

and in several instances repeated incisions and drainage were carried out prior to the correct diagnosis. The tumors arising at the lid margin in Zeis glands may show an ulcerated surface and create confusion

TABLE 57–5 SEBACEOUS CARCINOMA OF EYELID, EYEBROW, AND CARUNCLE*

Site of Origin	Number
Meibomian gland	24
Zeis gland	9
Meibomian and Zeis glands	9
Eyelid, exact site undetermined	36
Caruncle	8
Eyebrow	2
	88

*Modified from Boniuk and Zimmerman: Trans. Am. Acad. Ophthalmol., 72:619, 1968.

with a basal cell epithelioma. Other clinical signs may be present, such as unilateral conjunctivitis or blepharitis.

On histopathologic examination of the tumor, varying degrees of sebaceous differentiation may be observed. The cells characteristically show foamy cytoplasm, and frozen sections with fat stains may be a helpful aid in diagnosis.

The clinical course of adenocarcinoma of the sebaceous glands is poor. Ten patients (13.5 percent died with probable or proven metastases in 74 cases with adequate follow-up (Boniuk and Zimmerman, 1968). Regional lymph node metastases (preauricular, submandibular, or cervical) were reported in 21 of these patients (28.4 percent). Orbital invasion ne-

cessitated an exenteration in 15 of 88 patients (17 percent) for treatment of direct extensions.

Adequate local excision is the recommended mode of therapy, followed by careful observation for local recurrence or regional lymph node metastasis.

Other Malignant Tumors. Several other types of malignant tumors occur in the lids. We have seen rhabdomyosarcoma on two occasions present as lid masses in children (Fig. 57–11). These tumors develop almost exclusively in the pediatric age group and arise deep in the interstitial tissues of the orbit superonasally. Rarely metastatic tumors to the lids have been reported (Riley, 1970). The breast and the gastrointestinal and geni-

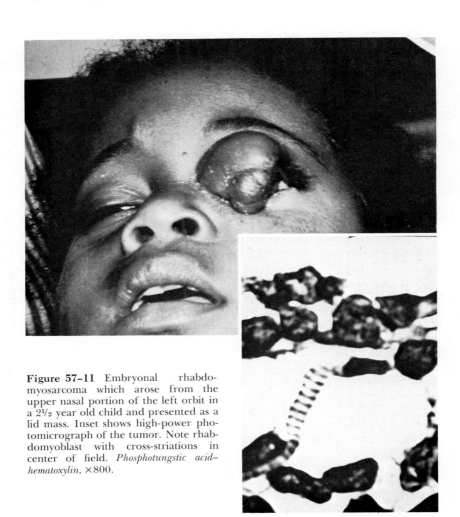

Figure 57–11 Embryonal rhabdomyosarcoma which arose from the upper nasal portion of the left orbit in a 2½ year old child and presented as a lid mass. Inset shows high-power photomicrograph of the tumor. Note rhabdomyoblast with cross-striations in center of field. *Phosphotungstic acid–hematoxylin,* ×800.

lesions are radiosensitive, the treatment of choice is complete excision.

Squamous Cell Carcinoma. Squamous cell carcinoma appears at the limbus as a highly vascular, papillary growth firmly affixed to the globe. Though similar in histologic appearance to lesions of squamous cell carcinoma appearing elsewhere in the body, those lesions arising at the limbus tend to remain superficial for a long period. Eventually, if they remain untreated, extension occurs, and the tumor spreads over cornea and sclera (Fig. 57–17) and may finally prolapse through the lids. Not infrequently, it may grow entirely around the cornea at the limbus. Though squamous cell carcinomas may reach a

rather large size, they are of a very low order of malignancy and frequently show minimal invasion. Metastasis to regional lymph nodes or distant sites is quite rare (Zimmerman, 1964). Thus conservative management, such as local excision rather than early enucleation, should be employed in eradication of these tumors.

Some Lesions of the Conjunctiva Which May Be Confused Clinically With Cancer

Dyskeratosis (Leukoplakia). An alteration in the character of corneal and con-

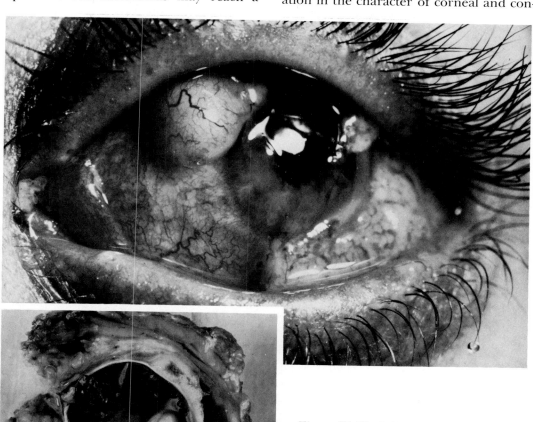

Figure 57–17 Orbital exenteration specimen of squamous cell carcinoma of the conjunctiva. Note the bulky, vascular masses at the limbus. The tumor (inset) surrounds the anterior segment of the eyeball.

junctival epithelium may appear, usually in the fifth or sixth decade. We conveniently classify these lesions clinically as "leukoplakia." These changes usually occur as localized opaque plaques at the limbus in the palpebral aperture (Fig. 57–18). Less commonly they appear on the bulbar or palpebral conjunctiva or on cornea. When present at the limbus, they may be associated with prominent feeder vessels but without an inflammatory element. They are freely movable over the underlying sclera and at times may extend onto cornea or over the bulbar conjunctiva. Histologically the changes are essentially those of epidermalization, acanthosis, and dyskeratosis.

Chalazion. A chalazion is a chronic inflammation of a meibomian or Zeis gland. These lesions are usually painless and slow-growing. They appear as a localized swelling in the conjunctiva (or overlying lid) (Fig. 57–19). Some associated hyperemia of the conjunctiva is often present. The characteristic histologic appearance is one of a lipogranuloma, often with a capsule around the lesion. In the early stage a vacuole lies in the center of the lesion surrounded by epithelioid cells, multinucleated giant cells, lymphocytes, and plasma cells. The lesions have on occasion been misinterpreted as the lesions of sarcoidosis or tuberculosis. They are treated with simple incision and curettage.

Papilloma. Papillomas of the conjunctiva are common and appear in all age

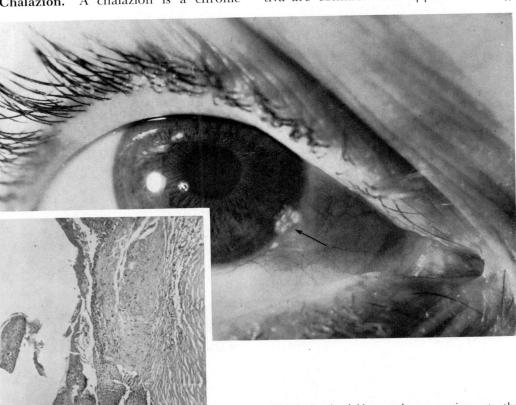

Figure 57–18 Leukoplakic patch presenting at the limbus, right eye. Histopathologic examination (inset) revealed acanthosis and epidermalization. This picture is quite characteristic of benign dyskeratosis.

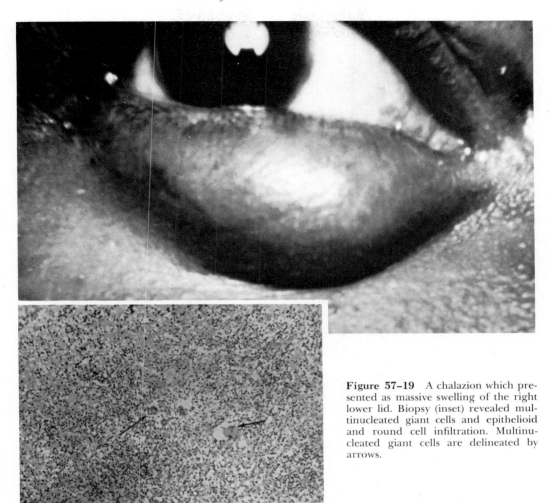

Figure 57-19 A chalazion which presented as massive swelling of the right lower lid. Biopsy (inset) revealed multinucleated giant cells and epithelioid and round cell infiltration. Multinucleated giant cells are delineated by arrows.

groups. They appear at the limbus, on the caruncle, and at the lid margin and are typically soft, pink, pedunculated, or sessile (Fig. 57-20). They have a raspberry-like appearance, and close examination reveals their characteristic fingerlike processes with a vascularized core. Recurrence, rather rapid at times, is common following incomplete excision. Recently cryotherapy has been added as a therapeutic modality, although we favor excision.

Pigmented Conjunctival Tumors

Nevi. Nevi are the most frequently found tumors in the conjunctiva. Approximately one-third are detected before age 9 and 90 percent by age 30 (Jay, 1965 and 1967). They are, for the most part, benign lesions which, after their initial appearance, usually grow slowly in childhood, arrest in adulthood, and atrophy in old age. Some nevi appear to undergo malignant transformation and become melanomas.

Nevi are frequently located at the limbus or on the bulbar conjunctiva in the interpalpebral fissure (Fig. 57-21). Limbal nevi tend to be flat and may extend onto the cornea. Bulbar nevi may be more bulky and elevated. Nevi may also be found on the plica and caruncle (Fig. 57-22). In the latter location they often appear cystic when examined with the slitlamp biomicroscope. Clinically, nevi usually present as dark brown or black spots, but apigmented or salmon-colored lesions are not rare, and

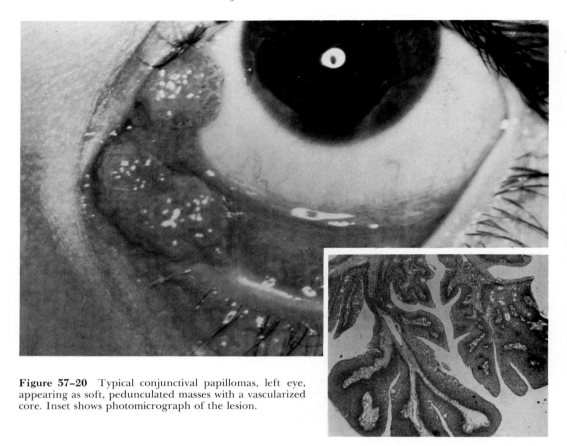

Figure 57–20 Typical conjunctival papillomas, left eye, appearing as soft, pedunculated masses with a vascularized core. Inset shows photomicrograph of the lesion.

about 30 percent lack pigment (Duke-Elder, 1965). Cyclical increases and decreases in pigmentation have been observed. Such changes have been described both at puberty and during pregnancy. Junctional nevi are a common finding in children. With aging, the nevus cell population tends to migrate to a subepithelial location. Intraepithelial cell nests of nevus cells are uncommon after the third decade and should be viewed with some suspicion. About one-half of conjunctival nevi have associated epithelial downgrowths (Fig. 57–22), and cystic change is not infrequent (Jay, 1965); this is unlike the situation in skin nevi, where such findings may suggest malignant change.

We routinely photograph and follow patients with conjunctival nevi. Indications for excision are progressive enlargement, increased vascularization, inflammation, excessive pigmentation, or poor cosmetic appearance. Excisional biopsy is the procedure of choice when it is elected to remove these lesions.

Precancerous Melanosis. This condition represents the conjunctival counterpart of Hutchinson's freckle of the skin (Fig. 57–23). Synonyms include malignant lentigo and intraepithelial melanoma (Jay, 1965). Precancerous melanosis is a lesion of the elderly, first appearing in the fifth and sixth decades. Characteristically, the lesion is unilateral, patchy, and widespread (Reese, 1966). Multiple, flat, brown or black pigmented areas are scattered in the conjunctiva. The skin of the lids and the corneal epithelium may also be involved. The melanosis has a variable and protracted course. It may remain stationary, regress, or progress to invasive melanoma. Probably less than a quarter of cases undergo malignant change, and only then after five to ten years. The development of malignancy is heralded by enlargement, increased pigmentation, and

del Regato, J. A.: Roentgen therapy of carcinoma of the skin of the eyelids. Radiology, 52:564, 1949.

Riley, F. C.: Metastatic tumors of the eyelids. Am. J. Ophthalmol., 69:259, 1970.

Robbins, P., Henkind, P., and Menn, H.: Chemosurgery for eyelid lesions. Trans. Am. Acad. Ophthalmol., 75:1228, 1971.

Russell, W., Wynne, S., and Loquvam, G.: Studies on bovine ocular squamous carcinoma. Cancer, 9:1, 1956.

Smith, B., and Cherubini, T. D.: Oculoplastic surgery: A compendium of principles and techniques. St. Louis, Mo., C. V. Mosby Company, 1970, p. 54.

Stetson, C. G., and Schulz, M. D.: Carcinoma of the eyelid: Analysis of 301 cases and review of the literature. New Engl. J. Med., 241:725, 1949.

Welch, R. B., and Duke, J. R.: Lesions of the lids: A statistical note. Am. J. Ophthalmol., 45:415, 1958.

Zimmerman, L. E.: Squamous Cell Carcinoma and Related Lesions of the Bulbar Conjunctiva. *In* Boniuk, M. (Ed.): Ocular and Adnexal Neoplasms. St. Louis, Mo., C. V. Mosby Company, 1964, p. 49.

Zimmerman, L. E.: Criteria for management of melanosis. Arch. Ophthalmol., 76:307, 1966.

58

Cancer of the External Ear Canal

John F. Daly, M.D.

Squamous cell carcinoma of the external ear canal is not common; the explanation may be in the special features the canal presents. The skin-lined tube is peculiarly suited to its functions: the transmission of sound and the protection of the delicate tympanic membrane located in its depths. The epidermis of the canal is of a special type; it is only two cells thick covering the drum, 0.1 mm. thick over the bony canal, and 1 to 1.5 mm. in the cartilaginous part. There are no hair follicles or sebaceous glands on the tympanic membrane, and only a few scattered hairs are found on the upper wall of the bony canal. Other unique features are the absence of sweat glands, and the ability of the squamous epithelium to migrate toward the external meatus before degenerating. The outer cartilaginous portion is generously supplied with hair follicles, sebaceous glands, and apocrine (ceruminous) glands, providing another protective barrier. These remarkable features for protecting the drum membrane, which lies 1½ inches deep to the surface of the head, also protect the canal from injury. It is protected from the actinic rays of the sun, from carcinogens, and from trauma to which structures covered by squamous epithelium are normally subjected.

These protective features are lost in the presence of irritating discharge from a chronic otitis media or chronic dermatoses, or when picks of various types are used to alleviate an itch.

The incidence of cancer of the external ear canal is usually determined by admissions to an otolaryngologic clinic. Parrott found 9 cases in 8500 admissions to an otolaryngologic clinic. Lewis (1960) reported that cancer of the external canal occurs in from 1 to 5000 to 1 in 15,000 otologic conditions, depending on the clinic's population, being higher in a cancer referral center.

Moreover, the reported incidence of cancer of the ear as it occurs in its three parts differs from author to author—a difference that reflects a difference in the selected population and not a difference in the disease. Generally the incidence decreases from the external ear (pinna), to the external canal, to the middle ear. Conley (1965) reported 50 percent inci-

1372

dence in the external ear, 30 percent in the ear canal, and 20 percent in the middle ear. However, Lewis (1960), reporting 143 advanced cancers of the ear, found 20 cases arising primarily on the external ear, 105 primarily in the external ear canal, and 18 on the middle ear and mastoid process.

AGE, SEX, AND RACE

Squamous cell carcinoma of the external ear canal is rare before the fourth decade. It is a condition of the aging process. Its highest incidence is in the sixth decade of life. Women are slightly more prone to develop cancer of the ear canal than are men; the reverse is true for cancer of the external ear. Tabb et al. (1964) reported 10 cases of cancer of the canal, all in white patients, from a clinic population that was 60 percent black, confirming other reports of its higher incidence in white patients.

PREEXISTING CONDITIONS

One-third to one-half of the patients have chronic middle ear infections or chronic dermatoses. Repeated trauma from toothpicks, match sticks, and other instruments used to relieve itching of an underlying dermatosis may be another contributing factor. However, in one-third of the patients a precipitating factor cannot be established, and one must conclude that the lesions arose de novo. Since discharge is also a common presenting symptom of cancer of the ear, in many instances it is difficult to determine whether it is an indication of a preexisting infection or of the cancer itself.

PATHOLOGY

Primary malignant neoplasms of the external ear canal are classified according to origin as epithelial (squamous cell carcinoma, basal cell carcinoma, melanoma), glandular (adenocarcinoma, including cerumenomas, malignant salivary gland tumors, and adenoid cystic carcinomas),

or mesenchymal tumors (sarcomas, rhabdomyosarcomas).

The squamous cell carcinomas tend to be moderately well differentiated and slow-growing; usually they remain locally invasive and metastasize late in the course of the disease. They occur more frequently in the bony portion of the canal.

The basal cell cancers follow the biologic pattern of basal cell cancer seen elsewhere. They appear first as a waxy, elevated growth near the external meatus, then develop to the ulcer stage with raised edges, and finally extensively invade the surrounding structures, becoming locally destructive. They are more common on the external ear.

Melanomas are uncommon in the external ear canal. Adenocarcinomas are rare. They may arise from the cerumenous glands (cerumenomas) or from salivary gland tissue—either as adenoid cystic carcinomas or malignant mixed tumors.

Embryonal rhabdomyosarcomas of the external ear canal occur in the pediatric age group and are aggressive, fast-growing tumors.

Tumors may involve the external ear canal by extension from contiguous structures, e.g., the pinna and middle ear and the parotid gland. Kidney and breast carcinomas metastasize to the temporal bone and present in the external canal.

Benign tumors of the external canal are many and include osteomas found along the suture lines, polyps, papillomas, eosinophilic granulomas, hemangiomas, and chemodectomas. Chemodectomas are locally destructive neoplasms arising from nonchromaffin paraganglioma tissue in the middle ear and in the jugular fossa.

Malignant granuloma may arise in the external auditory canal. Because its presentation and clinical course resemble those of a malignant neoplasm, it must be considered in a differential diagnosis. Malignant granuloma should be mentioned here even though it is not a neoplastic process. Clinically it resembles malignant disease in its destructive course and thus is a problem in the differential diagnosis before a definitive microscopic diagnosis of cancer has been made.

ANATOMY

The anatomic features of the canal determine the course of the disease, set limitations on its treatment, and influence its
prognosis. The external ear canal penetrates deeply into the temporal bone,
bringing it in contact with the surrounding
structures (Fig. 58–1). Its outer third is
cartilaginous and fibrous; it contains the
ceruminous glands, hair follicles, and sebaceous glands. The cartilage forms the
anterior and inferior walls and is incomplete posterosuperiorly where it abuts the
mastoid process. The cartilage is split anteriorly by the clefts of Santorini. The
inner two-thirds is the bony portion; the
tympanic plate of the temporal bone comprises the inferior and anterior wall, and
the squama and mastoid process make up
the superior and posterior wall. The
neighboring structures are, superiorly,
the middle fossa; anteriorly, the temporomandibular point; inferiorly, the parotid
gland and the soft tissue of the neck; and
posteriorly, the mastoid process and the
vertical portion of the facial nerve. Medially the middle ear is separated by the
thin drum membrane. Laterally it is continuous with the concha of the external
ear.

Its sensory nerve supply is from the
auriculotemporal branch of the trigeminal
nerve, the auricular branch (Arnold) of

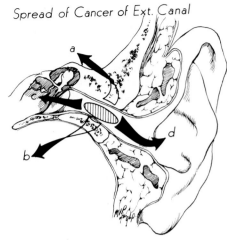

Spread of Cancer of Ext. Canal

Figure 58–2 Pathways of spread of cancer of external ear canal: *(a)* middle fossa; *(b)* neck and
pterygoid muscles and temporomandibular joint; *(c)*
middle ear, inner ear, facial nerve, eustachian tube,
and jugular bulb; *(d)* external meatus and pinna.

the vagus, and the glossopharyngeal
nerve. The skin of the canal receives a
generous nerve supply and is very sensitive. The facial nerve courses through the
middle ear on its medial wall, and in its
vertical course through the mastoid portion it is only a few millimeters from the
external canal.

The middle ear may be invaded by
cancer arising in the external canal, thus
providing additional pathways of extension along the facial nerve and eustachian
tube to the parapharyngeal space, into the
petrous portion of the temporal bone,
through the thin tegmen tympani into the
middle cranial fossa, into the inner ear,
posteriorly into the mastoid and inferiorly
into the jugular fossa (Fig. 58–2).

The great venous channels of the head
surround the temporal bone, the lateral
sinus, the jugular bulb, and the petrosal
sinuses. On the anterior medial wall of the
middle ear, the internal carotid courses in
a thin-walled bony canal. These vascular
channels provide additional routes of extension; they are sources of massive hemorrhage and are major factors limiting the
operative procedures for cancer of the
temporal bone.

The lymphatic vessels of the external
canal drain anteriorly into the preauricular nodes, posteriorly into the postauricu-

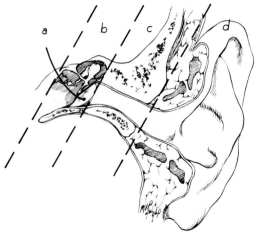

Figure 58–1 Anatomic divisions of ear: *(a)* drum
membrane; *(b)* middle ear; *(c)* osseous canal; *(d)*
cartilaginous canal and pinna.

lar nodes, and inferiorly into inferior auricular and subdigastric nodes.

CLINICAL COURSE

Chronic discharge (usually serous or serosanginous), pain (usually constant), a blocked sensation, swelling of the external auditory meatus, and loss of hearing are symptoms common to infections of the middle and external ear canal and also to cancer of the external canal (Fig. 58–3). Since infection is by far the more common disease of the ear, carcinomas are frequently not suspected when first seen. This is particularly true when the patient has had a chronic ear discharge for from 10 to 20 years. Delays of six months or more may occur before a biopsy is taken and correct diagnosis established.

Constant deep ear pain, a bloody discharge, and failure to respond to antibiotic therapy finally warn the unsuspecting otolaryngologist that another disease process has arisen in a relatively innocuous chronic ear condition.

The severity of the pain is due to the pressure of the swelling of the tissues confined within the bony cartilaginous walls, to secondary infection, and to invasion of bone and nerve sheaths.

These symptoms occurring in a patient

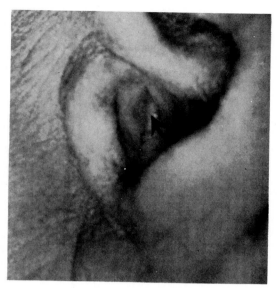

Figure 58–4 Complete obstruction of external ear canal by squamous cell carcinoma.

over 50 years of age who has had a chronic ear discharge for many years should prompt a presumptive diagnosis of cancer. Ulcerations, granulomas, polyps which bleed when manipulated, and a stenotic swelling of the canal are definite indications for biopsy (Figs. 58–3 and 58–4). Tissue for histologic diagnosis can easily be obtained. The skin of the meatus can be infiltrated with an anesthetic agent, and the tissue can be obtained painlessly with a small punch biopsy forceps.

Swelling in the preauricular region or mastoid area in part may be due to infection but commonly is due to extension through the cartilage or metastasis to the pre- and postauricular lymph nodes (Fig. 58–5). Relief of symptoms and a decrease in the swelling of the canal, which follow administration of antibiotics, should not be taken as evidence that the process is simply infectious in nature. Biopsy of a suspected lesion in the canal should not be delayed. Facial nerve paralysis, partial or complete, may be due to extension into the middle ear or invasion posteriorly into the mastoid, where the facial nerve in its vertical course lies only a few millimeters away.

Vertigo is a late and ominous sign. Deep boring pain on the temporal area and behind the eye signals intracranial extension and involvement of the dura as

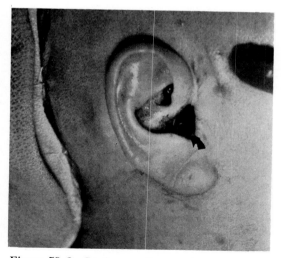

Figure 58–3 Carcinoma of external ear canal extending to and involving external meatus and infiltrating the concha of the pinna with upper cervical lymph node metastases.

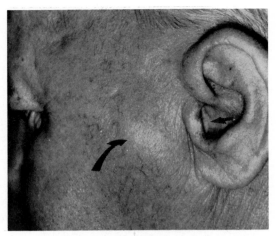

Figure 58–5   Carcinoma of cartilaginous portion of external canal; positive metastatic preauricular lymph node.

well as the trigeminal nerve and its branches. Extension anteriorly involves the temporomandibular joint, the parotid gland, and the pterygomaxillary space. Trismus is an indication of infiltration of the pterygoid muscles. The tumor may extend along the eustachian tube, invading the base of the skull. Invasion of the parapharyngeal space may present as a smooth bulge of the lateral nasopharyngeal wall.

Involvement of 9th, 10th, and 11th cranial nerves occurs late in the course of the disease when the tumor has invaded the jugular fossa and base of skull.

Roentgenograms are helpful in determining the extent of the disease. Routine mastoid and skull films and tomography of the temporal bone should be done. Angiography of the carotid vessels and jugulograms give additional information about involvement of these structures or their displacement by the tumor. The clinical findings and the roentgen studies help to define the extent of the disease upon which a judgment of its resectability can be made.

Distant metastasis of squamous carcinoma of the external ear is uncommon. The tumor tends to remain localized, producing death by invasion of the intercranial cavity. Only 20 percent of the tumors have distant metastasis.

DIFFERENTIAL DIAGNOSIS

Two lesions of a progressively destructive nature which present in the external canal are the glomus jugular and malignant granuloma.

Glomus jugular tumors may present in the floor of the canal near the drum. The bluish color of the tumor, covered by a thin layer of the skin, and its definite pulsation indicate the nature of the tumor. They occur in a younger age group.

Malignant granuloma of the external canal may present with symptoms of serosanguineous discharge, pain, swelling of the canal, hearing loss, and, later in the course, facial paralysis. The patients are usually in the sixth and seventh decades, are diabetic, and have had a chronic ear infection. Several biopsies may be necessary to confirm the diagnosis.

Neurilemmomas of the middle ear, cholesteatoma primary or secondary to middle ear disease, osteomas, meningiomas, and metastatic carcinoma to the temporal bone should also be considered in the differential diagnosis.

In children, rhabdomyosarcoma runs a rapidly fatal course.

CLASSIFICATION OF SQUAMOUS CELL CARCINOMA OF EXTERNAL EAR CANAL

Staging of cancer of the external ear canal according to the TNM system has not been feasible. The anatomy of the area does not lend itself readily to this type of classification. A simple classification is the division into (1) cancers localized to the external canal and not extending widely; (2) advanced cancers extending beyond the canal that are resectable; and (3) advanced cancers extending widely that are not resectable. This simple classification separates the cancer that can be resected with adequate margins from the advanced cancers, in which resection is doubtful or impossible and the prognosis is poor. Miller (1955) has analyzed a group of cancers of the external canal and found no significant difference in prognosis based on the location in the canal, the size of the presenting lesion, the quadrant of the canal in which the tumor was located, and its relation to the lymphatic drainage; nor does the histologic classification significantly determine the course of the disease and its prognosis.

The far advanced lesions are those that have invaded, superiorly, the intracranial cavity; anteriorly, the eustachian tube, parapharyngeal space, and jugular bulb; and medially, the inner ear and internal auditory meatus, the posterior fossa, or occipital bone. These are surgically not resectable.

TREATMENT

Radiation therapy and radical surgery have been used as primary forms of treatment of cancer of the external ear with disappointing results. Cure rates are low, ranging from 20 to 25 percent and lower. The reasons for the poor results are: (1) the tumor is diagnosed late, and (2) its extent is greater than judged clinically. The technical difficulties of the anatomic site are considerable, both for radiation therapy and surgery. These factors account for the limited success of either method. The growing trend is to combine both modalities. Some authors prefer preoperative radiation, others postoperative radiation. Although the theoretic advantages and disadvantages of each combination can be stated, the superiority of one regimen over the other is yet to be proved.

Preoperative radiation has the obvious advantage of delivering radiation when the blood supply has not been disturbed by surgery and is theoretically more effective. The cancer cells at the periphery are destroyed, thereby removing one of the limitations of surgery; moreover, the chance of seeding the surgical field with viable tumor cells is diminished and the bulk of the tumor is reduced. The principal disadvantage is the osteonecrosis and secondary infection attendant on radiation. The pain due to the reaction to the radiation may place limits on the administration of radiation in the full amount planned. The effect of radiation on brain

tissue in the wide fields employed carries with it a calculated risk and may also become a limiting factor.

Radical Surgery and Planned Postoperative Radiation

Radical surgery as the primary treatment has the advantage of encompassing the potential cancer field and delineating the actual extensions of the cancer. Thus the critical areas of extension of the tumor beyond the surgical field can be definitely identified for the radiation therapist. The resection of bone and cartilage invaded by tumor relieves the patient of pain. By removal of bone and cartilage, the problem of radiation necrosis is eliminated. The possible effect of radiation on brain tissue must still be considered.

The so-called sandwich technique of radiation therapy delivered in two courses, one before surgery and one following surgery, has been recommended by other therapists as a compromise.

Because the number of cases is small, even in the experience of large tumor clinics, the question of which regimen is to be preferred may be unanswerable for some time. What is evident is that no one is satisfied with the result of either radiation or surgery alone in the advanced cancers of the external ear canal. Faced with these realities, the surgeon and radiation therapist must develop a combined regimen for the management of cancers of the ear canal. It is worth repeating at this point the well-established aphorism of cancer treatment, "Success in management of cancer depends upon the adequacy of the first treatment." This holds true in cancer of the external ear canal, where the regimen must be planned in advance by both the radiation therapist and the surgeon.

If we divide cancers of the ear canal into (1) the early cancers limited to the canal or with limited invasion of the bony and cartilaginous walls; (2) advanced but resectable cancers of the canal; and (3) far advanced cancers that extend beyond the surgical field, involving vital structures, e.g., carotid artery, with intracranial invasion, invasion of deep neck spaces, occipi-

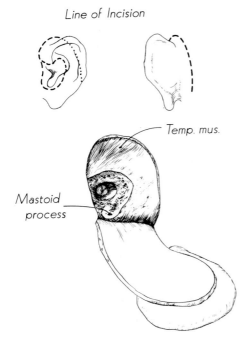

Figure 58–6 · Incision for resection of external auditory canal. (*Modified from* Tabb et al.: Laryngoscope, 74:634, 1964.)

tal bone, atlas, and axes, then a plan of therapy can be outlined.

Early Cancers Limited to the External Ear Canal

These lesions are surgically resectable with an adequate margin encompassing

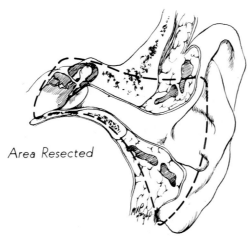

Figure 58–7 · Area resected. (*Modified from* Tabb et al.: Laryngoscope, 74:634, 1964.)

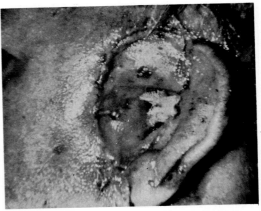

Figure 58–8 · Defect covered by split-thickness graft: packing in osseous canal. Drain and middle ear preserved.

the cancer field. The operation is known as the sleeve operation; it combines a radical mastoidectomy with a wide resection of the ear canal and the preservation of the external ear and facial nerve. The sacrifice of hearing, with or without the destruction of the inner ear function, is a calculated risk of the procedure and will depend upon whether the middle ear is involved.

Although there are many modifications of the procedure, the operation described by Tabb et al. (1964) gives the essential features of the sleeve operation.

An incision is made which includes the conchal cartilage, the tragus, and a portion of the anterior area of the helix. The incision across the helix is continued over and behind the ear as the classic postauric-

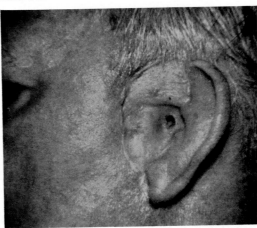

Figure 58–9 · Postoperative appearance following partial resection of pinna, external canal, and parotid.

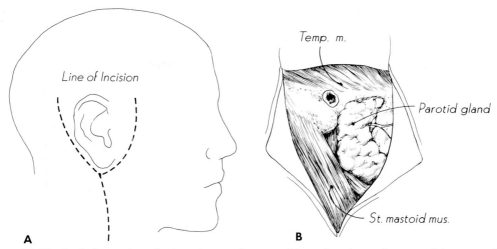

Figure 58–10 Radical resection of external ear and temporal bone for advanced cancer of the external ear. *1*, External ear turned upward as a superiorly based flap. *B*, Exposures after developing three flaps.

ular incision. This allows the external ear to be retracted downward, now attached at the antitragus and lobule. The conchal cartilage and tragus remain attached to the external canal (Figs. 58–6 and 58–7).

An alternate procedure is to raise the external ear as a flap attached superiorly, as in the radical block dissection of the temporal bone (Fig. 58–8).

The mastoid is exenterated down to the facial canal; the bony posterior wall and floor of the canal are outlined with cutting burs. The tympanic membrane and ossi-

cles are usually taken with the canal. The cartilaginous and anterior bony wall are widely resected; chisels are used to complete the resection.

Tabb et al. (1964) destroyed the inner ear by injection of 0.1 ml. of 99 percent alcohol into the oval and round windows. This prevents persistent vertigo experienced by patients following radical surgery of the middle ear.

The wound is packed with a synthetic sponge and allowed to granulate. Healing is sufficiently advanced at the end of

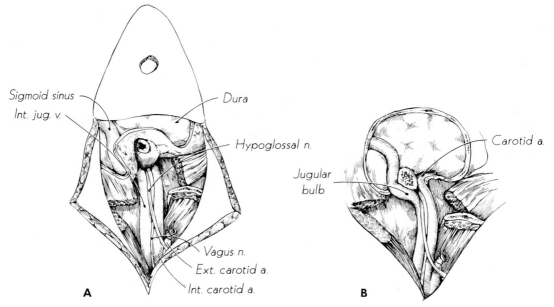

Figure 58–11 Radical resection of external ear and temporal bone. *A*, Resection completed. *B*, Temporal bone exposed.

the fourth week to start radiation therapy. Tabb advocated a dosage of 5000 roentgens.

Modification of the procedure consists of application of skin grafts to the mastoid cavity to hasten healing. The grafts take well (Fig. 58–9) and survive postoperative radiation. If the margins of the resection are adequate and are checked by frozen section and paraffin sections, radiation therapy may not be needed. However, this would apply to only those lesions entirely contained in the external canal.

Advanced Cases

Resection of the temporal bone by a combined intracranial and extracranial surgical en bloc dissection, as described by Parsons and Lewis and Page (1966), is the procedure of choice when the cancer has extended into the middle ear structure or invaded the middle cranial fossa (Figs. 58–10 to 58–16). The intracranial approach to the middle fossa, with removal of cerebrospinal fluid or shrinking of brain or both, provides an adequate exposure of the temporal bone from above. At this point an assessment of the extent of the tumor is made. If the tumor has

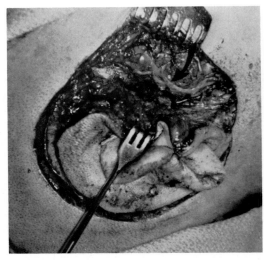

Figure 58–13 Block dissection of external ear and canal and parotid superficial lobe showing facial nerve dissected.

not extended intracranially and is limited to the temporal bone, the resection of the bone is carried out using the Stryker saw and chisels placed lateral to the carotid canal and the internal auditory meatus. Hemorrhage from venous sinuses is brisk.

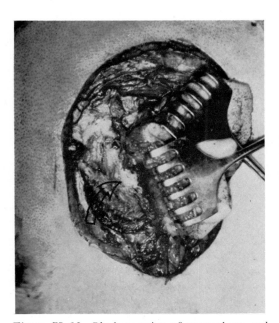

Figure 58–12 Block resection of external ear and canal. Mastoid exposure.

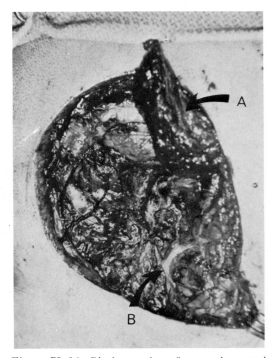

Figure 58–14 Block resection of external ear and canal. Temporal muscle graft *(A)* developed to cover defect. Facial nerve *(B)*.

Hypotensive technique (the systolic pressure to 60 mm. of mercury) reduces blood loss during the procedure. Injury to the dura is repaired by suturing or by temporal fascia graft. The temporalis muscle and fascia are used to cover the dura, and split-thickness grafts are laid over the surgical defect (Figs. 58–8 and 58–9). A neck dissection is not included as part of the initial surgical procedure.

COMPLICATIONS AND SEQUELAE

1. Facial nerve paralysis. This requires a tarsorrhaphy to protect the cornea.
2. Vertigo. This gradually subsides over a 2- to 3-week period and is not disabling.
3. Infection and meningitis are a risk because of exposure and injury of the dura during the surgical procedure and postoperative wound infection.

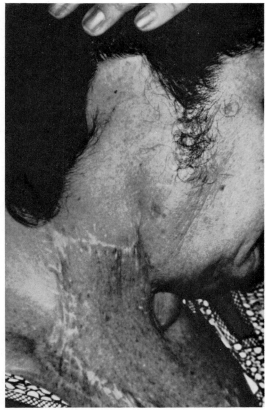

Figure 58–16 Postoperative appearance.

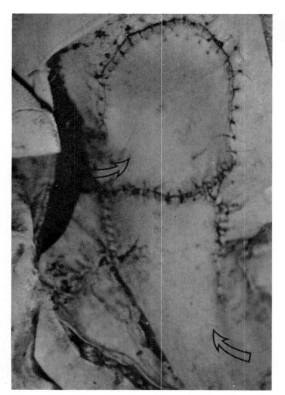

Figure 58–15 Cervical and chest sliding flaps developed to cover defect.

4. Hemorrhage and thrombosis of the venous sinuses and carotid are more common if surgery follows radiation therapy.

FAR ADVANCED CANCERS

These are the cancers which extend either intracranially, producing destruction of the base of the skull, or into the parapharyngeal spaces of the neck. In the advanced lesion palliation should be the objective. Radiation and chemotherapy may give relief of pain for many months.

CURE RATE

The overall cure rate of all regimens is about 25 percent. Lewis (1960) reported an overall salvage rate of 28 percent (26 cases of 92 resected).

REFERENCES

Conley, J.: Cancer of the middle ear. Trans. Am. Otol. Soc., 53:189, 1965.

Conley, J. J., and Novack, A. J.: The surgical treatment of malignant tumors of the ear and temporal bone. Part I. A.M.A. Arch. Otolaryngol., 71:635, 1960.

Friedmann, I., and Osborn, D. A.: Metastatic tumours in the ear, nose and throat region. J. Laryngol. Otol., 79:576, 1965.

Kuilman, J.: Cancer of the auditory canal. Pract. Otorhinolaryngol. (Basel), 24:119, 1962.

Lederman, M.: Malignant tumours of the ear. J. Laryngol. Otol., 79:85, 1965.

Lewis, J. S.: Cancer of the ear: A report of 150 cases. Laryngoscope, 70:551, 1960.

Lewis, J. S., and Page, R.: Memorial. Radical surgery of malignant tumors of the ear. Arch. Otolaryngol., 83:114, 1966.

Miller, D.: Cancer of the external auditory canal. Laryngoscope, 65:448, 1955.

Nelms, C. R., Jr., and Paparella, M. M.: Early external auditory canal tumors. Laryngoscope, 78:986, 1968.

Tabb, H. G., Komet, H., and McLaurin, J. W.: Cancer of the external auditory canal: Treatment with mastoidectomy and irradiation. Laryngoscope, 74:634, 1964.

59

Tumors of the Umbilicus

Bernard Duperrat, M.D., and Gabrielle Noury, M.D.

ANATOMY

The anatomic connections of the umbilicus are complex because of the embryologic development of this "crossroads."

Vitelline Duct

The vitelline duct is connected to the upper part of the intestinal loop. It narrows down and resorbs into a fibrous cord. Sometimes a finger-shaped vestigium remains: Meckel's diverticulum, located about one meter away from the ileocecal valve, sometimes connected to the distal face of the umbilicus and sometimes not.

Allantoic Duct

The persistent portion of the allantoic canal, which goes from the umbilicus to the remnants of the vesical embryo, is reduced to a median, azygous, fibrous cord which follows the peritoneal face of the anterior abdominal wall.

Umbilical Arteries

Each umbilical artery becomes a primitive iliac artery so that, in the space between the umbilicus and the iliacs, they become atrophied into fibrous cords located on each side of the urachus: the lateral vesicoumbilical ligaments.

Umbilical Vein

It is known that umbilical blood feeds the fetus through two channels: (a) the direct way—umbilical vein, Arantius' canal, common afferent hepatic vein, vena cava; and (b) the indirect way—umbilical vein, umbilical afferent vein, hepatic capillaries, subhepatic vein, vena cava. The placental circulation stops at birth, making the umbilical vein useless. It becomes atrophied, becoming a fibrous cord between the umbilicus and Arantius' canal, which undergoes a similar transformation. Thus is formed a fibrous cord between umbilicus and vena cava: the "round" or "falciform" hepatic ligament.

1383

OMPHALOMESENTERIC MALFORMATIONS

The remnants of the vitelline canal can cause a whole range of lesions, which vary from direct communication between the intestinal lumen and the outside to the formation of simple cysts. Thus one can observe (a) exceptionally, direct communication; (b) sometimes, the total eversion of the mucosa of a diverticulum which is open only on the umbilical side (Lexer's diverticulum); (c) more often, the adenoidal diverticular tumor, a small tumor which appears after the cord has been shed. The work of Forgue and Riche on this tumor is considered a classic. Fêvre and Huguenin give an excellent description:

The tumour is as a rule very small in size (a grain, a pea, a cherry). It is club-shaped, rounded or pear-shaped, with a pedicle located in the umbilical region which is seldom cylindrical in shape. Its main characteristics are the bright red colour, the smooth, shining, moist, varnished aspect resembling that of an intestinal mucosa. Resilient and elastic to the touch, the adenoidal tumour does not give under pressure. The surface oozes a viscous sticky liquid which in Sheen's case had an alcaline reaction.

From the anatomo-pathological point of view, the intestinal origin of these small tumours is evident. They comprise: a connective center, a digestive-type external mucosa, usually intestinal. It is often striated, the grooves corresponding to glandular tubes which remind one of Lieberkühn's glands. This glandular abundance explains why Lannelongue and Fremont called them diverticular adenoidal tumours.

It appears obvious that the origin of these tumors is an omphalomesenteric tissue inclusion. These tumors are not to be confused with a simple telangiectatic granuloma; the latter is a fleshy bud, soft and bloody, which causes a purulent discharge curable by the use of silver nitrate.

However, when confronted with a resistant or recurrent umbilical granuloma, one must consider the possibility of an adenoidal diverticular tumor.

To proceed to simple resection would be a serious mistake: the case calls for radical and delicate surgery, which may lead to the discovery of deep-seated malformations of the intestine and a possible Meckel's diverticulum.

Umbilical cysts occur less frequently than diverticular adenoidal tumors (Fig. 59–1). Sometimes superficial, sometimes deep, they can be closed, emit pus, or be fistulized. In the latter case the discharge, through the fistula, of digestive enzyme can lead to the appearance of periumbilical sores.

HYPERTROPHIC UMBILICAL SCARS

There is a great variety of umbilical scars, and their appearance can be used in

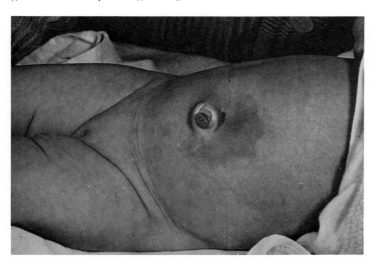

Figure 59–1 Adenoidal diverticular tumor with enzymatic oozing dermatitis in a one month old baby.
(See also Color Plate X–E.)

forensic medicine for the purpose of body identification. To describe them all would be an endless task. The two extremes are represented by, on the one hand, smooth, depressed scars, forming a hole, and, on the other hand, hypertrophic scars or even a keloid, which can reach the size of an egg and have the appearance of a tumor. The latter type of scar occurs more often.

URACHUS

The remnants of the allantoic vesicle can cause cysts of the urachus. These are normally subumbilical rather than umbilical. They are located in the abdominal wall. Their distal face is located under the peritoneum. Wilmoth described a fistula of the urachus which discharged, through the umbilicus, a liquid which was not urine but a secretion mixed with pus.

The probe travels downwards when it enters the fistula. The x-ray contrast material gathers in a retromuscular, anteperitoneal, oblong, downward sinus.

UMBILICAL HERNIA

The diagnosis of umbilical hernia is generally easy owing to the reducibility of the swelling. This is not the case when dealing with a strangulated hernia. In several personally observed cases, we noticed that strangulation does indeed arise in practice. It may be that the strangulated tissues are neoplastic.

The following is a case in point: Mrs. T., aged 57, obese, has had an umbilical hernia for a long time. When the hernia becomes painful, Dr. Huchet decides to operate. He finds a strangulated epiplomphalocele and adds: "I believe there is a neoplasic metastasis in this epiploon (omentum)." Several sections are made (Fig. 59–2) which show numerous cylindrical, glandular, epithelioma tubes, which are undoubtedly gastrointestinal in origin. This is a case in which the strangulation of an epiplomphalocele leads to the discovery of a peritoneal carcinoma. This observation must be compared with that made by Canuet in 1892.

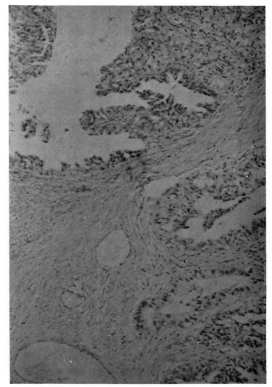

Figure 59–2 Metastatic carcinoma in umbilical hernia.

BENIGN UMBILICAL TUMORS

Sometimes the most common lesion can mimic umbilical tumors: Mrs. M., an Algerian of uncertain age, speaking no French, shows her umbilicus, which bears a coal-black, hazelnut-sized mass set in a patch of scabby dermatitis. This is a case of umbilical concretion, the removal of which brings about a complete cure.

As is known, a fleshy bud may appear on the umbilicus quite frequently. It is often sanious and smelly and can reach the size of a large strawberry. We have observed many such cases.

Although papillomas and epidermal cysts occur in the umbilicus, they will not be discussed here.

ANGIOMA

The umbilical angioma is far from exceptional, constituting up to 1 percent of tumors, according to Goetschel. Most often it takes the form of a widespread capillary angioma, sometimes discrete and hardly noticeable. We observed with Dr. Goetschel several cases of red or purple tuberous angioma the size of a pea or cherry; treatment with carbon dioxide "snow" was successful. *It must be noted that, in patients with sores and purulent discharge, there may be deep-seated pain in the subhepatic region, which is due to the localization of lymph ducts leading, in the ligamentum falciforme, to the liver.*

Lymphangiomas are rare; they consist of small, light-colored, translucent vesicles.

BENIGN NEVUS

The benign melanocytic nevus of the umbilical fossa occurs frequently (Figs. 59–3 to 59–5). It is not serious, but when it is removed by electrocoagulation, the resulting small wound can become inflamed. In such cases we have witnessed the appearance of slight fever accompanied by nausea, abdominal swelling, and subhepatic pain due to the path followed by lymph ducts.

UMBILICAL ENDOMETRIOSIS

This is by no means an infrequent condition, and the diagnosis can be very

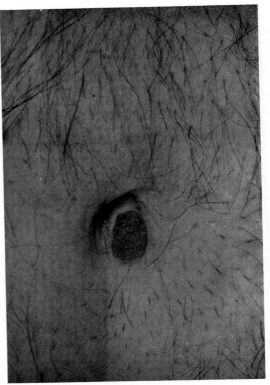

Figure 59–4   Benign nevus of the navel. (See also Color Plate X–F.)

tricky. There are over 200 published cases. We have personally observed four cases.

Case No. 1

Mrs. D., under the care of Dr. Forget of Dinard, develops a purplish umbilical nodule. Endometrioma is suspected because of congestive catamenial outbreaks. The histologic section is typical of endometrioma: the glandular cavities are filled with blood. They have a high cylindrical lining. The cytogenous chorion can be seen all around.

Case No. 2

A woman, aged 42, has a small, well-delineated, firm tumor showing no particular coloring; nevertheless there are periods of painful stress. The examination of the histologic section gives cause

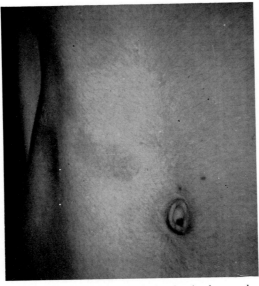

Figure 59–3   Small benign lentigo in the navel.

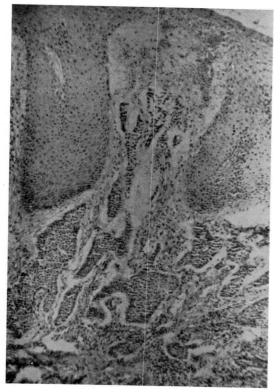

Figure 59–13 Umbilical metastasis of ileal carcinoid.

Stomach	50 cases	= 33%
Indeterminate origin	40 cases	26%
Intestine and colon	20 cases	13%
Ovary	15 cases	11%
Uterus	5 cases	4%
Bile duct	9 cases	6%
Pancreas	9 cases	6%
Miscellaneous	3 cases	

The pathogenesis of these metastases raised many questions. The embryologic and anatomic peculiarities of the umbilical crossroads were often considered to be the explanation of their mechanism:

(a) Direct propagation through the chorda venae umbilicalis
(b) Direct propagation through a remnant of the urachus
(c) Propagation through the retrograde lymph ducts
(d) Arterial embolism
(e) Contiguous extension
(f) Implantation of "floating" cells in the tip of an umbilical hernia or in a dehiscence of the retroumbilical fascia.

umbilical metastasis led to the discovery, for instance, of a plastic linitis of the pylorus. The sections show the invasion of the various levels of the umbilicus, from the deeper part towards the surface, by more or less differentiated neoplastic tubes.

The origin of the neoplasm is difficult to determine. In certain cases, it is impossible to define it precisely (for instance, when surgery reveals profuse carcinosis). Our 20 cases can be subdivided as follows:

Stomach	9 cases, of which 4 were Brinton's disease
Intestine and colon	4 cases, of which one was carcinoid
Ovary	3 cases
Indeterminate origin	3 cases
Bile duct	1 case

Joining our 20 cases to the 131 published cases, the protocol of which were available to us, we obtained the following statistics:

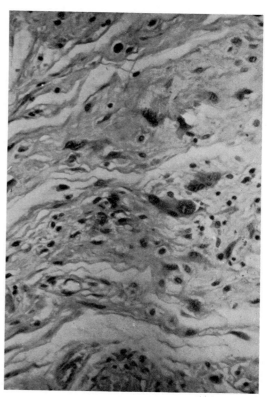

Figure 59–14 Peritoneal myxosarcoma.

In fact, the problem varies with each case, and the question sometimes remains unanswered. The absence of cancer of the bladder from the statistics is to be noted, as it appears to militate against the urachian path, Chuquèt's case remaining isolated.

UMBILICAL METASTASIS OF PERITONEAL TUMORS

This condition is rarely seen. However, we have observed a case in a woman, aged 65, who showed abdominal dropsy, the cause of which was unknown. On the spread-out umbilicus, she developed a hard, reddish, hazelnut-sized node. Following biopsy, the histologic sample showed a fibromyxosarcoma. Laparotomy led to the discovery of numerous sarcomatous nodes in the peritoneum.

REFERENCES

Anglesio, B.: Carcinome dell'ombilico. Minerva Méd., 3:413, 1913.

Assued, A.: Pathologie de l'ombilic. E.M.C., Paroi Abdominale, 1957.

Begg, R.: The urachus. J. Anat., 64:170, 1930.

Berardi, P.: Tumore metastatico dell'ombilico. Clinica Bologna, 2:133, 1962.

Bernstein, J. S., Perlow, V., and Brenner, J. J.: Ascite et endométriose ombilicale et intra-abdominale. Am. J. Dig. Dis., 6:1, 1961.

Beurey, J., and Rousselot, R., Vadot, J., and Barbier, J. M.: Tumeurs de l'ombilic. Bull. Soc. Fr. Dermatol. Syphiligr., 68:953, 1961.

Brocq, P., and Varangot, J.: Les Endométrioses. Rapport au 48ème Congrès Français de Chirurgie, Paris, 1939.

Caresano, G.: Métastases ombilicales des tumeurs ovariennes et intestinales. Ann. Ostet. Ginecol., 87:446, 1965.

Clements, A. B.: Metastatic carcinoma of the umbilicus. J.A.M.A., 150:556, 1952.

Cordie, A.: Contribution à l'étude de l'endométriose. Thèse, Paris, 1954, No. 256.

Cueno, M.: Lymphatiques de l'ombilic. Bull. Soc. Anat. Paris, 1901, p. 580.

Cullen, T. S.: The Umbilicus and Its Diseases. Philadelphia, W. B. Saunders Company, 1916.

Danil, C., and Babes, A.: Métastases of cancer of female genitals. Ann. Med. Clin., 1:35, 1927.

Delarue, J.: Le Problème Biologique du Cancer. Paris, Masson, 1947.

Del Gaudio, A.: Metastasi ombelicale de neoplasie dei genitali feminini. Cancro, 6:690, 1964.

Desforges, G.: Adéno-carcinome primitif de l'ombilic. Arch. Pathol., 42:635, 1946.

Desjacques, R.: Sur les tumeurs de l'ovaire. Lyon Chir., 43:559, 1948.

Dina, M. A.: Metastasi cutanee da carcinoma vesicale. Arch. Ital. Anat. Istol. Patol., 22:182, 1946.

Donati, E., and Borghi, A.: I. Tumori ombilicali metastatici. Oncologia, 19:475, 1965.

Duperrat, B., and Noury, G.: Les métastases ombilicales. A propos de 20 pièces personnelles. Bull. Soc. Fr. Dermatol. Syphiligr., 75:638, 1968.

Dvorak, H.: Implantation malignancy of the abdominal wall. Surg. Gynecol. Obstet., 50:912, 1930.

Ewing, J.: Neoplastic Diseases. Philadelphia, W. B. Saunders Company, 1928.

Feltmann, J.: Les métastases cutanées de la linite plastique. Thèse, Paris, 1944, No. 498.

Fèvre, M., and Huguenin, R.: Malformations tumorales et tumeurs de l'enfant. Paris, Masson et Cie, 1954, pp. 288–292.

Fialho, F.: Adéno-cancer de l'ombilic (canal omphalomésentérique). Rev. Brasil Cirurg., 36:237, 1958.

Finochietto, R.: Patologia umbilical y uraco. Prensa Med. Argent., 46:940, 1959.

Franchini, A.: Il carcinoma metastatico dell'ombelico. Ann. Ital. Chir., 30:739. 1953.

Franchini, A., and Del Gaudio, A.: Metastasi all'ombelico. Omnia Med., 42:1, 1963.

Galliani, A.: Tumori metastatici dell'ombelico. Chir. Ital. 1:1, 1960.

Gates, O.: Cutaneous metastases of malignant disease. Am. J. Cancer, 30:718, 1937.

Gauthier-Villars, P., and Ameline, P.: Métastases à l'ombilic. Arch. Mal. App. Digestif, 41:599, 1952.

Goebel, F.: Sitzungsberichte aus chirurgischen Gesellschaften, Zentralbl. Chir., 62:2915, 1935.

Hartman, P.: Epithélioma de l'ombilic consécutif à un néoplasme gastrique. Rev. Gen. Clin. Thèse, 41:311, 1927.

Head, J. R.: Cancer of the umbilicus secondary to cancer of the coecum. Surg. Gynecol. Obstet., 42:356, 1926.

Hugues, J.: Melanoma of the umbilicus. J. Ir. Med. Assoc., 53:94, 1963.

Kirmisson, R.: Les tumeurs de l'ombilic. Rev. Gen. Clin. Thérap., 21:726, 1907.

Konjetzny: Der Magenkrebs. Stuttgart, 1938.

LaPiere, S., and Castermans-Elias, S.: Epithéliomas cutanés secondaires. Xème Congrès des Dermat. de Langue Française, Alger, 1959. (Paris) Masson, 1961, pp. 331–353.

Latcher, J. W.: Endométriose de l'ombilic. Am. J. Obstet. Gynecol., 66:161, 1953.

Le Coniac, F.: Métastases ombilicales utéro-ovariennes. Thèse, Bordeaux, 1898.

Levan, E. N.: Carcinoma of the bowel metastatic to skin 10 years post operation. Arch. Dermatol., 83:857, 1961.

Lombardi, L. E., and Parsons, L.: Metastatic umbilicus carcinoma from carcinoma of the stomach (38 cases all gastric). Ann. Intern. Med., 22:290, 1945.

Mechin, W. A.: Formations malignes se développant sur des restes du canal omphalo-mésentériques. Virchows Arch. Pathol. Anat., 41:553, 1933.

Mondor, H., and Mazingarbe, R.: Endométriose ombilicale. Mém. Acad. Chir., 65:988, 1939.

Neveu, C.: Contribution à l'étude des tumeurs malignes secondaires de l'ombilic. Thèse, Paris, 1890, No. 50.

Nicolas, J., and Rousset, J.: Epithélioma ombilical non ulcéré. Bull. Soc. Fr. Dermatol. Syphiligr., 34:718, 1937.

Noury, G., and Duperrat, B.: Les métastases ombilicales. Thèse, Paris, 1968.

Novak, E.: Umbilical endometriosis. *In* Gynecologic Pathology. Ed. 3. Philadelphia, W. B. Saunders Company, 1938, p. 485.

O'Leary, J. L., and O'Leary, J. A.: Carcinoma of the umbilicus. Ann. J. Obstet. Gynecol., 89:136, 1964.

Pinheiro: Carcinome primitif de l'ouraque. Thèse, Rio de Janeiro, 1926.

Poinso, R., Calas, E., and Sauve, M.: Les métastases cutanées et sous-cutanées du cancer de l'estomac. Presse Méd., 61:1188, 1953.

Prior, C.: Metastasi cutanee e viscerali multiple conseguenti ad un carcinoma duodenale. Riv. Anat. Patol., 3:214, 1950.

Puccini, C., and Nocentini, P.: La cisti ad i tumori dell'ombilico. Arch. De Vecchi, 12:58, 1949.

Quenu, J., and Longuet, Y. J.: Les tumeurs de l'ombilic. Rev. Chir., 16:97, 1896.

Rochet, F., and Francillon, M.: Tumeur de l'ombilic. Lyon Méd., 167:239, 1942.

Rouviere, H.: Anatomie de l'ombilic. *In* Traité d'Anatomie. Vol. II. Paris, Masson et Cie, 1954.

Scalfi, A.: Di un raro tumore dell'ombelico: l'adenocarcinoma primitivo da resuidi del dotto omfalomesenterico. Boll. Soc. Med. Chir. Pavia, 53:1211, 1939.

Schiebel, W.: Metastatic carcinoma of the umbilicus. J.A.M.A., 157:1489, 1955.

Scott, R. B., and Te Linde, R. W.: External endometriosis. Ann. Surg., 131:697, 1950.

Scott, R. B., Nowak, R. J., and Tindale, R. M.: Umbilical endometriosis and Cullen sign. Obstet. Gynecol., 11:556, 1958.

Silva De Assis, F.: Adenocancer mucipare de l'ouraque. Hospital, 36:913, 1943.

Steck, W., and Helwig, E.: Cutaneous endometriosis. J.A.M.A., 191:167, 1965a.

Steck, W., and Helwig, E.: Tumors of the umbilicus. Cancer, 18:907, 1965b.

Teinturier, B.: Métastase ombilicale révélatrice d'une tumeur du tube digestif. Maroc Méd., 1956, p. 125.

Thiers, H., Colomb, D., and Fayolle, J.: Cancer de l'ovaire révélé par les métastases ombilicales et ganglionnaires. Bull. Soc. Dermatol. Lyon, 6 Février, 1958.

Trimingham, H., and MacDonald, J. R.: Congenital anomalies in the region of the umbilicus. Surg. Gynecol. Obstet., 80:152, 1945.

Varangot, J., Giraud, J. R., and Bignon-Schnirer, J.: Etiologie, pathogénie de l'endométriose génitale. Bull. Soc. Gynecol. Obstet., 17:239, 1965.

Verriotes, C.: Riv. Obstet. Milano, 34:447, 1952.

Viars, S.: Physiopathologie des endométrioses. Thèse, Paris, 1955, No. 733.

Villars, F.: Tumeurs de l'Ombilic. Thèse, Paris, 1886.

Walters, W.: Carcinoma and other malignant lesions of the stomach. Philadelphia, W. B. Saunders Company, 1942.

Walther, H. E.: Krebsmetastasen. Basel, Schwabe, 1948.

Warner, F.: Carcinoma of the umbilicus with report of two cases. Surg. Gynecol. Obstet., 27:204, 1918.

Wechsler, P.: Les aspects dermatologiques de la pathologie ombilicale. Thèse, Paris, 1962.

Williams, C.: Unusual surgical lesions of the umbilicus. Ann. Surg., 124:1108, 1946.

60

Cancer of the Anal and Perianal Areas

Bradley Bigelow, M.D.

Although relatively rare, cancer of the anal and perianal regions warrants a separate discussion for several reasons. In the first place, anal cancer is frequently associated with benign or inflammatory conditions, and the diagnosis is often delayed. A variety of histologic types of cancer has been described, and confusion has arisen as to their significance. Finally, the proper management of anal cancer has been controversial.

ANATOMIC CONSIDERATIONS

The location of the upper limit of the anal canal is poorly defined in most papers dealing with this region. Walls (1958) performed a gross and microscopic study of the anatomy of the anus and rectum and stated that the anorectal ring, formed by the insertion of the puborectalis portion of the levator ani muscle, forms the upper margin of the anus (Fig. 60–1). Simple columnar mucosa of colonic type lines the rectum above, covers the anorectal ring, and extends below it for 0.5 to 1.5 cm. Thus, according to Walls,

the upper portion of the anal canal is lined by colonic mucosa and there is no histologically defined border between anus and rectum. Reflecting this point, the term "anorectal" is often used in the literature dealing with this region. Proceeding downward, the cloacogenic zone appears at about the level of the dentate line. This zone, also known as the transitional, intermediate, or membranous zone, was described by Tucker and Hellwig (1935) and was further studied by Grinvalsky and Helwig (1956). It is an area of transitional or stratified columnar epithelium which closely resembles the bladder neck or prostatic urethra (Fig. 60–2). It varies from 0.3 to 1.1 cm. in width and forms a band between columnar epithelium above and squamous epithelium below. It usually lines the anal crypts (sinuses of Morgagni) and may cover the anal valves, but it is discontinuous, so that columnar (colonic) mucosa and squamous (anal) mucosa may meet. From the anal crypts arise the anal ducts, or glands, which Herrmann described in 1880. They penetrate the internal sphincter muscle and usually extend in a

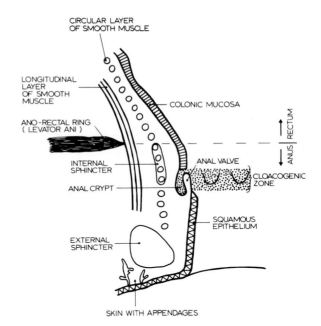

Figure 60–1 Schematic diagram of the anorectal region as described by Walls (1958). Note that the upper portion of the anatomically defined anus is lined by colonic mucosa. As described in the text, cloacogenic and squamous epithelium line it further down.

caudad direction, although their course may be cephalad (Figs. 60–3 and 60–4). Below the transitional zone the anal canal is lined by stratified squamous epithelium which is, in reality, modified skin containing occasional appendages and melanin pigment, which appear a short distance below the anal valves. These skin constituents increase as the anal orifice (verge) and the true skin of the perianal region are reached.

This variety in histology, from columnar mucosa above to skin below, forms the basis for the variety of anal tumors to be discussed.

TYPES OF TUMORS

The main primary tumors encountered in the anal and perianal areas are as follows:

1. Adenocarcinoma of colonic mucosal origin
2. Carcinoid tumor
3. Epidermoid (squamous cell) carcinoma
4. Cloacogenic carcinoma
5. Bowen's disease
6. Basal cell epithelioma
7. Paget's disease
8. Melanoma

Both adenocarcinomas and carcinoid tumors arise in colonic mucosa and do occur in the upper portion of the anal canal, as defined anatomically by Walls (1958). Since they pertain more properly to the colon and rectum than to the anus, they will not be discussed in detail. It should be emphasized, however, that colonic adenocarcinomas are by far the most frequent tumors of this region, comprising 94 percent of 1171 neoplasms of the anorectal canal below the rectosigmoid (Klotz et al., 1967). Carcinoid tumors represent approximately 1 percent of tumors in the same series.

EPIDERMOID AND CLOACOGENIC CARCINOMA

If colonic adenocarcinomas are excluded, the great majority of anal cancers are either of epidermoid or cloacogenic type. These two forms are best discussed together, since they are generally similar from clinical and therapeutic standpoints.

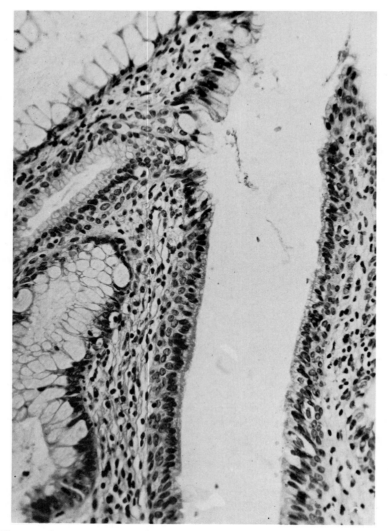

Figure 60–2   Cloacogenic mucosa, adjacent to mucus-secreting colonic mucosa at top and left. Note the transitional appearance of the cloacogenic epithelium. ×*200.*

As will be mentioned, they often overlap histologically. Certain variants, such as basaloid cancers and anal duct tumors, show distinct features which will be described.

Clinical Description

Epidermoid-cloacogenic tumors occur at peak frequency at age 55 to 60 years. The sex incidence shows a predominance of females by ratios varying between 1.5:1 and 2:1. There appears to be no racial predisposition. By far the commonest pre-senting symptoms are bleeding and pain, one or both of which occur initially in over 80 percent of patients in most series. Constipation is less common, occurring in 26 percent of Stearns' and Quan's (1970) large series of 234 cases. The most infrequent initial complaint is the sensation of a mass, documented in 7 percent of Stearns' and Quan's series; this symptom more often accompanies tumors arising in the lower anal area and anal margin. The correct diagnosis is often delayed; Kuehn et al. (1964) reported that cancer was unsuspected for six months or longer after onset of symptoms in 37 of their 157 cases

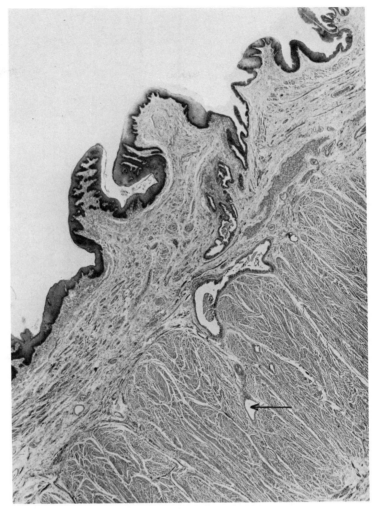

Figure 60–3 Anal ducts penetrating anal sphincter muscle to point indicated by arrow. The surface epithelium lining the anal canal is mainly squamous, with areas of transitional (cloacogenic) epithelium near origin of anal duct and at upper right. *Low power.*

(24 percent). There are many reports of unsuspected anal cancers which are only discovered at tissue examination after the unsuccessful treatment of clinically benign conditions, such as hemorrhoids, fistulas, fissures, abscesses, condylomas, and lymphogranuloma venereum. This will be discussed further under differential diagnosis.

Location

The exact location of anal tumors is often poorly established in the literature. As already mentioned, according to Walls' (1958) study, the border between upper anal canal and rectum is not defined histologically. Most discussions encompass "anorectal" tumors and relate the location of lesions to the dentate line above and to the anal orifice (verge) below. The anal canal is usually said to be between the dentate line and anal orifice, and the anal margin to be at or below the orifice.

In three series of cases of epidermoid carcinoma, totaling 388 cases, the location of the tumor was described precisely (Morson, 1960: 141 cases; Richards and Woolner, 1962: 58 cases; Kuehn et al., 1968: 189 cases). Combining these series, the tumor was entirely below the dentate line in 111 out of 388 cases (29 percent), entirely above it in 51 out of 388 (13 percent), and extended to or across it in 226 out of 388 (58 percent). In the report of Klotz et al. (1967) on 373 cases of transitional cloacogenic carcinoma, the respec-

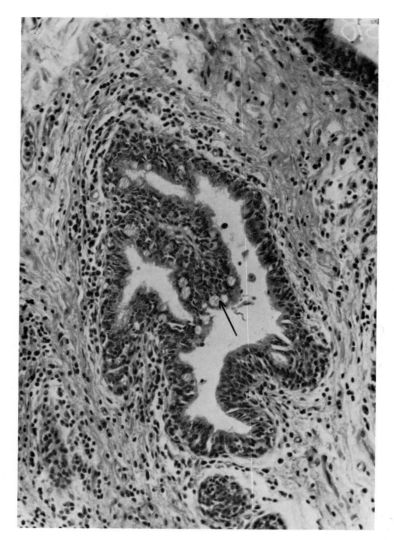

Figure 60–4 Magnification of anal duct shown in Figure 60–3. Note the mucus-containing cells (arrow) within the epithelium. ×200.

tive figures for tumor location were 46 percent below, 13 percent above, and 41 percent involving the dentate line.

Tumor location relative to the circumference of the anal canal is sparsely reported. Anterior location predominates slightly, and annular lesions are rare, in contrast to colonic adenocarcinoma. Of 26 tumors of the anal canal reported by Gabriel (1941), 14 (54 percent) were anterior and only two were annular. Klotz et al. (1967) reported that, of their precisely located tumors, 37 percent were anterior, 23 percent posterior, and 12 percent circumferential.

Gross Appearance

The majority of tumors present as an ulcerated mass (Figs. 60–5 and 60–6) and measure about 4 cm. in diameter at time of diagnosis. There are no gross features to distinguish epidermoid-cloacogenic tumors from the commoner colonic adenocarcinomas.

A minority of cases have no intraluminal mass and may present as draining areas in the perianal skin. Zimberg and Kay (1957) described three such cases, all adenocarcinomas microscopically, and suggested origin in anal ducts. Because of marked extension, they advocated very wide resection. Rundle and Hales (1953) reviewed 17 cases of fistula in ano, most of long duration and refractory to treatment, in which the diagnosis of carcinoma was eventually made. Anal ducts have long been incriminated in the etiology of fistula in ano and may also be the source of these supervening cancers. It is problematical, however, whether fistula in ano and cancer are pathogenetically related.

Those anal ducts which extend in a cephalad direction, the minority, may give rise to unusual cancers of epidermoid-cloacogenic type which appear in the rectal mucosa and apparently do not involve the lining of the anal canal (Grinvalsky and Helwig, 1956).

Microscopic Description

The variety of types of mucous membrane encountered within the anus is reflected in the multiplicity of histologic types of tumors which have been described. Within the broad category of epidermoid-cloacogenic carcinomas, the following terms are found in the literature, divided into three closely related groups:

1. Epidermoid; squamous

2. Cloacogenic; transitional cloacogenic; transitional; mucoepidermoid; cylindromatous; adenoid cysts

3. Basosquamous; basaloid squamous; basaloid; basaloid small cell; undifferentiated small cell; oat cell

For the most part they are clinically

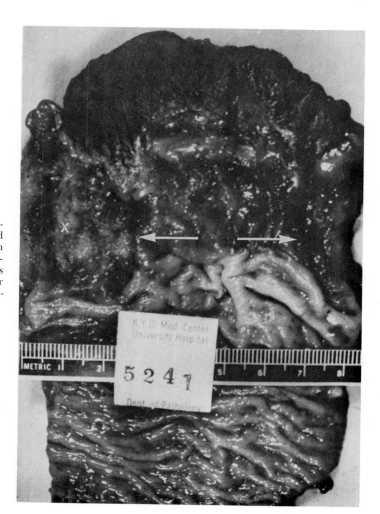

Figure 60–5 An epidermoid carcinoma of the anus, which occurred in a Negro patient. The specimen has been opened through the ulcerated tumor, whose lateral margins are shown by the arrows. The center of the tumor is at *X*. Pigmented perianal skin is at top.

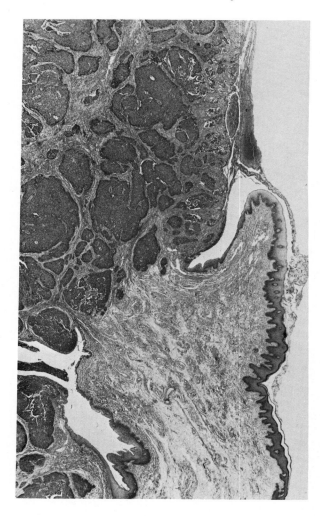

Figure 60–6 The ulcerated surface of an anal cancer sectioned at its lower margin. The squamous mucosa of the anal canal overhangs the edge of the tumor. An anal duct, at lower left, is involved. *Low power.*

indistinguishable, and, as pointed out by Stearns and Quan (1970), most types should be considered as variants of epidermoid carcinoma as far as choice of therapy is concerned. Two groups of tumors, however, deserve special note: the basaloid tumors of group 3, and tumors of probable origin in anal ducts. These will be discussed separately below.

A review of anal cancers encountered at New York University Medical Center reveals that the majority show squamous differentiation and have been classified as epidermoid type (Fig. 60–7). Considerable histologic variation is found, however, not only between individual tumors but also in different areas of a single tumor (Fig. 60–8).

Transitional cell histology is often encountered (Fig. 60–9). Here there is a re-

semblance to cancers of the urinary bladder, and we have occasionally seen apparent origin in the cloacogenic surface mucosa. We have usually found that such tumors also show squamous differentiation and most have been classified as such. Since 1956, when the term "transitional cloacogenic carcinoma" was proposed by Grinvalsky and Helwig (1956), a few papers have appeared on anal tumors designated as such. The reported frequency has been about half that of squamous cell carcinoma. The 373 cases of transitional cloacogenic carcinoma described by Klotz et al. (1967) were selected on the basis of predominance of transitional pattern, and the authors reported a frequency equal to that of squamous cell carcinoma. They described varying degrees of squamous differentiation, as well

coexisted with cancer in 5 of their 39 patients. Forty-nine cases of associated lymphogranuloma venereum and anal cancer were described by Rainey (1954). Most patients were Negro females in the fifth decade of life with long duration of lymphogranuloma venereum and rectal stricture. Ackerman and Rosai (1974) illustrated an ulcer of granuloma inguinale which clinically mimicked cancer.

Treatment and Prognosis

Most authors advocate abdominoperineal resection for cancers of the anus and emphasize the need for a wide perineal excision to avoid recurrence. It is generally recommended that local excision be reserved for small tumors which are circumscribed and not fixed to underlying tissue. Most papers urge that this procedure be limited to low-lying tumors of the anal margin or perianal skin.

Irradiation therapy was formerly advocated as the primary means of treatment by Roux-Berger and Ennuyer (1948), among others. Irradiation has also been used as an adjunct to surgery, but the lack of improved survival with this method as compared with surgery alone and the resulting morbidity, and especially the pain, have generally led to limitation of its use to inoperable or recurrent tumors.

It is often necessary to excise the posterior vaginal wall because of tumor extension, and it may also be necessary to remove the uterus or prostate. In addition to the resection of mesenteric lymph nodes as part of the abdominoperineal procedure, Stearns and Quan (1970) perform a dissection of pelvic lymph nodes, obturator and hypogastric, in good risk patients.

The advisability of inguinal node dissection has long been debated in the literature. Cattell and Williams (1943) were among those who advocated groin dissection, in addition to abdominoperineal resection, as part of the primary treatment. The extremely bad prognosis (see below) of patients presenting with involved inguinal nodes at the time of diagnosis led Turell (1958) to condemn groin dissection as either useless, if nodes were positive, or

unnecessary, if negative. Stearns (1958) took the intermediate position, now generally advocated, that the procedure is of value if inguinal node metastases develop following the primary surgical treatment. He reported the 100 percent mortality of 15 patients who presented with involved inguinal nodes and underwent simultaneous abdominoperineal resection and groin dissection. This group contrasts with 12 other patients who presented with clinically negative nodes at the time of abdominoperineal resection. They subsequently developed groin metastases, underwent inguinal dissection, and 5 of the 12 patients survived over five years. Other authors have since confirmed Stearns' position and advocated groin dissection only for secondarily involved nodes. Prior to radical groin dissection, Kuehn et al. (1968) performed a laparotomy to check for abdominal extension or metastases to periaortic nodes or liver.

The prognosis of anal cancer of epidermoid-cloacogenic type depends primarily on the size and on the degree of extension or metastasis of the tumor at the time of diagnosis.

These considerations are more important for deciding proper therapy and gauging prognosis than are the histologic type and degree of differentiation of the tumor. As already mentioned under microscopic description, epidermoid and transitional types apparently have similar prognoses, while the course of basaloid tumors is controversial. There is little evidence that the behavior of a given tumor is related to its degree of differentiation. In fact, Dillard et al. (1963) reported poorer results with better differentiated tumors treated by local excision than with their radically resected tumors, most of which were less differentiated (see below). Although Klotz et al. (1967) do suggest that poorly differentiated tumors have a worse prognosis, their minimal follow-up of only one year renders this conclusion questionable.

The five-year survival of patients treated for cure by abdominoperineal resection is reported to be approximately 50 percent in most of the more recent reports. The majority of reported cases are treated by radical surgery. The minority, usually those with small, circumscribed, and low-lying tumors, are treated by local excision, and their five-year survival is generally about 65 percent. One report, however (Dillard et al., 1963), contrasted a 58 percent five-year survival after radical surgery with a figure of only 28 percent after local excision. This occurred despite the presence of smaller tumors in the latter group. The authors join those who urge radical procedures for most anal cancers.

The effect of node involvement on prognosis has been alluded to in relation to inguinal nodes. Initial involvement of the groin when the anal cancer is discovered is extremely ominous; secondary involvement is less so. Kuehn et al. (1968) reported that, for all patients with metastases to inguinal nodes, including those with far advanced disease, the prognosis is reduced to an absolute five-year survival of less than 5 percent.

Mesenteric node involvement, demonstrated microscopically after abdominoperineal resection, was reported by Dillard et al. (1963) to not significantly alter the prognosis. Their 32 cases with negative mesenteric nodes had a five-year survival of 56 percent, while 18 cases with positive nodes had a 50 percent figure. This similarity in prognosis may reflect the greater importance of local extension of tumor and of pelvic recurrence, the frequency of which is emphasized by many authors.

OTHER ANAL TUMORS

Four other anal tumors will be briefly discussed: Bowen's disease, basal cell epithelioma, Paget's disease, and melanoma. All four are rare.

Bowen's Disease

Intraepithelial squamous cell carcinoma (Bowen's disease) is rare in the anal region. Grodsky (1954) described three cases and emphasized the necessity to rule out invasive cancer by biopsy. The recommended treatment is wide local surgical excision.

Basal Cell Epithelioma

The histologic similarity of some epidermoid-cloacogenic carcinomas of the anus to true basal cell tumors of the skin has been mentioned. In contrast to the female sex predominance of the former, basal cell epitheliomas are commoner in the male by a ratio of 2:1 to 3:1. The reported location of true basal cell tumors at a lower level in the anus than the "basaloid" ones (Wittoesch et al., 1957) has been mentioned. Thirty-one basal cell epitheliomas of the anus, reviewed by Matt and Dilger (1956), had a long duration which averaged four years. Two-thirds of patients complained of a mass, in contrast to the rarity of this complaint with epidermoid-cloacogenic cancers, and the treatment of choice was local excision.

Paget's Disease

Extramammary Paget's disease is a rare tumor which may involve the anus. Of 40 cases of anogenital Paget's disease (Helwig and Graham, 1963), 15 occurred in the anal region. Most patients complained of long-standing itching and presented with elevated, papillary, scaly lesions. An associated underlying carcinoma, apparently of apocrine gland origin, was found in one-third of cases. The majority of these adnexal cancers metastasized, usually to inguinal and pelvic lymph nodes. One-sixth also had a primary cancer elsewhere, involving rectum, breast, or urethra. Surgical excision is the treatment of choice. Of the total group of 40 cases, 15 died as a result of either the adnexal or the separate internal cancer. The perianal skin is primarily involved by Paget cells. Extension of the process from skin up the anal canal to just below rectal mucosa has been described (Hutcheson et al., 1960), as well as apparent anal duct involvement (Rabson et al., 1958).

Melanoma

Although melanoma is relatively rare in the anus, this site is said to rank third in frequency after skin and eye. Mason and Helwig (1966) discussed the literature and described 17 cases. About one-half presented with either rectal bleeding or hemorrhoids. In several of the remainder, the tumors were discovered incidental to the investigation of unrelated conditions. Most of the tumors were polypoid, in contrast to the usual gross appearance of anal cancers. The melanomas appeared to originate in the squamous epithelium of the anal canal, as demonstrated by the finding of junction change in seven tumors. In nine cases the columnar mucosa above was also involved, apparently by the upward spread of a tumor originating below. The prognosis is extremely bad, and in the above series it appeared unrelated to the extent of the surgical treatment, which included both local and radical excisions. Of 13 patients followed after varied treatment, all died after an average interval of 15 months. Several cases showed metastases to lymph nodes and distant organs at autopsy.

CONCLUSIONS

The diagnosis of anal cancer is often delayed. Intractable fistulas in ano should be scrutinized for an associated tumor.

If anal cancer is present, it is most often adenocarcinoma of colonic mucosal origin.

Epidermoid and cloacogenic carcinomas are a poor second in frequency. Although the histology of these tumors is extremely varied, their behavior does not seem to show a comparable variation; the prognosis of so-called basaloid tumors, however, needs further evaluation. The selection of cases for conservative local excision is a difficult and controversial problem, which was recently discussed by Eby and Sullivan (1969). Most anal cancers should be treated by abdominoperineal resection performed widely to avoid local recurrence. Inguinal node dissection should be reserved for groin involvement manifest after the primary surgical therapy.

Four other anal tumors have been discussed briefly. They are rare and of widely varying prognosis.

REFERENCES

Ackerman, L. V., and Rosai, J.: Surgical Pathology. Ed. 5. St. Louis, Mo., The C. V. Mosby Company, 1974, p. 492.

Berg, J. W., Lone, F., and Stearns, M. W.: Mucoepidermoid anal Cancer. Cancer, 13:914, 1960.

Brennan, J. T., and Stewart, C. F.: Epidermoid cancer of the anus. Presented to New York Surgical Society, January 13, 1971.

Buckwalter, J. A., and Jurayj, M. N.: Relationship of chronic ano-rectal disease to carcinoma. Arch. Surg., 75:352, 1957.

Bunstock, W. H.: Basal cell carcinoma of the anus. Am. J. Surg., 95:822, 1958.

Cattell, R. B., and Williams, A. C.: Epidermoid carcinoma of the anus and the rectum. Arch. Surg., 46:336, 1943.

Dillard, B. M., Spratt, J. S., Ackerman, L. V., and Butcher, H. R.: Epidermoid cancer of anal margin and canal. Arch. Surg., 86:772, 1963.

Eby, L. S., and Sullivan, E. S.: Current concepts of local excision of epidermoid carcinoma of the anus. Dis. Colon Rectum, 12:332, 1969.

Fisher, E. R.: The basal cell nature of the so-called transitional cloacogenic carcinoma of anus as revealed by electron microscopy. Cancer, 24:312, 1969.

Gabriel, W. B.: Squamous cell carcinoma of the anus and anal canal: An analysis of 55 cases. Proc. R. Soc. Med., 34:139, 1941.

Grinnell, R. S.: An analysis of forty-nine cases of squamous cell carcinoma of the anus. Surg. Gynecol. Obstet., 98:29, 1954.

Grinvalsky, H. T., and Helwig, E. B.: Carcinoma of the ano-rectal junction. I. Histological considerations. Cancer, 9:480, 1956.

Grodsky, L.: Bowen's disease of the anal region (squamous cell carcinoma in situ). Am. J. Surg., 88:710, 1954.

Helwig, E. B., and Graham, J. H.: Anogenital (extramammary) Paget's disease. Cancer, 16:387, 1963.

Herrmann, G.: Sur la structure et le développement de la muqueuse anale. J. Anat. Physiol., 16:434, 1880.

Hutcheson, J. B., Gordon, J. B., and Fuqua, W. N.: Extramammary Paget's disease of the ano-rectal junction. Arch. Pathol., 69:728, 1960.

Kay, S.: Mucoepidermoid carcinoma of the anal canal and its relation to the anal ducts. Cancer, 7:359, 1954.

Keyes, E. L.: Squamous cell carcinoma of the lower rectum and anus. Ann. Surg., 106:1046, 1937.

Klotz, R. G., Pamukcoglu, T., and Souilliard, D. H.: Transitional cloacogenic carcinoma of the anal canal: Clinicopathologic study of 373 cases. Cancer, 20:1727, 1967.

Kuehn, P. G., Beckett, R., Eisenberg, H., and Reed, J. F.: Epidermoid carcinoma of the perianal skin and anal canal: A review of 157 cases. New Engl. J. Med., 270:614, 1964.

Kuehn, P. G., Eisenberg, H., and Reed, J. F.: Epidermoid carcinoma of the perianal skin and anal canal. Cancer, 22:932, 1968.

Lone, F., Berg, J. W., and Stearns, M. W.: Basaloid tumors of the anus. Cancer, 13:907, 1960.

Mason, J. K., and Helwig, E. B.: Ano-rectal melanoma. Cancer, 19:39, 1966.

Matt, J. G., and Dilger, J. T.: Basal cell carcinoma of the anus. Am. Surg., 22:886, 1956.

Morson, B. C.: The pathology and results of treatment of squamous cell carcinoma of the anal canal and anal margin. Proc. R. Soc. Med., 53:416, 1960.

Pang, L. S. C., and Morson, B. C.: Basaloid carcinoma of the anal canal. J. Clin. Pathol., 20:128, 1967.

Rabson, A. S., Van Scott, E. J., and Smith, R. R.: Carcinoma of the ano-rectal junction with "extramammary Paget's disease." Arch. Pathol., 65:432, 1958.

Rainey, R.: The association of lymphogranuloma inguinale and cancer. Surgery, 35:221, 1954.

Richards, J. C., and Woolner, L. B.: Squamous cell carcinoma of the anus, anal canal, and rectum in 109 patients. Surg. Gynecol. Obstet., 114:475, 1962.

Roux-Berger, J. L., and Ennuyer, A.: Carcinoma of the anal canal. Am. J. Roentgenol., 60:807, 1948.

Rundle, F. F., and Hales, I. A.: Mucoid carcinoma supervening on fistula-in-ano, its surgical pathology and treatment. Ann. Surg., 137:215, 1953.

Sawyers, J. L.: Squamous cell carcinoma of the perianus and anal canal. *In* Turell, R. (Ed.): Diseases of the Colon and Anorectum. Philadelphia, W. B. Saunders Company, 1969.

Stearns, M. W.: Epidermoid carcinoma of the anal region. Surg. Gynecol. Obstet., 106:92, 1958.

Stearns, M. W., and Quan, S. H. Q.: Epidermoid carcinoma of the anorectum. Surg. Gynecol. Obstet., 131:953, 1970.

Tucker, C. C., and Hellwig, C. A.: Anal ducts: Comparative and developmental histology. Arch. Surg., 31:521, 1935.

Tucker, C. C., and Hellwig, C. A.: Proctologic tumors. J.A.M.A., 111:1270, 1938.

Turell, R.: Colonic and anorectal function and disease—Collective review. Surg. Gynecol. Obstet., Int. Abst. Surg., 107:417, 1958.

Walls, E. W.: Observations on the microscopic anatomy of the human anal canal. Br. J. Surg., 45:504, 1958.

Winkelman, J., Grosfeld, J., and Bigelow, B.: Colloid carcinoma of anal-gland origin. Am. J. Clin. Pathol., 42:395, 1964.

Wittoesch, J. H., Woolner, L. B., and Jackman, R. J.: Basal cell epithelioma and basaloid lesions of the anus. Surg. Gynecol. Obstet., 104:75, 1957.

Zimberg, Y. H., and Kay, S.: Anorectal carcinomas of extra-mucosal origin. Ann. Surg., 145:344, 1957.

61

Cancer of the Skin of the Male Genitalia

Robert S. Hotchkiss, M.D.

THE PENIS

Cancer of the penis is one of the oldest known neoplasms. Celsus, Sapata, Hildanus, and other ancient writers have described tumors of the penis and the operations used to treat such lesions. Although cancer of the penis is relatively rare in the United States, it is well to heed the words of Jonathan Hutchinson, who delivered a lecture on cancer of the penis in London in 1889. He effectively paraphrased the importance of knowledge of the disease when he said, "It is such rare afflictions which are worthy of study because it is their rarity which leads to mistakes in diagnosis at a time when treatment might be successful."

The management of the patient afflicted with penile cancer evokes from the physician every measure of sympathy and compassion that can be rendered. There are few, if any, malignant lesions which provoke emotional repercussions equal to those of cancer of the male genitalia. Disfigurement or mutilation of the sex organs was the most feared combat injury, as testified by many physicians serving in the Armed Forces. Those individuals who

have the misfortune of developing cancer of the penis not only are subjected to the alarm of a destructive disease but also often are confronted with horrendous decisions relative to the required surgery. The despondent patient needs all the support that a kind physician can muster for him.

Geographic Considerations

Cancer of the penis is directly related to the religious customs of the peoples of the world. The high incidence in certain areas, as compared to rarity in other districts, gives strong support to the belief that cancer of the penis is a preventable disease. The incidence of cancer of the penis in India varies from 2 to 10 percent of all malignant neoplasms in the male (Paymaster and Gangadhavan, 1967; Thomas and Small, 1968). The Hindus, Christians, and Parsis are far more susceptible than are the Moslems, who practice circumcision at some time between the ages of 3 and 10 years, or the Jews, who circumcise at birth and are therefore almost immune. The Tate Hospital in

1409

India has treated 500 men for carcinoma of the penis. In Siriray Hospital in Siam there were 231 admissions for cancer from 1927 to 1931. Fifty-two (22 percent) were for cancer of the penis (Noble, 1933). Likewise, in Africa, the disease is not uncommon, for 12 percent of men admitted to hospitals in Uganda had penile cancer (Dodge and Linsell, 1963), and it is regarded there as one of the commonest malignant lesions, exceeded in frequency only by malignant lymphoma and carcinoma of the cervix. In Kenya, however, carcinoma of the penis accounts for only 1.9 percent of all cancers in men. In the latter country, circumcision is universally practiced by all but two tribes, whereas ritualistic circumcisions are not done in Uganda. Shabad (1964) stated that in Vietnam over 15 percent of all cancers in men are found on the penis and estimated the incidence in China to be 18 percent. Tan (1963) found that in Macassar one case of penile cancer occurs among each 20,000 Mohammedans who practice late circumcision (5 to 10 years). The Chinese in the same area are not circumcised, and the incidence is one in every 10,000. Sanjurjo and Flores (1960) stated that in Puerto Rico 90 percent of the male population is uncircumcised, yet only 0.2 percent of the hospital admissions from 1946 to 1959 had the disease. In the United States carcinoma of the penis is a rare disease, estimated as from 1 to 3 percent of all malignancies, whereas on the European continent the incidence is about 5 percent of all malignancies (Buddington et al., 1963; Dean, 1935).

The records of the New York University Medical Center yield the following information relative to the incidence of cancer of the penis:

Three hospitals comprise this complex, each drawing from different socioeconomic groups. The Universal Hospital is primarily a private patient hospital. The Manhattan Veterans Hospital receives veterans and has almost exclusively a male population. Bellevue Hospital receives the vast majority of its patients from the underprivileged segment of the inhabitants of the city and has the largest proportion of Negroes and Puerto Rican citizens. These economic factors are considered, for carcinoma of the penis is often regarded as predominantly a disease of the underprivileged.

Etiology

Overwhelming evidence points to the accumulation of carcinogenic irritants within the confines of the preputial space as the common cause for cancer of the penis. Smegma sterols have been accused of having this effect, and efforts have been made to induce penile cancer in rabbits by anthracine applications, but with limited success. The data on religious practices, however, are most convincing. Prophylaxis against cancer is almost completely assured by circumcision at birth. There are, nevertheless, seven cases of carcinoma of the penis in Jews so circumcised (Kaufman and Sternberg, 1963; Paquin and Pearce, 1955; Marshall, 1953; Ledlie, 1956; Amelar, 1956; Reitman, 1953). If circumcision is delayed until age 5 to 10 years, the protection is far less complete. Under the intriguing title "Jewish Penile Carcinoma," Licklider (1961) reviewed, according to religion, 152 cases of penile cancer (Table 61–2).

The prepuce is not the only source of

TABLE 61–1

Hospital	Bed Capacity	Years	Cases of Carcinoma of Penis	Average Yearly Admission	Incidence
University	600	1940–1968	56	11,950	1 per 5957 admissions
Manhattan Veterans	1000	1956–1969	31	9646	1 per 3422 admissions
Bellevue	2200	1939–1969	40	12,370	1 per 9277 admissions
Totals:	3600		127	11,322	1 per 6218 admissions

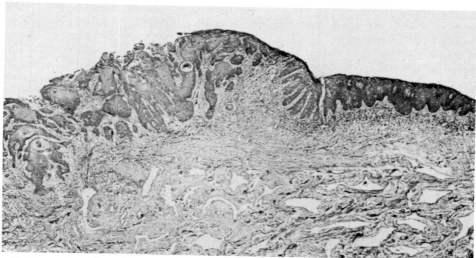

Figure 61–3 Low-power photomicrograph of erythroplasia of penis and adjoining carcinoma. ×25. Note hyperplastic epithelium on right, invading tumor cells with pearl formation on left, and inflammatory reaction in supporting tissues. *(From* Buddington et al.: J. Urol., 89:442, 1963.)

of the probable interrelationship of dermatologic lesions and malignancy. Erythroplasia of Queyrat has received ample attention in this regard, over 260 cases having been reported in the literature, with an incidence of 2:1 in males over females. Montgomery (1939) estimated that 20 percent or more of these cases develop into carcinoma. Moreover, coexisting cancer and erythroplasia of Queyrat have been reported (Fig. 61–3) (Wechler et al., 1955; Friedman, 1953; Merricks and Cottrell, 1953).

Benign Tumors of the Penis. The paraffinomas of the penis present as firm, nodular areas which are difficult to diagnose because of the usual reluctance of the patient to admit their cause. Men have injected paraffin and oils into the penile subcutaneous tissue to enlarge the organ (Zolar et al., 1969; Quenu and Perol, 1948). One such individual admitted to 200 injections of Depo-testosterone (oil) into the penis for psychosexual reasons.

The fibrolipomas may develop without known cause (Fig. 61–4). One the size of a golf ball was removed from the penis of a 14 year old boy (Gernon and McKenna, 1937).

Hirsutoid papillomas form around the coronal margins as white or yellowish elevations and are not apt to be confused with cancer, but their common incidence

in men (8 percent) makes them worthy of mention (Winer and Winer, 1955; Tanenbaum and Becker, 1965). The very rare tumors of congenital origin are mentioned for their curiosity. Herman and Fleicher (1962) removed a large cauliflower tumor, which had been present since birth, from an 8 month old child.

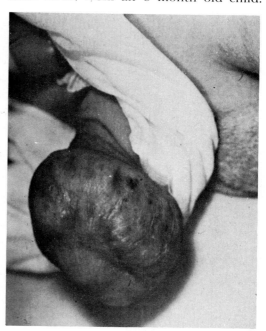

Figure 61–4 Giant keloid of penis in boy 8 years of age. (Courtesy of Bellevue Hospital, New York.)

Many diagnoses were made, but the tumor was finally classified as a mixed mesenchymal benign tumor.

Sarcomas. These rare tumors appear in numerous reports in the literature and are important more from an academic than a practical point of view. Ashley and Edwards (1957) collected and reviewed 54 cases in the world literature, and since then others have added to this collection. Among the varieties described are neurosarcoma (schwannoma), appearing as nodules along the shaft (Mecenas and Woodruff, 1962), and embryonal rhabdomysarcoma of the penis, occurring in a 2 year old child (Ramos and Pach, 1966). Hemangioendotheliomas usually arise in the corpora cavernosa but are also described as a painful nodule on the dorsum of the penis (Kovacs and Crouch, 1958; Barnett and Low, 1960). In 1968 Hutcheson et al. collected nine cases of leiomyosarcoma of the penis which were usually situated in the shaft. They may grow slowly and may recur as late as 24 years after excision (Fagundis et al., 1962). Fibrosarcomas (Wheelock and Clark, 1943) are also described by Tripathi (1968).

Kaposi's sarcoma appearing as multiple purplish blue spots on the penis of a man, aged 20 years, has been reported by Low et al. (1954).

Primary malignant melanomas are very rare. Gupta and Grabstald (1965) noted that, of 1200 cases of melanoma admitted to the Memorial Hospital for Cancer and Allied Diseases, only two occurred in the penis. Schneiderman et al. (1965) collected 18 cases of penile malignant melanoma. The longest survival after amputation was 11 years.

In general, sarcomas of the penis, with the exception of the fibrosarcoma, are rapidly fatal, but one should be aware of their possible occurrence.

Metastatic or Secondary Tumors of the Penis. Abeshouse (1958 and 1961) found a total of 140 patients having the site of the primary tumor in the kidney, prostate, rectum, lung, bronchi, bone, or skin, with subsequent metastasis to the penis. The corpora cavernosa were usually involved, and consequently 38 percent of the patients had priapism. Wilson et al. (1954) noticed that the nodular lesions in one case resembled a chancre.

Treatment of Epithelial Cancer of the Penis

An appraisal of the efficacy of the various methods of treatment of cancer of the penis is difficult for a number of reasons. The number of cases in each series is too small for an accurate analysis of one type of treatment as compared to another. Those reports which include a larger number of patients extend over a period of 15 to 20 years. Consequently, several individuals have been involved in the management, and therapeutic policies

TABLE 61–6

Reporter	Years Involved	Cases
1. Hanash et al. (1970)	1945–1965	169
2. Colon (1952)	1941–1952	145
3. Hardner and Woodruff (1967)	1944–1964	135
4. Jackson (1966)	1942–1957	130
5. Dean (1935)	1915–1935	120
6. Buddington et al. (1963)	1928–1963	104
7. Spratt et al. (1965)	1940–1961	88
8. Furlong and Uhle (1953)	1921–1946	88
9. Basset (1952)	no specific years	78
10. Young (1931) and Lewis (1931)	1916–1931	70
11. Horn and Nesbit (1934)		37
12. Fegan and Persky (1969)	1955–1967	35
13. Dean and Dean (1935)	1947–1950	29
14. Sanjurjo and Flores (1960)	1946–1959	24
15. Harlin (1952)	10 years	21
16. Melicow and Ganem (1946)	1928–1944	19

have varied according to the convictions of several surgeons. Furthermore, analyses are hampered by ambiguity relative to spread to the lymph nodes. The prognosis obviously is worse if metastasis has occurred. In 50 percent or more of the cases involving palpable inguinal lymph nodes, the enlargement is due to an inflammatory process, and unless the nodes are removed the true incidence of metastasis remains uncertain. This information is often lacking in the reports, and the effectiveness of treatment, whether or not metastases are present, cannot be accurately determined. Finally, the value of a certain mode of treatment depends upon satisfactory post-treatment evaluation. This has proved to be difficult in many series. To illustrate these important points, some of the larger series are listed in Table 61–6.

NONSURGICAL TREATMENT

Chemotherapy. Ichikawa et al. (1969) announced the use of a new antitumor antibiotic, known as bleomycin, for the treatment of epithelial tumors of the penis and scrotum (Fig. 61–5). Eight men with penile cancer were given 15 to 30 mg. of the drug intravenously twice a week, for a total of 300 mg. within 5 to 10 weeks. Six of the patients responded with spectacular shrinkage and disappearance of the cancer. Two others with condylomata acuminata were cured by local applications. The drug may be administered either intramuscularly or intravenously, but it is capable of producing serious complications, such as nausea, vomiting, pyrexia, depilation, stomatitis, lung complications, and sclerotic changes in the skin.

Erythroplasia of Queyrat has been treated topically with 5-fluorouracil and has shown prompt resolution. Huessar and Pugh (1969), Jansen et al. (1967), and Cheng and Veenema (1965) used thio-TEPA in the form of a local bath with no effect on squamous cell cancer of the penis, but after 21 soaking treatments of two hours each some condylomata disappeared.

Irradiation. X-rays have been employed by external radiation, radium plaques, and seeds alone or in conjunction with surgery (Overhof, 1935). Jackson (1966) reported using a combination of surgery and x-ray in the form of molds or

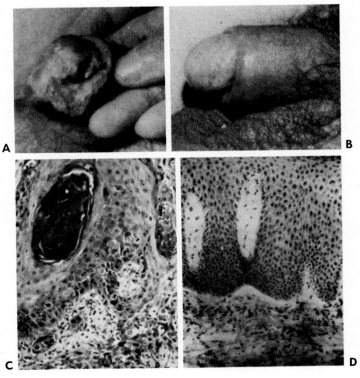

Figure 61–5 Bleomycin for treatment of carcinoma of the penis. *A*, During treatment, 12/22/66. *B*, During treatment, 2/27/68. *C*, Photomicrograph before treatment. *D*, Photomicrograph after treatment. (*From* Ichikawa: J. Urol., 102:699, 1969.)

TABLE 61–7*

Method	Cases	Five-year Survival	Disease Sterilized† 1 to 5 Years
Radiation only	39	22–56%	31–79%
Radiation and surgery	40	26–65%	30–75%
Surgery only	51	27–53%	34–67%
Totals:	130	75–58%	95–73%

*From Jackson: Br. J. Surg., 53:33, 1966.

†Sterilization is interpreted as survival for one year or more with clinical healing and no evidence of spread.

external irradiation. His results are summarized in Table 61–7.

Jackson believed that with grade I tumors (confined to glans penis or prepuce), "there is no real difference in results between surgery and irradiation" but suggested that, if the primary lesion is not cured in six months, surgery is indicated.

Most of the reporters, however, take the attitude that only very small primary lesions (2 cm. or less) be treated with x-ray or rely on surgery for all lesions. There is general agreement that irradiation of metastatic lymph nodes is not curative and has little value. Buddington et al. (1963) reported on 12 patients treated by irradiation alone, eight of whom had extensive disease; all died within five years. Three men with small lesions refused surgery and received 6000 R., but all suffered severe painful irradiation effects requiring penectomy for relief of pain. Harlin (1952) summarized the inherent disadvantages of irradiation as follows:

1. The tumor itself is radioresistant.

2. Concomitant infection at the site of the lymph nodes lowers tolerance for x-rays.

3. Skin over the groin has low tolerance for irradiation because of moisture.

4. Perilymphatic fat prevents adequate response.

In summary, it would be fair to report that a trial of irradiation for small, superficial, primary penile cancer less than 2 cm. in diameter is consistent with current thought. It has been estimated that less than 5 percent of all patients would come under this category. Others who refuse surgery or who have very extensive lesions are candidates for x-ray as a palliative measure.

SURGICAL TREATMENT

Anatomy. The surgical treatment of carcinoma of the penis is predicated on anatomic structures and the routes by which metastasis occurs.

Buck's fascia surrounds the corpora and forms a barrier, of sorts, against invasion into the blood spaces of the corpora and thence dissemination by the venous system to the vertebral areas. The lymphatic channels and nodes are, by far, the favorite routes of extension beyond the confines of the penis to the inguinal nodes (Fig. 61–6). The excellent monograph by Spratt and his associates (1965), entitled Anatomy and Surgical Technique of Groin Dissection, gives superb instruction and many essential details that will serve the reader well. The basic features of the lymphatic system involved herewith are as follows:

A. At about the depth of the sweat glands, lymphatic channels of sufficient size are found to accept malignant cells.

B. There are three principle intercommunicating lymphatic systems within the penis:

(a) The prepuce, frenulum, and skin of the shaft drain into the superficial and deep inguinal nodes.

(b) The glans penis and corpora cavernosa drain into a lymphatic plexus lying in front of the symphysis pubis and thence to the deep inguinal nodes.

(c) The urethra and corpus spongiosum drain partly into the deep inguinal nodes and partly into the external iliac nodes within the pelvis.

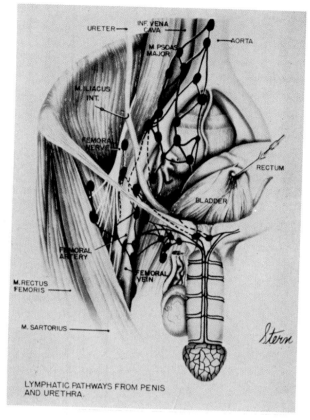

Figure 61-6 Lymphatic pathways from the penis and urethra. *(From* Hotchkiss and Amelar: J. Urol., 72:1181, 1954.)

C. The regional lymph nodes consist of:
(a) Pelvic lymph nodes, which lie in the retroperitoneal space above the inguinal ligament. These are arranged in three groups; median, lateral, and anterior to the iliac vessels. They are 8 to 10 in number and drain the deep sublingual nodes. The common iliac glands are 4 to 6 in number and lie posterior and medial to the iliac artery.

(b) Inguinal lymph nodes, which lie below the inguinal ligament and are subdivided into two groups:
1. The superficial inguinal nodes, which are 12 to 20 in number, situated in the femoral triangle (Fig. 61-7). They form a general line parallel to the inguinal ligament and extend along both sides of the saphenous vein.
2. The deep inguinal nodes, which are 1 to 3 in number,

lying below the fascia lata (Fig. 61-8). One is in the femoral canal, one below the junction of the saphenous and femoral veins, and one in the lateral part of the femoral ring.

All these various groups of glands have intercommunicating channels furnishing avenues for cancer cells to pass to another group, once one group becomes involved. Furthermore, it is important to note that the pre-symphysis group furnishes a communication between the right and left inguinal nodes, so that cancer cells may pass over the midline to establish bilateral inguinal node residence.

This elaborate intercommunicating system furnishes the basis for surgical procedures to be considered herewith.

SURGICAL PROCEDURES

The extent and type of operative procedures are based upon (1) the degree of in-

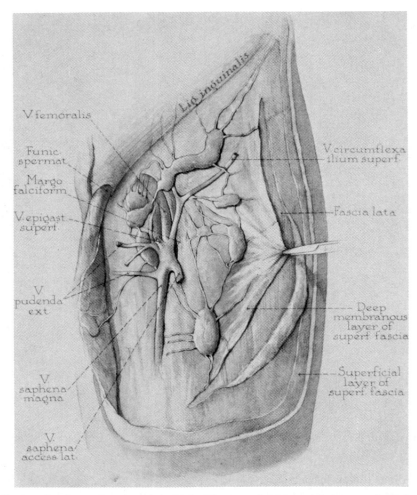

Figure 61–7 Anterior femoral region—left thigh. The superficial layer of the superficial fascia has been removed to reveal the deep layer with its contained inguinal lymph glands and the veins of the saphenous system to which the glands are intimately related. The deep layer has been incised and partially freed from the subjacent fascia lata. *(From* Daesler et al.: Surg. Gynecol. Obstet., 87:679, 1948. By permission of Surgery, Gynecology & Obstetrics.)

volvement, (2) the age of the patient, and (3) the ability of the patient to withstand surgical endeavors, often of some magnitude.

The degree of involvement is categorized as follows:

Grade I: disease limited to the distal one-third of the penis (Fig. 61–9)

Grade II: disease involves the entire penis (Fig. 61–10)

Grade III: disease involves the penis and lymph nodes (Fig. 61–11)

For grade I and II lesions, amputation of the penis proximal to the cancer is all that is theoretically required, with or without transplantation of the urethra into the perineum. Grade III lesions require, in addition, the removal of the cancer-bearing nodes.

It is vital to ascertain whether the regional lymph nodes contain cancer cells; unfortunately, this is difficult to establish without their removal. All authors agree that if the regional nodes are enlarged, only 30 to 50 percent or less actually contain tumor cells. Inflammatory lymphadenopathy commonly accompanies the primary lesion. If the grade of the primary tumor is high, as denoted by the biopsy, and if no infection is present, the probabilities are high that palpable inguinal nodes are involved with tumor.

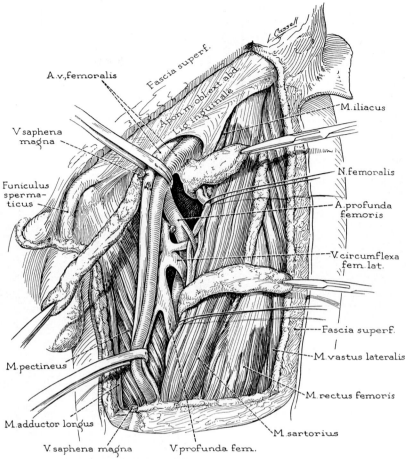

Figure 61–8　The deep inguinal glands. *(From* Daesler et al.: Surg. Gynecol. Obstet., 87:679, 1948. By permission of Surgery, Gynecology & Obstetrics.)

Furthermore, if the nodes do not regress in two to four weeks following the complete removal of the primary tumor, the inference is that they contain metastatic deposits. Hardner and Woodruff (1967) advocates bilateral inguinal lymphadenectomy as the only way to determine whether or not metastasis has occurred, for in his series 12 percent of cases without palpable adenopathy had metastatic deposits when the nodes were excised and examined. Experience has also shown that some very extensive penile tumors do not metastasize and that there is poor correlation between enlarged inguinal nodes and metastatic deposits. Lymphangiography has not been accurate in identifying involved nodes.

If metastatic cancer has involved the inguinal nodes, the amputation of the penis alone must then be regarded as inadequate for a cure. Accordingly, if the patient is able to undergo groin surgery, a bilateral node dissection is a necessary procedure to determine if all cancer cells have been removed.

Conservative Penile Amputation. A partial penectomy 1.5 to 2 cm. proximal to a small lesion has proved to be curative. A tourniquet is applied at the base of the penis and a guillotine amputation is done, leaving the urethra 1 cm. longer than the stump. The dorsal blood vessel is tied, and a double ligature is passed between the septum of the corpora cavernosa and tied around each (Fig. 61–12). The tourniquet is released, and mattress sutures are used to control any bleeding points. The urethra is then spatulated, and the entire cut edges are sutured to the skin

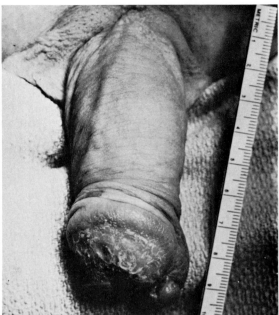

Figure 61–9   Carcinoma of the penis, involving distal one-third of the penis; grade I. (Courtesy of Bellevue Hospital, New York.)

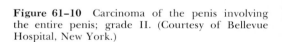

Figure 61–10   Carcinoma of the penis involving the entire penis; grade II. (Courtesy of Bellevue Hospital, New York.)

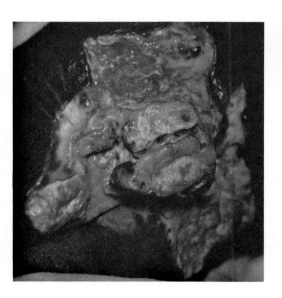

Figure 61–11   Carcinoma of the penis; grade III. There is complete destruction of the penis with extension to the abdominal wall and inguinal area. (Courtesy of Bellevue Hospital, New York.)

mg. per kg.) to a total of 72 mg., together with inguinal and iliac node dissection. MacKenzie and Whitemore (1968) resected the pubic rami in two patients with advanced penile carcinoma, but both died within seven months; they regarded the extension of surgery as having "a narrow range of usefulness." External irradiation has also been used to supplement surgery by many authors.

Edema of the lower extremities and scrotum requires elastic bandages and scrotal support until it subsides. Diuretics and limited activity may also be required.

Results of Treatment

The mortality from node dissection ranges from 1 to 4 percent before the patients leave the hospital. The disturbing fact is that many patients undergo node dissection without the benefit of removing metastatic nodes. The operation has questionable advantages unless cancer cells are removed. The experiences of the following surgeons indicated the incidence of positive inguinal nodes when such were removed:

Hardner
41 patients   53% had metastasis
Buddington
11 patients   3 had positive nodes
Furlong
88 patients   23% had positive nodes
Dean
"50% with adenopathy have metastasis"
Spratt
88 patients   35% had positive nodes
Sanjurjo
16 patients   2 had positive nodes
Young and Lewis
34 patients   13 had positive nodes
Basset
78 patients   26 (33%) had metastasis

Thus it is apparent that a majority of patients subjected to lymphadenectomy do not have metastasis.

The survival rates of patients who have had partial penile amputation or total penectomy with and without regional lymph node dissection have been presented by various authors. For reasons previously given, it is extremely difficult to draw conclusions from these reports.

Rough information is recorded in Table 61–8 for what judgment and conclusions are warranted.

Conclusion

The incidence of carcinoma of the skin of the penis varies widely according to geographic areas and, more particularly, to the custom of circumcision practiced within the areas. The disease is one that is more prevalent among the lower socioeconomic groups but not exclusively so. There is a considerable lag period between onset and treatment. Small superficial lesions are treated with a high success rate either by x-ray or amputation. Lymphadenopathy is common, but most enlarged nodes are the result of inflammatory reaction rather than metastasis. The differential diagnosis between inflammatory lymphadenopathy and metastatic deposits cannot be made with certainty except by excision and examination of the nodes. Until reliable tests are devised to differentiate between inflammatory reactions and tumor metastatic nodes, it would appear that inguinal node resection is necessary if complete extirpation of all cancer is to be achieved with reasonable certainty. Inguinal node excision is an operation attended by some morbidity but low mortality in selected cases if performed with pre- and postoperative precautions. If the inguinal nodes are involved with tumor, the survival rate is definitely lower than if they are uninvolved.

Carcinoma of the skin of the penis is preventable by circumcision at birth but less so if the operation is performed in later years. Cases diagnosed and treated early have a high cure rate. Delay in diagnosis favors extension to the lymphatic system, and the prognosis is thereupon relatively poor for survival.

CANCER OF THE SKIN OF THE SCROTUM

A special interest in cancer of the scrotum has developed because of historical connotations that appear to the biblio-

TABLE 61–8

Reporter	Cases	Five-year or Less Survival
Brady Institute	70	55% alive without tumor 31% alive with tumor
Sanjurjo	24	35% survived 5 years, providing no metastasis to lymph nodes
Buddington	45	21 partial amputation 50% alive, 5 years

		24 total amputation with and without lymph node dissection
		  10 of 24 alive and well 5 years
		    3 with positive nodes have 2 survivors 5 years or more

Dean (1935)	40	75% survival, superficial tumors, partial penectomies
		60% survival, extensive tumors without metastasis
		5% survival, metastatic tumor

Hardner	41	partial penectomy and node dissection:
		18 had positive nodes:
		  8 free of tumor, 2 years
		  2 alive with tumor
		  1 died free of tumor

		23 with negative nodes: none died, 1 alive with tumor

Spratt and Beggs	88	35% with inguinal lymph node had metastasis
		72% with negative nodes, 5-year survival
		19% with positive nodes, 5-year survival
		  7 too far advanced or refused surgery, all died
		  8 initial radiotherapy
		    1 controlled, 5 years
		  5 local excision
		    3 living, 6 mos. to 10 yrs. free of cancer
		37 subtotal penectomy; 8 died, cancer
		31 amputation and groin dissection
		    45% survival, 5 years
		no difference if nodes removed early or late

Overhoff	22	4 patients—primary surgery plus irradiation
		  3–5 year survival
		4 patients—primary surgery with radiation for recurrence
		  1–2 year survival
		8 radiation only, 5 had 2–5 year survival
		6 radiation followed by surgery, 3 had 2–6 year survival

philes of the Dickens era when chimney sweeps plied their trade. But also, the implications of the cause of scrotal cancer stimulated investigators to use allied chemical substances at a later date to produce the first experimental skin cancer in laboratory animals.

It has been related that nomadic tribesmen living in Persia and Turkistan were subjected to scrotal skin cancer because of the custom of carrying a pot of charcoal under their skirtlike garments for warmth. Graves and Flo (1940) credited Bassius in 1731 as the first to report upon scrotal cancer, but the classic report "Cancer Scroti" by Percival Potts in 1775 has established him in the annals of history as the originator of the term "chimney sweep's cancer." Thus he wrote:

...this distemper was peculiar to a certain set of people which has not, at least to my knowledge, been publicly noticed; I mean chimney sweeper's cancer. They are treated with great brutality and almost starved from cold and hunger; are thrust up narrow and sometimes hot chimneys where they are some-

TABLE 61–8 *(Continued)*

Reporter	Cases	Five-year or Less Survival
Harlin	21	70% cure with early lesions 5% with metastasis 　　only 1 alive, 5 years (nonoperative)
Furlong	88	40 inoperable, 34 died within 1 year 48 treated "with some chance of cure" 　　26 died of disease 　　11 died unrelated causes 　　13 (27%) alive 5 years, 2 with tumor 　　14 had penectomy and inguinal node dissection, 　　　cure rate 21%
Colon	29	with groin dissection, with and without x-ray, 20 alive 　　6 years or more (70%)
Paymaster	500	survived 5 years: 　　53% partial amputation 　　　no treatment of nodes 　　59% negative nodes 　　　partial amputation and groin dissection 　　11% positive nodes 　　　partial amputation and groin dissection 　　　9% radiation to groin node 　　55% radiation to primary only 　　70% negative nodes 　　　total amputation and groin dissection 　　10% positive nodes 　　　total amputation and groin dissection
	(of 500 patients)	42% alive, 5 years 26% dead, 5 years 21% lost to follow-up
Fegan	35	stage I　　　93% stage II—invasion corpora 　a—no nodes　　33% 　b—with nodes　50% total of 31 patients followed 　21 survived 80%
Basset	78	26 patients had metastasis 　19 proved histologically 　6 suspected 　1 alive, 5 years
Hanash	169	overall 10-year survival 67% 　if metastatic lymph nodes present, 10-year survival 11% 40% recurrence after simple excision of lesions on glans

times bruised and burned and sometimes almost suffocated and when they get to puberty, are peculiarly liable to a most noisome, painful, and fatal disease.

He advocated prompt removal of "the distempered part for the loss of the part is attended with a small degree of inconvenience." Others in the early 19th century described scrotal cancer and its treatment by salves and surgery. In 1876 Bell wrote of "paraffine epitheliomas of the scrotum," also linking the disease to an oc-

cupation—the paraffin workers. Chimney sweeps had almost vanished by this time.

Thus scrotal cancer remained associated with these two occupations until 1910, when Wilson described 40 patients with scrotal carcinoma. Of these patients 80 percent were wool spinners, most of whom had spent 14 to 20 years in this trade. These spinners attended a pair of machines called "mules." When the yarn would break, they would climb over the machine to splice the ends; in the warm, humid atmosphere their trousers would become soiled with lubricating oils. The oils penetrated the trousers, irritated the scrotum, and caused cancer. Mule spinner's disease, as it then came to be known, chimney sweep's cancer, and paraffin worker's cancer all had certain common factors: mechanical irritation, dust, grit, and exposure to tar, pitch, and oils. Enterprising investigators were quick to use fractions of mineral oils to produce experimental skin cancers in animals, sometimes called "tar cancers." The higher distillations of oils were soon found to be more carcinogenic, which probably explained why coal miners were not subject to the disease, for oxidation seemed necessary for carcinogenic potentials.

Kennaway and Kennaway (1946) made an exhaustive study of cancer of the scrotum as related to occupation. From 1911 to 1935 in a population of 14,000,000 there were 1752 deaths due to scrotal cancer recorded. Among these, 723 were individuals exposed to tar, pitch, and lubricating oils, leaving 1029 patients having nonoccupational disease. However, only one case of scrotal cancer was from "the highest professional class." Henry (1937) analyzed the reports of the Registrar General for England and Wales from 1911 to 1935 and collected 1487 fatal cases of scrotal cancer. In this group there were 147 fatal cancers in chimney sweeps, 44 of which were in sites other than the scrotum. From 1921 to 1935 there were 669 scrotal cancer deaths among the mule spinners. Even as late as 1944 to 1957, Avellan et al. (1967) of Goteberg, Sweden, described 8 cases of scrotal cancer among 250 automatic lathe operators.

In contrast to the European statistics, cancer of the scrotum in the United States is a very rare disease. The Brady Urological Clinic in Baltimore had only 2 cases in 12,000 admissions, and the Massachusetts General Hospital admitted only 4 patients with scrotal cancer in a 25-year period. Kickham and Dufresne (1967) found that 28 men with this disease were admitted to the Pondville Hospital in Massachusetts between 1930 and 1936, Dean (1948) reported that only 27 patients with scrotal cancer were seen at the Memorial Hospital in a period of 21 years; 22 of these patients were exposed to crude wool, tar, or lubricating oil.

Other authors have presented small groups of patients with carcinoma of the scrotum: Higgins and Warden (1949), 6 cases in 20 years at the Cleveland Clinic; Tucci and Haralambdis (1963), 2 cases; Ross (1928), 5 cases; and Carteaud (1964), 4 cases.

It is apparent that cancer of the scrotal skin is almost wholly dependent upon environment and hygiene and, as such, is a preventable disease, providing precautions are taken to avoid repetitious contact and to keep clothing and skin clean.

Clinical Descriptions

Epithelial cancer of the scrotum may be multiple or single, usually appearing on the dependent area of the scrotum. A long history of an indolent ulcer or sore precedes the development of a malignancy. Coexisting skin disorders are not uncommon and may deter suspicion and the diagnosis of cancer, thus requiring care not to overlook this possibility in connection with chronic skin diseases. Inguinal node enlargement may or may not be found, yet the same factors are to be considered in relation to enlarged lymph nodes as were outlined in detail in the section on cancer of the penis. A biopsy is essential for diagnosis.

Pathology

The squamous cell carcinomas are often described as poorly differentiated epitheliomas, but many descriptions include typical invasive cell nests. Basal cell tumors are rare.

Differential Diagnosis

Epithelial tumors of the scrotum must be differentiated from a variety of benign and malignant lesions, such as sebaceous cysts, cutaneous nevi, testis tumors eroding through the skin, and the rare sarcomas. The latter tumors, which were reviewed by Waller (1962), include three spindle cell sarcomas, one neurofibrosarcoma, one fibrosarcoma, and one rhabdomyosarcoma, and he added one liposarcoma. Immergut et al. (1965) described one fatal case of leiomyosarcoma of the scrotum. There are also several reports on sclerosing lipogranulomas which may easily be confused with scrotal cancer (Smetana and Bernhard, 1950; Best et al., 1953; Carlson, 1968; Arduino, 1959). About 15 instances of these curious tumors have been reported. The causes of this lipid tumor are thought to be trauma, mineral oil injected into the scrotal skin, and repeated applications of medical salves to the skin. They appear as nodular lesions, one of which weighed 158 g. These lesions consist of areas of hyaline necrosis, with numerous vacuoles lined by giant cells and separated by fibrovascular septa. Special stains demonstrate the spaces to be filled with lipids. The report of Hausfeld (1961) mentioned a 5 year old boy who developed a large scrotal mass which proved to be sarcoidosis (Boeck's sarcoid), and he stated that there were 20 cases of genital sarcoidosis in the world literature, the skin being part of a generalized process affecting the reticuloendothelial and lymphoid-hematopoietic systems.

Treatment

The method of treating carcinoma of the skin of the scrotum vary considerably with the authors and in accordance with the extent of the disease, the age of the patient, and unrelated but coexisting disease. The paucity of clinical material prohibits statistical analysis, but the report of Kickham and Dufresne (1967) on 28 men seen between 1930 and 1966 at the Pondville Hospital is one of the most informative.

28 patients:
operative measures	25
no other therapy	12
local excision	9
groin dissection, 11 of these bilateral	16

x-ray was given to 13 as last resort was ineffective

results:
2 postoperative deaths

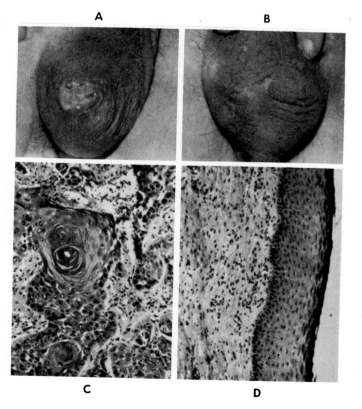

Figure 61–19 Carcinoma of the scrotum treated by bleomycin. *A,* Before treatment, 5/17/67. *B,* After treatment, 10/19/67. *C,* Photomicrograph before treatment. *D,* Photomicrograph after treatment. *(From* Ichikawa et al.: J. Urol., 102:699, 1969.)

3 died of disease independent of the malignancy

of remaining 23, only 1 alive at time of report (1967)

9 patients died of cancer within two years

9 patients died of cancer within five years

of 5 survivors:

1 died 8 years later without recurrences

1 died 12 years later with recurrence

3 survived 7–10 years and 20 years without demonstrable disease

Avellan et al. (1967) operated upon eight men, resecting the scrotal wall and reconstructing the area by skin graft; five had inguinal node surgery; one patient died of the disease 1½ years later.

Of 27 patients treated at the Memorial Hospital, only 8 lived five years or more (Dean, 1948). Tucci and Haralambidis (1963), Higgins and Warder (1949), and Ross (1928) also reported on smaller groups. If the lesion is small the prognosis is reasonably good; later recurrences occur despite initial removal. X-ray has been used with unimpressive results.

Long periods of palliation between initial treatment and late recurrences offer encouragement for surgical treatment.

Ichikawa et al. (1969) used bleomycin on two patients having squamous cell carcinoma of the scrotum (Fig. 61–19). One received 900 mg. of the drug in 78 days; one of the scrotal lesions healed, while the other remained and was removed surgically. Metastatic nodes present prior to treatment were negative on biopsy following therapy. The second patient had complete healing of a 2 × 2 cm. cancer after three courses of bleomycin were given intravenously.

Carcinoma of the scrotum is a rare disease in the United States, but the incidence in European countries in the 18th and 19th centuries, as well as in the early years of the 20th century, marks this type of malignancy as one of considerable importance. Cancer of the scrotum is closely related to the occupations that expose the individuals to soot, tar, dust, grit, pitch, oil, and sweat. The avoidance of such contacts and good hygiene afford a great measure of protection.

The lesions are primarily indolent and slow in development. The treatment consists of surgical excision and removal of the inguinal lymph nodes when such appear to be involved with metastatic lesions. Late recurrences may occur years after the initial treatment.

REFERENCES

Abeshouse, B. S.: Primary and secondary melanoma of genitourinary tract. South. Med. J., 51:994, 1958.

Abeshouse, B. S., and Abeshouse, G. A.: Metastatic tumors of the penis. J. Urol., 86:99, 1961.

Amelar, R. D.: Carcinoma of the penis due to ·trauma occurring in male patient circumcized at birth. J. Urol., 75:728, 1956.

Arduino, L.: Sclerosing lipogranuloma of male genitalia. J. Urol., 82:155, 1959.

Ashley, D. S., and Edwards, E. E.: Sarcoma of penis. Br. J. Surg., 45:170, 1957.

Avellan, L., Breine, J., Jacobsson, B., and Johanson, B.: Carcinoma of scrotum induced by mineral oil. Scand. J. Plast. Reconstr. Surg., 1:135, 1967.

Barnett, C. P., and Low, R.: Hemangio-endothelioma of corpus cavernosum penis. J. Urol., 83:160, 1960.

Barringer, B. S.: Inguinal gland metastasis in cancer of penis. J.A.M.A., 106:21, 1935.

Basset, J. W.: Carcinoma of the penis. Cancer, 5:530, 1952.

Beggs, J. H., and Spratt, J. S.: Epidermoid carcinoma of the penis. J. Urol., 91:166, 1964.

Best, E., De Weerd, H. L., and Dahlin, D. C.: Sclerosing lipogranuloma of male genitalia produced by mineral oil. Proc. Staff Meet. Mayo Clinic, 28:623, 1953.

Block, N. L., Rosen, P., and Whitmore, W. F.: Hemipelvectomy for advanced penile cancer. J. Urol., 110:703, 1973.

Boyd, H. L.: Metastatic carcinoma of penis secondary to carcinoma of rectum. J. Urol., 71:82, 1954.

Buddington, W. T., Kickham, C. J., and Smith, W. E.: An assessment of malignant disease of the penis. J. Urol., 89:442, 1963.

Burns, E., and Thompson, I.: Infections and inflammations of male genital tract. In Campbell, M. F. (Ed.): Urology. Vol. I. Ed. 2. Philadelphia, W. B. Saunders Company, 1963, p. 489–535.

Burns, E., and Thompson, I.: Penis and urethra. In Campbell, M. F., and Harrison, J. H. (Eds.): Urology. Vol. I. Ed. 3. Philadelphia, W. B. Saunders Company, 1970, pp. 513–553.

Carlson, H. E.: Sclerosing lipogranuloma of penis and scrotum. J. Urol., 100:656, 1968.

Carteaud, R.: Cancer of scrotum due to coal tar or derivatives. Press Med., 72:3355, 1964.

Cheng, S. F., and Veenema, R.: Topical applications of thio-TEPA to penile and urethral tumors. J. Urol., 94:259, 1965.

Colon, J. E.: Carcinoma of penis. J. Urol., 67:702, 1952.

Daselar, E. H., Anson, B. S., and Reimann, A. F.: Radical excision of inguinal and iliac glands. Surg. Gynecol. Obstet., 87:679, 1948.

Davis, C. M.: Granuloma inguinale. J.A.M.A., 211:632, 1970.

Davis, S. W.: Giant condyloma acuminata: Incidence among cases diagnosed as carcinoma. J. Clin. Pathol., 18:142, 1965.

Dean, A. L.: Epithelioma of penis. J. Urol., 33:252, 1935.

Dean, A. L.: Epithelioma of penis in Jew circumcized in infancy. Trans. Am. Assoc. Genitour. Surg., 29:493, 1936.

Dean, A. L.: Epithelioma of scrotum. J. Urol., 60:508, 1948.

Dean, A. L.: Conservative amputation of the penis for carcinoma. J. Urol., 68:374, 1952.

Dean, A. L., and Dean, A. L., Jr.: Tumors of the penis, urethra, scrotum, and testes. *In* Campbell, M. F. (Ed.): Urology. Vol. I. Ed. 2. Philadelphia, W. B. Saunders Company, 1963, pp. 1227–1283.

Dodge, O. G., and Linsell, C. A.: Carcinoma of penis in Uganda and Kenya Africans. Cancer, 16:1255, 1963.

Fagundis, L. A., Hampe, O., Brenland, L., and De Jalma, J.: Leiomyosarcoma of the penis. J. Urol., 88:803, 1962.

Fegan, R., and Persky, L.: Squamous cell carcinoma of penis. Arch. Surg., 99:117, 1969.

Fowler, H. A., and Dorman, H. N.: Transitional cell carcinoma of penis. J. Urol., 41:575, 1939.

Friedman, S. J.: Queyrat's erythroplasia with carcinomatous invasion. J. Urol., 69:813, 1953.

Furlong, R. R., and Uhle, C. A.: Cancer of penis — A report of 88 cases. J. Urol., 69:550, 1953.

Gernon, J. T., and McKenna, C. M.: Fibrolipoma of penis. J. Urol., 38:500, 1937.

Gersh, I.: Condylomata acuminata of the penis. J. Urol., 69:164, 1953.

Grabstald, H.: Carcinoma of the penis involving skin of the base. J. Urol., 104:438, 1970.

Grauer, R. C., and Burt, J. E.: Glomus tumors of prepuce. J.A.M.A., 112:1806, 1939.

Graves, R. C., and Flo, S.: Carcinoma of Scrotum. J. Urol., 43:309, 1940.

Gupta, T. D., and Grabstald, J. H.: Melanoma of the genitourinary tract. J. Urol., 93:607, 1965.

Haines, C. E., and Garvey, F. K.: Neurosarcoma of penis associated with multiple neurofibromatosis (Von Recklinghausen's disease). J. Urol., 63:542, 1950.

Hanash, K. A., Furlow, W. L., Utz, P. C., and Harrison, E. G., Jr.: Carcinoma of penis: A clinicopathologic study. J. Urol., 104:291, 1970.

Hardner, G. J., and Woodruff, M. V.: Operative management of carcinoma of penis. J. Urol., 98:487, 1967.

Harlin, H.: Carcinoma of penis. J. Urol., 67:326, 1952.

Hausfeld, K. F.: Primary sarcoidosis of scrotum. J. Urol., 86:269–272, 1961.

Henry, S. A.: Fatal scrotal cancers. Am. J. Cancer, 31:28, 1937.

Herman, R. R., and Fleicher, R. L.: Congenital penile tumor. J. Urol., 87:701, 1962.

Higgins, C. C., and Warden, J. G.: Cancer of scrotum. J. Urol., 62:250, 1949.

Horn, K. W., and Nesbit, R. H.: Carcinoma of penis. Ann. Surg., 100:480, 1934.

Hotchkiss, R. S., and Amelar, R. D.: Primary carcinoma of the male urethra. J. Urol., 72:1181, 1954.

Huessar, J. N., and Pugh, R. P.: Erythroplasia of Queyrat treated with topical 5-fluorouracil. J. Urol., 102:595, 1969.

Hutcheson, J. B., Whittaker, W. W., and Fronstin, M. H.: Leiomyosarcoma of penis: Case report and review of literature. J. Urol., 101:874, 1968.

Hutchinson, J.: A clinical lecture on epithelioma of the penis and its treatment. Lancet, 1:1071, 1899.

Ichikawa, T., Nakana, I., and Hirokawa, T.: Bleomycin treatment of the tumors of penis and scrotum. J. Urol., 102:699, 1969.

Immergut, S., Epstein, S., Levy, S., and Cottler, Z. R.: Leiomyosarcoma of scrotum. J. Urol., 93:479, 1965.

Jackson, S. M.: Treatment of carcinoma of the penis. Br. J. Surg., 53:33, 1966.

Jansen, G. T., Pillaha, C. J., and Honeycutt, W. M.: Erythroplasia Queyrat treated with topical 5-fluorouracil. South. Med. J., 60:185, 1967.

Kaufman, J. S., and Sternberg, T. H.: Carcinoma of the penis in a circumcized man. J. Urol., 90:449, 1963.

Kennaway, E. L., and Kennaway, N. W.: Social distribution of cancer of scrotum and cancer of penis. Cancer Res., 6:49, 1946.

Kickham, C. J. E., and Dufresne, M.: An assessment of carcinoma of the scrotum. J. Urol., 98:108, 1967.

Kovacs, J., and Crouch, R. D.: Sarcoma of penis. J. Urol., 80:43, 1958.

Kuehn, C. A., and Roberts, R. D.: Amputation and radical lymph gland dissection in carcinoma of the penis. J. Urol., 69:173, 1953.

Ledlie, R. C. B., and Smithers, D. W.: Carcinoma of penis in man circumcized in infancy. J. Urol., 76:756, 1956.

Lewis, L. G.: Young's radical operation for cure of cancer of the penis. J. Urol., 26:295, 1931.

Licklider, S.: Jewish penile carcinoma. J. Urol., 86:98, 1961.

Low, H. T., Coakley, H. E., and Shonts, W. C.: Kaposi's sarcoma of penis. J. Urol., 72:886, 1954.

Mackenzie, A. R., and Whitemore, W. T.: Resection of pubic rami for urological cancer. J. Urol., 100:546, 1968.

Mark, E. G.: Sarcoma of penis. J. Urol., 15:611, 1926.

Marshall, V.: Typical carcinoma of the penis in a male circumcized in infancy. Cancer, 6:1044, 1953.

McAninch, J. W., and Moore, C. A.: Precancerous penile lesions in young men. J. Urol., 104:287, 1970.

Mecenas, H. J., and Woodruff, M. W.: Hemangioendothelioma of the male genitalia. J. Urol., 87:560, 1962.

Melicow, M. M., and Ganem, E. J.: Cancerous and precancerous lesions of the penis. J. Urol., 55:486, 1946.

Merricks, J. W., and Cottrell, T. L. S.: Erythroplasia of Queyrat. J. Urol., 69:807, 1953.

Montgomery, H.: Precancerous dermatosis and epithelioma in situ. Arch. Dermatol. Syph., 39:382, 1939.

Morgan, G., Jr.: Bone formation in penis associated with neoplasm. J. Urol., 96:229, 1966.

Noble, T. B.: Carcinoma of the penis in Siam. Br. J., 5:242, 1933.

Organ, C. H., Jr., and Carnazzo, A. J.: An extended method of the treatment of carcinoma of the penis. J. Urol., 93:396, 1965.

Overhof, K.: Cancer of the penis. Rontgenpraxis, 7:466, 1935.

Parra, C. A.: Solitary neurinoma of glans penis. Dermatologica, 137:150, 1968.

Paquin, A. J., and Pearce, J. M.: Carcinoma of the penis in man circumcized in infancy. J. Urol., 74:626, 1955.

Paymaster, J. C., and Gangadharan, P.: Cancer of penis in India. J. Urol., 97:110, 1967.

Pond, H. S., and Wadt, J. C.: Urinary obstruction secondary to metastatic carcinoma of the penis. J. Urol., 102:333, 1969.

Quenu, J., and Perol, E.: Paraffinomas of the penis (abstract). Surg. Gynecol. Obstet., 86:174, 1948.

Ramos, J. S., and Pach, G. T.: Primary embryonal rhabdomyosarcoma of penis in a 2 year old child. J. Urol., 96:928, 1966.

Riveros, M., and Cabanas, R.: Lymphography and cancer of the penis. Semaine Hop. Paris, 44:1616, 1968.

Reitman, P.: An unusual case of penile carcinoma. J. Urol., 69:547, 1953.

Ross, J. C.: Cancer of the scrotum. Liverpool Med. Chir. J. (Part 2), 42:170, 1934.

Sanjurjo, L. A., and Flores, B. G.: Carcinoma of penis. J. Urol., 83:433, 1960.

Schneiderman, C., Simon, M. A., and Levine, R. M.: Malignant melanoma of the penis. J. Urol., 93:615, 1965.

Shabad, A. L.: Some aspects of etiology and prevention of penile cancer. J. Urol., 92:696, 1964.

Shelley, H. S., and Wilderanders, R. E.: Case of carcinoma of the penis treated without phallectomy and showing no recurrence in nine years. J. Urol., 82:659, 1959.

Smetana, N. E., and Bernhard, W.: Sclerosing lipogranuloma. Arch. Pathol., 50:296, 1950.

Spratt, J. S., Shieber, W. S., and Dillard, B. M.: Anatomy and Surgical Technique of Groin Dissection. St. Louis, Mo., C. V. Mosby Company, 1965.

Sundell, B.: Polymorphous-called sarcoma of the penis. J. Urol., 86:612, 1961.

Tan, R. E.: Observations on frequency of carcinoma of penis at Macassar and its environs (South Celebes). J. Urol., 89:704, 1963.

Tanenbaum, M. H., and Becker, S. W.: Papillae of corona of glans penis. J. Urol., 93:391, 1965.

Taylor, J. A.: Penile horn. J. Urol., 52:611, 1944.

Thomas, J. A., and Small, C. S.: Carcinoma of the penis in southern India. J. Urol., 100:520, 1968.

Tripathi, V. N. P., and Dick, V. S.: Primary sarcoma of urogenital system in adults. J. Urol., 101:898, 1968.

Tucci, P., and Haralambidis, G.: Carcinoma of the scrotum. J. Urol., 89:585, 1963.

Waller, J. T.: Liposarcoma of the scrotum. J. Urol., 87:139, 1962.

Wattenberg, C. A.: Unusual tumors and secondary carcinomas of the penis. J. Urol., 52:169, 1944.

Wechsler, H. W., Spivack, L. L., and Dean, A. L.: Erythroplasia of Queyrat with invasive carcinoma with coincidental carcinoma in situ of urethra. J. Urol., 73:697, 1955.

Wheelock, M. C., and Clark, P. J.: Sarcoma of penis. J. Urol., 49:478, 1943.

Whitmore, W. F.: Tumors of the penis, urethra, scrotum, and testes. *In* Campbell, M. F., and Harrison, J. H. (Eds.): Urology. Vol. II. Ed. 3. Philadelphia, W. B. Saunders Company, 1970, pp. 1190–1229.

Wilson, M. E., Horton, G. R., and Horton, B. I.: Secondary tumors of the penis. J. Urol., 71:721, 1954.

Wilson, S. R.: Cancer of cotton mule spinners. Br. Med. J., 2:993, 1927.

Winer, J. H., and Winer, L. H.: Hirsutoid papillomas of coronal margins of glans penis. J. Urol., 74:375, 1955.

Wolbarst, A. L.: Circumcision and cancer. Lancet, 1:150, 1932.

Young, H. H.: A radical operation for cure of cancer of the penis. J. Urol., 26:285, 1931.

Zolar, J. A., Knode, R. E., and Mir, J. A.: Lipogranuloma of the penis. J. Urol., 102:75, 1969.

62

Malignant Tumors of the Hand

Robert W. Beasley, M.D., and
Bruno von B. Ristow, M.D.

Fortunately, malignant tumors of the hand are relatively uncommon, but their optimal management requires such special surgical knowledge, attitudes, and refined techniques as to merit separate consideration.

The hand is our primary tool for manipulating the environment. It also is a basic sensory organ which in many circumstances exceeds even the eye in gathering information. Impairment in either its sensory systems or complex prehensile mechanisms results in a serious loss and handicap. The loss is great for anyone, but it is especially great for the laboring man whose hands are virtually his only capital.

Interest in surgery of the hand has increased chiefly through increased interest in trauma, as the hand is by far the part most frequently injured. The principles learned through the surgical treatment of hand injury result in better care of the hand with a tumor. A few years ago it was taught that surgery of the hand should be divided clearly into the acute and reconstructive phases. With so few surgeons trained in the field, this was a practical and logical concept. However, it

is giving way to the realization that the initial care determines to a great extent the final outcome, and secondary procedures cannot always put things in good order, regardless of the initial treatment. Much the same is true of tumor surgery of the hand. Optimal results require projection of an ultimate plan from the start of treatment.

Cosmetic considerations cannot realistically be ignored. The term "function" is usually used to refer to prehensile capabilities of the hand. Yet if a man will not take a mutilated hand from his pocket, he is almost as much of a cripple as if the hand had been amputated—perhaps more of one, as the psychologic response reflects on all his other activities. Function must be thought of in terms of how well the person performs totally, rather than in the classic limited sense. The hand is constantly exposed to scrutiny in ordinary activities and is exceeded only by the face in portraying personality. It is apparent that in our competitive society both the manipulative abilities of the hand and its appearance bear a very real relation to socioeconomic well-being. The treatment of cancer of the skin of the hand requires extraordinary judgment in weighing the biologic factors of the tumor against the biomechanical and esthetic considerations.

PRECANCEROUS LESIONS OF THE HAND

Epitheliomas are the most frequent cancers of the hand. It is of fundamental importance to realize that in almost every instance *the malignancy has been preceded by a long-standing, precancerous, specific skin lesion.* The most common of the premalignant skin lesions is the solar keratosis, while radiation and arsenical and chemical dermatosis are less frequent. The duration of these premalignant lesions offers ample opportunity for their eradication by simple and nonmutilating treatment, emphasizing the importance of early, accurate diagnosis and awareness of the potential hazard of the premalignant skin lesions.

Solar Keratosis

Solar keratosis, often referred to as senile or actinic keratosis, has a high rate of malignant transformation. Cooley (1964) estimated this to be between 20 and 25 percent. Lund (1957) stated emphatically that the solar keratosis can be looked upon as an evolving carcinoma. Solar keratosis develops exclusively on the dorsal surfaces, being essentially unknown on the palmar skin.

Clearly chronic exposure to the sun is a fundamental etiologic factor, although there are great variations in individual susceptibility. Blum (1941) has demonstrated that it is the ultraviolet spectrum of light to which the basic damage can be attributed. The variation in individual susceptibility is related to the ability of the skin to develop, in response to the exposure, protective pigmentation which subsequently screens out the damaging rays. Thus people of fair complexion with minimal pigmentation are most susceptible. The incidence increases with age, as the damage from the exposure is cumulative.

The solar keratosis can be effectively treated by surgical excision, as well as by simpler measures, such as curettage, electrodesiccation, or topical application of 5-fluorouracil. Should there be induration at the base of the lesion or any other signs suggesting that malignant transformation may have already occurred, excisional therapy is required.

Arsenical Keratosis

In the last century when arsenic was commonly incorporated into medications, Hutchinson (1888) made the astute observation that it bore a relation to the development of cancer. The response could be from either systemic or topical administration of the drug. Currie (1947) reported a high incidence of carcinoma among people whose drinking water contained substantial levels of arsenic. *In contrast to solar keratosis, these lesions characteristically develop on the palmar surfaces of the hands or soles of the feet* (Fig. 62–1). There is controversy concerning the relationship between handling industrial inorganic arsenic and the eventual development of cancer, but evidence for this appears unconvincing. When carcinoma develops in an arsenical keratosis, it is invariably of the squamous cell type. In the patient who develops a carcinoma without a preexisting keratosis at the site, either squamous or basal cell type may be found (Lund, 1957). The malignancy of these tumors tends to be greater than that of those developing from solar keratosis. They should be surgically excised, the less aggressive modalities of treatment being unsuitable for these dangerous lesions.

Other Chemical Carcinogens

Many chemicals clearly cause dermatosis of the hand, but convincing demonstration of their etiologic relation to the development of cancer is rare. Chronic exposure to tar or cutting oil has been implicated (Lund, 1957), as well as to printer's ink (Conway et al., 1966), but the incidence is extremely low generally and virtually unknown among Black people. Like other chronic dermatosis with irreparable skin damage, excision of the skin of the area with resurfacing is required.

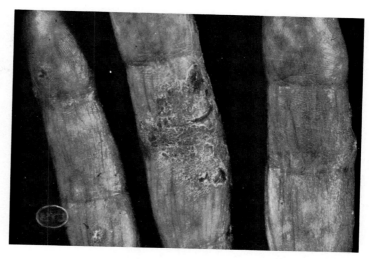

Figure 62–1 Arsenical keratosis, characteristically appearing on the palmar surface.

Radiation Dermatosis

The deleterious effects of ionizing radiation are so well established and severe that one must fully consider their implication in prescribing radiation for the treatment of any benign lesion. The radiation affects indiscriminately all cell structures, severely deranging their molecular configurations. A major deterrent to the general recognition of the potency and hazard of this destructive agent lies in the relatively small initial response of the tissue, while *the peak of destruction becomes evident only many years following the exposure.* The greatest factor determining the damage is the dosage. In general, damage is slightly less with divided doses and increased intervals between administration of each (Lund, 1957).

Malignant tumors resulting from roentgen irradiation are usually squamous cell carcinomas with a very bizarre microscopic cellular pattern. The development of basal cell carcinoma is rare. A massive, high-voltage dose may result in the development of fibrosarcomas, referred to often as irradiation pseudosarcomas or carcinosarcomas because of their erratic histologic appearance. There are also malignant tumors capable of both local extension and distant metastasis.

The treatment of radiation dermatosis with or without tumor is adequate surgical excision followed by repair of the defect with transplanted healthy tissues (Fig. 62–2). The clinician treating areas of irradiation injury must be keenly aware of the severe effect it has had on the vascular system, with thrombosis and permanent obliteration of the normal intercommunicating network of vessels. As with other changes, this obliteration is progressive for many years subsequent to the exposure. *It appears that there may also be a permanent change in the tissues which favors abnormal thrombosis to subsequent trauma.* This is seen in elevating even the smallest flap, which will bleed freely at the time of surgery but invariably will undergo progressive thrombosis thereafter, resulting in its necrosis. Realization of this is of extreme clinical importance, precluding the use of local flaps. These changes consistently have extended into the adjacent tissues over a wide area, even though they show absolutely no clinical evidence of having received any irradiation. Thus it is mandatory that tissues required for the repair of a defect resulting from irradiation injury be taken from an area which is a great distance from an exposed area. Many disasters have resulted from violation of this principle.

CANCERS OF THE HAND

Basal Cell Epithelioma

Basal cell epitheliomas are uncommon on the hand. Lawrence et al. (1953) re-

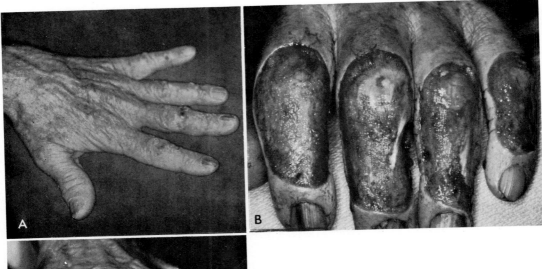

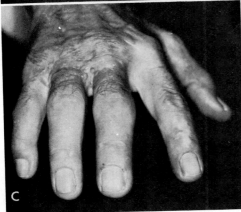

Figure 62–2 *A,* Radiodermatitis with squamous cell carcinoma of the middle finger. *B,* Margins of excision carried to the mid-axial lines to avoid troublesome contractions. *C,* Defects repaired with medium-thickness split skin grafts.

ported the incidence of squamous cell carcinoma of the hand to be 10 times greater than that of basal cell epithelioma. In discussing this tumor the term "epithelioma" is preferred, as it defines its malignant nature but implies a much less aggressive behavior than does the term "carcinoma." Metastasis of basal cell epithelioma is virtually unknown. Lattes and Kessler (1951) reported the incidence to be 0.09 percent with a 50 percent mortality in a series of 9050 cases. Therefore, in the treatment of basal cell epitheliomas, it is essential only to eradicate the local lesion, which may be done in many ways. Surgical excision has the advantage of permitting examination of serial sections of the specimen for residual tumor, as does Mohs' chemosurgical technique, but small lesions are satisfactorily managed by other locally destructive techniques, such as curettage and electrodesiccation. The minimal margin of surgical excision should be 5

mm. These tumors certainly can be destroyed by roentgen irradiation, but they also can be caused by this irradiation along with other problems.

Bowen's Disease

Bowen's disease is intraepithelial squamous cell carcinoma (Fig. 62–3). It is a malignant tumor having a tendency for lateral spread through the epidermis rather than for early deep invasion. The incidence of deep tissue invasion has been reported to vary between 5 and 20 percent (Conway et al., 1966). Metastasis may occur but is uncommon.

There is a possible relation between Bowen's disease and arsenical keratosis. In a series of patients with Bowen's disease, 82 percent were demonstrated to have abnormally high concentrations of arsenic in their tissues (Graham and Helwig, 1961).

Histologically the two lesions frequently are indistinguishable.

There is also evidence implicating a relation between Bowen's disease and other, internal malignancies, especially carcinoma of the lung and the genitourinary or gastrointestinal tracts. Graham and Helwig (1961) found this incidence to be 68 percent, while Conway et al. (1966) found it to be 19.3 percent.

The treatment of Bowen's disease is essentially that of removal of the lesion, which is best accomplished by surgical excision and repair of the defect. The extension of the tumor is well defined, so that surgical margins of only 3 to 5 mm. are planned. Many of the lesions occur on the working surfaces of the hand. Local flaps frequently are used in repair of the defect for optimal restoration of these functionally important areas.

Squamous Cell Carcinoma

Squamous cell carcinoma is the most common malignant tumor of the hand. The anticipated clinical behavior of the

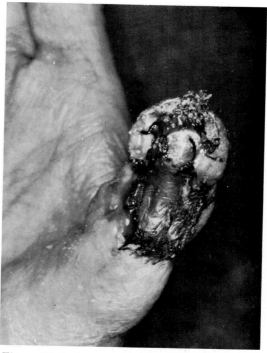

Figure 62–4 Squamous cell carcinoma of the thumb arising "de novo." In this case the lesion was eradicated by Mohs' chemosurgery, followed by amputation of the distal phalanx.

tumor and the prognosis bear a relation to its origin. In general, squamous cell carcinoma arising in a preexisting keratosis has a low incidence of metastasis, reported to be 0.1 percent (Conway et al., 1966). These tumors are highly differentiated histologically. In contrast to this behavior, squamous cell carcinoma arising in apparently healthy skin is prone to a high incidence of metastasis, which frequently occurs early in the course of the disease.

Moreover, with squamous cell carcinoma of the hand there is a correlation between the clinical behavior of the tumor and its histologic characteristics. In Broders' histologic classification of these tumors, grade I is highly differentiated and associated with an excellent prognosis, while grade IV is poorly differentiated and carries a correspondingly poor outlook (Broders, 1959).

The treatment of squamous cell carcinoma of the hand is surgical excision followed by repair. In selected cases Mohs' chemosurgery may be a useful method of ablation of an advanced tumor with deep

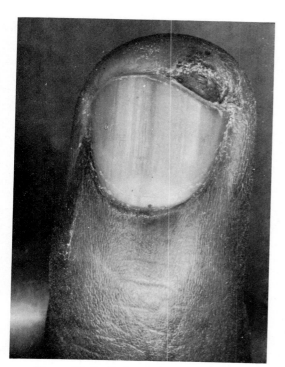

Figure 62–3 Periungual Bowen's disease.

invasion where involvement of vital structures by tumor is not readily apparent (Fig. 62–4). Squamous cell carcinoma arising in a keratosis is a problem of local control, and it is managed with a correspondingly conservative attitude. Surgical margins of about 1 cm. are recommended for the excision. For carcinoma arising "de novo," a more aggressive treatment is required, with 1.5 to 2.0 cm. surgical margins of excision. To achieve this, partial or complete amputation may be necessary, and consideration must be given to an elective axillary node exenteration for the poorly differentiated tumors, even in the absence of clinical lymphadenopathy. Metastasis to the epitrochlear nodes is extremely rare. Obviously an axillary node dissection is indicated in the presence of lymphadenopathy without evidence of pulmonary, hepatic, or other uncontrollable metastasis. A patient who, long after control of the primary lesion, develops a solitary pulmonary metastasis in the absence of other evidence of persistent tumor may still have a rsasonable prospect of cure by pulmonary resection. The axillary node dissection may be deferred for about three weeks. This is based on the assumption that tumor cells in transit at the time of resection of the primary lesion will then be entrapped in the lymph nodes.

Sarcoma

Sarcomas of the skin of the hand are rare, although a wide variety of types have been described. They all share a common mesodermal origin but little in terms of clinical behavior and degree of malignancy.

At the lower end of the malignancy spectrum is fibrosarcoma. Most often it arises on the extremities and frequently within an existing scar. Its presence must be considered when a firm nodule develops in a scar of long standing. Typically there is very slow but progressive invasion of adjacent tissues, with a very low incidence of metastasis which occurs to regional lymph nodes late in the course. At the other extreme of the malignancy spectrum is the angiosarcoma, which metastasizes very early, with a correspondingly poor prognosis. Lying between these two extremes are the myxosarcomas and the hemangiopericytomas, which, like the others, are very rare.

Treatment of sarcomas of the skin of the hand varies with the anticipated degree of malignancy. Fibrosarcomas require a relatively limited excision, with about 1 cm. of skin margins (Fig. 62–5) while the more malignant sarcomas necessitate much greater margins of excision which often can be achieved only by partial or total amputation. With lymphadenopathy, dissection of the regional lymph nodes should always be done. It is generally indicated with the more malignant sarcomas, even in the absence of clinical evidence of their involvement.

Kaposi's Sarcoma

Frequently the first evidence of Kaposi's sarcoma is found on the hands, usually manifested as elevated purple plaques (Fig. 62–6). Histologic diagnosis of the disorder is often very difficult and can be made only by correlation with clinical information. This peculiar disorder clinically resembles a dermatosis more than a serious sarcoma, although it usually progresses over a long period to a fatal termination. Its eventual generalized involvement of internal organs appears to be due to multicentric origin of tumor rather than to metastatic spread. Occasional spontaneous regressions of the tumor have been reported, as well as cures by excision of the primary lesion. Solitary lesions are best treated by excision, while radiotherapy is used for generalized disease.

Melanoma

Melanomas are common, constituting about 15 percent of skin cancers. Of these about 7 percent occur in the hand, one-third of which will be subungual in location.

As in other areas of the body, this

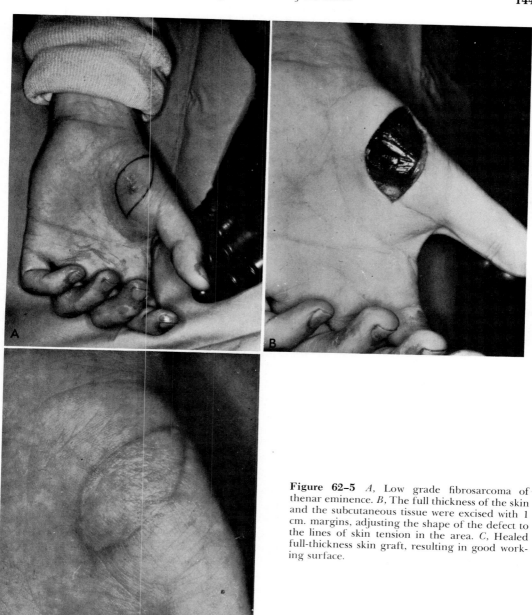

Figure 62–5 *A,* Low grade fibrosarcoma of thenar eminence. *B,* The full thickness of the skin and the subcutaneous tissue were excised with 1 cm. margins, adjusting the shape of the defect to the lines of skin tension in the area. *C,* Healed full-thickness skin graft, resulting in good working surface.

treacherous lesion must be suspect with any pigmented skin lesion showing changes of color, size, or crusting, especially with a friable lesion which is prone to bleeding with trivial trauma. Recurrent bleeding is frequently the complaint which first brings the patient to the physician (Fig. 62–7).

The key to diagnosis is a high index of suspicion with confirmation depending on biopsy of the lesion. Excisional biopsy is the technique of choice, but in the hand

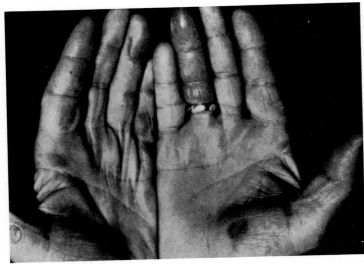

Figure 62–6 Kaposi's sarcoma, which most often appears first on the hands.

possible damage to functionally important structures frequently imposes limits on this technique. In such cases incisional biopsy is justified. If melanoma is clinically suspected, a single negative biopsy should not be considered conclusive. Under such circumstances one is obligated not only to keep the lesion under surveillance but also to repeat the biopsy, taking specimens from several areas of the lesion.

The treatment of melanoma is surgical. Of primary consideration in formulating a plan of treatment is the depth of the lesion—the greater the depth, the poorer the prognosis. Therefore, the greater the depth of the lesion, the more radical the resection required. Removal of very wide margins of apparently normal tissue around the lesion is indicated for all melanomas because of the high incidence of local recurrence. Pack et al. (1945) reported an incidence of local recurrence of the tumor of 64 percent, which is in keeping with Adair's earlier report of 61 percent (Adair, 1936). Local recurrences tend to be in the direction of the regional lymph nodes, with the vast majority occurring within 10 cm. of the site of the original lesions (Petersen et al., 1962). This implies that surgical margins should be at least 10 cm. on the side of regional lymph nodes and 5 cm. on all other sides, but obviously this cannot always be achieved in the hand without its total amputation. Since a high proportion of melanomas metastasize by

the bloodstream, which is not controlled by wide margins of excision, one is not always justified in performing the total amputations necessary to achieve the ideal margins of excision. Usually the involved digit is ablated by a total amputation which causes minimal derangement of the hand and still approaches the ideal surgical margins (Fig. 62–7). Such resection should be in conjunction with exenteration of the axillary lymph nodes, even if there is no clinical lymphadenopathy.

PRINCIPLES OF TREATMENT

Surgical excision of malignant and premalignant skin tumors of the hand is the treatment of choice in the vast majority of cases. Very small lesions may be satisfactorily eradicated by any means of destruction, such as curettage and chemical or electrosurgery. Radiation has been too frequently employed and probably should be reserved for radiosensitive sarcomas. One of the problems of treating tumors of the hand is the very limited amount of tissue that can be extirpated without resulting in some functional impairment. Surgical removal of the tumor, always performed in a bloodless field maintained by a pneumatic tourniquet, permits a precision in control of the margins of resection that is unobtainable by any other technique. This precise control is essential in order to assure that structures whose

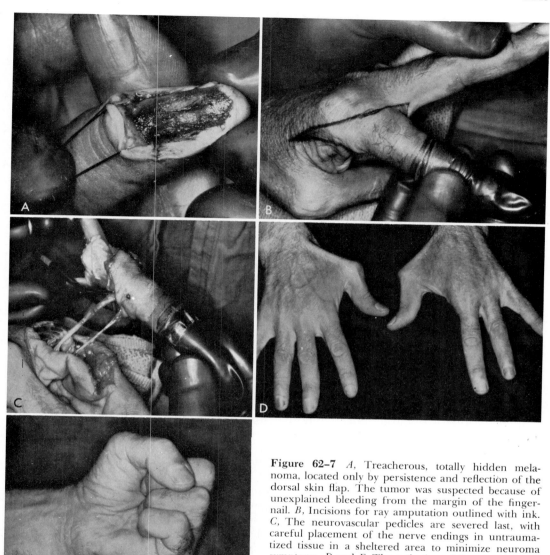

Figure 62–7 *A*, Treacherous, totally hidden melanoma, located only by persistence and reflection of the dorsal skin flap. The tumor was suspected because of unexplained bleeding from the margin of the fingernail. *B*, Incisions for ray amputation outlined with ink. *C*, The neurovascular pedicles are severed last, with careful placement of the nerve endings in untraumatized tissue in a sheltered area to minimize neuroma symptoms. *D* and *E*, The esthetic and functional result of the ray amputation.

preservation has been elected will not be inadvertently damaged. It also provides the pathologist with an unmutilated specimen so that he may study fully the extension of the neoplasm and the adequacy of the excision. Surgical excision usually results in a wound which may be promptly closed to minimize inflammatory reaction; this is a prime factor in preventing stiffness of adjacent small joints.

Anesthesia for Skin Lesions of the Hand

Excisions are done with local, regional, or general anesthesia. General anesthesia is required for children and when multiple operative sites are to be used, as in taking a large skin graft for repair of a defect on the hand. The excellent local anesthetic agents currently available with high potency and rate of diffusion have displaced "brandy and the silver bullet." There is little place for local infiltration anesthesia, its use being only for biopsy or excision of very small lesions. When infiltration anesthesia is administered, it must be deposited in the dermis where the nerve endings are located if anesthesia is to be consistently complete. Its placement in the subcutaneous tissues usually results in incomplete loss of sensibility in the area. With its placement in the dermis remarkably little anesthetic is required, especially if a small syringe and No. 30 gauge needle is employed. The volume of anesthetic used is too often determined by the size of the needle and syringe rather than by the task presented.

The hand lends itself admirably to regional block anesthesia. When this is chosen, preoperative sedation must be mild and without narcotics, as the patient's full cooperation in eliciting paresthesias is necessary. Once the nerve block has been completed, more sedation is given, usually intravenously, to permit full relaxation and sleep if the patient so desires. In the absence of pain, surprisingly little medication is required, but in almost every case blood gas determinations show a slight hypoxia. In the patient in whom this is of concern, it is readily corrected by the intranasal catheter administration of oxygen at a flow of 6 liters per minute, as demonstrated by Abadir (1970). Hypoxia is notably due to the sedation, but often to a greater extent it is due to oral secretions or positioning of the head in flexion, which narrows the airway across the pharynx. Since most of the skin cancer patients are of the older age group, there should be an awareness of the potential, subclinical hypoxia.

Digital nerve or ring blocks of fingers are not done, as the risk of gangrene, even using anesthetics free of epinephrine, is too high. Digital nerve blocks in the palm are safe. Median and ulnar nerve blocks at the wrist are safe, simple, and reliable in giving excellent anesthesia to the palmar surface of the hand. Ulnar nerve blocks at the elbow should never be done, as the risk of neuritis is unacceptably high. Anesthesia of the dorsal skin results from blocking the superficial branches of the radial and ulnar nerves, but technically this is difficult, as their positions are variable and often they have divided into multiple branches. For dorsal skin lesions brachial plexus blocks are preferred, either by the supraclavicular route or by the safer axillary route. The placement of a fine catheter in the axillary sheath permits reliable, prolonged, excellent anesthesia with minimal complications (Abadir, 1970).

The intravenous regional anesthesia technique is unsatisfactory. There is a constant oozing of solution into the wound, impeding critical dissection; anesthesia is gone when the tourniquet is released for hemostasis, and the distal tourniquet is too low on the arm.

Use of a Tourniquet

A tourniquet to maintain a bloodless field is essential for all but the simplest of surgical procedures on the hand. The pneumatic type with precisely controlled pressure delivered to a wide cuff for even distribution is safe and in standard use today. For adults a pressure of 250 to 300 mm. Hg is selected. The cuff must be as proximal on the arm as possible in an effort to occlude all major nutrient arteries to the humeral canal to assure a bloodless field. For tumor surgery the arm is not exsanguinated by compression with a rubber bandage but only by elevation for a few minutes before inflation of the pneumatic tourniquet. There will be surprisingly little blood remaining in the hand if this method is used.

If blood is first drained from the arm, the tourniquet still may be used for 30 to 50 minutes with local infiltration or distal regional nerve blocks without pain. Otherwise most patients find the inflated tourniquet to be intolerable after about 10 minutes.

Placement of Incisions

Incisions in the hand must be carefully planned if troublesome contractures are to be avoided. All incisions result in a scar. All scars contract. There is no essential difference between the behavior of scars on the volar surface of the hand and that of scars on the dorsal surface. The well-known greater latitude in the placement of dorsal incisions is due to the mobility of the dorsal skin, permitting shifting to compensate for the shortening of contracture. In contrast, the skin of the volar surfaces is firmly fixed to the skeleton by fibrous septa. This is essential for a working surface but results in a strict limitation of the degree of contracture tolerated without functional restriction.

The common denominator of satisfactory incisions is that they are along lines which undergo no change in length with any motion of which the part is capable. For example, the mid-axial incision so frequently recommended for opening a finger lies precisely midway between flexion and extension. An incision along this line results in a scar which contracts the same as any other scar but limits neither flexion nor extension. Skin creases are the hinges of the skin. They lie at right angles to the underlying joints. Incisions in them or parallel to them undergo no change in length with motion of the joint, and contracture of the resulting scar is no problem. When it is necessary to cross a skin crease, this should be done as obliquely as possible. In practice, one outlines incisions precisely with pen and dye. Then the parts are passively moved to confirm that the lines are in neutral zones undergoing no change of length with these motions.

The scar at the junction between a flap or graft and the normal skin behaves in the same way the scar of the incision does. Therefore, the margins of the defect of tumor incision must be planned in accordance with the same principles that govern the placement of elective incisions.

Closure of Wounds of Excision

Direct Closure. Defects resulting from excision of small lesions on the dorsum of the hand may be closed by direct approximation of the skin margins because of the mobility of the skin of this area. Usually the defect is made elliptical in shape to minimize puckering of the tissues. In areas where the lines of skin tension are not clearly defined, one may initially make a circular excision. The resulting defect will distort into an oval shape, indicating the skin tension in the area. It is then converted into an ellipse along these lines for closure. In practice, rarely can the wound of tumor excision from the volar surfaces be directly closed. Wounds of the volar surface require vertical mattress sutures for closure to prevent inversion of the margins when the hand is cupped in a functional position.

Grafts vs. Flaps. Soft tissue defects which cannot be satisfactorily closed by direct approximation of the wound margins are closed by grafts or flaps. A graft is tissue that is totally severed from the donor site and placed in the recipient site. Its survival is dependent on the rapid ingrowth of vessels from the recipient bed into it. A flap is tissue that remains attached either temporarily or permanently to the donor site by a pedicle through which its blood supply is maintained. In general, the simplest method of repair giving a good result is the best. Usually this is a graft, and it is preferred, especially in cancer surgery, when the thick flap might conceal an otherwise detectable early tumor recurrence.

The general indications for a flap are:

1. When the recipient wound surface is unfavorable for the rapid vascularization of a graft required for its survival.

2. When subcutaneous tissues are needed along with skin for planned reconstruction.

3. When certain vital structures will be better preserved by coverage with the subcutaneous tissues

The second indication for a flap is not frequently applicable in cancer surgery, especially when one is dealing with tissues with a high incidence of local recurrence. In these cases reconstruction usually is deferred until a reasonable period of observation for tumor recurrence has passed.

Skin Grafts. The use of full-thickness skin grafts is limited to the repair of small wounds in the working surfaces. Successful transplantation requires optimal conditions in the recipient site and the utmost attention to all technical details. As with other grafts, care with the dressing is paramount. There must be absolute immobilization to prevent sheering action at the interface between graft and recipient bed and to avoid rupture of the delicate capillary buds growing into the graft.

Full-thickness grafts up to 1 cm. in width may be taken from the volar wrist crease without disfigurement or functional impairment. Suture marks are avoided by wound closure with a continuous intradermal monofilament suture. The antecubital fossa is not an acceptable graft donor site. Larger full-thickness grafts are best taken from the hairless skin of the inguinal fold. The secondary disfigurement is minimal, as is the mobility following closure of the wound with a continuous intradermal suture.

The graft is cut to fit the defect exactly. Fixation is secured with fine sutures following complete hemostasis, which is critical. The graft is further fixed by a precisely fitting small dressing, which is taped in place. A bolus dressing is never used, as it puts tension on the sutures. Immobilization is completed by application of a padded outer dressing covered with a light plaster shell. The wrist joint must be included for adequate immobilization. Unless there are specific indications for inspection of the graft, the dressings are not disturbed for five to eight days. Prior to this, evaluation of the progress of vascularization of full-thickness grafts is very difficult.

Complications at the graft's donor sites, including hypertrophy of the resulting scars, increase proportionally with the depth. Therefore, any graft donor site deeper than 0.016 inch should be immediately covered with a graft of 0.008 or 0.010 inch. Both wounds usually heal uneventfully in a period of 10 to 12 days. The noticeable reduction of the patient's discomfort with this technique is a bonus. The donor site of choice for large split-thickness skin grafts to be used in the hand is high on the contralateral buttock, directly below the belt line. This is an area of relatively hairless skin which matches the hand well. The disfigurement is greatly reduced, and the minimal motion of the area favors rapid and kind healing. Often the thigh is selected as a convenience to the surgeon. The

wounds of very thin grafts heal well, but usually the area is hairy and subjected to more motion, and scar hypertrophy is more common.

The key to trouble-free donor sites lies in drying them rapidly. The wound is covered with fine-mesh gauze, beneath which epithelialization occurs. After 24 hours the outer dressings are removed down to the level of the Xeroform, and an electric fan is directed on the wound until drying is complete. Once this is accomplished, the wound is almost pain-free, and complications are exceedingly rare. When large defects are to be grafted, the delayed technique is indicated. The wound of excision is protected with a sterile dressing for 24 to 72 hours, at which time it is closed by application of the graft. The graft may be cut at the time of tumor excision to avoid a second anesthesia. Storage of the graft may be in a refrigerator at 4° C., or it may be reapplied to the graft donor site (Shepard, 1972). The graft is fixed to the recipient wound with strips of tape and immobilized with a dressing.

Amputations

In certain situations the necessary treatment of the tumor can be achieved only by amputation of the part involved. This involves two fundamental considerations: the resulting physical impairment and the psychologic impact of the loss. Too often concern over the physical handicap is unrealistic and disproportionate. Even following a total arm amputation, one can accomplish about 90 percent of the activities necessary for daily living without difficulty with the other normal hand. For the younger patient vocational re-training appropriate to his abilities is readily available, and with lesser amputations the problems are proportionately diminished. Loss of a single digit, with the exception of the thumb, results in almost no handicap. In the latter case thumb reconstruction can be offered (Fig. 62–8). In consideration of the physical impairment, persistent pain is of paramount concern. This is much more of a problem in crushing injuries than in elective amputations.

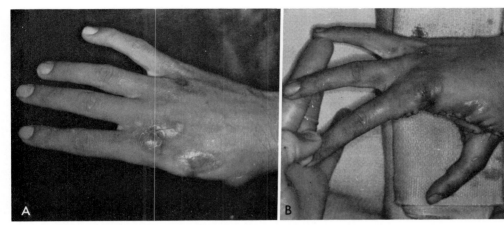

Figure 62–8 Amputation of the thumb imposes a severe handicap, which can be significantly reduced by thumb reconstruction (*A*). *B*, The index finger is isolated on its neurovascular systems and transferred to the base of the first metacarpal. This preserves normal sensibility and results in a good functional and esthetic restoration.

Its presence is usually associated with neuromas of the severed nerves being entrapped in cicatrix or poor soft tissue coverage. Symptomatic neuromas are uncommon if the nerves are severed with a sharp knife and their endings are permitted to retract or are purposely placed in untraumatized soft tissues (Fig. 62–7C). Treatment of the severed nerves with ligation, cauterization, or any of the many other treatment modalities recommended for painful neuromas has no place. The patient should be warned that he must expect to experience a "normal phantom," that is, the persistent sensation of presence of the part but without pain.

Special attention should be given to the psychologic impact of amputation, for it is ever present. Yet the patient and the surgeon often find it awkward to approach the problem. Aside from the anxieties derived from realization of the presence of a cancer, the patient may be overwhelmed by unrealistic views of the socioeconomic consequences of the amputation. It is the surgeon's responsibility to recognize that these ideas always exist to some extent and to deal with them.

The esthetic results of the amputation are psychologically important, a conspicuous loss being a social handicap to all except the unusually mature personality. Conspicuousness of the amputation depends to some extent upon the resulting form, scars, and so forth, but in reality it depends to a much greater extent on the manner in which the part is used in activities. In this lies the difference between the artist's most beautifully executed cosmetic hand prosthesis and a good reconstruction, even though alterations in form and numbers may have been necessary.

REFERENCES

Abadir, A.: Anesthesia for hand surgery. Orthop. Clin. North Am., 1:205, 1970.

Adair, F. E.: Treatment of melanoma; report of 400 cases. Surg. Gynecol. Obstet., 62:406, 1936.

Blum, H. F.: Photodynamic Action and Diseases Caused by Light. New York, Reinhold Publishing Corporation, 1941.

Broders, A. C.: The microscopic grading of cancer treatment. *In* Pack, G., and Ariel, I. (Eds.): Cancer and Allied Diseases. New York, Paul B. Hoeber, Inc., 1959.

Conway, H., Norman, E. H., and Tulenko, J. F.: Surgery of Tumors of the Skin. Ed. 2. Springfield, Ill., Charles C Thomas, Publisher, 1966, pp. 250–259.

Cooley, S. G. E.: Tumors of the hand and forearm. In Converse, J. M. (Ed.): Reconstructive Plastic Surgery. Vol. IV. Philadelphia, W. B. Saunders Company, 1964, p. 1740.

Currie, A. H.: The role of arsenic in carcinogenesis. Br. Med. Bull., 4:402, 1947.

Graham, J. H., and Helwig, E. B.: Bowen's disease and its relation to systemic cancer. Arch. Dermatol., 80:133, 1959.

Graham, J. H., and Helwig, E. B.: Bowen's disease and its relationship to systemic cancer. Arch. Dermatol., 33:76, 1961.

Graham, J. H., and Helwig, E. B.: Cutaneous precancerous conditions in man. Conference of Cutaneous Cancer. Natl. Cancer Inst. Monogr., 10:323, 1963.

Graham, J. H., Mazzanti, G. R., and Helwig, E. B.: Chemistry of Bowen's disease: Relationship to arsenic J. Invest. Dermatol., 37:317, 1961.

Hutchinson, J.: Arsenic cancer. Br. Med. J., 2:1280, 1888.

Lattes, R., and Kessler, R. W.: Metastasizing basal cell epithelioma of the skin; report of 2 cases. Cancer, 4:866, 1951.

Lawrence, E. A., Dickey, J. W., and Vellios, F.: Malignant tumors of the soft tissues of the extremities. Arch. Surg., 67:392, 1953.

Lund, H. Z.: Tumors of the Skin. Ed. 1. Washington, D.C., Armed Forces Institute of Pathology, 1957.

Pack, G. T., Sharnagel, I. M., and Morfit, M.: Principle of excision and dissection in continuity for primary and metastatic melanoma of skin. Surgery, 17:849, 1945.

Pack, G. T., Perzik, S. L., and Sharnagel, I. M.: Treatment of malignant melanoma, report of 862 cases. Calif. Med., 66:283, 1947.

Petersen, N. C., Bodenham, D. C., and Lloyd, D. C.: Malignant melanomas of the skin. Br. J. Plast. Surg. , 15:49, 1962.

Shepard, G. H.: The storage of split-skin grafts on their donor sites. Plast. Reconstr. Surg., 49:115, 1972.

63

Cancer of the Nipple

Leopold G. Koss, M.D.,
and Guy F. Robbins, M.D.

ANATOMIC AND HISTOLOGIC CONSIDERATIONS

The nipple is a pigmented papillary protuberance on the anterior surface of the skin of the breast wherein converge the 12 to 20 principal breast ducts. The nipple is surrounded by an approximately round area of pigmented skin—the areola. The areola contains a number of modified apocrine glands of Montgomery and numerous sweat and sebaceous glands. For the purposes of this discussion, the entire area of the nipple and the areola will be considered as a single entity.

The dermis of the areola and the nipple is provided with a layer of smooth muscle, accounting for the contractility of this area.

The epidermis presents several features of note: the number of the epithelial cell layers is somewhat greater than that of the surrounding skin, although the general make-up is similar. The rete pegs are often longer. The deep layers of the epidermis contain melanin pigment. The epithelium frequently contains a variable number of cells with clear cytoplasm occurring singly and in small clusters (Fig. 63–1). Toker (1970) observed the clear cells in 12 percent of 190 nipples in autopsy material in the absence of breast cancer. The clear cells may be observed in all layers of the epithelium; they are ovoid or spherical in shape and have a dark nucleus of a size comparable to that of the surrounding epithelial cells. This latter point is of considerable importance in the differential diagnosis of Paget's disease. The identity of the clear cells is not known at the time of this writing (1972). They resemble Langerhans' cells or melanophores found elsewhere in the epidermis (Zelickson, 1963).

PAGET'S DISEASE OF THE NIPPLE

In 1874 Sir James Paget described a "disease of the mammary areola preceding cancer of the breast." Paget described 15 cases of the disease and noted that "... in every case which I have been able to watch, cancer of the mammary gland has followed within at the most two years and usually within one year." The cancer was located "in the substance of the mam-

1449

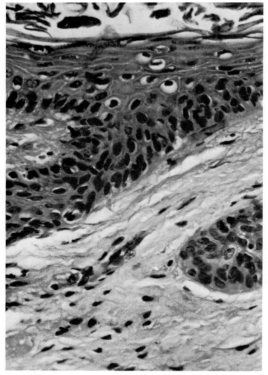

Figure 63–1   Clear cells in nipple epithelium. ×350.

mary gland, beneath or not far from the diseased skin and always with a clear interval of apparently healthy tissue." Paget noted further that there was nothing peculiar about the breast cancer itself.

Graham (1939) pointed out that the first case of Paget's disease in the male was recorded by John of Ardenne in the first part of the 14th century. Treves (1954) and Cheatle and Cutler (1931) quoted Velpeau, who described the lesion of the female nipple in 1841.

Clinical Presentation

The disease occurs primarily in middle-aged women. The youngest patient observed at the Memorial Hospital for Cancer in New York was 28 years of age, the oldest 82. The average age for 214 patients was 54 years (Ashikari et al., 1970).

The lesion, affecting as a rule a single nipple, presents as a sharply demarcated area of redness involving a part or all of the nipple and the areola (Fig. 63–2). In a fully developed form the lesion is "intensely red . . . finely granular as if nearly the whole thickness of the epidermis were removed, like a surface of very acute diffuse eczema," and has a "clear, yellowish, viscid exudation. In some of the cases, the eruption presented the character of an ordinary chronic eczema . . . or psoriasis. [In such cases] I have seen the eruption spreading far beyond the areola in widening circles, or, with scattered blotches of redness, covering nearly the whole breast." Little can be added to the masterful description of Sir James Paget except that in some instances the lesion may be indurated. Bloody nipple discharge may occur. In spite of an enormous literature on the topic of Paget's disease, little is known about the clinical presentation of the very early stages, perhaps because biopsies of the nipple are rarely taken when only slight changes occur. However, incidental histologic findings of Paget's disease with other forms of breast cancer suggest that the disease need not be associated with any visible clinical changes. This was noted in about 10 percent of all cases of Paget's disease observed at the Memorial Hospital (Ashikari et al., 1970) and in the Philadelphia study (Maier et al., 1969).

Clinically palpable masses within the underlying breast are observed in about

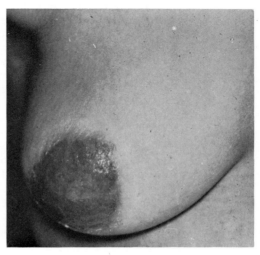

Figure 63–2   Paget's disease.

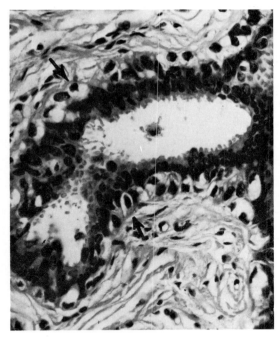

Figure 63–9 Breast duct showing permeation of periductal lymphatics with cancer cells (arrows). The lumen is clear of cancer. This duct was found midway between the nipple shown in Figure 63–6 and the duct carcinoma located beneath. ×350.

spite of clear-cut clinical evidence of a major, life-threatening disorder, significant delays in treatment were encountered. The delays in treatment were from 6 to 11 months in the Memorial Hospital group (Ashikari et al., 1970) and 13 months in the Philadelphia experience (Maier et al., 1969).

The generally recommended treatment is radical mastectomy with axillary lymph node dissection, even in the absence of a palpable mass; lymph node metastases were observed in 13 percent of such patients in the Memorial Hospital experience (Fig. 63–10).

Prognosis

The overall five-year survival of patients with Paget's disease of the breast was 52 percent in the Philadelphia experience (Maier et al., 1969). An overall survival of 60 percent at 10 years was recorded at the Memorial Hospital. Both reports are in agreement that the presence of a palpable mass prior to surgery

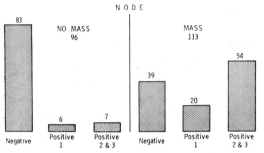

Figure 63–10 The relationship of clinical findings (palpable breast mass) to lymph node metastases in 209 cases of Paget's disease of the nipple. Included in the 83 cases with "no mass—negative nodes" are 6 cases in which breast carcinoma was not demonstrated. "Positive 1, 2 and 3 ' refers to metastatic carcinoma in lymph nodes at the 3 axillary levels; level 1 is the most proximal and level 3 the most distal to the breast (see text). (*From* Ashikari et al.: Cancer, 26:680, 1970.)

has an unfavorable prognostic significance: the 5-year survival of this group of patients at the Memorial Hospital was 42.5 percent and, at 10 years, 37.9 percent (Fig. 63–11).

Lymph node metastases also have an ominous prognostic significance, although there is a marked difference according to the nodes involved: metastases to nodes proximal to the breast (level I) have less impact on survival than those to nodes in the mid-axilla (level II) or in the apex of the axilla (level III) (Fig. 63–11).

The best therapeutic results were observed in patients without palpable masses whose cancer on histologic examination was still confined to the ducts or lobules.

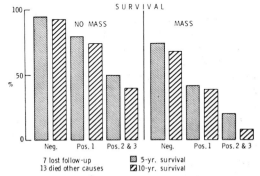

Figure 63–11 The relationship of lymph node metastases and palpable breast mass to survival in 189 cases of Paget's disease of the breast. It may be noted that in the absence of a palpable breast mass and absence of lymph node metastases the 5- and 10-year survival is close to 100 percent. (*From* Ashikari et al.: Cancer, 26:680, 1970.)

Of the 63 patients in this category (including six with no breast cancer demonstrated) seen at Memorial Hospital, all survived five years without evidence of recurrent disease. The Philadelphia study (Maier et al., 1969) suggested that the overall prognosis was better in the postmenopausal than in the premenopausal patient.

These results clearly suggest that early and aggressive treatment of Paget's disease is fully warranted.

Paget's Disease in the Male

There are sporadic reports of Paget's disease in the male breast, always accompanied by infiltrating breast cancer. A summary of the historical data may be found in the excellent paper by Treves (1954), who reported two cases. Sarason and Prior (1952) recorded five cases, and Adam et al. (1956) one case. Undoubtedly there are other case reports scattered throughout the literature. The extreme rarity of the disorder is well illustrated by the fact that there was only one male to 213 females with Paget's disease observed at the Memorial Hospital from 1950 through 1968.

The clinical presentation and treatment are those of breast cancer.

Differential Diagnosis of Paget's Disease

Breast Cancer Invading the Nipple. Breast cancer may invade the nipple and cause ulceration without evidence of Paget's disease. This may also occur in the presence of so-called inflammatory carcinoma with extensive involvement of superficial lymphatics by cancer.

Florid Papillomas (Adenomas) of the Subareolar Ducts. This is a distinct benign lesion of the terminal ducts of the breast, first clearly identified by Jones (1955), which may clinically imitate Paget's disease. The lesion is usually relatively voluminous, often measuring more than 1 cm. in diameter, and is located in the ducts immediately beneath the nipple (Fig. 63–12). Because of pressure on the

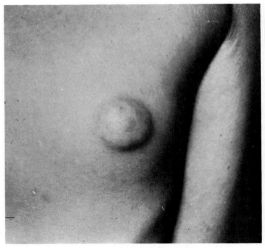

Figure 63–12   Intraductal papilloma. (See also Color Plate XI-B.)

nipple, ulceration, erosion, fissurization, or scaling is commonly observed, and in the majority of cases the clinical diagnosis of Paget's disease is made. The disease is usually unilateral and occurs most often in the 30 to 50 year old age group. This clinical presentation, coupled with a palpable mass, has led to numerous unnecessary mastectomies.

The histologic presentation may also be misleading to an uninitiated observer: the lesion is characterized by a florid growth of ductlike structures, with formation of numerous papillary and solid areas of cell proliferation. On close inspection the nuclei are uniform, and the distinction between myoepithelial and duct cells is readily made. As is often the case in duct papillomatosis, hyaline connective tissue may separate the proliferating ducts, and this appearance may mimic duct carcinoma.

The nipple shows no lesions except for those due to pressure and surface necrosis. Paget's cells are absent.

By unanimous consent (Jones, 1955; Handley and Thackeray, 1962; Taylor and Robertson, 1965), florid duct papillomatosis is benign and should be handled conservatively. However, Handley and Thackeray (1962) observed a carcinoma elsewhere in the breast with florid papillomatosis. McDivitt et al. (1967) recorded three cases of cancer of the homolateral breast, one in-continuity with florid duct papillomatosis. A similar case was recently observed by one of us (LGK): a classic infiltrating duct carcinoma was observed incontinuity with an equally classic florid papilloma of a nipple duct.*

It is evident, therefore, that the presence of florid duct papillomatosis should not preclude a careful histologic examination of the entire specimen.

Malignant Melanoma of the Nipple. Three such lesions were studied: two of them were advanced infiltrating melanomas with abundant pigment production. The third lesion was a melanoma of the superficially spreading variety (Mihm et

al., 1971) which, in its noninvasive portion, closely resembled Paget's disease (Figs. 63–13 and 63–14). Yet subtle differences could be observed: the melanoma cells displayed a greater variability in size than did Paget's cells, and their cytoplasm was opaque rather than clear (compare Figs. 63–4 and 63–6 with Fig. 63–14).

Nests of melanoma cells displayed central necrosis. Not shown in the photographs was abundant pigment present in the invasive portion of the tumor.

Melanomas do not display any of the histochemical reactions characterizing Paget's disease, described above.

Other Tumors Involving the Nipple. Common benign and malignant tumors of the skin may be occasionally observed in the nipple. Thus benign nevi (Fig. 63–15),

*This and two additional such cases were published by Bhagavan, B. S., Patchefsky, A., and Koss, L. G.: Hum. Pathol., 4:289, 1973.

Fig. 63–13

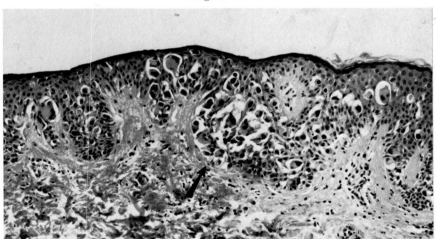

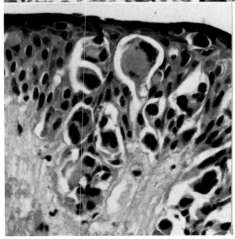

Figure 63–13 Malignant melanoma of nipple. Note the nest of loosely arranged melanoma cells (arrow). ×150.

Figure 63–14 Malignant melanoma of nipple. A higher power view of a segment of the lesion shown in Figure 63–13. There is a general and superficial similarity in the distribution of melanoma cells and Paget's cells within the epidermis (see Fig. 63–4). Yet the melanoma shows a much greater variability in cell sizes and a greater tendency to formation of nests of cells. At times the differential diagnosis may prove very difficult. ×350.

Fig. 63–14

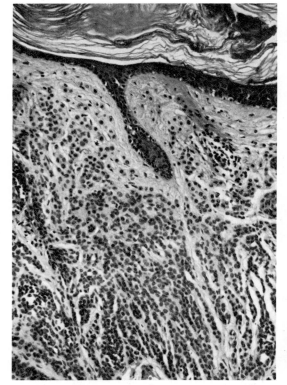

Figure 63–15   Benign nevus of nipple. ×*150.*

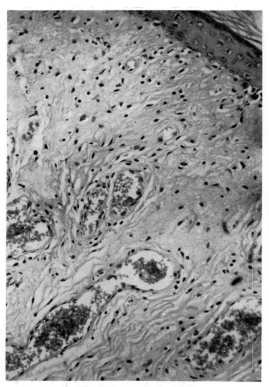

Figure 63–16   Fibroangioma of nipple. ×*150.*

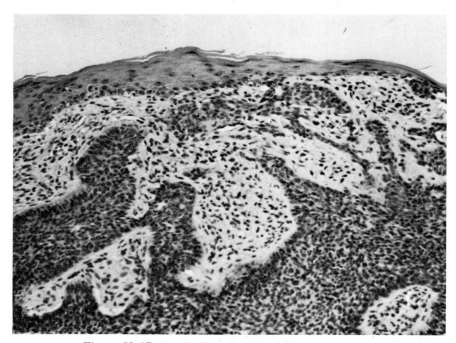

Figure 63–17   Basal cell carcinoma involving nipple. ×*150.*

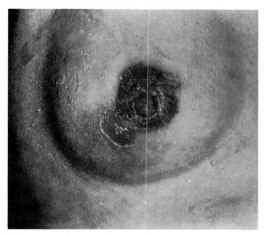

Figure 63–18 Eczema.
(See also Color Plate XI-C.)

fibroangiomas (Fig. 63–16), and other benign neoplasms may occur.

Basal cell carcinomas (Fig. 63–17) and squamous cell carcinomas have been recorded. Cheatle and Cutler (1931) recorded a case of sweat gland carcinoma; however, the histologic differentiation of this lesion from breast cancer was not possible. The same reservation may be expressed about some of the primary carcinomas of the nipple described by Congdon and Dockerty (1956).

Inflammatory Lesions. Eczematoid

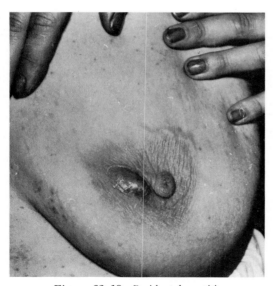

Figure 63–19 Periductal mastitis.
(See also Color Plate XI-D.)

dermatitis (Fig. 63–18), contact dermatitis, and psoriasis may affect the skin of the nipple and imitate Paget's disease. In most instances the disease is bilateral. Occasionally a periductal abscess may affect the nipple (Fig. 63–19). In case of doubt a biopsy is strongly indicated to rule out Paget's disease.

REFERENCES

Adam, W., Nikolowski, W., and Wiehl, R.: Uber Ca. mammae virile spontaneum. Arch. Klin. Exp. Dermatol., 203:1, 1956.

Arud, W.: Über die Pagetsche Erkrankung der Brustwarze. Virchows Arch., 261:700, 1926.

Ashikari, R., Park, K., Huvos, A. G., and Urban, J. A : Paget's disease of the breast. Cancer, 26:680, 1970

Cheatle, G. L., and Cutler, M.: Tumours of the Breast. London, Arnold, 1931.

Congdon, G. H., and Dockerty, M. B : Malignant lesions of the nipple exclusive of Paget's disease. Surg Gynecol. Obstet., 103:185, 1956.

Graham, H. (pseudonym for Flack, I. H.): The Story of Surgery. New York, Doubleday, Doran & Company, Inc., 1939.

Handley, R. S., and Thackeray, A C.: Adenoma of nipple. Br. J. Cancer, 16:187, 1962.

Helwig E. B., and Graham, J. H.: Anogenital extramammary Paget's disease; a clinicopathological review. Cancer, 16:387, 1963

Jones, D. B : Florid papillomatosis of the nipple. Cancer, 8:315, 1955.

Koss, L G., and Brockunier, A., Jr.: Ultrastructural aspects of Paget's disease of the vulva. Arch. Pathol., 87:592, 1969.

Koss, L G., Ladinsky, S , and Brockunier, A , Jr.: Paget's disease of the vulva. Report of 10 cases. Obstet. Gynecol., 31:513 1968.

Maier, W. P., Rosemond, G. P., Harasym, E. L., Al-Saleem, T. I., Tassoni E. M., and Schor, S. S : Paget's disease in the female breast. Surg. Gynecol. Obstet., 128:1253, 1969.

McDivitt, R. W., Stewart, F. W., and Berg, J. W.: Tumors of the breast. Atlas of Tumor Pathology, Series 2 Fascicle 2. Washington, D.C., Armed Forces Institute of Pathology, 1967.

Mihm, M. C., Clark, W. H., and From, L.: The clinical diagnosis, classification and histogenetic concepts of the early stages of cutaneous malignant melanomas. New Engl. J. Med., 284:1078, 1971.

Montgomery, H.: Dermatopathology. New York, Harper & Row, 1967.

Paget, J.: On disease and mammary areola preceding cancer of the mammary gland. St. Bart. Hosp. Rep., 10:87, 1874.

Sagebiel, R. W.: Ultrastructural observations on epidermal cells in Paget's disease of the breast. Am. J. Pathol., 57:49, 1969.

Sarason, E. L., and Prior, J. T.: Paget's disease of the male breast. Ann. Surg., 135:253, 1952.

Taylor, H. B , and Robertson, A. G.: Adenoma of the nipple. Cancer, 18:995, 1965.

Toker, C.: Some observations on Paget's disease of the nipple. Cancer, 14:653, 1961.

Toker, C.: Further observations of Paget's disease of the nipple. J. Natl. Cancer Inst., 38:79, 1967.

Toker, C.: Clear cells of the nipple epidermis. Cancer, 25:601, 1970.

Treves, N.: Paget's disease of the male mamma. Cancer, 7:325, 1954.

Velpeau, A.A.L.M.: Leçons orales de clinique chirurg-icale faites à l'Hôpital de la Charité recueillies et publiées par Gustave Jeanselme. Vol. 2. Paris, Germain-Baillier, 1841.

Winkelman, R. K : Histochemistry of the skin. *In* Montgomery, H.: Dermatopathology. New York, Harper & Row, 1967.

Yates, D. R., and Koss, L G.: Paget's disease of the esophageal epithelium: Report of first case. Arch. Pathol., 86:447, 1968.

Zelickson, A. S.: The Langerhans cell. J. Invest. Dermatol., 44:201, 1963.

64

Carcinoma of the Vulva
The Radical Surgical Approach

E. Mark Beckman, M.D., F.A.C.O.G.

This chapter is concerned with the technique of radical vulvectomy in the treatment of squamous cell carcinoma of the vulva. The discussion will also center on other modes of therapy and will attempt to show why we feel that the radical surgical approach is, undoubtedly, the best method of treatment.

Diagnostic methods will not be discussed, as they have been presented in another chapter in this text. As an introduction to this topic, it should be noted that squamous cell carcinoma is, by far, the most common malignancy of the vulva, accounting for approximately 90 percent of all cases. The disease itself is rare, with an incidence of less than 1 percent of all cancers and approximately 4 percent of all gynecologic cancers. Other malignant tumors of the vulva include basal cell carcinoma, carcinoma of the Bartholin's gland, sarcomas, and melanomas.

The symptoms encountered most frequently are pruritis or a lump or both. Other presenting symptoms are ulceration and bleeding. One of the more discouraging factors in an approach to this disease is the delay between onset of symptoms and definitive diagnosis. In most series, the patient had had symptoms varying in duration from six months to 3½ years, with a 12-month delay in seeking treatment extremely common.

Squamous cell carcinoma of the vulva is a disease of the aged. Its incidence has been shown to increase as the age of the population increases. Green et al. (1958), in an analysis of 238 cases, found that 70 percent of patients were over 60 and 36 percent over 70, with an average age of approximately 62. We have had similar experience, and this will be presented later in this article.

METHODS OF TREATMENT OF CARCINOMA OF THE VULVA

Prior to 1940, with few exceptions, there was no definite approach to therapy. In the 1930's, the most popular modes of therapy were either local excision, radiotherapy, or electrocoagulation (Berven, 1949). All these methods had very poor results. Way (1951) reported that 87 patients treated between the years of 1908

1461

and 1943 with simple vulvectomy showed only a 24 percent five-year survival rate. Of 32 patients treated prior to 1938 reported by McKelvy (1955), the survival rate was approximately 19 percent.

In earlier days, radiation therapy was a prime mode of treatment because of the high mortality in operative cases. The usual mode of treatment was the use of radium needles, giving approximately 5500 R. total tumor dose with the needles implanted directly into the tumor. External beam, as orthovoltage, or recently, cobalt 60, was used for the inguinal and deep pelvic nodes, with a total tumor dose of approximately 5000 R. to a 15 × 15 cm. pelvic portal.

The main difficulty in using this procedure is that, while the area radiated is always radiosensitive, the tumor itself may be radioresistant, causing extreme pain, ulceration, erythema, and mucositis without curative results. Sloughing of the entire area radiated also might occur, and the patient would have an extremely uncomfortable post-treatment course, causing great problems to the physician, as well as to the patient. Therefore, most radiotherapists will prefer the use of surgery as the prime mode of treatment for vulvar carcinoma. In our hands, radiation therapy is reserved for those cases that are inoperable because of medical contraindications, or for palliation of far advanced, inoperable metastases.

In the 1940's when surgical treatment was coming into play, most commonly various surgical techniques were used for treatment of vulvar carcinoma. Hemivulvectomies, local excision, and simple vulvectomies were all used at this time. However, the overall survival rates ranged only from 20 to 35 percent. Studies by Eichner et al. (1954) and Twombly (1953) have shown that the vulva is rich in lymphatics and there is commonly cross-drainage. Therefore, contralateral metastatic disease has been reported in up to 10 to 15 percent of patients undergoing surgery. Other workers have shown that ipsilateral groin metastases are found in approximately 30 percent of all cases. This includes palpable and nonpalpable preoperative inguinal disease. Recently Collins and his coworkers (1971) found

regional lymph node metastases in 31 percent of their cases. Another point to be made prognostically is that, if the lesion is smaller than 3 cm. in diameter, the rate of node metastases falls. For these reasons, we feel that the best approach to the treatment of vulvar carcinoma is a radical vulvectomy with a bilateral superficial and deep groin dissection and bilateral retroperitoneal iliac and obturator node dissections. The first large series in which this type of procedure was introduced was that of Taussig (1940). He stressed that wide excision with node dissections markedly improved the five-year survival rate. In 1946, Watson and Gusberg showed that, even though the patients had a markedly mutilating operation, the survival rate, both from the surgery and the disease, increased with proper surgical technique and postoperative management. This will be discussed later under the section dealing with complications and their treatment. The procedure being performed today (as discussed above) is long and tedious. However, we feel that, if proper surgical technique is used, the patients do well, and thus the procedure can be done as a one-stage operation, whereas earlier workers had done the node dissection separately from the vulvectomy. The oldest patient in our experience was 96 years old and had a large vulvar lesion with gross inguinal node metastases; she survived the one-stage operation with no complications and is now alive and well, approximately 18 months later.

Since the newer techniques described in this section have been employed, the five-year survival rate has gone from the region of 30 percent to close to 80 to 85 percent in those cases with no node metastases. The five-year survival rate decreases with the extent of inguinal and deep pelvic metastatic disease; the survival rate correlates very well with whether or not the metastatic disease is on the ipsilateral or contralateral side. For instance, ipsilateral superficial nodal disease decreases the survival rate to about 70 percent. Once we have contralateral superficial metastatic disease, the survival rate falls in most cases to well below 50 percent. When the deep pelvic nodes are involved, the literature indicates a 21 percent five-year survival rate. We also learn from these studies that, in addition to getting increased survival rates from radical surgery, we are more able to outline the prognosis of the disease in terms of five-year survival once the pathology report is in our hands.

TECHNIQUE

In discussing the technique, one must keep in mind that this is a long and tedious procedure that requires meticulous care, both in removing all nodal tissues and in avoiding damage to the major vessels and nerves that are encountered. The procedure usually lasts about four hours.

In addition to routine work-up, the preoperative preparation consists of making sure the patient is well hydrated and typing and cross-matching the patient's blood, keeping four units of whole blood available. In our clinic, there is no further work-up unless indicated, i.e., cytoscopy,

if there is urethral involvement. We have found that other screening tests, such as bone survey, lymphography, and liver scan, are of little or no help.

In Figure 64–1*A*, the limits of the skin incision for the groin dissections can be seen. All the skin overlying the dissection is excised. Superiorly the dissection is carried down to the external oblique aponeurosis and laterally down to and including the fascia lata, exposing the medial portion of the sartorius muscle. The lower pole of the incision is the inferior apex of the femoral triangle, which then continues superiorly along the lateral edge of the adductor longus muscle. The actual groin dissection is then carried out from lateral to medial.

In Figure 64–1*B*, the completed dissection on one side is shown. After exposing the sartorius muscle and continuing medially, branches of the femoral nerve are encountered lying over the muscle and in the adiposonodal tissue in the femoral triangle. The branches may be cut; however, one must be extremely careful not to

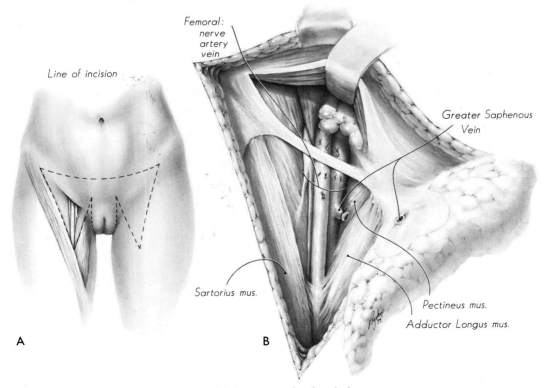

Line of incision

Femoral:
nerve
artery
vein

Greater Saphenous
Vein

Sartorius mus.

Pectineus mus.

Adductor Longus mus.

A   B

Figure 64–1 See text for description.

sever the femoral nerve itself. The femoral artery is then exposed and dissected free from the nodal tissue. We find that, by using sharp dissection in a vertical fashion along the wall of the artery and vein, one is less likely to injure the major vessels. The femoral vein is then carefully exposed, and the node-bearing tissue medial to the vein is now dissected free. This is probably the area with the most abundant nodes, and it must be carefully dissected. The lower end of the saphenous vein is usually encountered near the medial portion of the lower apex of the triangle and is doubly ligated and cut. Hemostasis is constantly checked, and bleeders are clamped and ligated or coagulated. In dissecting the tissue off the aponeurosis, one comes upon the round ligament, which is ligated and cut. With the groin dissection now completed, all the tissue is attached over the pubis. This is wrapped in a wet lap pad and held there. The same procedure is carried out on the opposite side.

The deep pelvic node dissection is begun by following the round ligament lat-erally and inferiorly, incising above Poupart's ligament, the external oblique aponeurosis, the internal oblique muscle, and the transverse fascia. Now by blunt dissection the retroperitoneal space is entered and the iliac vessels exposed. The inferior epigastric vessels are identified just inside the femoral canal, and they are then ligated and cut. An assistant, holding a Deaver retractor medially, will keep the peritoneum with the ureter coursing it out of the operating field. The nodal tissue along the external iliac vessels, the obturator fossa, and the hypogastric vessels are then excised and submitted as one specimen.

In Figure 64–2, on the right, one can see the pelvic area free of nodal tissue. On the left, the defect has been closed with a technique similar to that used in a herniorrhaphy. Here both groins have been fully dissected, with the tissue lying medially on the pubis. The patient is now placed in the lithotomy position and redraped.

In Figure 64–3*A*, the line of incision around the vulva is shown. Note that the

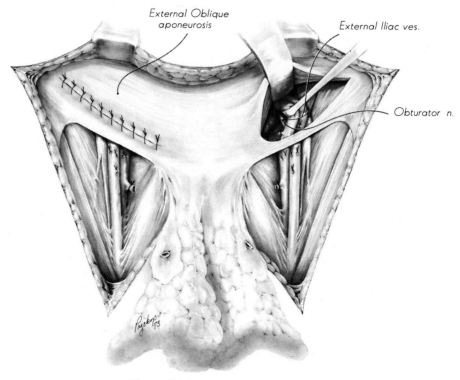

External Oblique aponeurosis

External Iliac ves.

Obturator n.

Figure 64–2 See text for description.

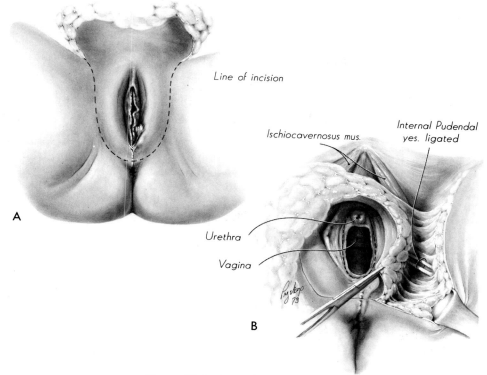

Line of incision

Ischiocavernosus mus.

Internal Pudendal
yes. ligated

Urethra

Vagina

A

B

Figure 64-3 See text for description.

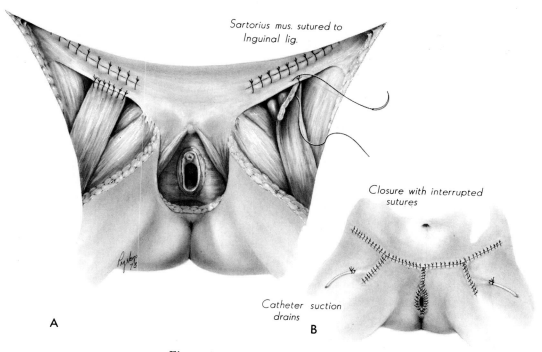

Sartorius mus. sutured to
Inguinal lig.

Closure with interrupted
sutures

Catheter suction
drains

A

B

Figure 64-4 See text for description.

lateral incision is in the fold between the labia majora and the thigh and is continued around the perineal body. The inner vaginal incision is then made (Fig. 64–3B). This, of course, can vary with the extent of the lesion. Care must be taken to preserve urethral integrity. The dissection is then continued laterally and the pudendal vessels exposed, ligated, and cut. The opposite side is done in a similar fashion. Now the entire mass of dissected tissue is draped over and peeled off the pubis by sharp dissection. The corpora cavernosa are identified, ligated, and cut, and the dissection is continued circumferentially down to the perineal muscles. The vaginal incision is then approached and the entire specimen excised. The urethra is suspended to the pubis in the midline and the levator muscles brought to the midline posteriorly.

In Figure 64–4A, one can see the dissection completed. As an added protection, the sartorius muscle is transected at its insertion in the anterior superior iliac spine and transposed over the femoral vessels and sutured to the inguinal (Poupart's) ligament. Hemostasis is thoroughly checked and ligatures placed where necessary. Catheter suction drains are then brought out through lateral stab incisions, and the entire defect is brought together with interrupted sutures (Fig. 64–4B). It is important that this be an airtight closure to facilitate the suction drainage. A foley catheter is put in place, and a light dressing is placed over the groins.

COMPLICATIONS AND THEIR TREATMENT

As stated earlier, because of the large amount of tissue that is excised in this procedure, the operative mortality formerly fell in the range of 20 to 30 percent. However, with recent improvements in anesthesia, parenteral therapy, and antibiotics, in most series the operative mortality has fallen to less than 10 percent. It is our opinion that the operative mortality should approach 0 percent. We have operated on approximately 50 patients and have had only one death resulting. It should also be noted that the operability

in more recent studies is around 90 percent (Shingleton et al., 1970). This indicates that approximately 10 percent of the cases have nonoperable metastatic disease or, because of medical complications, are considered extremely poor operative risks.

The most frequent post-operative complication has been necrosis of the skin overlying the area of wide dissection, especially in the groin. Many workers do not excise the overlying skin in the groin dissections but rather undermine the area and lay the skin back. Following this procedure, collections of serosanguineous fluid separate the skin flaps, with resulting necrosis. Two newer therapeutic techniques have decreased this complication, although it is still seen today to a lesser extent. The first of these new techniques is the employment of constant suction to the operative site by the use of Hemovac (Zimmer, U.S.A.) plastic suction catheters. This decreases the problem, because the overlying skin is held closely adherent to the underlying musculature, allowing for greater improvement in circulation to the skin. The second development, described by Nelson in 1969 and used in very recent cases, is a technique which we use, in which the skin is excised and the borders brought together for primary closure. We do run into an occasional problem of tension and breakdown when this procedure is employed; however, it is our feeling that there is less necrosis than had been seen previously. Also, one must consider primary grafting at the time of the original procedure. In those cases in which widespread breakdown occurs, grafting by half-thickness or pinch grafts when the field is clean and granulating gives good results. It should be noted that, even if the wound is left wide open, it will heal. The only problem in allowing this healing process to take place is the time element, for it takes many weeks, and one would find this financially prohibitive for the patient when one considers today's hospital costs.

A recent approach to the treatment of wound breakdown is the use of honey by local application (Cavanagh et al., 1970). The honey was thought to be a nonirritating agent, and its use was felt to promote the rapid growth of healthy granulation tissue. "The patient's acceptance of the method was excellent, once she overcame her initial surprise at the apparently ridiculous method of treatment." We have not had any experience with this technique.

Another common problem is postoperative wound infection. Our technique is to culture drainage from the constant suction, as described above, within the first 24 hours and treat the patient with the appropriate antibiotic, or one might use prophylactic antibiotic therapy. Both techniques markedly decrease the infection rate.

Hemorrhage in the postoperative period has also been seen in rare instances. In one recent case seen in consultation at another institution, a patient had a severe problem of blood loss ten days postoperatively because a tie on the femoral artery came loose. Fortunately, a resident was present in the room when this occurred. Here again, a meticulous technique when performing surgery will prevent this type of problem. We doubly ligate the saphenous insertion to the femoral vein with a transfixing suture and the distal portion of the saphenous muscle over the exposed femoral vessels, with the hope that any postoperative trauma will thus be prevented.

Because of the extensive dissection, the lymphatic drainage of the legs is usually affected, and very frequently postoperative leg edema is encountered. In our experience, the edema usually subsides gradually over one to three years. Elastic support plays an important role in the alleviation of symptoms and in allowing for collateral drainage to develop. Elevation of the legs with a wedge-shaped pillow while the patient is asleep has also improved lymphatic drainage.

Another problem that should be mentioned is serous collection in the groin after the primary healing has occurred. This is probably related to the lymphatic obstruction from the groin with collection of fluid. We have handled this problem simply by using a syringe and a No. 20 gauge needle for drainage every few days. Cultures have usually been negative, and the problem usually subsides after two to three months, when the skin is completely

adherent to the underlying tissues. We believe that incision and drainage is not indicated, because of the possibility of the development of a chronically infected, draining lymphocyst.

Recurrences are not very common, but when they do occur, they should be treated by wide excision. It is worth noting that the incidence of other squamous cell carcinomas of the female genital tract is greater in these patients than one would expect to occur by pure chance. For this reason, one should look for these tumors with special care and should note whether the supposed recurrence is really a recurrence of the vulvar lesion or a new primary lesion of independent origin. Multicentricity of squamous cell tumors of the female genital tract plays an important role in this disease. This is an important consideration in alleviating the problem of recurrences along the surgical margins.

OUR EXPERIENCE

Between the years 1963 and 1970, 30 cases of invasive vulvar squamous cell carcinoma were treated at our institution. The average age of the patients was 63.4 years. The youngest patient was 35 years old and the oldest 83.

Treatment

As can be seen from Table 64–1, 84 percent (25) of the patients had some form of node dissection. Of the remaining five patients, three had radical vulvectomies without node dissection, only be-

TABLE 64–1

Procedure	Number of Cases
Radical vulvectomy, bilateral inguinal and pelvic nodes	23
Radical vulvectomy, bilateral inguinal nodes	1
Radical vulvectomy, bilateral inguinal nodes; AP resection	1
Radical vulvectomy (no node dissection)	3
Simple vulvectomy	1
Local excision	1
Total:	30

TABLE 64–2 NODAL DISEASE VS. SURVIVAL

Pathology	No. of Cases	No. Done >5 Yrs. Ago	No. Alive & Well @ 5 Yrs.	% 5 Yr. Survival
Negative inguinal*	1	1	1	100
Negative inguinal and negative pelvic	15	12	10**	83†
Positive inguinal and negative pelvic	5	2	2	100
Positive inguinal and positive pelvic	4	4	0	0
Negative inguinal and positive pelvic	0	0	0	0
Total:	25	19	13	68%‡

*No pelvic node dissections.
**One patient died at 4 years from CVA, no evidence of tumor.
†Corrected to 91%.
‡Corrected to 73%.

cause of overwhelming medical diseases with histologically small lesions. These cases are all alive and well at between three and four years. The patient who had undergone local excision only, as well as the patient who had a simple vulvectomy, was lost to follow-up soon after the procedures were performed.

Technique

Further discussion will be limited to the patients who had node dissections. We had no operative mortalities in the 25 cases. All save one of the operations were performed as one-stage procedures, following the techniques previously described by Twombly (1953, 1966). The four most recent cases were done by the technique described in this chapter.

Results

Table 64–2 compares the results with reference to nodal disease. As can be readily seen, none of the patients with positive deep pelvic and inguinal nodes survived (4/4). Interestingly, two of these patients had been previously treated with radiation therapy and because of poor results were referred to our institution. We had no cases with positive pelvic nodes and negative inguinal nodes. As mentioned previously in this text, there is a very high survival rate with negative nodes. If one includes the patient who died at four years from a CVA with no evidence of tumor, our corrected five-year survival rate increases to 91 percent. Another important factor is that fully 36 percent of our patients (9/25) had positive nodes.

Table 64–3 gives our overall five-year survival rate, which is 68 percent. This can be corrected, if one includes the patient who died of a CVA, to 73 percent. Our figures generally agree with the literature.

SUMMARY

The importance of treatment of vulvar carcinoma cannot be understated. Even if

TABLE 64–3 OVERALL FIVE-YEAR SURVIVAL RATE WITH NODE DISSECTIONS

No. Patients Operated On >5 Years Ago	No. Patients Alive & Well @ 5 Years	No. Patients Dead of Cancer	No. Patients Dead Without Cancer	Lost to Follow-up	Percentages
19	13	4	1	1*	13/19 = 68% corrected % 14/19 = 73% (see Table 64–2)

*One patient developed transitional cell cancer of the bladder with vaginal invasion at four years and had anterior exenteration, then was lost to follow-up.

the disease remains localized for some time, there will develop an ulcerating, fungating mass, which will destroy the vulva, urethra, and anus, causing painful fistulas and/or death from ulceration of large blood vessels or from sepsis. This process is painful, as well as fatal, and can happen before widespread metastases occur.

In reviewing the literature and our small series, it is evident that the treatment of choice for vulvar squamous cell carcinoma is radical surgery with inguinal and pelvic node dissections. This may be done as a one-stage procedure with little or no operative mortality or morbidity, even though patients are, for the most part, over 60 years of age. If meticulous technique and good postoperative management are used, there is no question that radical vulvectomy with bilateral groin and pelvic node dissections markedly increases the survival rate.

REFERENCES

Berven, E. G. E.: Carcinoma of the vulva. Br. J. Radiol., 22:513, 1949.

Cavanagh, D., Beazley, J., and Ostapowicz, F.: Radical operation for carcinoma of the vulva—a new approach to wound healing. J. Obstet. Gynecol. Br. Commonw., 77:1037, 1970.

Collins, C. G., Lee, F., and Roman-Lopez. J.: Invasive carcinoma of the vulva with lymph node metastases. Am. J. Obstet. Gynecol., 109:446, 1971.

Eichner, E., Goldberg, I., and Bove, E. A.: In vivo studies with direct sky blue of the external genitalia of women. Am. J. Obstet. Gynecol., 67:1277, 1954.

Eichner, E., Mallin, L., and Anjell, M.: Further experiences with direct sky blue in the in vivo study of gynecic lymphatics. Am. J. Obstet. Gynecol., 69:1019, 1955.

Green, T. H., Jr., Ulfelder, H., and Meigs, J. V.: Epidermoid carcinoma of the vulva: An analysis of 238 cases. Am. J. Obstet. Gynecol., 75:834, 1958.

Gusberg, S. B., and Frick, H. C.: Corscaden's Gynecologic Cancer. Ed. 4. Baltimore, The Williams & Wilkins Company, 1970.

McKelvey, J. L.: Carcinoma of the vulva. Obstet. Gynecol., 5:452, 1955.

Nelson, J. H., Jr.: Atlas of Radical Pelvic Surgery. New York, Appleton-Century-Crofts, 1969.

Plentl, A. A., and Friedman, E. A.: Lymphatic System of the Female Genitalia. Philadelphia, W. B. Saunders Company, 1971.

Rutledge, F., Smith, J., and Franklin, E. W.: Carcinoma of the vulva. Am. J. Obstet. Gynecol., 106:1117, 1970.

Shingleton, H. M., Fowler, W. C., Palumbo, L., and Koch, G. G.: Carcinoma of the vulva; influence of radical operation on cure rate. Obstet. Gynecol., 35:1, 1970.

Taussig, F. J.: Cancer of the vulva—An analysis of 155 cases. Am. J. Obstet. Gynecol., 40:764, 1940.

Twombly, G. H.: The technique of radical vulvectomy for carcinoma of the vulva. Cancer, 6:516, 1953.

Twombly, G. H.: Surgical treatment of vulvar cancer. *In* New Concepts in Gynecological Oncology. Philadelphia, F. A Davis Company, 1966.

Watson, B. P., and Gusberg, S. B.: Prevention and treatment of carcinoma of the vulva. Am. J. Obstet. Gynecol., 52:179, 1946.

Way, S: Malignant Disease of the Female Genital Tract. Philadelphia, The Blakiston Company, 1951.

Way, S.: Carcinoma of the vulva. Am. J. Obstet. Gynecol., 79:692, 1960.

Part
IV

Therapy

65

Reconstructive Plastic Surgery

Thomas D. Rees, M.D

The general surgeon and the dermatologist, and the plastic surgeon face similar problems in reconstructing defects created by ablation of skin cancer. They are working more closely together now because of (1) recognition on the part of the plastic surgeon that there are instances in which the general surgeon and dermatologist are obliged to exercise skills in the area of reconstructive surgery, and (2) recognition on the part of the general surgeon and dermatologist that they need an understanding of reconstruction as their own field broadens. The principles of restorative surgery should be grasped by all disciplines concerned with the treatment of skin malignancy.

Both the surgeon and the dermatologist must apply the same principles to the excision of skin lesions. These include adequate excision, atraumatic technique, wound repair, and aftercare. The methods of repair when skin must be replaced or revised—grafts, flaps, Z-plasty—often apply to the treatment of skin cancer.

Skin loss can result from mechanical, infective, or postsurgical causes. The treatment of premalignant and malignant growth is probably the most common cause of postsurgical skin loss. One is nec-essarily committed to extricating the lesion first, then to considering the type of restoration to use. This is not to say that consideration of all reconstruction possibilities should be overlooked in planning the surgery.

EXCISION OF THE LESION

When surgery is the modality of treatment selected, simple excision and primary repair are preferable when feasible. Atraumatic technique is a primary principle in the success of any restorative effort. Trauma causes necrosis of the skin edges, potentiating the incidence of delayed healing and subsequent infection and scarring.

MATERIALS OF REPAIR

Hemostats cause localized tissue necrosis by crushing, with spilling of lymph, blood, and protoplasm into the interstitial spaces. This can subsequently create the necessary circumstances for more tissue destruction through extension of necrosis or infection, since all the surrounding cells are served by the same system of lymph

1473

and blood circulation. Hemostats used in skin surgery should therefore have the finest precision points possible. Every attempt should be made to grasp only the bleeding point.

The use of overly hot gauze sponges, inviting capillary bleeding, venous and lymphatic congestion, and infection, is another neglected source of trauma. Excessive heat promotes necrosis and also helps to incubate microorganisms. There is no place in restorative surgery for the use of hot sponges. Warm sponges can be used sparingly.

Bracing the surgeon's elbow against his own body or on an operative arm rest can help reduce tremor while doing fine work. This is analogous to the way in which a hard surface serves as a brace to the hand when writing. Tremor can increase microtrauma to the wound.

The instrumentation used in the operative procedure is also crucial to the prevention of trauma. The finest, sharpest instruments available for a given situation are mandatory for the best result. The use of skin hooks is advantageous because they produce less trauma than forceps, which tend to crush tissue. Only fine dissecting forceps should be selected, and care should be taken to avoid undue squeezing or crushing. Scissors should be fine, sharp, and of two types—sharp straight for use at the edge of the wound and blunt curved for undercutting. The latter are often double-edged like a saber. Some surgeons prefer the needle holder combined with scissors for suturing, and it is usually better to ligate with instruments which make possible more delicate movements than the fingers. Detachable No. 11 or No. 15 knife blades are usually used in skin surgery. Suture needles should be of the smallest caliber possible with cutting rather than round edges.

PATIENTS AND LOCATION OF SURGERY .

Other factors to be considered in obtaining the best operative results in skin surgery are age, body region, type of skin, and the presence or absence of general-ized skin disease. Adults generally have a shorter postoperative period of erythema and hypertrophy than children. Time is required to determine the final result. An elevated red scar may blanch to the point of almost becoming invisible over a period of weeks or months. In children, the process may take years. As a general rule, the thicker the skin of the body area, the greater the possibility of hypertrophy or spreading of the scar. Eyelid scars are usually finer than scars of the trunk or lower extremities, for example. People who have oily skin with highly active sebaceous glands are more likely to form depressed and irregular scars than people with dry skin. Abnormalities in the elastic or fibrous tissues frequently lead to severe wide scars following surgery. For example, patients with "cutis hyperelastica" (Ehlers-Danlos syndrome) almost always form stretched or wide scars.

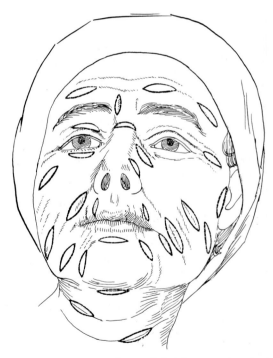

Figure 65–1 The lines of facial expression (not Langer's lines) provide the best guide for planning the direction of excisions so that the final scar will be of optimal cosmetic acceptability. The lines of expression lie roughly at right angles to the direction of the underlying muscle pull. The illustration demonstrates elliptical excisions in many of the common areas of the face.

The lines of facial expression, the lines of dependency, and the contour of the body can be used to advantage in planning incisions so that the scars will be least evident. Figure 65–1 shows the location of some of these reference points on the face.

Lines of Expression

The lines of facial expression comprise the system of wrinkles which develop on the face as a result of the animation of smiling, laughing, frowning, and other commonly repeated facial motions. Muscular contraction of the muscles perpendicular to the line of wrinkling causes these skin creases. They are best observed by having the patient contract or extend the facial muscles or by lifting the skin with thumb and finger to see where the wrinkles fall. The most familiar facial lines are horizontal forehead lines, vertical glabellar lines with associated frown lines, horizontal folds at the nasal base, wrinkles running lateral to the nose, the wrinkles of the lids which extend outward from the canthus, and the nasolabial folds near the inferior border of the mandible. The area of least expression is where the skin lies close to the underlying cartilage without intervening musculature.

The lines of expression (Fig. 65–1) are optimal for the placement of scars and should not be confused with Langer's lines, which were long considered to indicate the proper direction for scars. Langer's lines are of little consequence in planning skin surgery.

Contour Lines

Contour lines occur at juncture points—where the lip skin meets the vermilion, where the scalp or cheek meets the ear, and where the cheek meets the nose. Other contour areas are where the neck joins the cheek in the submandibular area, and the inframammary fold where the inferior portion of the breast joins the chest.

Lines of Dependency

Loose skin and fatty tissue evident with aging produce the so-called lines of dependency. Submandibular and submental lines are typical of this. These lines may mesh with lines of facial expression in some older people to form a crisscross diamond-shaped pattern of wrinkles.

Hairlines

For cosmetic purposes, the proper placement of scars in the hairline should not be overlooked. The incision in this case should be parallel to the hair follicles, so that a hairless scar resulting from a sectioning of the follicles can be avoided. It should be kept in mind that scars may become evident in the hairline as hair becomes sparse with aging or in patients prone to alopecia. Tension on the incision and the extent of excision should be carefully considered to avoid misalignment of the hairline.

PROCEDURE

There are three basic types of simple skin excision—elliptical, wedge, and circular.

Elliptical Excision

In making an elliptical incision, the long axis should be about four times the length of the short axis and parallel to a line of expression, contour line, or line of dependency (Fig. 65–2). If the ellipse is too short, bunching of the skin will occur at the points of the ellipse. These are referred to as "dog ears" or "pig's ears" by surgeons (Figs. 65–3 and 65–4). This bunching may flatten over a period of time, but it is best avoided because subsequent correction may be required if it persists. When it is necessary to make a slightly curved ellipse, the surgeon may increase the curve on the side closest to the skin line he is following, while making the other side as straight as possible.

The surgeon outlines the incision with a

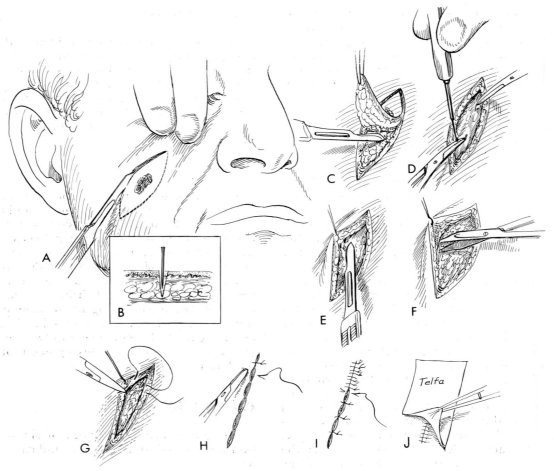

Figure 65–2   The technique for simple primary (elliptical) excision of a small skin malignancy. *A,* The borders of the excision should extend at least 5 mm. from the clinical edges of the tumor. *B,* The skin should be excised at right angles to prevent beveling. *C,* The depth of excision should be adequate without undue sacrifice of subcutaneous tissue; however, when in doubt "go deeper." *D,* All bleeding points are grasped with fine hemostats and coagulated. *E* and *F,* The wound edges are undermined with scalpel or fine-pointed scissors. Suturing can be accomplished by several different techniques; however, the edges must be everted. A subcuticular closure is shown in *G.* Interrupted suture of fine suture material, taking small bites and placing the sutures closely together, is shown in *H* and *I.* A nonadherent dressing is usually applied (*J*), or the wound is left exposed altogether. Some surgeons utilize such taping instead of skin sutures after obtaining accurate approximation of the deep dermal edges with buried sutures.

suitable ink or dye and places tension on the skin to stretch it so that the outline can be followed more exactly (Fig. 65–2*A*). The initial incision is made at right angles (Fig. 65–2*B*) with a No. 15 blade, and a No. 11 blade is used vertically at the tips of the incision for best precision. If the incision is not made at right angles, beveling results, which can cause an irregular or "stair-stepping" effect because of the unequal contraction of the wound edges. Undermining through the superficial subcutaneous tissue should be done

either by employing the use of one sweep of a No. 15 blade or by using sharp scissors (Fig. 65–2*E, F*). This will encourage a smooth closure of the wound without tension. Fine plain catgut, vicryl (polyglycol), or mersilene is used to make inverted sutures in deep tissue, while fine nonabsorbable sutures may be used on the skin as either interrupted, continuous, or subcuticular sutures (Fig. 65–2*H, I*). It is important to evert the skin edges and to secure a careful approximation of the deep dermis with these sutures to prevent post-

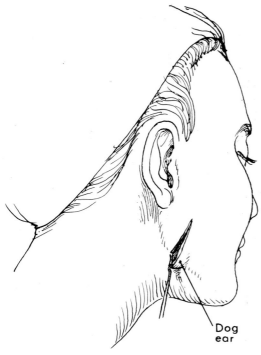

Figure 65-3 A "dog ear" or "pig's ear" frequently results at the ends of an ellipical incision during closure

operative spreading of the scar and to achieve an exact wound closing.

The multiple excision technique may be used in excising large benign lesions. In such large lesions, elliptical excision under tension can be done. After healing, the skin becomes lax again with the passage of time. This allows excision in stages. It is important to plan well so as not to create a shortage of skin and poor approximation. The scalp is a good example of a location where this method is applicable. Because of its relative inelasticity, primary excision and closure of lesions larger than 3 cm. are impracticable. In the initial stage, an incision is made between the lesion and normal tissue down to loose areolar tissue beneath the galea aponeurotica. The undermined scalp is pulled over the area to be excised, which has been marked with methylene blue. After the marked area is removed, the wound is closed. When the scalp has loosened enough to permit it, the same procedure is repeated on the side opposite to the lesion. After sufficient repetition of the procedure, the two healthy segments of scalp are fully approximated. This method is often used for burn scars and can be used to correct radiation dermatitis, scars, hemangioma, nevi, and certain other lesions. It is applicable to the repair of malignancy only in affecting wide scars or skin-grafted areas after primary excision.

Wedge Excision

Wedge excision is applicable when one edge of the wound is an open full-thickness area, such as the edge of the lip, ear, or eyelid. Primary closure of the lower lip can be made after wedge excision when as much as a third of it has been removed, and the same is true for the upper lip. A flap from the lower lip to the upper lip and vice versa (Fig. 65-5) are useful for closure of larger defects. These are referred to as lip-switch flaps or often by their eponym, Stein-Estlander-Abbe flap. Additional tissue in the area of lymphatic drainage may need to be removed in treating certain carcinomas, such as those of the lip. The restoration of symmetry of the vermilion cutaneous border is important for cosmetic reasons. As in elliptical excision, the area is outlined with methylene blue. The No. 11 and No. 15 blades are used similarly, and the wound is closed in three layers.

A circular excision may be used in ablating large skin cancers or removing lesions over cartilage, such as those of the nose and ear. The position assumed by the tissues after excision will tend to show the natural facial lines if these were not evident before. The circular excision can then be converted to a linear wound or closed with appropriate local flaps by further tailoring the wound, or by skin grafting.

HEMOSTASIS

The importance of hemostasis cannot be overemphasized in any surgical procedure, and it is most certainly vital to successful results in reconstructive surgery. Hematoma is the commonest cause of delayed normal healing and poor surgical results in skin surgery. There are six basic

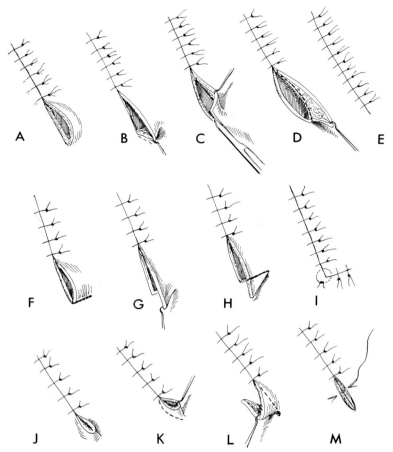

Figure 65–4 Various methods for trimming redundant skin tags that occur at the extreme ends of the wound when an elliptical or round wound is closed by direct approximation—the so-called "dog ear." Ingenuity is the best guide.

methods of obtaining hemostasis: ligatures, electrosurgery, topical vasoconstrictors, fibrin or gelatin foam, clamping and twisting small vessels, and pressure.

Ligature

To use ligature, the surgeon either ties the suture material around the vessel directly after applying the hemostat or passes the suture through adjoining tissue with a needle to add stability to the ligature. Catgut is usually used for ligation, but nonabsorbable sutures must be used on large vessels to avoid early absorption and recurrence of bleeding.

Electrosurgery

Electrosurgery is another effective method. A high frequency, high amperage current is combined with low voltage. The use of high frequency current negates the convulsive reaction caused by low frequency electricity. Cycles of 2 to 18 million per second are usually used in cautery. When electrocoagulation is used, every effort should be made to apply pinpoint coagulation to prevent destruction of adjacent normal tissue which impedes wound healing. A small hemostat on the vessel is usually brought into contact with the electrode to reduce trauma, or a fine-tipped electrode may be applied directly

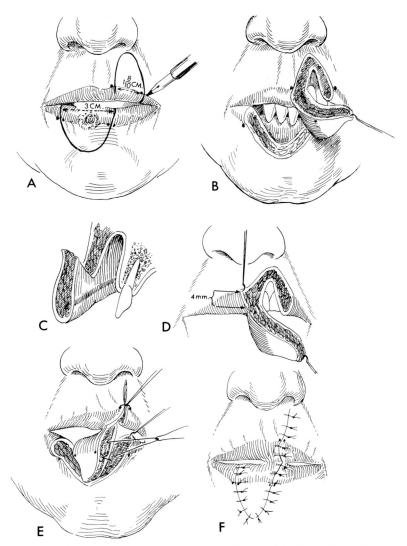

Figure 65–5 A popular method of reconstruction of a large defect of the lip and sometimes eyelid is the use of a full-thickness wedge flap, which is attached and nourished by a very small pedicle containing the arterial supply. This is "robbing Peter to pay Paul." The flap need be only one-third to one-half the size of the defect. In this way very large blocks of tumor excision can be repaired and the circumoral musculature reestablished (or full-thickness of the lid). The arterial pedicle is cut and trimmed 10 days later. Lesions of the lip requiring full-thickness excision of less than one-third of the lip can be closed primarily in layers.

(Fig. 65–2D). Although some trauma arises from the slight burning of the vessel tip, it is not believed to be any more extensive than ligatures and is probably the most rapid and effective means for hemostasis.

The high frequency electrosurgery with a dampened wave current is preferred by most. Monoterminal units are usually used in hemostasis, although biterminal ones are also available. Explosive materials should not be used near the electrosurgical unit.

Topical Vasoconstrictors

Some capillary and small vessel bleeding may be controlled by applying sponges containing 1:100,000 epinephrine solution.

Either of two varieties of foam may be used; both are particularly good for packing small, oozing cavities. Fibrin foam made of human fibrinogen and thrombin is one type, and the other is absorbable gelatin. Although neither of these causes significant tissue reaction, they should not be used on a graft bed because they prohibit close union of the graft and its recipient area.

Clamping

Clamping and twisting small vessels is sometimes done, but it is not a method of choice.

Pressure

Direct pressure on the wound is a good method of hemostasis for capillary oozing, but it should be remembered that the time element is important—pressure should be applied for at least five minutes to achieve an effect.

SKIN CLOSURE

The four methods of skin closure are sutures, skin clips, skin tapes, and wound adhesive.

Sutures

Absorbable or nonabsorbable sutures may be used. In general, absorbable sutures are used in the deeper tissues, and fine nonabsorbable material is used to close the skin. In the selection of suture material, one considers tensile strength, ease in use, and tissue reaction. Reconstructive surgery usually demands the finest suture which is strong enough to achieve the wanted effect.

Plain or chromic catgut and polyglycol (vicryl) are the common absorbable sutures. The catguts are collagens from the serous layer of sheep intestine or from the flexor tendon of cattle. The variety made from cattle tendon is stronger and more pliable. Absorption time ranges between two weeks and six months for two reasons: plain catgut is absorbed more rapidly than chromic; serous or mucous membranes absorb the suture more rapidly than does other tissue, such as muscle. Tissue reaction is initially less from chromic catgut than from plain, but the chromic type produces reaction after the chromium is gone.

Research on collagen as a buried suture is promising, although this material is not yet perfected.

Synthetic absorbable sutures, such as polyglycol (vicryl) and Dexan, are in wide use at present. These sutures seem less reactive than catgut, yet they absorb slowly enough to allow sufficient tensile strength to develop in the wound.

Silk, cotton, nylon, proline, and stainless steel are varieties of nonabsorbable suture which are stronger than catgut and which cause less reaction. Silk has the advantages of being easy to handle, of holding the knot well, and of being pliable enough to allow the ends of the suture to lie flat after knotting. However, both silk and cotton cause more wound reaction than does nylon or steel wire.

Tension, the length of time the suture is left in, the proximity to the wound edge, and the region of the body determine the likelihood of suture scarring. Infection and tendency to keloid formation also are important factors.

To achieve the proper amount of tension, the surgeon must acquire the skill of suturing the wound tightly enough to approximate it well without undue pressure. The natural surgical edema which arises adds to the initial tension. One advantage of fine suture used in reconstructive surgery is that it produces less tension than a heavy one. Tension is also caused by muscles which pull at right angles to the wound. Of course, tension also increases in proportion to the size of the segment excised. Subcutaneous sutures help to reduce pull on the skin sutures, as does placement of the excision parallel to skin lines.

The length of time in which the sutures remain may be as important in preventing scars as the type used. Usually, alternate skin sutures should be removed on the third day following surgery, and the rest

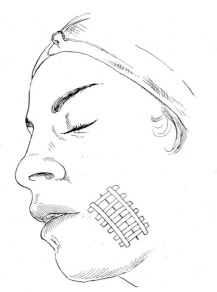

Figure 65–6 Cross-strips of sterile paper tape are most useful in splinting fresh wounds during the immediate postoperative period. Such tape splints permit early removal of sutures so that suture marks do not result across the wound. They may also be applied at night for several months during wound maturation to prevent excessive spreading of the scar.

removed on the fifth day. Support can be given for several more days with skin tape or collodion on fine mess gauze. Paper tape or "steristrips" are particularly useful for wound support (Fig. 65–6). About seven days are required to prevent wound disruption in the case of sutures on the trunk or extremities. Some sutures must remain for from 10 days to two weeks, for example, those on the back or extremities, where wound healing is slow and permanent suture marks may remain.

Proximity of suture to wound edge can govern the degree of scarring to some extent. The larger the distance between suture entry and skin edge, the greater the possibility of scarring.

As well as being a consideration in determining the length of time sutures should be left in, body region also is a factor in determining the likelihood of scarring. The skin of the eyelids and mucous membrane heals with finer scars than does the skin of the trunk and extremities.

Infected sutures should be treated by prompt removal of the sutures and the application of warm, wet dressings. Ke-

loids may form at suture sites in patients with a keloid tendency.

The subcutaneous and deeper tissues must be sutured to relieve skin tension and to avoid dead space, but small sutures should be used where possible, and as few sutures as possible should be used in order to achieve the desired result. As a general rule, the less foreign material necessary, the better the healing.

Inverted wound edges often will create a depressed scar, while everted edges will smooth out to a flat surface. The methods of making an everted suture line include vertical mattress sutures, suturing subcutaneous tissue to reduce skin tension, undermining, and incising so that the skin edges slightly overhang the perpendicular. Z-plasty can be used to correct a depressed scar (this technique will be defined later); an elliptical cut and closure around the denuded scar also may correct it. Undermining or redistribution of subcutaneous tissue can help in closing a wound of unequal thickness.

Different suture techniques may be used. Each layer must be carefully closed. Subcutaneous sutures should be tied on the underside of the suture away from the skin with 4–0 or 5–0 catgut or a synthetic suture, either absorbable or nonabsorbable. Interrupted suture, vertical mattress suture, half-buried horizontal mattress suture, subcuticular suture, and continuous suture all may be used, provided the dermis is approximated and the skin edges everted. Inclusion cysts are best prevented by the removal of skin sutures as early as it is prudent to do so. Excellent light is a necessity for suture removal, and the suture should be removed by pulling toward rather than away from the wound.

Skin Tape

Sometimes skin tape may be used to close the wound, and it can be applied and removed more easily than can sutures. It also produces less scarring.

Skin Clips

Skin clips are a poor second choice to sutures. When used, they should be of the sharp-toothed type rather than blunt, and care must be taken to place the clips consistently.

Wound Adhesive

Wound adhesive may be used, but it will hold only on a dry wound. Also, there is no solvent available if it adheres to gloves or linen. In certain instances, paper tape may replace the use of skin sutures altogether, provided the deep layers are closed in accurate proximation.

METHODS OF REPAIR

Once a defect of the skin is made, the surgeon must decide on the best method of repair. The choices available to him, depending on the size and location of the defect, are (1) direct or primary closure, (2) closure by local flaps, (3) closure by free skin grafting, and (4) closure by migration of a flap from a distance.

It is always best to use the most simple technique available; therefore, a graft or a flap is never used if primary closure can be accomplished easily without tension. In the treatment of skin malignancies, however, the complexities of wound closure

should never influence the surgeon in his judgment as to how much normal tissue margin is to be removed with the tumor. He must not compromise his excision because he is concerned with the technique of closure: the defect is created, and then it is repaired. This is not to rule out thoughtful preoperative planning and preparation, however, as it is usually possible to make a fairly accurate appraisal of what probable size and shape the defect will encompass. This appraisal is accepted after careful examination and clinical judgment.

If it is not possible to close the wound easily by primary repair without excess tension or distortion of adjacent structures, such as the mouth or eyelids, the surgeon must decide whether to employ some type of local flap or a free skin graft.

Local flaps are frequently used; however, in the treatment of malignancy, the surgeon should be as secure as possible in his belief that all of the tumor has been removed. Otherwise, foci of malignant cells could be covered by flaps and remain undetected until a recurrence becomes quite sizeable and often invasive.

Many believe that free skin grafts are always preferable to repair wounds created by cancer ablation. Such grafts may be removed subsequently and more

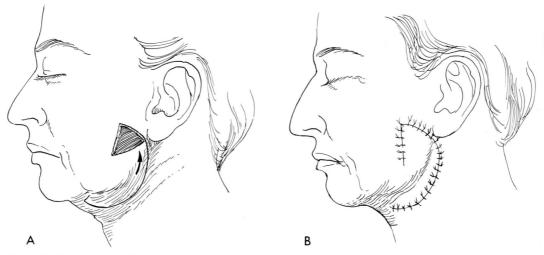

A   B

Figure 65–7 A rotation flap can be used to close defects too large for direct closure, provided the surgeon is reasonably certain that the tumor has been adequately excised. Such flaps are nourished by the uncut vascular pedicle, which also provides venous and lymphatic drainage. This is a one-step maneuver. Many pedicle flaps, such as tubed flaps and others, are more complicated and require multiple procedures both to prepare the flap and to transfer it. Such preparatory procedures are known as "delays." They promote increased vascularization of the flap through its pedicle.

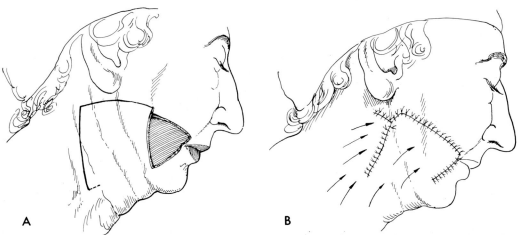

A   B

Figure 65–8 Sometimes it is necessary both to rotate a flap and at the same time to advance it. Such a flap is shown here. Small areas of skin redundancy incurred by this maneuver must be excised and sutured, as represented in this illustration by the horizontal suture line beneath the ear lobe.

definitive flap closures initiated after a suitable passage of time to be reasonably sure that the tumor is cured. A time interval of at least one year is preferred by most. However, there are no hard and fast rules and certainly no substitutes for sound clinical judgment which takes into consideration all the many factors that determine when the clinician feels quite secure about his treatment.

Flaps

If the surgeon elects to use a local flap, he must design one from adjacent tissue.

The simplest type of local flap is undercutting or undermining of the wound edges to relieve tension so that they can be advanced and sutured (Fig. 65–2). This is known as an advancement flap. Also adjacent tissue can be rotated or even doubly rotated into the defect (Fig. 65–7 to 65–10), or it can be "jumped" over a bridge of normal tissue when necessary and be interpolated into the defect (Fig. 65–9). A flap sometimes may bridge intact skin adjacent to its pedicle; it is then called a bridging flap. Another flap is the bilobed flap. Full-thickness flaps of the lips or eyelids can be rotated almost 180° on small vascular pedicles (Fig. 65–6).

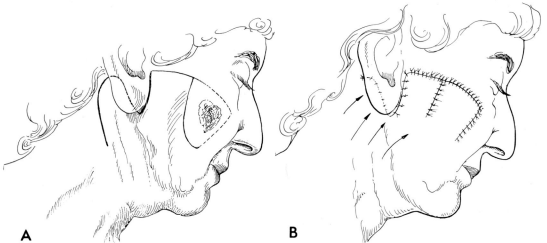

A   B

Figure 65–9 Larger flaps require ingenuity on the part of the surgeon. In the problem represented here, an additional flap of tissue from behind the ear was required to close the defect. Such a flap bridges or "jumps" areas of normal tissue, in this case the ear, and is therefore known as an interpolation flap.

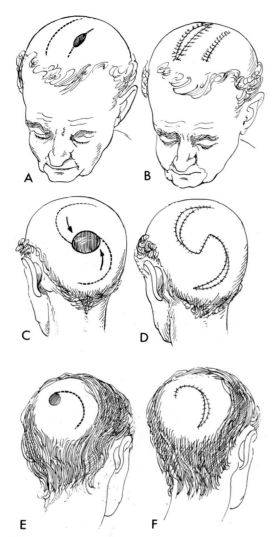

Figure 65–10 Defects of the scalp may require closure by a relaxing incision and shifting of a double pedicle flap (*A* and *B*). It may be necessary to utilize a free graft to relieve tension. Larger defects may require double rotation flaps (*C* and *D*) with or without free split-thickness grafts to relieve tension. Sometimes a simple rotation flap (*E* and *F*) suffices. The scalp poses special difficulties because of its inelastic nature. Even small defects may require sophisticated closures. The surgeon should be wary of excising even small tumors of the scalp without planning a flap closure.

These survive because they are fed by single, strong arteries, although they usually survive as composite grafts even if the pedicle is cut, provided they are not too large. Composite grafts (Fig. 65–21) depend on the rapid formation of vascu-

lar anastomoses and revascularization by capillary ingrowth.

The Z-plasty (Fig. 65–11) is actually a type of local double transposition flap which facilitates closure where contracture is apt to occur. The Z-plasty will be discussed separately.

The surgeon must not violate the principles of dimensions when designing flaps. The face and neck region, however, permits more latitude in designs because of the very rich blood supply of this region. Local flaps described and widely used in facial repair often violate accepted rules of dimension and would most certainly fail if similarly designed on the trunk or extremities.

Local flaps are almost always single pedicled, depending for their survival on the vascular supply and lymphatic and venous drainage through the pedicle. Larger flaps that are prepared at a distant site and migrated to the wound must be designed with a more rigid set of rules concerning shape and dimensions. They also may be of a double pedicle design during their preparation in order to maintain sufficient blood supply. Adequate blood supply is the key to survival of all types of grafts or flaps, but it is a much more critical factor in the preparation and transfer of flaps than it is in free skin grafts.

Skin Flaps. A skin flap provides restoration of lost skin and at the same time the added protection of a cushion of subcutaneous tissue and a vascular supply supported by its pedicle, provided the rules of dimension are not violated. Thus the flap is used instead of the skin graft when the area to be covered would present vascularization problems, when reconstruction of a full thickness of skin and subcutaneous tissue is required, or over deeper defects which uncover bone, tendon, cartilage, and other critical structures with little or no vascular supply.

Primary considerations in planning the flap are size and location, when it can be moved, and how blood supply may best be maintained. The larger the flap, the better the circulation required. A large flap can best be considered when the procedure can be done in several stages or when large axial blood vessels supply the

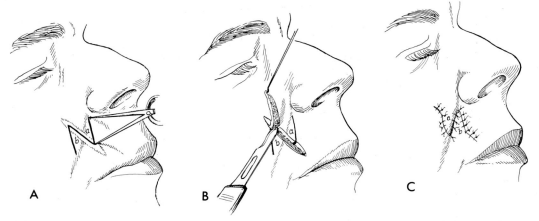

Figure 65–11 The Z-plasty principle is widely used in reconstructive surgery to relieve contracture lines, to cross flexion creases, and to shift tissue from less needy to more needy areas. The principle is generally the same with minor variations depending upon the size, shape, and location of the defect. The Z-plasty is essentially a double interpolation flap. The usual ideal angle of the apices of the flaps is 60 degrees. The Z-plasty must not be considered a substitute for tissue loss, however. It is sometimes used in conjunction with free skin grafts.

area (Figs. 65–12 to 65–16). Arteriosclerotic changes and fibrotic skin or subcutaneous tissue are relative contraindications for using a flap and may well present problems to the surgeon.

Skill in knowing when to "delay" a flap, that is, to move it in stages, is vital for assuring its survival. Since transfer can produce a kink in the flap, causing the circulation to move against gravity, or increase tension on the flap, it is sometimes prudent to move the flap in stages to develop better longitudinal circulation and to con-

dition the flap to withstand limited degrees of hypoxia.

The skin and subcutaneous tissue may be incised on three sides of the outlined single pedicle flap without undermining; then the edges are resutured. Such an operation constitutes a "delay." This method can be used to special advantage in the forehead and scalp, because the blood vessels there run longitudinally in the subcutaneous tissue without perforating branches. Flap preparation in other areas, such as the chest or abdomen,

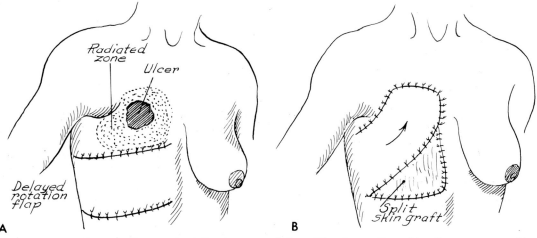

Figure 65–12 The use of a large local flap to cover a defect of the chest wall resulting from surgery and irradiation is shown. Such a flap must be "delayed" because of its dimensions and because it is not based on optimal segmental blood supply. Note in *B* that the donor site of the flap is grafted with a free split skin graft.

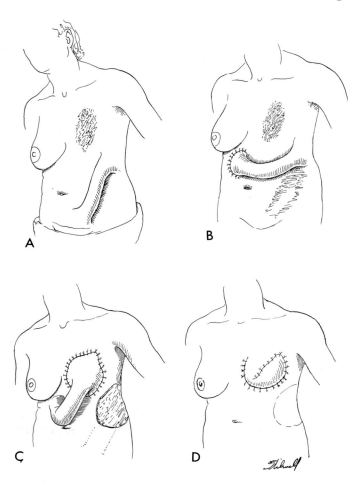

Figure 65–13 It is sometimes necessary to roll or tube a pedicle flap to facilitate its transfer to distant areas so that closed wounds can be maintained. Such tubing also facilitates contour restorations, as shown on the reconstruction of the breasts in this illustration.

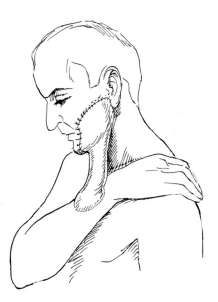

Figure 65–14 Pedicle flaps, particularly tubed flaps, can be carried from the site of formation, such as the abdomen or chest wall, by means of the extremities to their final site of insertion. The forearm and wrist have been particularly useful as carriers.

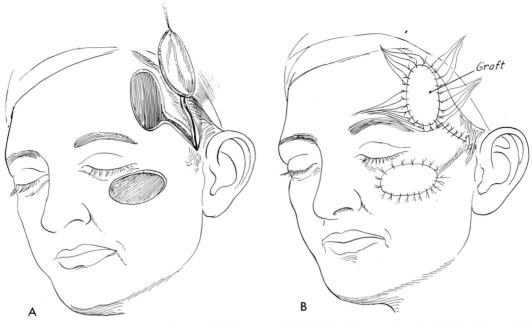

Figure 65–15 A special flap which is useful in covering difficult full-thickness losses is the island flap, which is transported on an artery pedicle. In the illustration the superficial temporary artery is the carrier. The artery supplying the block of tissue must be carefully dissected out and not injured in the process. The island along with its artery is tunneled beneath the skin to the recipient site. Often it is necessary to cover the donor site with a free skin graft.

requires additional undermining of the subcutaneous tissue for the distal one-third to one-half of the flap.

An alternative to undermining three sides is to incise two sides of the flap, undermine them after a waiting period of three weeks, and incise the third side (Fig. 65–12). This constitutes a second "delay." Longer flaps may be made safely in this way, provided that a bridge is maintained in the central portion. Then the remaining surgery can be accomplished in three or four stages. Any failure in development of satisfactory vascularization is reason for delay, and staging the procedure may help to ensure the viability of the flap. Undermining beneath the subcutaneous tissue preserves and enhances the rich vasculature of subdermal vessels lying at the union of the dermis and subcutaneous tissue in most areas of the body. However, large vessels can be found deep in the subcutaneous tissue of the trunk and often must be severed during these staged procedures.

Arteries in the flap change very little, but venous pathways may enlarge. Four to five days after transfer, the venous portions of the flap are seen on microangiography, and the anastomosis of arteries is seen approximately seven days afterward.

The terms "skin flap" and "pedicle" are synonymous. There are two types of pedicle flap: single pedicle and the bipedicle tube (Figs. 65–12 and 65–13). The bipedical type allows larger segments: a length to width ratio of 1:1 is usual for a single pedicle, while 2.5:1 can be safely done in one stage for bipedicle graft.

When there is excellent vascularity in the pedicle of the flap and the length to width ratio does not exceed safe limits, a flap can be transferred immediately. When larger amounts of flap tissue are required, it may be necessary to prepare the flap by "delay" operations and to do the definitive transfer subsequently, sometimes by way of a mobile "carrier," such as the wrist. A three-week interval is usually required between stages to allow for reorientation of the blood supply.

Vascular Competence. Certain tests of vascular competence of flaps are available for surgeons. These include the his-

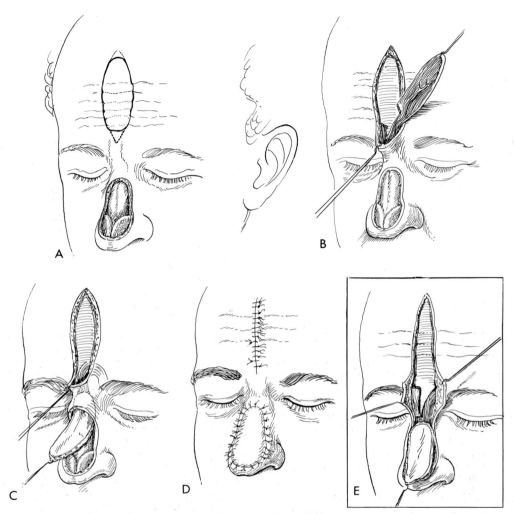

Figure 65–16 Of special use in reconstructing significant tissue loss on the nose is the forehead flap. The illustration shows a midline vertical flap, although there are many other different designs available to fit the needs of the individual problem. Such flaps are transported and nourished by narrow pedicles containing nutrient vasculature and may be tunneled through a bridge of skin as shown here.

tamine wheel test, radioactive isotope uptake studies, and others. However, these tests are never substitutes for clinical judgment.

Flaps are particularly useful in covering open cavities over the maxilla or skull. Thus they are important in considering how to repair lips, nose, ears, eyelids or brows, cheeks, and scalp or forehead. Reconstruction by flaps has the added advantage of withstanding subsequent operations in the same area, while the skin graft does not support such repetitive procedures.

Radioactive sodium (^{24}Na) clearance and plethysmography have been used to study the circulation in a flap. These tests showed that the flap undermined on three sides ultimately retains better circulation, and that a relatively small amount of blood (1.2 ml. per minute for every 100 ml. of tissue) will sustain the skin.

The capillaries at the end of the flap should refill on digital pressure as rapidly as those in the adjacent unoperated area, and this test helps to determine the extent of the undermining necessary, as well as the postoperative condition of the vasculature later.

The histamine wheel test is more sophisticated and possibly the most commonly used test of circulatory efficiency in the flap. Histamine acid phosphate (1:1000) is applied to scarified areas of the graft in two or three spots. Transudation of plasma produces a wheal. A rubber-shod bowel clamp may be applied to one end of the bipedicle flap and the histamine test performed at the distal margin. It is applied to a control area on the opposite side of the body as well. Wheals should appear in eight minutes, and simultaneous appearance on both flap and control area indicates that it is safe to divide the flap.

Problems that can arise include kinking, tension, hematoma, pressure, and infection. Kinking or tension may be corrected by repositioning. Hematomas must be evacuated and hemostasis restored. Pressure may be external and alleviated by altering the dressing, but internal pressure is more difficult to correct and may require surgery to return the flap to its donor area.

The importance of planning the flap preoperatively and the use of a pattern for each step of the procedure cannot be overemphasized. Planning is one of the most important elements in any successful reconstructive surgery. Patterns should be slightly larger than the area they cover to help avoid tension on the operative site later and to allow for contraction and shrinkage of the flap.

Various ways of creating flaps are shown in Figures 65-6 to 65–16. The local skin flap is similar in that it usually requires few stages. The donor area is usually covered with a split-thickness skin graft, except in the case of the interpolation flap or island flap, which may have the donor site closed primarily. Whenever primary closure is used, the surgeon must be very sure that this will not create undue postoperative tension.

The flap usually maintains its original color, and hair and sebaceous areas are, of course, transferred with it. The excess fat should be removed to avoid excessive bulk.

Within six weeks to three years, sensation and sweating can be expected to return to the flap. Painless ischemia can occur in the interim from lack of sensation, and the surgeon must watch for this possibility.

Z-plasty. Z-plasty is another commonly used procedure in reconstructive surgery. The Z-plasty is a maneuver designed to add length to a scar and thus avoid or correct scar contractures in vital areas such as the eyelids, the lips, over joint creases, and so forth. Such contractures can be unsightly and can inhibit joint function. The Z-plasty is also useful in breaking up straight line scars to make them conform to normal facial lines discussed previously. It is really a type of transposition flap (Fig. 65–11).

One of the most important things to remember in planning the Z-plasty is that the center arm of it must be equal in length to each of the other two arms. The angle of the Z-plasty should approximate 60°. It is a particularly effective method for correcting scars at flexion points or U-shaped scars. Also it is used to release circular scars at body orifices. Multiple Z-plasties may be used when indicated.

Skin Grafts

Free skin grafts are the most common method of wound repair following extirpation of skin malignancies where it is difficult to obtain primary wound closure because of the size or location of the wound.

There are two types of skin grafts, each with advantages and disadvantages: split-thickness skin grafts and full-thickness skin grafts. The split-thickness skin graft is composed of a partial thickness of skin. It is of different thicknesses, depending on the level at which it is cut through the dermis (Fig. 65–17).

Full-Thickness Skin Grafts. The full-thickness or whole-thickness graft is, as the name implies, the complete thickness of skin, including all of the dermis but not the subcutaneous fat (Figs. 65–18 to 65–20). The fat is actually trimmed from the graft so that it will not act as a barrier between the rich vascular plexus of the deep dermis and the vessels of the bed of the recipient wound (Fig. 65–18).

Another technique to promote bulk or

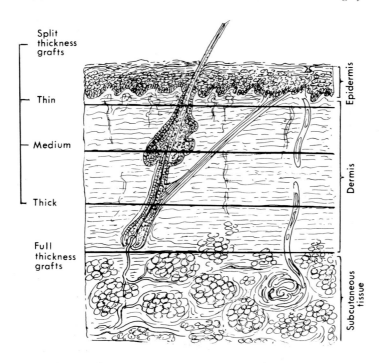

Split
thickness
grafts

Thin

Medium

Thick

Full
thickness
grafts

Epidermis

Dermis

Subcutaneous
tissue

Figure 65–17 Free skin grafts are of different thicknesses, depending upon the requirements of the graft. Split-thickness grafts are thin. medium, or thick. A full- or whole-thickness graft includes the entire thickness of the skin without subcutaneous tissue. These thicknesses of free grafts are represented by this diagram. See text for further discussion of the indications and uses of these different types of free skin grafts.

padding by supplying layers of skin over unstable scars is called overgrafting. The epidermis is removed by shaving or abrasion from the recipient area, and a split-thickness skin graft is applied on this open surface.

Split-Thickness Skin Grafts. Split-thickness skin grafts survive more easily than do full-thickness grafts, and the thinner the graft, the higher the incidence of "take' or success. This is because the split-thickness graft probably survives shortly after transfer by the exchange of extracellular fluid. It is invaded rapidly by new capillaries from the wound bed and probably becomes vascularized by the second to the fourth day.

Full-thickness grafts, being thicker, are more demanding on the recipient wound. They require a very adequate, if not rich, blood supply and are associated with minimal scarring and the absence of infection. These grafts contain their own vasculature intact. Early vascularization occurs both from the wound edges and from the bed to the undersurface of the graft. It is possible that vascular anastomoses are established within a few hours after transfer. Such anastomosis may precede the ingrowth of new vessels into the graft, which occurs from the second post-transfer day onward.

Nutrition by extracellular fluid exchange probably plays less of a role in the survival of full-thickness grafts than it does in split-thickness grafts.

From the foregoing description of free skin grafts, it is not difficult to understand why split-thickness grafts are favored as temporary dressing grafts in large defects or for use in irradiated tissue, infected or potentially infected wounds, granulating wounds, or large wounds where it would be difficult to provide full-thickness grafts of sufficient size.

The full-thickness skin graft is always preferred for facial reconstruction. It provides a better cosmetic result than the split graft in texture, bulk, and color. Sometimes it is very difficult to detect a well-placed full-thickness graft several months after transfer.

Composite Graft. A composite graft is one that is composed of two or more different tissues. The term usually refers to the chondrocutaneous auricular graft, which is most useful in reconstructing full-thickness defects of the nasal tip or ala nasi (Fig. 65–21). When tumor resection of the nose sacrifices full-thickness tissue, an exact pattern of the defect is made, and a suitably shaped donor area of the ear is selected. Such grafts may be

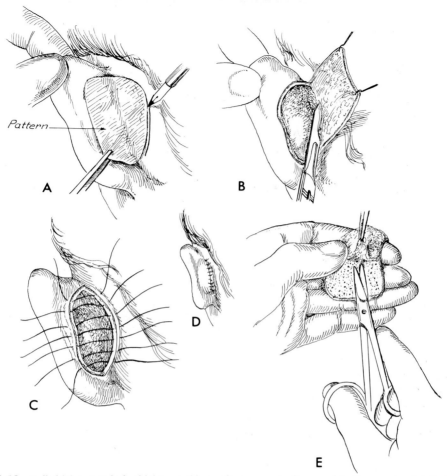

Figure 65–18 Full-thickness (whole-thickness) skin grafts are most often used in the repair of defects of the facial region following tumor ablation. They are superior because they do not contract to a significant degree and are of excellent color match. The postauricular skin is a choice donor area. The technique of cutting a postauricular skin graft is shown. Note the all-important step of trimming away the subcutaneous fat (*E*).

Figure 65–19 Another excellent donor site for whole-thickness skin grafts is the supraclavicular area. The redundancy of skin in this region permits primary closure of the wound even when large grafts are taken. It is of second choice in a woman, however, because of the visible scar that is left in the neck.

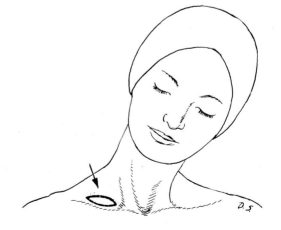

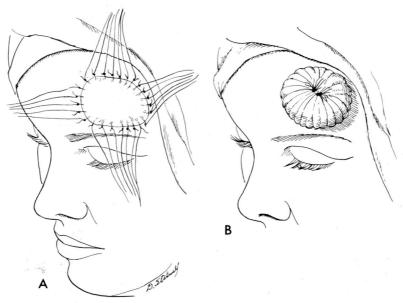

Figure 65–20   Whole-thickness skin grafts require early vascularization for survival. Such grafts should be immobilized, and the bandage should provide even pressure for the first few days. Tie-over dressings are most useful for this purpose.

of full thickness of the ear or skin-cartilage skin, or if all layers are not required, then one layer of skin attached to cartilage suffices.

Composite grafts must be handled atraumatically. They should be handled not by instruments but, rather, gently by the surgeon's hands or the employment of traction sutures. They are sutured exactly into the defect with fine sutures and extremely sharp needles. These grafts probably survive by direct vascular anasto-

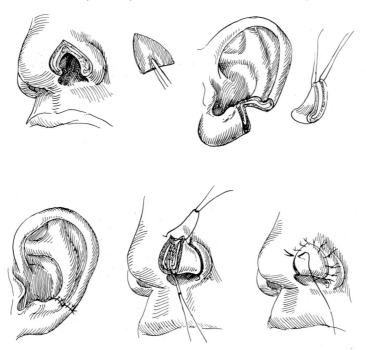

Figure 65–21   The chondrocutaneous composite graft is most useful in reconstructing defects of the nasal tip. The donor site on the ear is easily closed with little resulting deformity. Composite grafts have also been used between the eyelids and the lips.

the border of the lesion itself. The specimen should include a border of the lesion along with normal tissue. For lesions suggesting keratoacanthoma, the paracentral fusiform incisional biopsy technique is advised. The specimen should be handled with fine forceps or skin hooks so that it is not crushed or otherwise mutilated, rendering it poor for histologic processing. Particular attention should be given to the use of atraumatic technique in order to minimize the possibility of tumor seeding and implantation. Prior removal of any crusting present on or about the lesion should be done. Many times a negative diagnosis will be obtained in the presence of a positive clinical lesion because only the crusts were removed with the biopsy specimen. The use of sharp instruments for a biopsy causes little distortion of the tissues and allows for accurate suturing of the margins so that healing can occur per primam and with the least amount of inflammatory reaction.

The following are relative contraindications for incisional biopsy: (1) lesions which have a definite angiomatous appearance; (2) pigmented lesions that are clinically suspected of being melanomas, unless they are of a size or in a location that precludes a total excisional biopsy; (3) intraosseous cystic lesions; and (4) lesions in patients on anticoagulant therapy, unless the prothrombin level is evaluated (also true for other biopsy techniques).

Excisional Biopsy

A biopsy may be both diagnostic and therapeutic, as exemplified by the total excisional type. An excisional biopsy implies the total gross removal of the lesion in breadth and depth, which serves as the biopsy specimen. This is the method of choice for lesions of such size and in such a location that they may be readily removed and the defect closed primarily without difficulty. It is indicated for both benign and malignant tumors and particularly for a lesion suspected of being a malignant melanoma. The total excision of a melanoma enables the surgeon and pathologist to define the type of melanoma and the depth of invasion, criteria

that help determine the extent of the definitive surgery as to wide excision and the need for elective regional lymph node dissection. Whenever there exists any question as to the extent of the margins or the depth of invasion of a lesion, the excisional biopsy should be considered as purely diagnostic.

There is a great temptation to place biopsy incisions in natural skin lines. For the clinically benign lesion and the small malignant tumor, the cosmetic result is more acceptable if incisions correspond to the skin lines. However, in dealing with tumors of the skin, particularly malignant lesions, the excisional biopsy may be the first in a series of operations designed for the cure of the patient. Biopsy incisions for these lesions, particularly for melanoma, should be placed in the direction of the suspected pathway of lymphatic drainage, and this often does not follow natural skin lines. Necessary subsequent surgery becomes more difficult to perform, and more tissue removal is required if biopsy incisions are poorly planned.

If total excisional biopsy is decided upon, closure should be accomplished per primam. The use of grafts and flaps in such a primary procedure is discouraged (particularly should it be necessary to later identify and subsequently resect the tumor bed, and should the pathologist report that the lesion had not been completely excised). The patient should be apprised of the fact that re-excision may be necessary, depending upon the operative findings and the pathologic report. This explanation not only will avoid any later difficulties but also will help the patient to understand the nature of his problem.

Punch Biopsy

By means of a punch biopsy instrument, small cylinders of tissue are removed from the center of a lesion. The real advantage lies in the fact that it is a procedure which may be used for obtaining a specimen from an otherwise inaccessible area. It also allows for sampling of questionably suspicious lesions of the skin. In some instances a small lesion may be entirely removed using this technique. The main disadvantages are that the tissue obtained is often extremely small, it may not be totally representative of the lesion, the normal tissue margins are not included in the specimen, and the tissues may be crushed, thereby distorting relationships.

Shave Biopsy

Dermatologists frequently use shave biopsies to obtain specimens for histopathologic examination. A saucerlike, practically horizontal incision is made with the scalpel, usually in a single sweep through the lesion. The depth of the incision may be easily varied once some degree of skill has been achieved.

The procedure serves to provide a biopsy specimen and at the same time levels the tumor down to the skin surface, leaving a flat scar, usually with an excellent cosmetic result. It can be performed expeditiously with little bleeding and is often used when the tumor is subsequently to be definitively treated by electrodesiccation and curettage.

Shave biopsies are not ordinarily applicable for deeply seated lesions in which pathologic evaluation of the margins and depths is essential.

Aspiration and Needle Biopsy

This form of biopsy has the immediate advantage of establishing whether or not a lesion is cystic or solid and, if solid, whether or not it is benign or malignant. These advantages are tempered by the intrinsic deficiencies of the technique. The sections of tissue obtained are very small and often too scanty for the planning of major surgery on the basis of this pathologic data alone. There is always the possible danger of seeding and implantation occurring along the needle tract. Should the diagnosis prove to be malignant, the needle tract should be removed with the excised specimen. This is probably the least desirable of all the biopsy techniques; its place may be in the large cystic lesions of soft tissue, bone, and lymph nodes.

Frozen Section Technique

Frozen sections have been a great aid in the management as well as diagnosis of cancer. Recently, with the introduction of the cryostat, there has been significant improvement, and the technique has proved to be of incalculable value in the epithelial carcinomas and adenocarcinomas. However, the accuracy of the technique is limited in cutaneous lesions. The hazards created by an unrepresentative portion of tissue and a resulting incorrect diagnosis on the part of the pathologist cannot be overstated. Diagnosis made wholly by frozen section technique rarely justifies any large operative procedure that would seriously interfere with function or appearance.

At the time of definitive surgery, frozen section examination of margins may be helpful to determine the adequacy of the excision. This is especially valuable for lesions with clinically indefinite borders.

"Chemosurgical Check"

Recently, the refinement of the technique of Mohs' chemosurgery and its application in the treatment of difficult neoplasms of the skin has made available to the surgeon another method for determining the adequacy of the surgical margins following excision. This method is known as the "chemosurgical check." Following excision, a thin layer of Mohs' zinc chloride paste is applied to the remaining tissues, and thus this tissue is fixed in situ. This fixed tissue is then removed and examined immediately using frozen section techniques. If necessary, the operative field may be extended at this time.

Curettage

As a biopsy technique, curettage is used most often in lesions of the medullary region of bone. It may be utilized on the skin in relatively inaccessible areas. The specimens obtained are usually disappointing because of the crushing and tearing effect caused by the technique.

SURGICAL APPROACH TO CANCER OF THE SKIN

In determining the surgical approach for cancer of the skin the following factors should be considered: (1) the anatomic location of the lesion; (2) the microscopic evaluation of the specimen; (3) the extent of invasiveness of the lesion; (4) the physical and psychologic status of the patient; and (5) whether or not the lesion is primary, recurrent, or metastatic.

Before embarking upon any surgical procedure, the anatomic location of the lesion itself must be considered. This includes the presence of adjacent and nearby structures, such as eyelid margins, motor and sensory nerves, and such underlying structures as bone, cartilage, arteries, and veins. Whenever possible, all important structures should be preserved. No tissue should be needlessly sacrificed; no tissue should be salvaged if it interferes with adequate surgery for the malignant disease. In the microscopic evaluation of the malignant lesion, the extent of invasion at the margins and depth of invasion are of utmost importance. The recurrent lesion necessitates taking wider and deeper margins than does a primary lesion of the same size and site.

In any surgical procedure selected for a suspicious lesion, the use of careful "tumor technique" is mandatory. This implies the most gentle handling of all tissues, the use of fine instruments, and the discarding of clamps and needles after initial use for resterilization before being used again at the same operation. Should the surgeon anticipate the need for a skin graft, the graft from a distant site should be taken first and before definitive excision is performed. If the need for a graft has been uncertain at the start of the procedure, then it is advisable for the surgeon and his assistants to change gowns, gloves, and instruments before proceeding from a tumor-bearing area to a non–tumor-bearing area of the body. Even with the most careful application of "tumor technique," circulating tumor cells have been demonstrated in the blood stream in patients undergoing definitive surgery. It has been shown that the presence of these cells does not necessarily

mean that metastases will develop at some distant site, but certainly all attempts should be made to keep the number of cells to a minimum.

It is most important that prior to operation the planned extent of the incision or excision be marked out with a dye, such as methylene blue. This should be done prior to the infiltration of local anesthetic agents in order to avoid distortion of the tissue. As the incision progresses, the deep surgical margin of the specimen is carefully palpated to be sure that it, too, has an adequate surgical border. It is the surgeon's responsibility to orient the specimen for the pathologist so that the most meaningful interpretation can be obtained, and so that subsequent observation can be directed to areas of questionable involvement. This is very easily accomplished by placing sutures at several margins of the specimen and properly identifying these margins.

Following microscopic examination, should the pathologist report that the lesion extended to the surgical border, then consideration should be given to performing a re-excision. If the surgeon feels that his surgical margins are doubtfully wide of the lesion, re-excision should be done. When re-excision of the incompletely excised area is required, it may be deferred until the operative site has healed. If the operative site was closed primarily without a graft, the entire area should be re-excised if the tumor reaches a surgical margin of the specimen. Re-excision of the entire area need not be performed if only one border is involved, if a free graft was used for the closure, and if the specimen was carefully oriented by the surgeon for the pathologist. On the other hand, if several borders are involved, there may be no advantage in waiting for the operative site to heal and the graft to take, since the entire area should be re-excised.

In many instances, primary closure of the surgical wound cannot be accomplished; therefore, the use of other forms of closure becomes necessary. In general, either a full-thickness or split-thickness skin graft is preferred to the use of flaps. Although the split-thickness skin graft may not produce the immediate good cosmetic result that a rotated flap affords, the use of a free skin graft allows the surgeon to observe the tumor area for any evidence of possible recurrence. A flap rotated over an area of excision not only will tend to obscure any recurrences but also will add to the operative risk of spreading tumor cells over the surgical field. If the pathologist subsequently reports that the lesion has been incompletely excised, then re-excision of the entire area, including the flap, may be required because of possible contamination with residual tumor cells. At some later date, when the surgeon is reasonably satisfied that there is no evidence of recurrence, a reconstructive procedure may be performed for cosmetic reasons. The propensity of malignant tumors of the skin to recur is well known and should be borne in mind by all physicians treating these diseases. This problem is best avoided by adequate initial treatment.

In surgical procedures performed for malignant melanoma, it is desirable to use suture material which is not dark in color in order that any retained sutures, either under a graft or at the excision site, will not be mistaken for recurrent disease.

When dealing with cancer of the skin, the malignant melanoma requires separate classification in regard to regional lymph node dissection because of the characteristic aggressiveness and unpredictable behavior of the melanoma, including that of the amelanotic variety.

In general, an elective regional lymph node dissection is performed in most instances of invasive malignant melanoma. The exceptions include a melanoma which is definitely classified as superficial (levels I and II); a melanoma arising in the melanotic freckle of Hutchinson; a melanoma with the primary site so situated that the lymphatic drainage may be to several different groups of regional lymph nodes; the presence of serious intercurrent disease; the presence of distant metastases; and a melanoma in the aged patient.

The approach to the regional nodes is somewhat different when considering other malignant skin lesions, chiefly squamous cell carcinoma. The incidence of regional node metastases in the latter has been reported to be approximately 10 percent; therefore, a regional lymph node dissection is performed therapeutically rather than before clinical involvement becomes apparent. Needless to say, the patient must be carefully followed in all instances, and the surgeon must act as early as possible. Our impression is that the possibility for control of the disease is still good using this approach for the squamous cell carcinoma, even when there is subsequent metastasis to the lymph nodes.

CONCLUSION

There is no single routine type of biopsy technique applicable to all neoplasms of the skin. Biopsy techniques include incisional, excisional, punch, shave, aspiration and needle, frozen section, "chemosurgical check," and curettage. They have specific applications in the management of tumors of the skin and are performed singly or in combination where necessary.

A properly performed and informative biopsy is the initial phase in the development of a well-planned approach to surgery for cancer of the skin. It should be mentioned that other modalities are available for the treatment of tumors of the skin, and often a combination of therapy is necessary to achieve the desired result.

REFERENCES

Ackerman, L. V., and Rosai, J.: The pathology of tumors. Part III. Frozen section, gross and microscopic examination, ancillary studies. CA, 21:270, 1971.

Agostino, D., and Clifton, E. E.: Organ localization and the effect of trauma on the fate of circulating cancer cells. Cancer Res., 25:1728, 1965.

Cole, W. H., McDonald, G. D., Roberts, S. S., and Southwick, H. W.: Dissemination of Cancer: Prevention and Therapy. New York, Appleton-Century-Crofts, 1961.

Epstein, E., Bragg, K., and Linden, G.: Biopsy and prognosis of malignant melanoma. J.A.M.A., 208:1369, 1969.

Epstein, E., Epstein, N. N., Bragg, K., and Linden, G.: Metastases from squamous cell carcinomas of the skin. Arch. Dermatol., 97:245, 1968.

Glass, R. L., Spratt, J. S., Jr., and Perez, C.: Fate of inadequately excised epidermoid carcinoma of skin. Surg. Gynecol. Obstet., 122:245, 1966.

for one to two weeks, after which time a dry Telfa dressing may be sufficient. It is wise to inform the patient that there will be exudation and later crusting. The presence of an erythematous halo around the crust should arouse suspicion about the possibility of secondary infection. If persistent granulation tissue impedes epithelialization, application of 10 percent aqueous silver nitrate solution is helpful at weekly or semiweekly intervals. Follow-up visits to observe the patient for recurrence of basal cell epithelioma are suggested every three months during the first year, every six months during the second year, and once yearly thereafter up to eight years. For squamous cell carcinoma, follow-up visits during the first and second years should be more frequent.

COMPLICATIONS AND DRAWBACKS

In contrast to excisional surgery, the technique of curettage and electrodesicca-

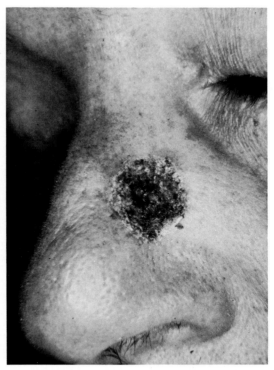

Figure 67–5 Basal cell epithelioma immediately following treatment by curettage and electrodesiccation. The procedure in this case was repeated a total of three times.

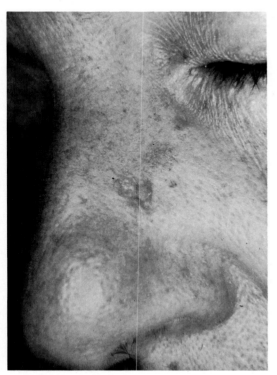

Figure 67–4 Basal cell epithelioma before treatment.

tion provides no specimen for the pathologist to determine the adequacy of borders. Instead, the operator must rely on his judgment and skill in deciding when sufficient curettage and electrodesiccation have been performed. However, the sense of feel and resistance to the scraping action of the curet help to provide the experienced clinician with this knowledge.

The healing time is prolonged, as compared with excisional surgery. Often healing requires two to four weeks, depending upon the size and extent of the lesion. The patient is inconvenienced only to a minor degree by this delay in healing—usually to the extent of daily dressing changes until a healing crust forms on the wound.

The appearance of the scar of curettage and electrosurgery improves with age (Figs. 67–4 to 67–8). However, it has drawbacks, as compared with the scar of excisional surgery (Figs. 67–9 and 67–10). Since many cases of skin cancer on the face occur in actinically damaged skin and may show telangiectasias and pigmentary oddity, the resulting scar of curettage and electrosurgery usually ends as a white patch (Figs. 67–11 to 67–13). This leukodermic end result is particularly pronounced when curettage and electrosurgery must be performed many times on a sun-damaged skin surface. By contrast, the scar of excisional surgery apposes sun-damaged skin, resulting in a linear type of scar which tends to become less conspicuous with the passage of time (Figs. 67–9 and 67–10).

As compared with radiation therapy, the curet and electrosurgical spark are less advisable in the special areas previously mentioned, i.e., the tip and ala of the nose, the vermilion border and commissures of the mouth, the eyelid margins, and the canthi. The appearance of the scar of radiation therapy, while good for the first few years, tends to deteriorate with the passage of time, developing telangiectasia and more pronounced atrophy in some cases.

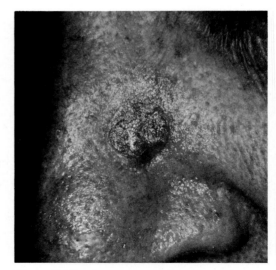

Figure 67–7   Appearance of treated site one month after curettage and electrodesiccation.

Complications of electrosurgery and curettage are few. One is delayed bleeding. When the treatment takes place in the vicinity of a small-sized arteriole, the later separation of tissue slough may result in vigorous and alarming bleeding. This complication can be managed by suture ligature at the time of the complication. The patient should be instructed to apply firm point pressure should this complication arise. If there is a strong likelihood of the complication occurring, preliminary suture ligature of the adjacent artery can be undertaken prior to beginning treatment, although this is rarely necessary. The author has seen this complication only twice in many thousands of cases. In both cases the complication occurred several days to one week after the electrosurgery and curettage.

Occasionally hypertrophic scars (Figs. 67–14 and 67–15) and keloids arise. The latter are more likely to be seen on the presternal or deltoid areas. Hypertrophic scars tend to subside spontaneously over a period of time, but their resolution may be hastened by the use of intralesionally injected triamcinolone suspension diluted to 2 to 5 mg. per ml. This may be done at intervals of one to two months until flattening of the hypertrophic scar is noted. Usually the injection of a few drops is sufficient. Contracture types of scars (so-called skin folds) are not infrequently

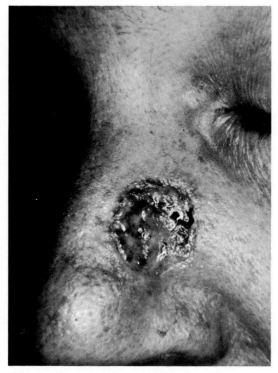

Figure 67–6   Appearance of the treated site one week after curettage and electrodesiccation.

Text continued on page 1510.

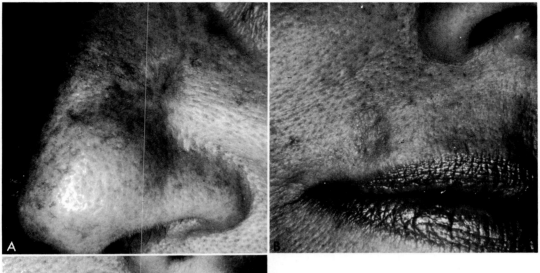

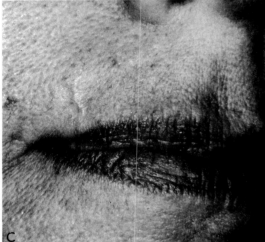

Figure 67–8 *A*, Healed end result one year after treatment of a basal cell epithelioma by curettage and electrodesiccation. *B*, Basal cell epithelioma. *C*, Excellent linear type of scar six months after treatment by curettage and electrodesiccation.

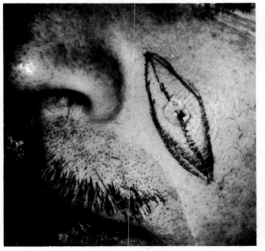

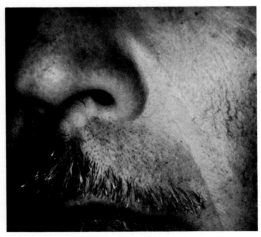

Figure 67–9 Basal cell epithelioma: projected excision outlined prior to local anesthesia infiltration.

Figure 67–10 Seven years after excision of basal cell epithelioma.

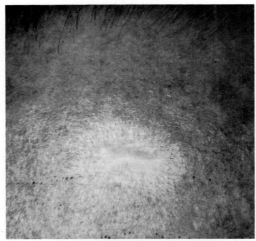

Figure 67–11 White scar following treatment of a basal cell epithelioma by curettage and electrodesiccation.

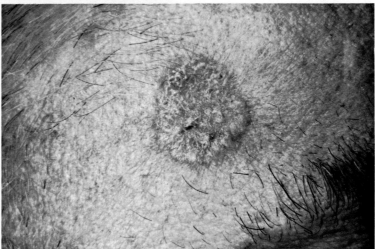

Figure 67–12 Basal cell epithelioma.

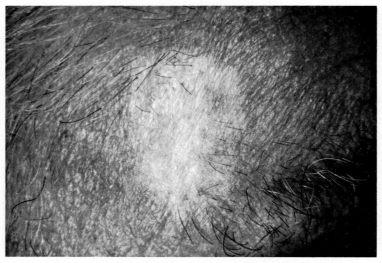

Figure 67–13 Scar several months after treatment of basal cell epithelioma by curettage and electrodesiccation. Hypopigmentation is not unusual against a background of actinically damaged skin.

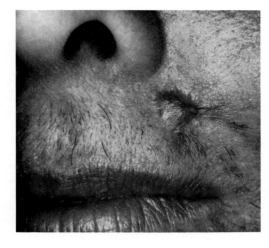

Figure 67–14 Hypertrophic scar after curettage and electrodesiccation of basal cell epithelioma.

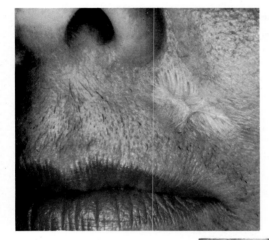

Figure 67–15 Hypertrophic scar two years later, showing considerable subsidence of hypertrophic aspects.

Figure 67–16 Basal cell epithelioma prior to treatment.

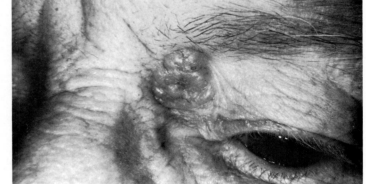

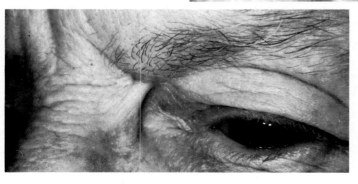

Figure 67–17 Skin fold type of scar following treatment by curettage and electrodesiccation. This is a complication seen on either side of the nose adjacent to the inner aspect of the eyelids.

seen after curettage and electrodesiccation of basal cell epitheliomas on either side of the nose adjacent to the inner aspect of the eyelids (Figs. 67–16 and 67–17).

For keloids, no completely satisfactory method of therapy has been devised. Administration of intralesional steroids, such as triamcinolone acetonide, at monthly intervals may help to reduce the keloid, particularly if it is a relatively new lesion. Often, however, the steroid suppresses the keloid growth. When the triamcinolone is absorbed, the intralesional injections must be repeated periodically as the keloid shows signs of becoming active. For treatment of keloids, excisional surgery combined with radiation therapy may yield success. However, schedules for such treatment vary, and patient response is highly unpredictable. Often the patient ends up with a new and larger keloid or must be satisfied with some degree of radiation sequelae replacing the keloid.

REFERENCES

Elliott, J. A.: Electrosurgery. Arch. Dermatol., 94:340, 1966.

Graham, J. H., and Helwig, E. B.: Precancerous skin lesions and systemic cancer. *In* Tumors of the Skin. Chicago, Year Book Medical Publishers, 1964, p. 209.

Jackson, R.: Basic principles of electrosurgery: A Review. Can. J. Surg., 13:354, 1970.

Popkin, G. L.: Curettage and electrodesiccation. N.Y. State J. Med., 68:866, 1968.

68

Radiotherapy from the Dermatologist's Point of View

Arthur H. Gladstein, M.D., and Earle W. Brauer, M.D.

INTRODUCTION

The use of radiation therapy in the management of many types of skin malignancies has been a recognized procedure since the early part of the century. Its popularity gained with advances in equipment, devices (e.g., shock-proof machines, beryllium window tubes), and techniques and waned with the improvement or introduction of other cancer-curing procedures—increasingly skillful plastic surgery, high frequency diathermy, topical cytotoxic agents, Mohs' chemosurgery, and related procedures.

There exists today a distinct and important position for roentgen radiation in the management of skin malignancies, as evidenced by the following:

1. Competent skill can be easily and rapidly acquired by the interested physician.

2. Experienced ancillary personnel, while helpful, are not necessary.

3. The outpatient clinic or private office regimen usually makes hospitalization of the patient unnecessary. There is rarely a hiatus in wage-earning capacity.

4. Pain and disability during treatment are minor or of no consequence.

5. Malignancies in selected sites often establish radiation therapy as the method of choice—for example, the eyelid, where skin tissue must be spared; the tip of the nose, where cosmetic factors are a paramount consideration; loci in and about the vicinity of vital structures, such as the ramus mandibularis or the facial nerve, where tissue sparing may prove exceedingly difficult with other modalities.

6. Patients whose overall medical status makes them poor surgical risks become candidates for radiation therapy.

7. Extensive malignancies, in which the goal is simply palliation, are best treated by radiation.

Naturally, there are disadvantages to the use of radiation therapy; these will be discussed as this chapter advances.

The principles expressed in the sections that follow reflect several decades of practice and experience with clinic and private patient populations. However, all data relating to recurrence and cure rates have been derived only from the extensive follow-up program conducted by the Oncology Section of our clinic, the electronically controlled data retrieval program of which has been described elsewhere.

An assumption is made that the reader has a basic knowledge of radiation therapy, for there will be little discussion relating to the equipment that produces ionizing radiation or to basic radiobiology. The election or rejection of this modality in the management of a skin malignancy becomes a matter of judgment on the part of the treating physician. The authors do not wish to convey the impression that skin malignancies *in general* are best treated with roentgen radiation.

In terms of pure technique, the major variables in the application of radiotherapy are:

1. *Quality.* Expressed as half value layer (HVL), half-dose depth (H-DD or $D\frac{1}{2}$), or occasionally peak kilovoltage (kvp.) with or without added filtration of the incident beam.

2. *Quantity.* Total dose of radiation administered, now expressed as rads, meaning "roentgen absorbed dose." This unit is more accurate than the older form of roentgen, R., (formerly r.), which denoted the ionizing energy potential in air. *N.B.:* When quantity of radiation is expressed throughout this chapter, virtually no difference is made between rad and R; consequently, these terms will be used interchangeably.

3. *Dosage schedule.* The number of R.'s delivered per dose and the time interval between treatments.

With the considerable latitude present in the variables listed above, inevitably an inordinately large number of differing treatment procedures have been published, taught, and practiced. Each regimen may yield success; some possess advantages over others. However, the diversity in techniques confounds comparison. Conclusions from long-term follow-up studies fail to meet requirements for statistical validity. The modality conveys an aura of hopeless complexity that seriously compromises the successful teaching of radiation therapy.

To mitigate the above, many years ago, one of us (EWB) established a "standard treatment program" at the New York Skin and Cancer Unit. It was derived from a

schedule suggested by the late Dr. Lionel C. Rubin.

This treatment schedule was selected because it gave every indication of successfully eradicating skin cancer (basal and squamous cell types) while being well tailored to the pattern of patient visits at the clinic or private office. It was never meant to be other than a teaching and research device. Once the physician trainee gained knowledge and confidence with the schedule, he was encouraged to vary it in his private practice to suit his own judgment and needs. Now, 25 years later, we are the beneficiaries of a wealth of carefully catalogued and easily retrievable data based on a single procedure. The goal has been fulfilled and the validity of the effort justified.

A STANDARD PROGRAM FOR THE TREATMENT OF BASAL AND SQUAMOUS CELL EPITHELIOMAS OF THE SKIN

Patient Selection

Only patients under the age of 40 years are excluded. This arbitrary age boundary was selected since the cosmetic appearance of radiation scars deteriorates with time. Advancing atrophy, alteration in skin color, and telangiectasia 8 to 10 years post-treatment may be of considerable severity but of small concern to a patient beyond the sixth decade of life. The patient with fair skin and blue eyes may be more susceptible to such sequelae. Skin exhibiting actinic damage need not be a contraindication to treatment. Previous radiation therapy in significant or unknown quantity deserves careful consideration.

Skin Site Selection

Any accessible area of the head and neck may be selected. While this radiation procedure will eradicate the epitheliomas of the trunk or extremities, it is not recommended for these loci. Early in our program a disproportionate number of successfully treated lesions in these areas produced painful, persistent, nonmalignant ulcers after several years. This has been attributed to the added friction, the weight-bearing insult, and the less favorable circulation typical of these acral sites. Permanent alopecia, a considerable cosmetic defect, occurs in hair-bearing areas.

Size of Lesion

The lesion should have a minimum diameter clinically determined to be not less than 1 cm. Lesions in excess of 10 cm. have been successfully treated; however, healing, particularly over the scalp, is considerably delayed.

Shielding of Lesion

With a skin-marking pencil, a border no less than 0.5 cm. from the clinically determined circumferential edge of the neoplasm is outlined. In lead foil sheeting 0.35 mm. thick, a template is cut with scissors to exactly conform to this pencil-marked border. The patient is then shielded in accordance with good medical practice (Cipollaro and Crossland, 1967).

Where the exit dose might affect tissue in apposition, such as the nasal septum and the gingiva, lead shielding is inserted into the nostril and beneath the lips to protect such surfaces.

Eye lesions demand special consideration (Kopf, 1971). Commercial shields of brass, graded for eye size, or specially fabricated shields (Gladstein, 1974) may be used. The mucosal surface of the eye is anesthetized with butacaine sulfate (Butyn) or a similar agent prior to insertion of the shield. At the conclusion of treatment, the shield is removed, ophthalmic antibiotic ointment is inserted, and an eye patch is applied immediately. The patch should not be removed for two to three hours to assure return of the corneal reflex.

Radiation Schedule

Reduced to its essentials, treatment planning for cutaneous malignancies in-volves selecting the quality of radiation (penetration) and the quantity (number of roentgens) (Table 68–1). Our "standard" procedure used in the past can be summarized as follows:

Quality of
  radiation: 0.9 mm. Al HVL

Quantity of
  radiation: Basal cell carcinoma, 3400 R.

                680 R. given every other day for five treatments

                Squamous cell carcinoma, 5440 R.

                680 R. every two or three days for eight treatments

Note that originally no real attempt was made to correlate the depth of the pathologic process with the quality of the radiation. It is a recognized principle in radiation therapy of neoplasms that the depth of the tumor should receive 50 percent of the surface dose. Recently, in conjunction with the acquisition of more modern roentgen apparatus, the same quantity of radiation is used, but the quality of the roentgen beam is selected in accordance with the established depth of disease. To understand how this is accomplished, a review of the following is in order. Half value layer (HVL) is the thickness of aluminum (Al) that reduces the intensity of a roentgen ray beam by one half. It is a standard means for identifying the quality of dermatologic roentgen radiation. Jennings in 1951 introduced the concept of half value depth (HVD or D $\frac{1}{2}$). Instead of aluminum being used as the index, skin or tissue is used. By definition, D $\frac{1}{2}$ is the depth in tissue at which the dose is 50 percent of the surface dose. The more penetrating ("harder") the roentgen beam, the greater the thickness of skin that will be required to absorb half the surface dose. In our department, we have modified the term "half value depth" to "half-dose depth" because we believe it more accurately describes the concept.

For the practical application of the half dose depth concept, the following must be accomplished:

1. The depth of the tumor under con-

TABLE 68-1. RADIATION SCHEDULE

Half value layer	0.9 mm. Al*
Voltage	100 kilovolts (peak)*
Added filtration	None*
Target-to-skin distance	20 cm.*
Current	5–10 milliamperes*
Dose per treatment	680 roentgens (air dose)
Total dose:	
Basal cell carcinoma	3400 roentgens (air dose)
Squamous cell carcinoma	5440 roentgens (air dose)
Number of treatments:	
Basal cell carcinoma	5
Squamous cell carcinoma	8
Interval	2–3 days
Time span	
Basal cell carcinoma	9–14 days
Squamous cell carcinoma	16–21 days
Minimum port diameter	2 cm.

*Factors utilized with original roentgen ray apparatus.

sideration is estimated. This is accomplished by examining mounted biopsy specimens with a microscope equipped with a micrometer.

2. The established depth of the tumor is then located on a calibration chart (Table 68–2), from which the treatment factors are established. For example, focus your attention on the D ½ mm. column of Table 68–2; for a neoplasm 8 mm. in depth, select the treatment factors corresponding with the figure 10 (Step 4), the closest calibration for this tumor depth. On our new apparatus, the equipment is set at 50 kv. with a filter of 1 mm. Al and a target-skin distance of 15 cm. For a tumor with a depth of 15 mm., the setting for Step 5 is utilized.

Radiation Response and Healing

At the time of the third scheduled treatment, redness and early swelling should be apparent. These will gain in intensity in succeeding days. Eventually a frank radiodermatitis *must* be observed, consisting of tenderness and a variable-sized surrounding zone of inflammation (edema and necrosis of tissue). If this acute radioreaction is not observed within 10 days of the last treatment, one, two, or more treatments must be immediately instituted to achieve this effect if a treatment failure is to be avoided. Complete healing usually occurs within six to eight weeks of the last treatment.

As the radionecrotic area heals, often a typical gray-brown crust develops that appears to be "pasted on" the ulcer surface. A thick gray discharge is beneath. This crust should be removed. An antibiotic cream or ointment may be prescribed for daily application.

During the early healing period of lesions treated on the nose, slight bleeding may be observed by the patient upon sneezing or upon forceful expiration through the nose. Lip lesions can be painful in the immediate postradiation period, and a bland diet is indicated.

Several weeks after the treated site has healed, especially about the nose and cheeks, a transient coronal zone of hyperpigmentation with dilated giant comedones is occasionally observed. This gradually disappears. However, the cosmetic effect is rapidly improved if the comedones are expressed manually. The time-dose relationship of this fractionated technique for basal-cell carcinoma (BCE) falls slightly below the curve offered by Strandqvist (1944), yet the cure rate in long-term follow-up is 93 percent.

Points for Special Consideration

1. The multicentric superficial basal cell epithelioma responds best to ultrasoft radiation and will be discussed in the section on grenz rays.

2. The morphea or sclerosing type of basal cell epithelioma is, contrary to general belief, radiosensitive and will respond well to the above procedure with one variation: the allowance for very liberal borders, no less than 1 cm. from the clinical edge, within the treatment port.

3. The adenocystic basal cell epithelioma is radiosensitive; however, a higher dosage schedule is required to achieve acceptable cure rates. Therefore, these lesions should receive the same dosage schedule as squamous cell epitheliomas.

4. The basosquamous or mixed cell type of epithelioma requires the same management as a squamous cell epithelioma.

5. Regional lymphadenopathy indicating metastasis or suspicion of metastasis in association with a primary squamous cell epithelioma (especially of the lip or auri-

TABLE 68–2. CALIBRATION FACTORS

	kv.	ma.	Filter	HVL (mm.) Aluminum	HDD D½mm. Tissue	TSD (cm.)	R./Min. Air	85 R. Min.	85 R. Sec.	100 R. Min.	100 R. Sec.	340 R. Min.	340 R. Sec.
Step 1	14	25	None	0.025	0.5	15	2360				2.5		
				0.032	0.9	30	350				17		
Step 2	29	25	0.3	0.1	2	15	430		12		14		48
						30	104		49		58	3	17
Step 3	43	25	0.6	0.35	6	15	448		11		13		44
					7	30	109		47		55	3	7
Step 4	50	25	1.0	0.85	10	15	408		13	1	15		50
					12	30	100		51			3	24
Step 5	50	25	2.0	1.3	13	15	195	1	26	2	31	1	45
					17	30	48		46		6	7	5
Teleroentgen Step 4	50	25	None	0.08	1.5	100	158	3	32	4	38	2	9
				0.17	2.0	200	20.5		55		52	16	40

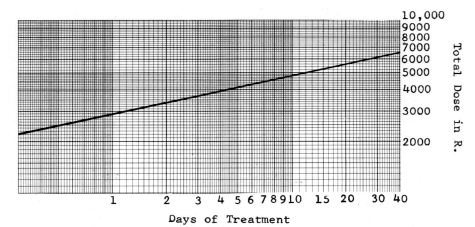

Figure 68–1 A practical average curve establishing equivalent total dose in relationship to fractionation for basal and squamous cell carcinoma of the skin, e.g., 2250 R. in a single massive dose is essentially equivalent to 4200 R. administered in equally divided doses every six days.

cle) considerably reduces the option for this dermatologic superficial radiotherapy.

6. A basal or squamous cell epithelioma situated over but not invading the cartilage of the ear or nose can be safely treated with this regimen.

Common causes for a radiation failure are:

1. Misdiagnosis and/or improper selection of a treatment schedule.

2. Too conservative an identification of the clinical margin of the neoplasm. This is especially true if tumor reappearance occurs at the edge of the radiated site.

3. Inadequate total dosage or selection of a schedule of fractionation that is too protracted. In such instances tumor reappearance will usually be near the center of the radiated site.

The success described previously with this standard program should be achieved by any practitioner. The following recommendations are made:

1. Have the calibration of the roentgen apparatus checked regularly by a physicist expert in such procedures.

2. Be certain that no variation occurs in total dosage delivered or in the period of fractionation.

3. Ascertain that a radiodermatitis occurs. See the patient in the post-treatment period every other day, if necessary, to observe this critical sign. If it fails to appear, inadequate tissue dosage has been achieved. This can be the result of equipment failure, inaccurate technique, or a

radioresistance (idiosyncrasy) on the part of the patient.

4. Check older patients during the radiation exposure period to make certain body movement has not altered the direction of the incident beam. This can easily take place when the apparatus is "coned down" to produce a beam of small diameter.

Hints for Special Problems

The skin surface to be treated should always be a plane, with the incident beam directed at its center. Often in order to achieve this, it may be necessary to exert and maintain pressure and tension with improvised splints and adhesive tape struts.

On occasion a concave or convex surface will present itself—e.g., the region near the inner canthus or the tip of the nose. Consider this unusual "multiplaned" site to be a clock face or a wheel. At each treatment, direct the axis of the incident beam to a different position on the imaginary clock face:

Treatment No.	Position in Clock Face to which Beam Is Directed
1	12 o'clock
2	3 o'clock
3	6 o'clock
4	9 o'clock
5	Hub or center

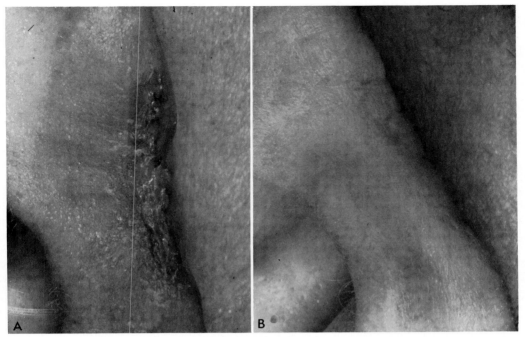

Figure 69–3 Basal cell carcinoma of the ear before (*A*) and one year following (*B*) radiation therapy. Apart from some slight loss of substance, the cosmetic effects are good. No chondritis is present.

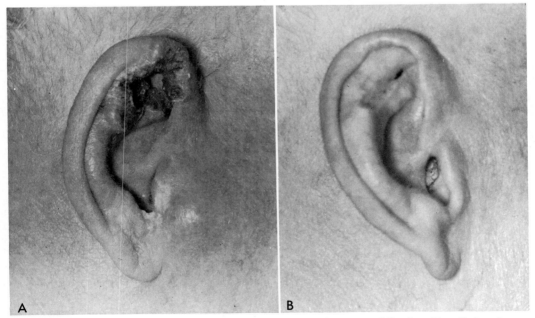

Figure 69–4 Squamous cell carcinoma of the ear before (*A*) and one year following (*B*) radiation therapy. The primary site is well healed without cartilage necrosis. In *A*, a preauricular lymph node is discernible. This was irradiated as well, with complete regression.

ence of Gooding et al. (1965), who found that clinical recurrences developed in only 35 percent of such patients. However, when follow-up may be difficult and in case of doubt, radiation should be given.

Squamous Cell Carcinoma

This lesion usually begins as a small growth above the skin surface having a tendency to ulcerate, the edge of which is irregular and lacks the well-defined border of the typical basal cell carcinoma. This lesion not only is locally invasive but also has the potential to spread to lymph nodes and eventually to distant sites. The incidence of lymph node metastases varies and has been variously reported as up to 12 to 15 percent. This figure is probably too high, and elective surgery or irradiation to the regional nodes is not necessary. However, careful follow-up examination of the nodes is mandatory.

There is no good evidence for a difference in radiosensitivity between basal and squamous cell carcinomas. It has been advocated that a smaller dose be used for the basal cell carcinoma on the grounds that the overriding principle of treatment is to obtain a good cosmetic effect and that any increased incidence of local failure which would be easily cured by excision is a small price to pay for a superior functional result. Whatever the merits of this approach to the management of the basal cell tumor, it has no place in the treatment of squamous carcinoma, and effective eradication of the tumor must be the fundamental principle of management. We use the same techniques and dose in the management of both basal and squamous cell carcinoma.

Keratoacanthoma

Keratoacanthoma has a characteristic history of a lesion developing over a few weeks and usually having a characteristic clinical appearance. Histologically it may be confused with squamous cell carcinoma, and when the clinical appearance is not absolutely typical, doubts may arise as to the correct management. The lesion will usually regress spontaneously without any treatment over a month or so, leaving a depressed scar. If there is doubt as to whether the lesion is squamous cell carcinoma or keratoacanthoma, it should be treated as the former. Radiation therapy will yield a minimum of untoward effects and avoid the potential dangers of a missed diagnosis of squamous cell carcinoma.

TECHNIQUES OF IRRADIATION

Three types of radiation are available in the modern radiotherapy department; x-rays of varying energy, radium and other radioactive isotopes in sealed form, and electrons. All play a part in the management of skin cancer, and each has specific indications.

External Irradiation

This is the most frequently used and generally most effective treatment modality. Although very superficial lesions may be successfully treated by beams of very low penetration, we believe for reasons already indicated that a standard technique be adopted using, for example, a minimum energy beam of 100 kv. to 120 kv. filtered by 1.0 to 3.0 mm. of aluminum. For lesions up to 1.0 cm. in maximum diameter, we use a treatment schedule of five sessions in five consecutive days. When the necessary field size exceeds 3.0 cm., it is necessary to individualize, depending on the site and characteristics of the lesion. In general, to obtain the best possible cosmetic result, treatment should be extended over longer periods. It is seldom necessary to treat over periods longer than three weeks, and then only if there is very extensive tumor destruction of bone. Adjacent sensitive structures must be protected from the beam, for example, by the use of silver-plated lead eye shields when treating lesions of the eyelids and inner canthus. Large and invasive skin cancers need not be considered beyond cure, and particularly when the required resection would be mutilative and require grafting and reparative procedures of magnitude, radiotherapy should be tried using, if necessary, more penetrating beams. Palliative therapy can be given in far advanced lesions with bone invasion in the hope of effecting growth restraint, control of bleeding, and relief of pain.

Treatment cones are available in varying sizes, and it is possible to treat these lesions by applying the applicator directly to the lesion. We believe, however, that to do so has disadvantages, in particular, the danger of movement during treatment, which results in part of the lesion being excluded from the beam. To avoid this, a lead mask of the appropriate size to accommodate the lesion should be prepared. The thickness of lead should be sufficient to filter out unnecessary radiation, and a cone of larger size than the diameter of the treated field should be used. For flat areas masks precut to a range of standard diameters can be used, but for difficult areas, such as the nasolabial folds, and when it is necessary to protect radiosensitive structures, such as the eyes, individually constructed masks should be used based on a plaster model of the patient. Details of the construction of such masks have been published by Paterson and Pointon (1963). Surprisingly one basic standard plaster model will frequently serve as a base for shaping the lead masks and may be a suitable compromise when the patient load is insufficient to support acquisition and development of the necessary mold-making skills.

With more deeply penetrating lesions, higher energy orthovoltage beams are necessary, and the shorter treatment times will not be used. Particularly in the case of bone invasion, the use of a megavoltage beam with a multiple field technique, when necessary, will have advantages. If the megavoltage beam is used, it must be remembered that the maximum energy build-up is deep to the skin surface (at a depth which varies with the beam energy), and suitable bolus must be used to ensure that the skin is fully irradiated.

Small lesions may be effectively cured by single treatments of 2000 to 2250 rads. The long-term cosmetic effects are poorer, however, and a higher incidence of late skin change and necrosis is found. Single treatments are therefore to be recommended only in exceptional circumstances.

Dose. Success in radiotherapy depends upon a favorable ratio between the dose necessary to destroy the tumor and that which allows recovery of normal tissues. Although results of treatment are satisfactory with regard to cure, treatment must be taken to levels approaching skin tolerance. The biologic effects of radiation for any given area or volume irradiated depend on the dose and the time over which the treatments are given, and these two factors cannot be considered separately. This relationship was examined by Quimby and MacComb in their classic paper (1937) and developed further by Strandqvist (1944). Time-dose curves for five-year cures of squamous cell cancer have been published by many authors in various forms (Ellis, 1969; Cohen, 1960). The slope of such a curve on a log-dose, log-time plot is 0.22. Figure 69–5 depicts such time-dose relationships for cure of squamous cell carcinoma, skin erythema, and normal tissue tolerance, respectively. The upper curve depicts one such finding for squamous carcinoma (Ellis, 1942), and the lower two graphs represent similar relations between skin tolerance and skin erythema. The skin tolerance line is based on data from Ellis (1942), Paterson (1948), and Jolles (1946) and the erythema line on the work of Reisner (1930) and Quimby and MacComb (1936). The two lower curves both have the same slope (0.33), suggesting that damage and repair in skin for such widely differing end points depend on the same mechanism, that is, cell killing, intracellular recovery, and homeostatically (extracellular) controlled repair. In Strandqvist's original work, he examined this relationship in 280 patients with cancer of the skin and lip and expressed it mathematically as follows:

$$D = kt^n$$

where D is the total dose administered in multiple increments in the time t, k is a constant having the value of the single dose for a specific response, and n is a positive

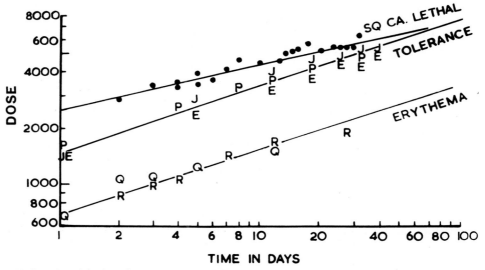

Figure 69–5 Time-dose iso-effect curves using different fractionation regimens for the cure of squamous cell carcinoma, the production of skin erythema, and normal tissue tolerance. The carcinoma line is derived from Ellis's (1969) work, and the tolerance line from the work of Jolles (1946), Paterson (1948), and Ellis (1942) (*J*, *P*, and *E*, respectively). The erythema line is derived from the work of Quimby and MacComb (1936) and Reisner (1930) (*Q* and *R*). (*From* Ellis: Clin. Radiol., 20:1, 1969.)

fraction which has been given the name of the recovery characteristic of the different cells. The equation illustrates to what extent the required dose is influenced by prolongation of the treatment time. Figure 69–6 depicts a summary of this work. The total accumulated dose for each case was plotted against overall treatment time using double log scales. When there was evidence of late radiation damage, the points tended to lie above the line, and when there were recur-

rences or persistence of tumors, the points lay below it. Strandqvist's curve really represents a zone for correct dosage and indicates the change in dose necessary for different overall treatment times. His results suggest that 3000 rads in four days is equivalent to 4000 rads in 11 days or 5000 rads in 25 days. Strandqvist's work is an important milestone in the development of modern radiotherapy, but it has limited usefulness when a specific lesion at a spe-

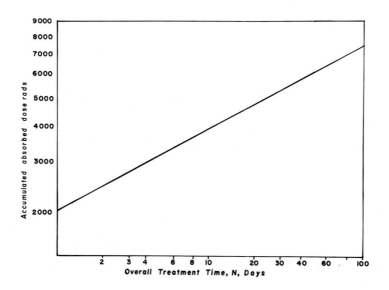

Figure 69–6 Dose curve for the cure of squamous cell carcinoma of the skin. (*Modified from* Strandqvist: Acta Radiol., Suppl. 55, 1944.)

cific site is considered, as his data include the average of skin lesions at many sites and of many sizes. He also included the results of cancers of unequal curability, so that the curve is not a true iso-effect curve. His work paved the way for others, however. Von Essen (1962) has also emphasized that it is not valid to derive a single iso-effect curve for a spectrum of tumors differing significantly in radiocurability. Allen and Freed (1956) confirmed the slope of Strandqvist's curve, but they concluded that the limits of safe dosage are great for small fields but diminish rapidly as the size of the field increases.

In a detailed study of the factors influencing the results of radiation treatment of 1355 carcinomas of the skin and lip, Von Essen (1962) found that, of 498 previously untreated lesions, 444 were small, and of those 17 recurred (3.84 percent). The equation of the extended iso-effect line expressing a 99 percent probability of a three-year cure was:

$$D = 2680 \times T^{0.14}$$

When the time-dose point fell below the line, the recurrence rate was 10.1 percent, whereas it was only 1.04 percent for those points above the line. The difference is statistically significant. He also attempted to analyze similar areas for large tumors, but the numbers were insufficient to yield significant results. Analysis of the incidence of necrosis following irradiation of small fields (less than 10 cm.^{2}) showed a significantly greater incidence when the time-dose points fell above the iso-effect line:

$$D = 1950 \times T^{0.27}$$

The number of cases of necrosis following the irradiation of large fields (greater than 10 cm.^{2}) was insufficient to construct a valid curve. If the points are plotted in relation to a curve of the same value as that for small lesions, the equation of the line displaced to incorporate the large field necrosis is:

$$D = 1700 \times T^{0.27}$$

Several very fundamental concepts of radiation therapy are evident from analysis of his results. They are:

1. Larger tumors are less radiosensitive. This finding is generally explained by the greater resistance to radiation of cells surviving in a condition of hypoxia. The large tumors presumably have a larger proportion of such cells.

2. Skin tolerance diminishes with increase in field size.

3. Fractionation assumes differential rates of recovery from radiation, with normal tissue recovering at a more rapid and predictable rate.

4. Larger tumors should be radiated to higher doses with a higher quality of irradiation over longer times.

Von Essen (1962) constructed a model incorporating the concepts of differential recovery of skin and tumor and differentiated radiosensitivity of tumor volumes and skin areas (Fig. 69–7). Only two of the iso-effect lines (small tumor recurrences and small field necrosis) were derived experimentally. The construction of the other curves parallel to these was hypothetical.

This study provides a theoretic basis for explaining the clinical phenomena and can serve as a guideline to the proper radiotherapeutic management of skin epitheliomas. It cannot be emphasized too strongly, however, that, for the proper management of skin cancer, a variety of treatment modalities must be available and due attention paid to the natural history of the tumor.

A summary of approximate external radiation techniques is shown in Table 69–1.

Radium and Other Sealed Radioisotopes

In any consideration of the place of radiation therapy in the management of skin tumors, attention must be paid to the use of techniques employing radium or other equivalent radioisotopes, such as radioactive cesium, cobalt, and so forth. Historically these have played an important part, but their role today is much more restricted for various reasons. Among

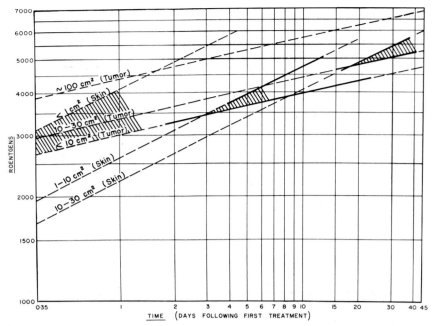

Figure 69–7 A hypothetical model based on the derived curves, assuming that k varies while m and n remain constant in the equations $D = k \cdot T_n$ and $D = k \cdot T_m$ for skin necrosis and tumor, respectively. The shaded areas represent favorable therapeutic regimens for particular treatment situations. (*From* Von Essen: Am. J. Roentgenol., 83:556, 1962.)

these are the problems of radiation exposure, the time and expertise necessary to construct the applicators, and, perhaps even more important, the equal efficacy at most sites, the simpler techniques, and the more ready availability of external irradiation.

Radium or its equivalent may be used either as an implant of sources within the tumor or as a surface applicator. The former method has been all but abandoned in the treatment of tumors of the skin and need not be considered further. The latter, however, has a real, albeit limited, place in treatment.

An applicator is constructed on which are mounted various radiation sources. The sources are placed thereby at a fixed distance from the lesion, which will vary according to the depth of penetration desired, with a usual distance of 1.0 cm. The appliance is worn for a fixed time daily until the necessary dose has been achieved in the tumor. Depending on the size of the area to be irradiated, doses of 6000 to 7000 rads in six to seven days are used.

The construction and use of such applicators has been fully described by Paterson and Gibb (1963). Although time-consuming, the method does give better cosmetic results. Because of the generally short treatment distance, the dose falls off rapidly, and consequently the underlying tissues are spared high doses. This, together with the lesser absorption by

TABLE 69–1 EXTERNAL IRRADIATION TECHNIQUES FOR BASAL CELL AND SQUAMOUS CELL CARCINOMA (100 KV – 2 mm. Al HALF VALUE LAYER)

Maximum Diameter Treated Dose	Given Dose	No. of Fractions	Overall Time
Less than 1.5 cm.	3500 rads	5	4 days
1.5 to 5.0 cm.	4500 rads	10	11 days
5.0 to 10 cm.	5500 rads	20	25 days

bone of the high energy gamma radiations, is a valuable consideration in the management of lesions affecting the scalp, the hands, and the feet, in which radium molds are the treatment method of choice.

Electrons

Beta-ray plaques have been used to treat superficial skin lesions but now are seldom used in this way. Electron beam therapy finds its major dermatologic role in the treatment of mycosis fungoides and will be considered at greater length there.

MALIGNANT MELANOMA

The radical treatment of malignant melanoma is based on the assumption that the tumor behaves as a metastasizing neoplasm arising from a primary site in the skin and spreading systematically to the regional lymph nodes. Because of the tendency of this lesion toward wide dissemination in the skin surrounding the tumor, the standard treatment is to excise the lesion with a wide margin of surrounding normal skin and the regional lymph nodes.

Evidence of the efficacy of radiation in the management of malignant melanoma is at best sketchy, and the widely held current belief in both the United States and Great Britain is that radiotherapy has little if any part to play in the curative management of the disease. Paterson and Gibb (1963) wrote that any malignant melanoma locally cured by radiotherapy is probably not a melanoma. From time to time, however, reports have appeared, particularly in the European literature, of the management of individual cases by radiation. This bibliography has been summarized by Sandeman (1966), who added his own experience. There seems little doubt that malignant melanoma does, on occasion, respond. Melanoma is undoubtedly a lesion of limited radiosensitivity, but this should not be regarded as being synonymous with unsuitability for radiation.

Although it is certainly not the prime

modality, there is a place for radiation therapy in the management of malignant melanoma. This may be considered from the following various viewpoints.

Curative Treatment—Radiation Therapy Alone. Reitman (1952) reported seven cases treated by radiation, including three cases of local cure of the primary lesion, one of which was associated with palpable regional nodes. Hellriegel (1963) described the cases seen at the University of Frankfurt Roentgen Institute over the period 1935 to 1960. Radiation therapy, either alone or in combination with surgery, was used to treat 342 patients. At the end of five years, 68 percent of patients without evidence of regional or distant metastases were alive. Unfortunately, in one-third of the patients the diagnosis was made on clinical grounds alone and not confirmed histologically.

The place of elective irradiation to the lymph nodes has been considered by Sandeman (1965). A small, unselected, retrospective series showed no benefits from such an approach, but planned studies have not been performed.

Curative Treatment—Combinations of Surgery and Radiotherapy. Dickson (1958) reviewed patients seen at the University of Toronto and the Johns Hopkins Hospital and compared the results of surgery alone with surgery and postoperative radiation. At the end of five years, 26 percent of the patients treated by the former method were alive, as compared to 41 percent of those treated by the latter. Although he concluded that these results appear to indicate that postoperative radiation improves prognosis, the series was not randomized and suffers from the defects of retrospective analysis.

It is clear that the true place of radiation therapy has not yet been properly evaluated. There is, however, sufficient evidence available to indicate that when surgery is refused or not possible, radical radiotherapy should be considered.

Palliative Radiation Therapy. Irrespective of the doubt concerning the place of radiation in the curative management of the disease, its efficacy in palliative therapy is established. Hilaris et al. (1963) described the cases involving radiotherapy of metastatic malignant melanoma at various sites seen at Memorial Hospital from 1956 to 1961. There were 73 patients in the series, and 57 percent showed either objective or significant subjective improvement in symptoms.

Therefore in situations in which incurable disease is causing local symptoms, radiation therapy may afford good palliation.

Technique and Dose

In view of the relative resistance of the lesion, it is important that adequate doses be given whether treatment is to be palliative or hopefully curative. This condition applies to the treatment of both the primary site and the regional lymph nodes.

Curative treatment should include the primary lesion and an adequate area of surrounding skin as well as the regional nodes whether or not they are clinically positive.

Primary Lesion. The dose to be given to the primary site should be of a similar level to that used for basal or squamous cell carcinomas and will approach skin tolerance. Hellriegel (1963), by means of contact therapy (60 kv., 5.0 cm. FSD), gave 6000 rads to the skin over two weeks, followed after a six- to eight-week interval by an additional 4000 to 5000 rads over two weeks. We should prefer to use rather more penetrating radiation and, with the factors previously noted (100 kv. to 120 kv., 1 to 3 mm. Al filter), would administer 5000 rads in 10 to 15 treatments, depending on the size of the lesion, with a 2.0-cm. free margin.

Surrounding Skin. Satellite recurrences around the primary lesion are a recognized complication of surgery. The incidence is difficult to evaluate but is probably in the region of 10 percent. It is therefore important to irradiate a further 5.0-cm band of normal skin surrounding the primary area. In view of the larger volume, however, the dose should be reduced to 4500 rads in three weeks.

Regional Nodes. The efficacy of radiation in controlling subclinical metastases to lymph nodes with doses of 4500 to 5000 rads in five weeks has been well documented for carcinoma arising from

various sites. If lymph nodes are clinically positive, the chance of eventual control is poor; a dose of 5000 to 5500 rads in five weeks delivered by megavoltage equipment is recommended.

An alternative approach to the management of metastatic regional nodes utilizes the techniques of lymphangiography. Edwards (1969) and Ariel (1971) have used this approach to administer radioactive isotopes endolymphatically. Large doses can be given by this means using isotopes emitting beta rays. Although the procedure must still be regarded as experimental, encouraging results have been obtained. Because of the limited penetration of beta rays, at least theoretically the method would seem to be of little value if used alone in the presence of clinically or radiologically detectable disease, and in such a situation administration of the isotope has been followed by excision of the nodes.

Palliative techniques would be those standard for the palliation of metastatic carcinoma of relative radioresistance and would depend on the site to be irradiated. In palliative circumstances a shorter treatment time is indicated.

MYCOSIS FUNGOIDES AND MALIGNANT LYMPHOMA OF THE SKIN

Radiation has long been used in the treatment of mycosis fungoides and other malignant lymphomas of the skin, particularly for the nodular stage of the disease. Although there is much debate as to the true nature and relationship of these entities, it has been our practice to consider them as one when planning treatment. Even in the early stages when the disease is apparently localized to the skin, mycosis fungoides is regarded as incurable, and treatment is therefore palliative. Locally the disease is usually highly radiosensitive, and small doses are effective in controlling local lesions. Friedman and Pearlman (1956) recorded the time-dose response of the lesions by a corroborated minimum dose technique. This technique is designed to establish the minimum tumor lethal dose necessary for local control, in contrast to the usual time-dose curves, which represent successful local treatment but in which the administered dose may have been much larger than necessary. Their analysis was based on the response of 63 separate lesions in two patients (28 and 35, respectively). They determined that the minimum single dose necessary to control individual lesions in the two patients was 250 rads and 800 rads. The marked radiosensitivity is apparent when one compares these levels to the necessary 2200 rads for skin carcinoma and 2000 rads for recurrent breast cancer found by the same authors.

Variation in sensitivity is seen and occasional radioresistant lesions are met, but there is no means available to predict such resistance, although Friedman and Pearlman attributed the difference in their two patients to different clinical types of presentation.

As has been noted, treatment to date has generally been considered palliative, with treatment of individual lesions as and when symptoms develop.

The feasibility of irradiating large areas up to and including the whole surface of the skin has been raised in recent years. Generally this has not been possible using orthovoltage x-ray apparatus, even that of low voltage, because of resulting damage to bone marrow. An advantage of the electron beam is its finite range in tissues, depending on the energy of the particle. By choosing the appropriate energy and therefore range, radiation could at least theoretically be confined to the skin. Such an approach has been adopted in several centers using different methods of electron production.

Smedal and his colleagues (1962) described their experiences with the use of electrons in treating 522 patients suffering from various forms of skin disease, including 220 with mycosis fungoides. They used a Van de Graaff electron generator, which yielded electrons with an energy range of from 1 to 4 Mev. Although localized areas were also treated, it is their experience with large-area irradiation that is most significant. Various techniques were tried, and a dose range of from 600 to 1200 rads, the most common being 600 to 800 rads, was used. The face,

eyelids, and axillary and perineal areas were shielded as necessary for most of the treatment but were exposed to the beam in separate single treatments of 400 rads. Alleviation of pruritus was obtained in 98 percent of the patients, and permanent control of local nodules was achieved in the majority.

Szur et al. (1962) used an 8-Mev. linear accelerator with reduced-energy electrons and achieved good palliation in nine patients, five of whom had mycosis fungoides. Similar results were obtained by Grollman et al. (1966), using a 6-Mev. linear accelerator in 29 patients, 16 of whom had mycosis fungoides.

Horwitz and Haybittle (1960) used radioactive strontium as the electron source to treat isolated skin lesions, and with the development of a second unit (Haybittle, 1964), they were able to treat large areas of skin. Strontium-90 decays to yttrium-90 and yields electrons of two energy levels, 0.6 Mev. and 2.0 Mev., in the process, the effective half value thickness of this electron beam in tissue being 2.0 mm. A dose to the skin of 2000 rads in 10 treatments has been used. Commonly, three to six months remission has been achieved, and multiple courses can be given. One patient has received a total of six courses. The advantage of this source and energy are real. Hair is not lost during treatment except in those areas involved by the mycosis. The fingernails are preserved and protection of sensitive structures achieved by simple measures (Bratherton, 1972). In all the above series, marrow damage has not been a problem. However, all accept the technique to be palliative.

Bagshaw (1961, 1968), using a linear accelerator at a 2.5-Mev. energy level, has described similar experiences but has postulated the concept of curative therapy. He has proposed total skin irradiation, even when the disease is in its earliest clinical stages. In 107 patients with mycosis fungoides of various clinical stages, recurrence-free survival for from 3 to 11 years after treatment was obtained in eight patients (Fuks and Bagshaw, 1971). Side effects of treatment include generalized erythema, epilation, skin edema, and loss of nails. Gynecomastia occurred in many male patients and was not prevented by shielding the scrotum.

Techniques

X-ray Therapy. As noted, the lesions are generally radiosensitive. Depending on the thickness of the nodules, the 100-kv. or the 250-kv. beam at short FSD is used. A generous margin of normal skin should be included in the field, the exact dimensions depending on the size of the lesion or lesions to be treated. A dose of 3000 rads in two weeks is generally adequate and can be modified according to tumor response, which is often rapid and early.

Electron Beam. For detailed descriptions of these techniques, the reader is referred to the original papers. Sometimes in patients following electron beam therapy, nodules remain, their persistence presumably due to inadequate penetration of the electrons. Additional kilovoltage therapy should then be used. It has been the experience of most workers, however, that lesions theoretically too bulky to respond do, in fact, on occasion regress.

KAPOSI'S SARCOMA

Like mycosis fungoides, Kaposi's sarcoma is generally considered to be a progressive, multicentric, and incurable disease, pursuing in the majority a rather indolent course. Usually the disease first presents as one or more isolated nodules, but with time and occasionally as the first presentation, visceral involvement is encountered.

Thus there are various well-defined forms of the disease for which radiotherapy might be considered as a primary or ancillary method of treatment.

Isolated Skin Nodules. At this stage, the disease is generally radiosensitive, and local superficial irradiation is effective in achieving local control. The patient should be kept under careful observation and further treatment given as and when lesions appear. Multiple contiguous nodules may be treated by the same approach. It will be appreciated that in this situation the approach has curative overtones.

Extensive Superficial Skin Involvement. An attempt can still be made at radical therapy by using superficial quality beams but of course treating large areas of the skin (Fig. 69–8).

Extensive Skin Involvement With Edema of the Limb. By this stage of the disease the nodules appear to be more fibrous, and they are certainly less radiosensitive. The edema generally is due to deep nodules. By now, treatment can only be considered palliative, not only because of the increased radioresistance but also because of the difficulty of treating the whole limb with a dose which can be considered as even approaching curative levels.

Disseminated Disease. Again the ap-

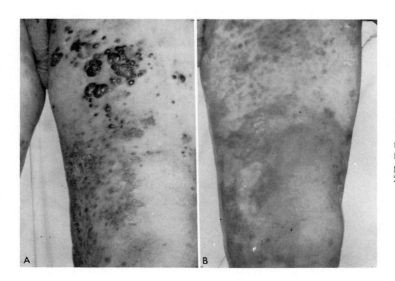

Figure 69–8 Extensive Kaposi's sarcoma before (*A*) and three months following (*B*) radiotherapy (250 kv., Thoreus filter, 30 cm. FSD 3000 rads given dose in 15 fractions over 21 days).

proach is palliative, with local treatment given to local symptomatic lesions.

Dose

Cohen (1962) has reviewed the dose-time-volume parameters in 38 cases of Kaposi's sarcoma with good local control of the disease. In small individual lesions he advocates a dose of 1000 rads in a single treatment. An alternative with less long-term changes would be 3000 rads in 10 treatments.

With more extensive and bulkier lesions, more penetrating irradiation may be necessary, but irradiation of the whole limb with either orthovoltage or megavoltage is unlikely to prove more than a temporary palliative procedure. Cohen found that 2500 rads in four weeks using orthovoltage was the maximum that a limb would tolerate, as figures higher than that resulted in a high incidence of complications, mainly vascular, including a 10 percent incidence of ischemic necrosis. If it is decided to use such an approach, the megavoltage beam should be used with a central dose not exceeding 3000 rads in four weeks. Bolus will be necessary to raise the dose to the skin to proper levels.

REFERENCES

Allen, K. D. A., and Freed, J. H.: Skin cancer. Correlation of field size and cancerocidal dose in roentgen treatment. Am. J. Roentgenol., 75:581, 1956.

Ariel, I. M.: Malignant melanoma: Its treatment by the endolymphatic administration of radioactive isotopes. Am. J. Roentgenol., 111:310, 1971.

Bagshaw, M. A., and Eltingham, J. R.: Observations on the electron beam therapy of mycosis fungoides. *In* Vaeth, J. M. (Ed.): Frontiers of Radiation Therapy and Oncology. Vol. 2. New York, Phiebig, 1968.

Bagshaw, M. A., Schneidman, H. M., and Farber, E. M.: Electron beam therapy of mycosis fungoides. Calif. Med., 95:292, 1961.

Borak, J.: The radiation biology of the cutaneous glands. Radiology, 27:651, 1936.

Bratherton, D. G.: Personal communication, 1972.

Cohen, L.: Ph.D. Thesis, University of Witwatersrand, 1960.

Cohen, L.: Dose, time and volume parameters in irradiation therapy of Kaposi's sarcoma. Br. J. Radiol., 35:485, 1962.

Del Regato, J. A., and Vuksanovic, M.: Radiotherapy of carcinomas of the skin overlying cartilages of the nose and ear. Radiology, 79:203, 1962.

Dickson, R. J.: Malignant melanoma. A combined surgical and radiotherapeutic approach. Am. J. Roentgenol., 79:1063, 1958.

Edwards, J. M.: Malignant melanoma: Treatment by endolymphatic radioisotope infusion. Ann. R. Coll. Surg. Engl. 44:237, 1969.

Ellis, F.: Tolerance dosage in radiography with 200 kV X-rays. Br. J. Radiol., 15:348, 1942.

Ellis, F.: Dose, time and fractionation: A clinical hypothesis. Clin. Radiol., 20:1, 1969.

Friedman, M., and Pearlman, A. W.: Time dose studies in irradiation of mycosis fungoides. Radiology, 66:374, 1956.

Fuks, Z., and Bagshaw, M. A.: Total-skin electron treatment of mycosis fungoides. Radiology, 100:145, 1971.

Gooding, C. A., White, G., and Yatsuhashy, M.: Significance of marginal extension in excised basal cell carcinoma. New Engl. J. Med., 273:923, 1965.

Grollman, J. H., Bierman, S. M., O'Homan, R. E., Morgan, J. R., and Horns, J.: Total-skin electron beam therapy of lymphoma cutis and generalized psoriasis: Clinical experiences and adverse reactions. Radiology, 87:908, 1966.

Haybittle, J. L.: A 24-curie strontium-90 unit for whole body superficial irradiation with beta rays. Br. J. Radiol., 37:297, 1964.

Hellriegel, W.: Radiation therapy of primary and metastatic melanoma. Ann. N.Y. Acad. Sci., 100:131, 1963.

Hilaris, B. S., Raben, M., Calabrese, A. S., Phillips, R. F., and Henschke, U. E.: Value of radiation therapy for distant metastases from malignant melanoma. Cancer, 16:765, 1963.

Horwitz, H., and Haybittle, J. L.: Whole body superficial irradiation with strontium-90 beta rays. (A report of cases treated with a moving couch technique.) Br. J. Radiol., 33:440, 1960.

Jolles, B.: Quantitative biological dose control in interstitial radium therapy. Br. J. Radiol., 19:143, 1946.

Parker, R. C., and Wildermuth, O.: Radiation Therapy of Lesions Overlying Cartilage. Cancer, 15:57, 1962.

Paterson, R.: The Treatment of Malignant Disease by Radium and X-rays. Ed. 1. London, Edward Arnold, 1948.

Paterson, R., and Gibb, R.: The skin. *In* Paterson, R. (Ed.): The Treatment of Malignant Disease by Radiotherapy. Ed. 2. London, Edward Arnold, 1963.

Paterson, R., and Pointon, R. S.: The preparation of radium applicators and beam direction shells. *In* Paterson, R. (Ed.): The Treatment of Malignant Disease by Radiotherapy. Ed. 2. London, Edward Arnold, 1963.

Quimby, E. H., and MacComb, W. S.: The rate of recovery of human skin from the effects of hard or soft roentgen rays or gamma rays. Radiology, 27:196, 1936.

Quimby, E. H., and MacComb, W. S.: Further studies on rate of recovery of human skin from the effects of roentgen or gamma-ray irradiation. Radiology, 29:305, 1937.

Reisner, A.: Untersuchungen uber die Veranderungender Hauttoleranz bie verschiedener Unterteilung der Strahlendosis. Strahlentherapie, 37:779, 1930.

Reitman, P. H.: Radiation therapy of malignant melanoma. Am. J. Roentgenol., 67:286, 1952.

Rubin, P., and Casarett, G. N.: Skin and adnexa. *In* Clinical Radiation Pathology. Ed. 1. Philadelphia, W. B. Saunders Company, 1968.

Sandeman, T. F.: Elective treatment of lymph nodes in malignant melanoma. Lancet, 1:345, 1965.

Sandeman, T. F.: The radical treatment of enlarged lymph nodes in malignant melanoma. Am. J. Roentgenol., 97:967, 1966.

Smedal, M. I., Johnston, D. O., Salzman, F. A., Trump, J. G., and Wright, K. A.: Ten year experience with ion megavolt electron therapy. Am. J. Roentgenol., 88:215, 1962.

Strandqvist, M.: Time-dose relationship. Acta Radiol., Suppl. 55, 1944.

Szur, L., Silvester, J. A., and Bewley, D. K.: Treatment of the whole body surface with electrons. Lancet, 1:1373, 1962.

Von Essen, C. F.: Skin and lip carcinoma. Am. J. Roentgenol., 83:556, 1962.

Wermuth, B. M., and Fajardo, L. F.: Metastatic basal cell epithelioma (review). Arch. Pathol., 90:458, 1970.

70

Mohs' Surgery in the Treatment of Basal Cell and Squamous Cell Carcinomas of the Skin

Perry Robins, M.D.

It is estimated that there are about 530,000 cases of basal cell carcinoma each year, making it the most common cancer to man and an entity familiar to all clinicians. There are a number of modalities that are effective in treating these tumors, such as conventional surgery, radiation therapy, and electrodesiccation and curettage. Many lesions, however, because of their type, site, or unexpected ramifications, resist the standard methods even under the best of conditions.

Another method of treatment, chemosurgery, developed by Mohs, has also been effective in eradicating these tumors. The essence of Mohs' chemosurgery is serial excisions and microscopic study of chemically fixed tissue suspected of harboring the malignant process. This technique results in total ablation of malignancy and at the same time sacrifices the least amount of normal tissue.

Chemosurgery was developed in 1932 by Dr. Frederic E. Mohs, Professor of Surgery at the Wisconsin Medical School.

As a medical student and research assistant at Wisconsin he developed a method to fix tissue in situ without altering the architecture of the tissue. In the presence of tumor tissue, the cancer cells were accurately visualized microscopically. The preservation of the tissue architecture was controlled by the use of paste which contained 40 percent zinc chloride in stibinite. These experiments led to the chemosurgical method by which cancer of the skin may be removed under microscopic control. Refinement of the technique now allows for the pinpoint location of a skin tumor so that it can be definitively removed.

A chemosurgical unit was established at New York University Medical Center *as a joint project* through the cooperation of Dr. Rudolf Baer, Professor and Chairman of the Department of Dermatology, and Dr. John Converse, Professor and Chairman of the Department of Plastic and Reconstructive Surgery. During the past nine years, more than 3,000 extensive tumors of the skin have been treated successfully by this method, the essence of which follows:

1. Fixation in situ of tissues suspected of being neoplastic by the application of zinc chloride paste.

2. Removal of this fixed tissue by scalpel excision.

3. Complete microscopic examination by a modified frozen section technique.

These steps are repeated as often as indicated by microscopic visualization of residual tumors, the ultimate being complete removal of the cancerous tissue with minimum sacrifice of normal tissue, a distinct advantage.

CHEMOSURGICAL TECHNIQUE

The steps required in the performance of chemosurgery are illustrated in Figures 70–1 to 70–7. The clinical extent of the tumor is first judged and measured by

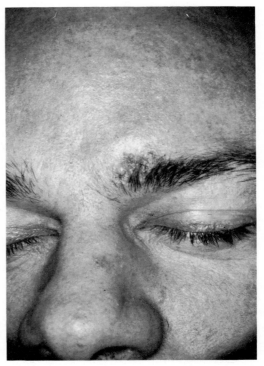

Figure 70–2   Dichloracetic acid coagulates epidermal proteins, enhancing absorption of zinc chloride paste.

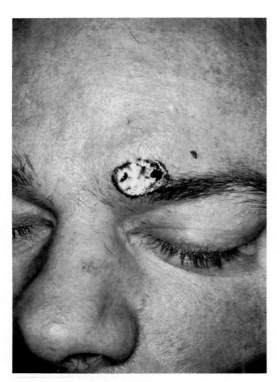

Figure 70–1   A basal cell epithelioma recurred twice following surgical excisions.

gross examination. Dichloracetic acid is then applied to the surface of the entire area, which coagulates epidermal proteins and enhances the percutaneous absorption of the zinc chloride fixative which is subsequently applied. Zinc chloride paste (a 40 percent solution of zinc chloride in stibinite paste) fixes tissue to a depth that depends upon the thickness of the layer of paste applied and the length of time it is permitted to act. A thin layer of paste (approximately 1 millimeter) is all that is required to fix to a depth of 2 mm. in a 24-hour period. The treated area is covered with an occlusive dressing in an effort to decrease absorption of water.

When adequate fixation has been achieved (a few hours to one day as judgment dictates), sections of tissue approximately 1 square cm. in area and 2 mm. in thickness are surgically excised in a saucerlike shape; there is no pain or bleeding if the excision is made within the fixed tissue. A map of the lesion site with a

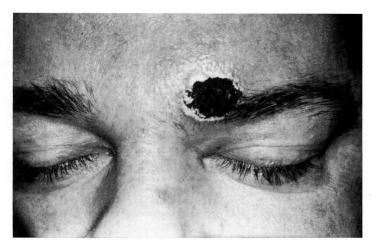

Figure 70–3 Zinc chloride paste fixes the tissue, with no destruction of histologic architecture.

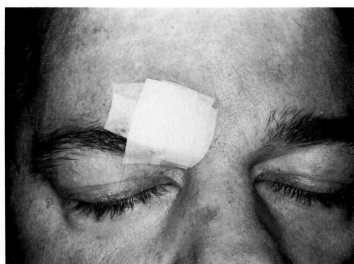

Figure 70–4 Fixation is accomplished over a 6- to 24-hour period.

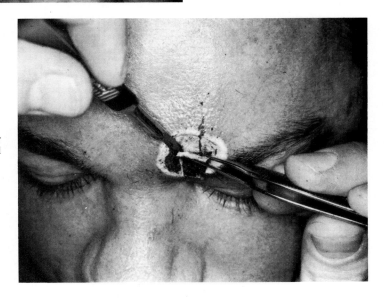

Figure 70–5 There is no pain or bleeding during excision of fixed tissue.

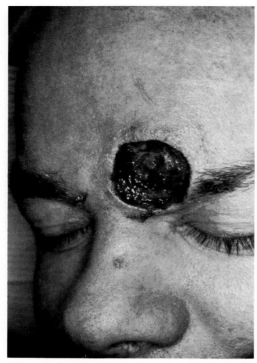

Figure 70–6 Extent of tumor following three stages of surgical excision.

number assigned to each section is drawn at the time of excision, and each section, as it is removed, is identified by its corresponding number. Indelible marks applied to two opposing edges of the tissue specimen are preserved during the histochemical staining process; when visualized microscopically, these marks allow the chemosurgeon to locate the exact position and location of any remaining malignancy.

This microscopic control enables the surgeon to trace out cancers of the skin, the columns of tumor cells that extend for a considerable distance beyond the apparent margins of the tumor into the surrounding tissue. In order to encompass these extensions, surgeons and radiologists will excise or radiate an extra margin of tissue. In the process, normal tissue is sacrificed without complete assurance of eradication. Chemosurgery minimizes the sacrificing of normal tissue.

Advantages and Disadvantages. The prime indication for this method is the advanced tumor which has recurred after previous treatment. It is equally effective in destroying those tumors found in locations where the maximum amount of normal tissue must be preserved, such as the eyelids, canthus, pinna, nasolabial fold, and ala nasi. Aggressive clinicohistopathologic types, such as morphea-like infiltrating and fibrotic basal cell carcinoma, should be included in this group. Chemosurgical technique is also indicated for tumors with poorly demarcated clinical borders and unusually large diameters.

In addition to the high cure rate, an ad-

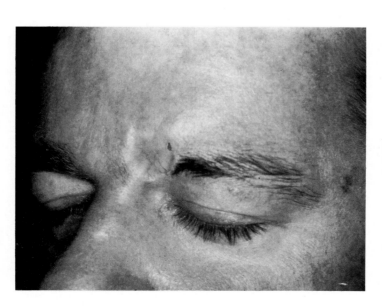

Figure 70–7 The surgical defect usually heals spontaneously and uneventfully.

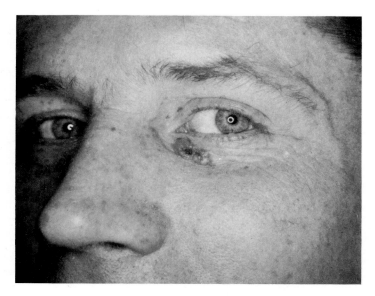

Figure 70–8 A 37 year old man shown with a 1.5-cm. recurrent basal cell carcinoma of two years' duration on the left lower lid.

vantage of chemosurgery is that the procedure does not require general anesthesia; thus it extends the benefit of cure to many people who are poor candidates for conventional surgery. Since the mortality rate is practically nil, elderly patients in poor health with respiratory and circulatory disorders are not precluded from treatment. Most of our patients, including many 65 year olds and some patients as old as 90, tolerate the procedure exceedingly well. Conveniently, patients undergoing chemosurgery are managed on an outpatient basis.

RECURRENT BASAL CELL CARCINOMAS

The skin cancer not totally excised in the initial treatment will recur and present greater therapeutic problems to the physician. It is a characteristic of recurrent lesions that their histologic architecture shows alteration. Instead of being solidly clustered within a mucinous stroma, tumor cells are now more widely dispersed in a dense scar tissue.

These changes make the boundaries and distribution of the malignancy difficult to detect by the usual clinical means. The danger lies in that unobserved and unpalpated pockets or extensions of tumor cells will escape the usual conventional treatment and re-seed new and deeper lesions.

NOSE

Chemosurgery is of significant value in the treatment of carcinomas of the nose, which often exhibit silent extensions not clinically detectable. They invade in a sur-

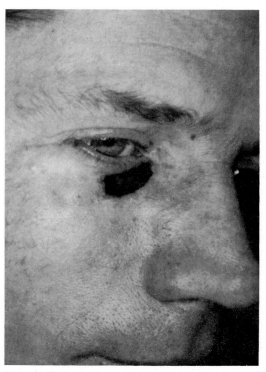

Figure 70–9 The extent of the tumor following three microscopically controlled stages of the fresh-tissue technique.

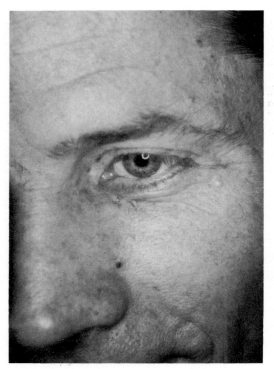

Figure 70–10   Follow-up six months later. Note the excellent cosmetic result.

should be observed, except when the tumor involves the upper lip. In the healing stage, one would see an upward retraction of the lip that is difficult to correct; therefore, use of a split-thickness graft at the onset of the granulating stage would partially alleviate this undesirable cosmetic result.

EARS

Cancer of the ear can also be safely excised by the Mohs' technique. Small lesions usually require no corrective surgery, while in large lesions the maximum amount of normal tissue is preserved as a basis for reconstruction. With basal cell carcinoma, the tumor rarely invades cartilage but will glide off and extend a considerable distance from its origin in a plane between the cartilage and epidermis. It is not uncommon to observe the tumor extending from the anterior to the posterior surfaces.

prisingly irregular and unpredictable manner, with a tendency to spread a great distance from the clinical border. The tumors rarely invade nasal bone or cartilage.

The nasolabial fold is an area that shows the greatest failure rate following initial treatment. Here one encounters more often the aggressive type of tumor—the morphea or sclerosing type of basal cell carcinoma. The direction of spread is unpredictable, the tumor having the ability to grow in depth, laterally along the cheek, or anteriorly along the nasal ala. Very frequently the surgeon is extremely reluctant to remove tissue from the nasal ala because of the deleterious effect on the patient's cosmetic appearance or because of the difficulty involved in the task of reconstruction. With complete microscopic control, the tumor can be extirpated with a high rate of cure, and a fairly good cosmetic result can be anticipated. If corrective surgery is indicated, a waiting period of six months to one year

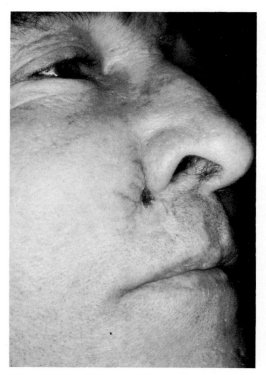

Figure 70–11   A 50 year old man with a 2-cm. recurrent basal cell carcinoma of the right nasolabial fold.

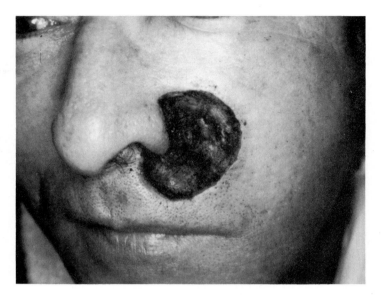

Figure 70–12 After the fifth stage, the tumor was still detected in depth and periphery.

EYE

Tumors on the lid and periorbital area are excised by a modified chemosurgical method with minimal complications. The chemical paste is not used because of the chance of damaging the cornea. This step is eliminated by excising fresh tissue and having frozen sections prepared. The sources of the specimen are recorded on a map. Following the removal of cancer from the lid margin, the surgical site usually heals spontaneously with a good cosmetic result.

Cancer of the medial and lateral canthi can be removed by the fresh tissue technique. It is possible to follow the tumor a considerable distance into the orbit and still leave a functioning eye.

Extensions of tumors from the eyelids deep into the inner and outer canthus are not a rare occurrence, especially in persistent or recalcitrant tumors. Bizarre tumor extensions must be considered each time a lesion is to be treated. Clinical judgment of extent of tumor by palpation and approximation is insufficient for the total extirpation of these more difficult tumors.

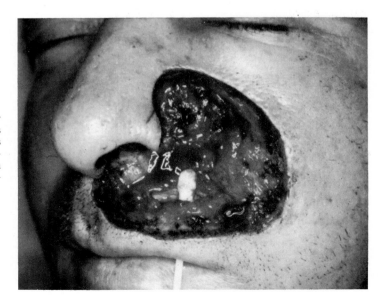

Figure 70–13 Further surgery was repeated for another six stages (total 11 stages) until the area was free of tumor. Reconstructive surgery will be commenced after a follow-up period has been observed.

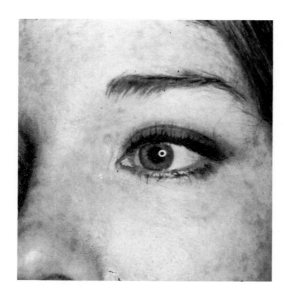

Figure 70–14 A 22 year old female developed a basal cell carcinoma on the left inner canthus. In the ensuing three years, the tumor was treated by curettage and electrodesiccation on four separate occasions without success.

Figure 70–15 Area following excision by the Mohs' technique after removal of three microscopically controlled stages of tissue.

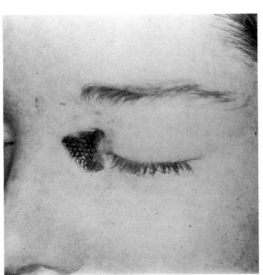

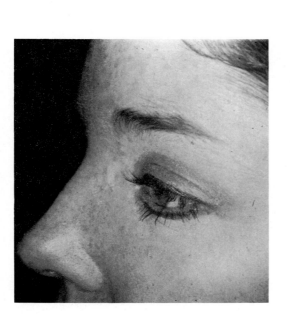

Figure 70–16 A revision of the scar tissue with Z-plasty was performed to improve the cosmetic appearance, and biopsies of the scar tissue and surrounding area at that time showed no evidence of tumor.

OTHER ORGANS

Of special interest is the treatment of squamous cell carcinomas and occasional basal cell carcinomas that involve the hands or fingers of physicians and dentists exposed to x-rays in their work. In many instances, without the presence of palpable nodes in the axilla, an amputation of the digit was recommended; however, after the tumors had been traced chemosurgically and the wound site allowed to granulate in, the individual could pursue his normal occupation.

Equally effective is the treatment of malignant lesions such as Bowen's disease, erythroplasia of Queyrat, or squamous cell carcinoma of the skin and glans of the penis, in which the tumor can be chemosurgically eradicated without sacrificing the organ or compromising its function.

Cancer of the vulva has been treated successfully and conservatively by chemosurgery.

FRESH TISSUE TECHNIQUE

The fresh tissue technique was first utilized when the Mohs' chemosurgical procedure was performed in areas involving the eyes, namely the inner canthus and upper and lower lids. Zinc chloride paste was not applied to these sites because of the possibility of the fixative causing irritation and damage to the globe. To avoid this possible complication, the tissue was excised without the use of chemicals. The excised specimen was then fixed in vitro, and frozen sections were cut through the undersurface of the fresh tissue specimens. The color coding of the edges and mapping of the tissue were performed as in the fixed tissue technique. The resulting fresh sections were of sufficiently fine quality and facilitated diagnosis.

The application of this technique to other areas of the body was first described by Theodore Tromovitch in 1970. The mechanics of the procedure became further developed, and the method was eventually applied to larger tumors on the body.

Procedure.   The clinical extent of the

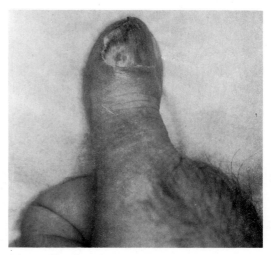

Figure 70–17   A 72 year old male with a recurrent squamous cell carcinoma of the distal portion of the thumb.

tumor is first judged by gross examination. The area is then anesthetized by the use of a regional or local block, and the patient is draped to allow for a sterile procedure.

A small curette is vigorously used to remove the necrotic tissue. Sections of tissue measuring approximately 1 square cm. in area and 2 mm. in thickness are excised in a saucerlike shape. After the tissue is examined microscopically, the location of the malignancy is marked on the original map, the area of the previously treated site is reanesthetized, and the additional tumor is surgically removed. This procedure is repeated until the entire area is found to be free of tumor.

Advantages.   The fresh tissue technique has been especially beneficial in treating areas where the minimal amount of tissue destruction is of major importance, such as the eyelids, inner canthus, nasal ala, and pinna of the ear. The application of this technique to other areas has the advantage of causing less discomfort than is experienced with the application of the paste while also saving a considerable amount of time, as subsequent layers of tissue can be removed without waiting for fixation. There can be an additional saving of tissue, as the final layer of tissue to be removed needs no fixation.

Wound healing is frequently facilitated

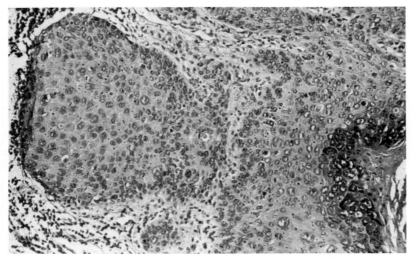

Figure 70–18   The lesion site confirmed by biopsy. Treatment recommendation was surgical amputation of the thumb. Mohs' surgery revealed the tumor extended into the bone of the distal phalanx. All other areas were free of tumor.

by the use of primary closures in the smaller treated sites. Larger sites granulate equally as rapidly and without infection.

Disadvantages.   The major problem is bleeding. However, most of the vessels encountered are relatively small and can be controlled by tying the bleeders, by electrocautery, or by use of hemostatic agents such as *Monsel's solution.* Orientation can become a problem when the treated site exceeds a few centimeters in diameter and depth. It is not unusual to commence on a large lesion with the fixative zinc chloride paste and terminate with the fresh tissue technique when the remaining tumor is localized to a small area.

It is too early to determine the five-year cure rate of the fresh tissue technique. However, preliminary reports by Drs. Mohs and Tromovitch reveal their findings to very much align with the success of the use of the paste.

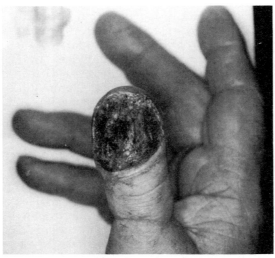

Figure 70–19   Extent of surgery prior to amputation of the distal phalanx.

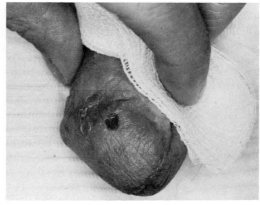

Figure 70–20   A 61 year old male with a 2-cm. squamous cell carcinoma of the glans penis. (Treatment recommended was surgical amputation.) Figure shows extent of lesion.

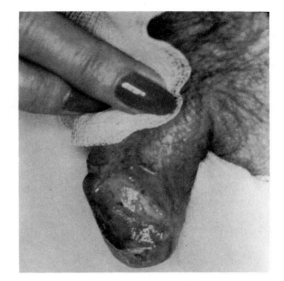

Figure 70–21   The extent of the tumor following removal by Mohs' chemosurgery.

RECONSTRUCTION

Where an extensive tumor has left a large defect, the surgeon, because of the reliability of the procedure, can consider an earlier repair than might normally be allowed. Frequently, the chemosurgeon works together with the ophthalmologist or plastic surgeon when extensive tumors of the upper lid involve the tarsal palate. Reconstructive surgery can be instituted upon showing that the final layer of tissue is free of neoplasm.

Frequently, selected cases have been handled jointly with the plastic surgeons, ophthalmologists, neurosurgeons, or otolaryngologists. An example of this would be tumor involving the auditory canal, in which the external portion can be handled effectively by the chemosurgeon. The internal aspect is then treated by an otolaryngologist, who repairs the canal to prevent stenosing of the orifice.

Approximately 20 percent of the cases require reconstructive surgery.

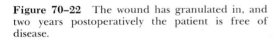

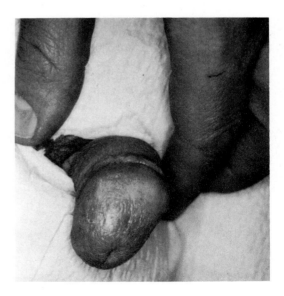

Figure 70–22   The wound has granulated in, and two years postoperatively the patient is free of disease.

TABLE 70–1 **CHEMOSURGERY, 1965–1971**

Basal Cell Carcinoma

Year	Number of Lesions	Recurrences	
1965	7	0	
1966	30	5	
1967	52	2	
1968	148	8	
1969	178	13	
1970	316	31	
1971	373	25	
TOTAL:	1,104	84	92.4%

Squamous Cell Carcinoma

1965–1971	42	2	95.2%

Prior to chemosurgery, approximately 50% of the above lesions had been previously treated an average number of 2.8 times by the standard modalities; many had been treated as frequently as ten times. The average size of the lesions was approximately 2 cm. in diameter, many being greater than 10 cm.

The primary cases that were referred for Mohs' chemosurgery were not the usual simple basal cell carcinomas but were complicated by the fact that there were extensive, poorly demarcated, and frequently poorly accessible areas. In view of this, we consider the cure rate achieved to be an outstanding figure.

CURE RATE

Chemosurgery offers the highest cure rate for malignancy of the skin.

From 1965 thru 1971 skin cancers were treated by the chemosurgical method at the New York University Skin and Cancer Unit. Of these, 657 had not been treated before and 618 were referred because previous standard treatments had failed to prevent recurrences. All of the latter were classified histologically as basal cell carcinomas, and the average number of previous treatments for these resistant lesions was 2.3; some had been treated five or more times.

Table 70–1 presents the recurrences to date following chemosurgery. Twenty occurred among lesions initially treated by us, representing a cure rate of 97 percent; 28 occurred among those referred to us after previous standard treatment, representing a cure rate of 95.5 percent. Among the recurrences in both groups,

75 percent involved tumors less than 4 cm. in diameter, and they were retreated with good results. Three patients treated chemosurgically had two or more subsequent recurrences. One of these, initially coming to us with a primary forehead lesion larger than 4 cm., required two separate treatment sessions. Another had undergone nine previous treatments for a nasal lesion prior to chemosurgery, and it was decided after the second chemosurgical recurrence to treat him with radiation therapy; there is no evidence of recurrence thus far after two years. The third patient, with a forehead lesion larger than 2 cm. previously treated once by conventional techniques, recently required his fourth session of chemosurgery.

The significant figure, of course, is that only 4.5 percent of the recurrent skin cancer patients subsequently returned after treatment by chemosurgery. This figure is only slightly above that for initial lesions, and it should be compared with the nearly 50 percent failure rate reported for other modalities for treating persistent skin cancers.

There were twice as many lesions of the nasolabial fold among those referred to us for continued treatment than among those we treated initially, which means that this site is exceptionally resistant to standard therapy. Conventional modes are apparently more successful with lesions of the eyes and ears, for there were substantially fewer such lesions among those referred than among those initially presented. The intractable lesion in the nasal groove apparently yields to chemosurgery, for there were no recurrences of such lesions among our patients thus treated in a primary way and only one among those referred. There were no recurrences of lesions on cheeks, whether initial or recurrent.

In a series of basal cell carcinomas followed for five years, Dr. Mohs reported a cure rate of 99.3 percent. In 2,030 squamous cell carcinomas followed for five years, there was a 94 percent cure rate.

CHEMO-CHECK

This is a modified one-stage chemosurgical procedure useful in confirming by microscopy whether a cutaneous cancer treated by surgery or electrodesiccation and curettage has been completely ablated. If there is any doubt that electrodesiccation and curettage or surgery has been absolutely successful, the patient can immediately—the earlier the better—be referred for this procedure.

The following steps are taken:

1. A thin layer of zinc chloride paste is applied to the fresh wound.

2. After two or three hours of fixation, a thin slice of fixed tissue in a saucer shape is removed by scalpel.

3. The excised specimen is then cut into several pieces, and frozen sections from the undersurface of each are stained for microscopy.

4. If no signs of malignancy are found under the microscope, the check is negative, and nothing more need be done. If malignancy is found in some or all of the sections, however, the chemosurgical steps are continued selectively or entirely until complete extirpation is achieved.

The advantages of the chemo-check are:

1. Certainty of cure.

2. Elimination of long, worrisome follow-ups for signs of recurrence.

THE CHEMOSURGERY UNIT

The chemosurgery unit should be an integral part of either the department of dermatology or the department of surgery within a university medical center.

Since chemosurgery deals with malignant tumors of the skin, specifically basal cell carcinoma, Bowen's disease, erythroplasia of Queyrat, and squamous cell carcinoma, it provides another modality of treatment for the more difficult of these lesions. The chemosurgeon would engage in the clinic and private practice of chemosurgery to satisfy the needs of those physicians in the city, state, and region of the country where the medical center is located.

At the New York University Medical Center, a one-year training program has been established to teach the chemosurgical procedure. This is one of six centers offering such a program, the goal of which is to train candidates in the skills of diagnosing and treating cutaneous malignancies of the skin. In addition to learning chemosurgery, the trainee receives instruction in surgery, electrosurgery, histopathology, radiotherapy, cryosurgery, and chemotherapy. Upon completion of this training, the chemosurgical fellow is truly a clinical cutaneous oncologist.

CONCLUSION

The skin cancer not cured by the initial therapy will return to present even greater difficulties to the therapist. It is characteristic of such recurrent lesions that their histologic architecture is changed; instead of being solidly clustered within a mucinous stroma, infiltrative tumor cells are now more widely dispersed in dense scar tissue or radiodermatitis. This change makes the boundaries and distribution of the malignancy extremely difficult to detect by the usual clinical means, and the danger becomes even greater than before that unobserved and unpalpated pockets and extensions of tumor cells will escape the scalpel and reseed new and deeper lesions.

The experience reported here indicates that the success rate in treating recurrent skin cancers can be raised to a level approaching that obtained by the initial therapy. The reason for chemosurgery's greater reliability in such cases lies in the microscopic control which enables the surgeon to identify and trace out tumor cells.

REFERENCES

Brodkin, R. H., Kopf, A. W., and Andrade, R.: Basal-cell epithelioma and elastosis: A comparison of distribution. *In* Urbach, F. (Ed.): Biological Effects of Ultraviolet Radiation with Emphasis on the Skin. International Conference of the Skin

Cancer Hospital. Temple University Sciences Center & International Society of Biometeorology. New York, Pergamon Press, 1969.

Crissey, J. T.: Curettage and electrodesiccation as a method of treatment for epitheliomas of the skin. J. Surg. Oncol., 3:287, 19xx.

Eade, G. G.: Basal-cell carcinoma. J.A.M.A., 229:23, 1974.

Menn, H., Robins, P., Kopf, A. W., et al.: The recurrent basal cell epitheliomas. Arch. Dermatol., 103:628, 1971.

Mohs, F. E.: Chemosurgery in Cancer, Gangrene and Infections. Springfield, Ill., Charles C Thomas, Publisher, 1956.

Mohs, F. E.: Prevention and treatment of skin cancer. Wis. Med. J., 73:85, 1974.

Robins, P., and Albom, M.: Recurrent basal-cell carcinomas in young women. J. Derm. Surg., 1:49, 1975.

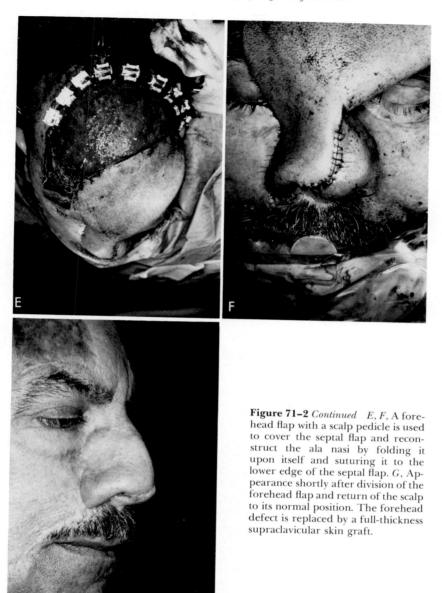

Figure 71–2 *Continued* *E, F,* A forehead flap with a scalp pedicle is used to cover the septal flap and reconstruct the ala nasi by folding it upon itself and suturing it to the lower edge of the septal flap. *G,* Appearance shortly after division of the forehead flap and return of the scalp to its normal position. The forehead defect is replaced by a full-thickness supraclavicular skin graft.

not encountered after conventional surgical excision. The principles of reconstructive surgery still apply, and three basic techniques, alone or in combination, are available for the repair of postchemosurgery defects—most of which are situated on the face. These are the skin graft (Fig. 71–2C), the local flap from the vicinity of the defect (Fig. 71–1B), and the employment of pedicle tissue. Because of the advanced age of many of the patients

affected with carcinoma of the skin, the simplest method compatible with an acceptable cosmetic and functional result should be chosen when planning reconstruction, and local anesthesia should be used when possible.

Mention has already been made of the dense fibrous tissue which develops in the treated area. For a satisfactory result, much of this fibrous tissue must be excised, together with the overlying scar

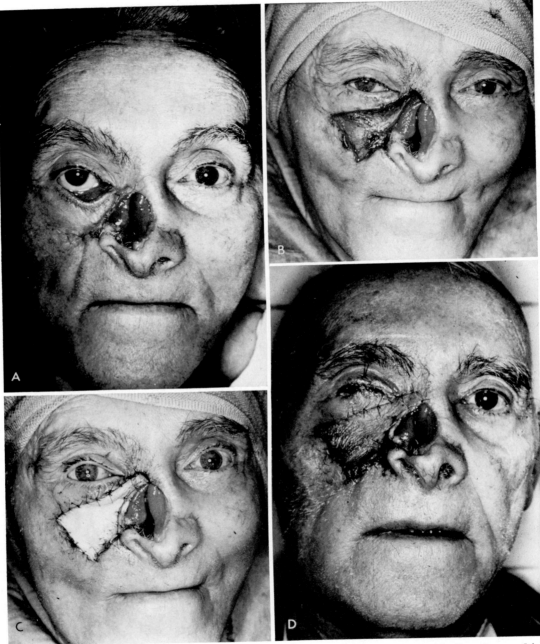

Figure 71–3   *A*, Appearance six weeks after chemosurgery for an extensive recurrent basal cell carcinoma of the nose and cheek; a cicatricial ectropion has developed. *B*, The original defect of the cheek is re-created by the removal of scar tissue under local anesthesia. *C*, The area of skin loss is now repaired by a full-thickness supraclavicular skin graft cut to the size of the defect and carefully sutured in place. *D*, Appearance at the first dressing change. The skin graft is well vascularized and the ectropion is corrected. Reconstruction of the nose is deferred for one year.

epithelium, re-creating to some extent the defect present at the termination of chemosurgery. This applies particularly to the patient undergoing early reconstruction, and undesirable postrepair contractures may be prevented to an acceptable degree by the aggressive removal of the immature fibrous tissue in and around the defect.

The distortion of contiguous structures as a result of these contractures, as seen on the lower eyelid (Fig. 71–3*A*) or the lip (Fig. 71–11), must also be corrected by undermining the surrounding skin and excising as much scar tissue as necessary to restore them to their correct relationship (Fig. 71–3*B*); only then is adequate replacement possible (Fig. 71–3*D*).

The Skin Graft

Large areas of the face may be resurfaced by full-thickness skin grafts; because of its simplicity, this method is recommended as the first choice for the repair of the postchemosurgical defect, whenever it is suitable (Fig. 71–2*B* and *C*). Technical success is dependent on meticulous hemostasis and careful dressing techniques, and to obtain the necessary control of bleeding in the larger defects, a delayed grafting technique is advised. At the first procedure, the scar epithelium, together with the underlying fibrous tissue, is excised. Deformities such as lower lid ectropion are then corrected by skin undermining and scar release, after which a nonadherent pressure dressing is applied for 24 to 48 hours. Bleeding is thus effectively controlled, and when the patient is returned to the operating room, a dry bed for the reception of a graft is present. An accurate pattern of the defect is then made, and a full-thickness skin graft is removed from the donor site or sites selected. After it is defatted and trimmed to fit the area to be grafted, the skin is carefully sutured in place, without fear of losing it because of a hematoma beneath. Although this technique has the disadvantage of requiring two operative procedures, which in most individuals may be performed under local anesthesia, (Fig. 71–3), it increases the success rate of large skin grafts. Full-thickness skin grafts are used almost exclusively because of the lesser tendency for them to contract, as opposed to the split-thickness skin graft, which has little benefit in the permanent reconstruction of defects of the skin of the face. The latter is useful to obtain a closure on the scalp, where it may be applied directly to the bony skull after removal of the outer table by an air-driven bur.

The preferred donor sites for full-thickness skin grafts are the retroauricular and supraclavicular areas, from which large pieces of skin may be removed and the defect closed by undermining and direct approximation. This skin provides the most acceptable color match for the skin of the face, unlike that removed from the buttocks and thighs, which develops a displeasing yellowish tan shade when transplanted to the face.

More elaborate methods are needed for the closure of mucocutaneous fistulas and for the reconstruction of the nose, lip, and ear. Among these, the most common site requiring repair after chemosurgery is the nose, and several techniques are available for this purpose.

The Composite Auricular Graft

For loss of the ala nasi (Fig. 71–4*A*), for the columella, and for small, full-thickness defects of the nose under 1.5 cm., a useful technique for repair is the composite graft taken from the ear (Maliniac, 1946). This type of graft, as its name implies, consists of two layers of skin between which is sandwiched the corresponding piece of ear cartilage. The size one is most often called upon to use varies from 1.0 to 1.5 cm., but larger grafts have been used with success (Rees et al., 1963). The edges of the defect are excised, and a pattern is made using dental compound to allow for both size and contour. A suitable donor site on the ear is then chosen and marked out with ink, after which the graft is carefully removed, using a nontraumatic technique. The graft is sutured in place using the same technique, and the ear donor site is closed by direct approximation, breaking the spring of the helix, if necessary, by undermining the skin and dividing the

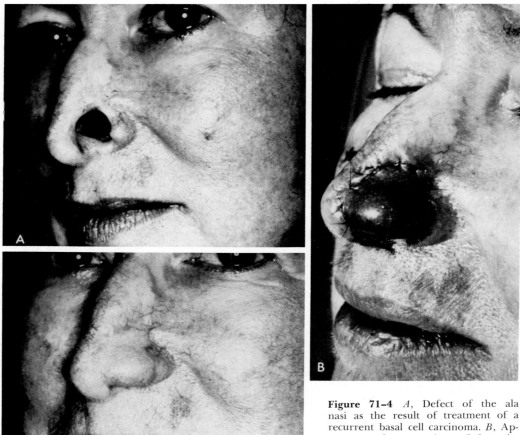

Figure 71–4 *A*, Defect of the ala nasi as the result of treatment of a recurrent basal cell carcinoma. *B*, Appearance of a composite graft from the ear, 1.5 × 1.8 cm. in size; on the third day, some vascularization is evident. *C*, Final appearance six months after grafting.

cartilage. During the postoperative phase, the graft is seen to undergo a series of color changes from dead white at the completion of surgery through purple to pink by the end of the fourth or fifth day, if the graft is to survive (Fig. 71–4*B*).

The success rate is determined by the size of the graft, careful surgical technique, and postoperative care. The last is perhaps the most important and includes the constant application of ice cold compresses for 48 to 72 hours, the rationale for this being the maintenance of tissue viability until revascularization takes place (Conley and VonFraenkel, 1956). Facial movements such as chewing and laughing are also restricted.

The successful composite graft gives a most satisfactory postoperative result without an additional scar on the face, provides an excellent color match, and shows little or no tendency to late shrinkage (Fig. 71–4*C*).

The Nasolabial Flap

The nasolabial flap (Fig. 71–5), more versatile and perhaps safer than the composite graft, is also used for reconstruction of defects of the ala nasi and the lateral wall of the nose (Fig. 71–6*A*). The method employs a superiorly based skin flap elevated from the nasolabial area that may measure up to 5 cm. in length and 2.0 cm. in width. Transposed to the nose,

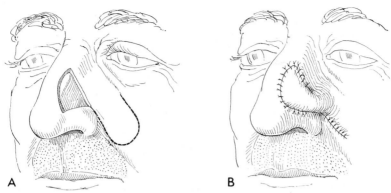

Figure 71–5   *A*, Outline of nasolabial flap to repair loss of skin of lateral wall of nose. *B*, Flap transposed into place and defect on cheek closed by direct approximation. (*From* Kazanjian and Converse: The Surgical Treatment of Facial Injuries. Ed. 2. Copyright 1959, The Williams & Wilkins Company, Baltimore.)

it may be folded on itself to repair alar defects (Fig. 71–6*A*, *B*, and *C*) or used in conjunction with a hinge flap turned in to provide lining if a full-thickness tissue loss is present. Any thickening at the base of the flap is corrected three to four months later by dividing it, defatting the flap, and excising any excess present.

The Median Forehead Flap

The forehead has been used for hundreds of years for reconstructing the nose; its use was first reported in modern medical literature in 1816 (Carpue, 1816). The technique has remained much the same (Fig. 71–7) (Kazanjian, 1946), and, despite the vertical scar it leaves on the forehead, excellent results may be obtained. Defects of the dorsum and lateral wall (Fig. 71–8*A*), too large for closure by a composite graft or a nasolabial flap, are readily repaired by the technique, and full-thickness losses may be reconstructed by a hinge flap turned in from one of the healed edges with the forehead flap rotated onto it. The flap is based inferiorly on the glabella and relies for its survival on a direct blood supply from the supratrochlear and frontal arteries. After the excision of the edges of the defect, the removal of scar tissue, and the development of a turn-in flap (if a full-thickness loss is present), a pattern of the final defect is made and placed upside down on the forehead. The flap is then raised

superficial to the frontalis, and as the nasion is approached, one side is chosen to provide the blood supply. The remainder of the flap is elevated just above the periosteum and rotated through 180 degrees into position and sutured in place (Fig. 71–8*B*). The donor site is closed by direct approximation and lateral undermining, with the pedicle of the flap being left open to avoid pressure on it by dressings. Some 12 to 16 days later, the pedicle is divided close to the forehead, whch is then sutured to close the defect completely. The flap itself is trimmed to fit the upper edge of the defect of the nose and sutured in place (Fig. 71–8*C*).

The Forehead Scalping Flap

Major defects of the nose (Fig. 71–2*B*) and those involving loss of the tip, both the ala nasi and the columella, require more tissue than is obtained by the previously described method. Again, the forehead provides the best source of tissue for this purpose, but instead of using the central part of the forehead where a skin graft replacement would be most conspicuous, the flap is elevated laterally and carried down onto the nose on a pedicle consisting of part of the scalp and the remaining forehead (Fig. 71–2*E*) (Converse, 1942; Converse and Casson, 1969; Converse, 1959). Lining is obtained by the use of local turn-in flaps, by a septal flap (Fig. 71–2*A*), or, if a very extensive

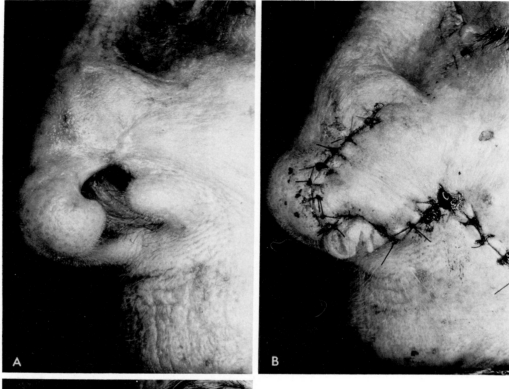

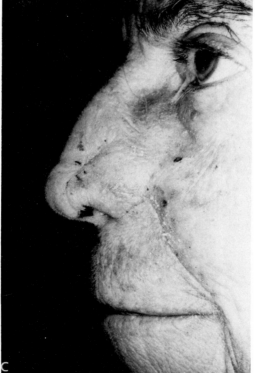

Figure 71–6   *A*, A defect of the ala nasi after treatment of a basal cell carcinoma by chemosurgery. The entire area was densely scarred and considered an unsuitable bed for a composite graft from the ear. *B*, A nasolabial flap has been elevated from the cheek and folded upon itself to reconstruct the alar rim after first closing the skin defect on the face. *C*, Appearance ten days after surgery.

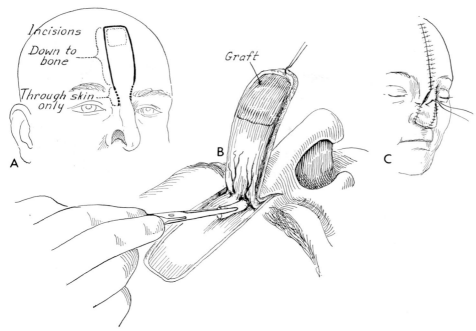

Figure 71–7 *A*, The median flap employed for a nasal defect. The forehead defect has been closed by direct approximation. *B*, At the root of the nose, the line of dissection is subperiosteal in order to avoid injury to the supratrochlear vessels. *C*, Median flap after transfer. (After Kazanjian.)

nasal loss is present, by a median forehead flap used in conjunction with the more laterally placed flap (Fig. 71–9) (Gillies and Millard, 1957; Converse, 1963). The flap is left in place for 16 to 21 days, at the end of which time the pedicle is divided and the scalp and the unused portion of the forehead returned to their normal positions, a full-thickness graft of retroauricular or supraclavicular skin replacing the forehead skin loss. Finally, the divided edge of the flap attached to the nose is trimmed and sutured into place.

Retouching operations to obtain symmetry and a bone or cartilage graft, if skeletal support has been lost, may be needed as later procedures after three months. The final results are most acceptable (Fig. 71–5*F*), and the procedure may be performed in individuals of advanced age.

Perioral and Lip Reconstruction

The treatment of tumors on and around the lips by chemosurgery is followed by rapid contraction and distortion of the soft tissues, which are indications for early reconstruction within days of the completion of treatment because of the difficulties encountered with mastication and the control of saliva. A variety of techniques have been described (Converse and Wood-Smith, 1964).

In the patient with only a superficial tumor in which the vermilion and lip mucosa are intact, scar tissue is excised and the skin and the mucosa undermined until the contracture is corrected. Replacement is then possible by the application of a full-thickness skin graft or an inferiorly based rotation flap from the nasolabial area. This method is also useful if the vermilion is intact in the presence of a fistula (Fig. 71–10*A*), and a full-thickness nasolabial flap with a mucosal lining based inferiorly provides adequate tissue replacement (Fig. 71–10*B* and *C*). For more extensive defects of the lower lip and upper chin, an undelayed cervical flap based posteriorly and advanced upward over the chin may be used, obtaining lining by turning in flaps from the edge of the defect (Fig. 71–1*A* to *D*).

In those full-thickness defects of the lip

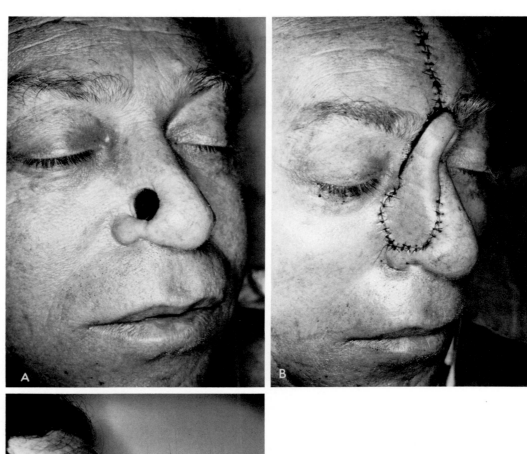

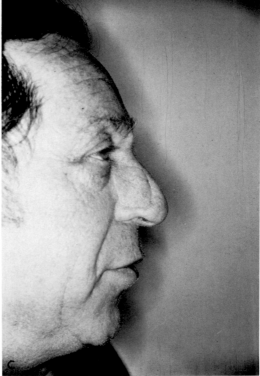

Figure 71–8   *A*, Full-thickness defect of the lateral wall of the nose six months after treatment of a basal cell carcinoma in the area. *B*, Hinge flaps have been turned in to provide a lining, over which a median forehead flap is placed. This is left in place for 16 to 18 days, when the pedicle is divided and the remainder of the flap sutured in place. *C*, Appearance six months after surgery. The color match is good.

72

*Cryosurgery**

Douglas Torre, M.D.

HISTORY

James Arnott (1851) of Great Britain used cryotherapy with a salt-ice mixture in special containers and applicators for palliative treatment of malignancies involving the skin (breast carcinomas) before 1850, but the first true cryosurgeon was the dermatologist Dr. A. Campbell White of New York, whose first publication on the use of liquid air appeared in the Medical Record in 1899. Although he used liquid air in spray form for treating other dermatologic lesions, for epitheliomas he used a swab method, dipping a cotton-tipped wooden applicator into the liquid air and then applying it to the epithelioma to be treated. In 1902 White reported on "Liquified Oxygen and X-ray Treatment of Malignant Growths." He used the term "liquified oxygen" instead of "liquid air," as he erroneously felt that as soon as liquid air was exposed to ordinary air, the nitrogen component immediately disappeared, leaving almost pure liquified oxygen owing to the more rapid evaporation rate of liquid nitrogen. In the early part of the year 1898, he began treating malignant growths. In the first two years only inoperable or recurrent cases were treated, but later operable

patients who refused to submit to the knife were treated. Repeated treatments were necessary. He preferred the use of cryosurgery over x-ray in treating superficial epitheliomas and ulcerated cancer of the breast but preferred x-ray for nonulcerated scirrhous carcinoma of the breast. He was particularly impressed by the effect of cryosurgery in controlling pain, hemorrhage, and disagreeable and malodorous discharge in cases of ulcerated cancer of the breast. Dr. White and his colleagues treated cancers of the lip and tongue as well as those on glabrous areas.

Whitehouse in 1907 described the technique used in treating epithelioma:

"In epithelioma firm pressure of considerable duration is essential. In those of the ordinary size that occur on various regions of the face the pressure should be exerted at the periphery rather than in the center or recurrences may be expected; the same interval rule applies here also. Exactly the same indications obtain for the superficial type of rodent ulcer. It is in this connection that the diagnostic value of the agent previously referred to is apparent. Formerly in curetting what seemed to be small pearly nodules at the periphery of a healed

---

*Based on studies supported in part by a grant from the John A. Hartford Foundation.

patch one frequently found some of them to be firm cicatricial tissue. Firm pressure with the liquid air applicator, covering several such nodules, freezes only the diseased nodules; no visible effect being observed on the others. I have found it a most valuable aid in this capacity. In treating indolent eroding epithelioma very firm pressure is required, particularly at the hard rolled edge, and in this type it generally requires several applications at intervals of two or three days before healing begins, but once commenced the same rule of waiting before making further applications should be observed. In rapidly advancing fungating epithelioma the remedy should be used with a very bold hand until recrudescence begins, after which the interval application should be adopted.

He reported on 15 cases, six of which needed only one treatment and the others two to over five treatments.

At about the turn of the twentieth century, research in cryosurgery was also going on. Max Juliusberg in 1905 described a method using carbon dioxide spray, adapted from the apparatus used with a freezing microtome. He wrote:

Instead of the microtome for the object, I had attached a sprinkler, such as used on a watering can, about 1½ cm. in diameter with several openings. By opening a valve using a lever one is able to let the carbonic acid spray out of the container—the duration of freezing was 30–60 seconds, opening and closing the valve at short intervals. The area remained frozen 1–2 minutes before thawing. Treatments were repeated at 5–10 day intervals.

Juliusberg stated that his experience was mainly with treating acne, psoriasis, sycotic processes, ulcus cruris, x-ray ulcerations, chancroid, lupus vulgaris, and lupus erythematosus, but he advocated the deeper destructive freezing for carcinomas as well as lupus vulgaris.

In his article he stated that Arnig reported to the medical society in Hamburg in 1903 on the use of ethyl-methyl chloride mixture (Bengue mixture) in the treatment of skin carcinoma. Arning's technique was to keep the area to be treated frozen for one minute and to repeat the treatment at three-day intervals. He also stated that Dethlefsen in Denmark and Saalfield in Berlin had been experimenting with freezing sprays in the treatment of skin lesions.

Dr. W. A. Pusey of Chicago started using carbon dioxide snow as a cryogen about 1905 and popularized it for dermatologic cryosurgery. However, Hockhaus had previously reported in 1898 on experimental work using solid carbon dioxide and ether in a copper vessel to freeze liver and kidney tissue in rabbits. Dr. Pusey described his method of making applicators:

The carbon dioxide snow is collected in a cloth or piece of chamois skin as it escapes from the cylinder. In order to collect it best the cylinder should be tipped up so that the opening is at the lower end. The carbon dioxide is deposited on the cloth in the form of a snow, which can be compressed and handled very much like ordinary snow. The liberation of gas is so rapid that unless the snow is firmly grasped there is a layer of gas between the solid mass and the skin so that it can be easily handled. The snow is pressed between layers of chamois skin into solid masses, as one would make a snowball, and then pared with a knife into whatever shape is desired. It is then held in forceps and applied to the surface. In treating lesions less than a centimeter square the snow can be melted, or pared between the fingers, into the shape of the lesion. In treating a larger lesion I have found that it is desirable to cut the snow in the shape of square sticks with an end surface not more than a centimeter square. In freezing, the end of the stick is applied. It is best to make the freezing surface of the snow rectangular, in order that adjacent areas when frozen may closely correspond to each other without overlapping.

Dr. Pusey used carbon dioxide sticks for treating premalignant lesions, such as actinic keratoses, freezing for 40 to 60 seconds, and for epitheliomas arising in actinic keratoses. Such lesions he froze with firm pressure for 60 seconds. Contemporaries of Dr. Pusey also treated superficial epitheliomas by freezing for from 30 to 90 seconds. Dr. Pusey preferred x-ray for treating deeper and thicker epitheliomas.

Many different types of apparatus for forming carbon dioxide applicators have been devised over the past half-century (Low, 1911). The one most widely used in the United States is a portable unit now manufactured by the Kidde Company, using miniature CO_2 cartridges and plastic forms for producing cylinders of different size. Dr. Carpenter (1942) described the prototype of this apparatus.

In more recent years Dr. Atkinson (1967) has been using CO_2 to treat basal cell epitheliomas following curettage.

In the 1920's, liquid oxygen became available, and Irvine and Turnacliff reported in 1929 on treatment of several epitheliomas with this cryogen using a swab technique such as Dr. White used with liquid air. They felt it to be of value in treating small epitheliomas.

In the 1940's liquid nitrogen became available and, since it was nonflammable, replaced liquid oxygen as the cryogen for dermatologic cryosurgery. Dr. Allington (1950) popularized this modality but did not recommend it for malignant tumors. However, liquid nitrogen has been widely used for treating premalignant lesions and, by some dermatologists, for treating epitheliomas, particularly the multiple superficial multicentric type. Dr. Jekel (1957) treated seven patients having between 1 and 100 or more lesions with this method. He used only a 10-second application (cotton swab technique) and used repeated treatments on all patients except one who had a single lesion.

Zacarian and Adham (1966) described the use of copper cylinder disks for use with liquid nitrogen. These disks were cooled in the liquid nitrogen and then applied to skin cancers. Deeper tissue destruction than that obtained by cotton swab application was accomplished. Although the disk is applied to the skin at approximately $-196°$ C., its temperature continuously rises as heat is extracted from the tissue. The limited heat sink capacity caused Zacarian to abandon this method in favor of a liquid nitrogen spray technique.

CURRENT INSTRUMENTATION

The apparatus that revolutionized cryosurgery was the closed-system liquid system first described by Cooper and Lee in 1961. This apparatus, manufactured by the Linde Division of Union Carbide, was capable of maintaining a cryoprobe tip at any preset temperature from about $-195°$ C. to $0°$ C. and provided a means of tissue destruction well beyond 1 cm. in depth. Although originally designed for neurosurgical operations, it was quite effective in treating skin tumors. Cahan (1965) improved the apparatus and devised cryoprobes for treating primary as well as metastatic malignancies of the skin. Several refinements of this system have been made, and the present models are now sold by Frigitronics, Inc., Shelton, Connecticut. These units are being used by surgeons and otolaryngologists to treat malignancies of the skin, particularly those involving the mucous membrane lesions of the mouth. This application is well described by Gage (1970).

I used the Cooper apparatus successfully in the treatment of skin tumors but found it (at least the early model) too bulky and expensive for use in the office practice of dermatology. Consequently since early 1965, with the help of Linde engineers, we have been developing a cryosurgical system (the Cryoderm System) which would be suitable for dermatologic use (Torre, 1967). To a much simplified version of the Cooper apparatus was added an interchangeable spray system which vaporized liquid nitrogen on the surface of the lesion. A spray is ideal for treating keratotic or irregular lesions, which constitute a large proportion of lesions suitable for cryosurgery in dermatology. Use of the spray also results in faster freezing and the capability for deeper destruction of tissue when needed.

The present model CE8, originally manufactured by the Linde Division of Union Carbide and now by Frigitronics, Inc., Shelton, Connecticut, consists of a withdrawal device, which can be inserted into either a 31-liter Dewar (Linde LD31) or a 17-liter Dewar (Linde LD17), and a flexible, insulated, metal delivery tube affixed to a handle to which cryoprobes or spray tips can be attached with Luer-Lok fittings. A heater attached to the distal end of the withdrawal tube is used to pressurize the liquid nitrogen to a working pressure of 10 to 21 p.s.i. A 12-p.s.i. safety valve prevents overpressurization (Fig. 72–1). The Dewar flasks are refilled at two- to four-week intervals, depending on Dewar size and rate of usage.

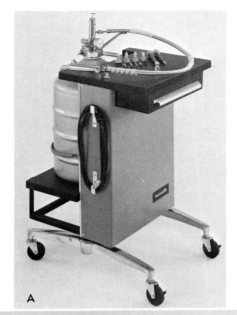

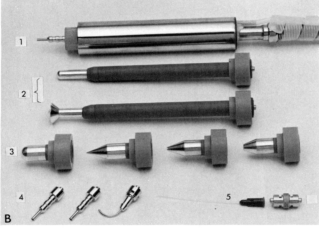

Figure 72–1 The Cryoderm System. *A*, CE8 unit utilizing 17-liter Dewar mounted on movable stand (Frigitronics, Inc., Shelton, Connecticut). *B*, 1. CE8 handle with coarse spray tip attached. 2. Extended closed-tip cryoprobes (for use in mouth or vaginal vault). 3. Various closed-tip cryoprobes for skin surface application. 4. Spray tips. 5. Luer-Lok adaptor for attaching various sized needles or needle hubs.

Portable spray units (refilled for treating each patient) are available from Brymill Corporation (Kryospray unit) and Frigitronics, Inc. (Zacarian C21 unit) (Fig. 72–2). These must be refilled from a larger liquid nitrogen source for treatment of each patient. Brymill also makes a large spray unit. Portable units using thermos bottle Dewars for liquid nitrogen storage and capable of treating a number of patients without refill are available from Medical Specialties, Inc., New Orleans, Louisiana (Foster Froster) and Physicians Products, Inc., Millbrae, California (TT32 unit).

Cryosurgical units using nitrous oxide for the cryogen (such as those made by Dynatech) are not recommended for treating malignant skin lesions.

CRYOBIOLOGIC BASIS OF CRYOSURGERY

The effect of cold on human tissue is dependent not only on the amount of temperature fall (minimum temperature reached) but also on the rate of temperature fall (cooling rate following freezing) and on the rate of temperature rise on rewarming (rewarming rate). Injury to the tissue is generally conceded to be due to damage by ice crystal formation and/or dehydration (chemical concentration of

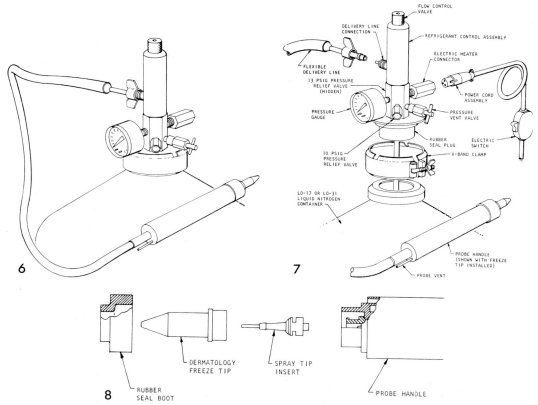

Figure 72–1 *(Continued)* 6. Diagram of unit inserted in Dewar. 7. Components of unit. 8. Method for interchanging spray tips and cryoprobes.

solute). Intracellular ice crystal formation is more damaging than extracellular ice crystal formation. Intracellular ice formation is increased with a rapid rate of cooling. With a slow rate of rewarming, cells are subject to dehydration over a longer period of time, which may be an important factor in the amount of damage done to cells. With very rapid freezing, relatively innocuous small crystals are formed intracellularly. On slow thawing these crystals grow to a damaging size by a process referred to as grain growth or recrystallization. For cryosurgical purposes then, tissue destruction is increased by a rapid rate of cooling and a slow rate of rewarming.

Merely freezing tissue is not lethal. A temperature below 0° is necessary. A temperature of −20° C. is given by many cryobiologists as a standard. There are many reasons for selecting this temperature (Torre, 1971). No cell is likely to remain supercooled (without intracellular ice crystals) at this temperature; it will be killed during the initial freezing or during the subsequent slow thawing when it is exposed to electrolytes during the time it takes the temperature to rise from 21.1° C. (the eutectic point of a sodium chloride solution) to about −4° C. (the point at which concentrations of unfrozen solution would be about one molar). The likelihood of cell lethality is also increased by repeating the freeze-thaw cycle.

In summary, in cryosurgical destruction of tissue, several factors are important, including (a) cooling rate, (b) rewarming rate, (c) minimum temperature reached, and (d) length of time the tissue is subjected to the below freezing temperature. Thus for clinical application of cryosurgery, the method used should provide for rapid cooling of the target tissue, extension of the ice ball beyond the target margins, so that the entire target becomes sufficiently cooled (−20° C. or below), slow thawing, and repetition of the freeze-thaw cycle if increased lethality is desired. For a broader understanding of the cryobiologic basis of cryosurgery, the texts by Von Leden and Cahan (1971), Meryman (1966), and Zacarian (1973 and 1975) are recommended.

In treating skin cancers, we generally use the $-20°$ C. goal because most other surgeons using the modality use this figure and thus we can compare our experience with that of other cryosurgeons. However, there is a great variation in the susceptibility of different tissues to cold. In our experience many basal cell epitheliomas have been apparently cured without the cells being subjected to $-20°$ C. of cold ($-10°$ C. to $-1°$ C. being the lowest temperature reached at the base of some lesions). The ideal minimum temperature for treating these lesions with maximum cure rate and minimum damage to surrounding tissue has not yet been established.

PATHOLOGY

Pathologic studies of the effects of cryosurgery on the skin have been published by several authors, including Grimmett (1961). Our own studies at Cornell (supported by a grant from the John A. Hartford Foundation and under the Direction of Dr. Farrington Daniels, Jr.) have shown that, following application of a copper block prechilled to $-196°$ C. for 15 to 30 seconds, edema and dermal blood vessel thickening occur in the early hours. Fluid exudes from the blood vessels, and the vessels become plugged with red cells. This corresponds with the clinical appearance of the lesion, which is urticarial. Later there is dermal-epidermal separation and vesicle formation, and the epidermis appears homogeneous with loss of nuclear staining. Acridine orange fluorochrome stain is useful in evaluating changes in DNA and RNA, since the orange fluorescence of RNA is increased during new protein synthesis (hyperplasia); moreover, this stain outlines the spindles of cytoplasm in fibroblasts that are not conspicuous with other stains.

During the first eight hours or more, there is a progressive loss of epidermal RNA starting in the basal layer and moving upward. Nuclear DNA fades more slowly, but fading also progresses upward from the basal layer. Dermal-epidermal

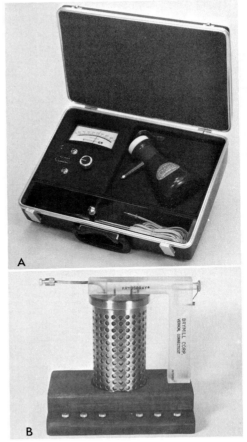

Figure 72–2 Portable units. *A*, C21 (Frigitronics, Inc.). *B*, Kryospray (Brymill Corporation).

separation is evident after the RNA has disappeared from the basal and lower spinous cells (Fig. 72–3). By 24 hours there are only small particles of fluorescent RNA and DNA in a few of the cells in the granular layer; the rest of the epidermis is blank (Fig. 72–4). However, the DNA and RNA of the fibroblasts is retained (Figs. 72–5 to 72–7), even though other stains show homogenization and injury to the upper dermis. The fibroblasts (or at least spindle-shaped cells) retain their RNA and DNA also in 48-hour biopsies (Fig. 72–8). If the fibroblast is, indeed, particularly tolerant of freezing, Dr. Daniels believes it may account at least in part for the relative lack of scarring.

Another possible factor in lack of scarring (at least in treating superficial lesions)

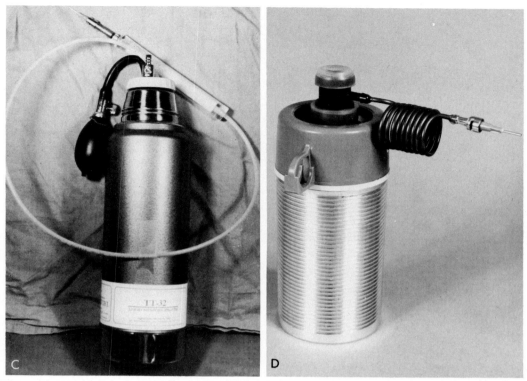

Figure 72–2 (*Continued*) *C*, TT32 (Physicians Products, Inc.). *D*, Foster Froster (Medical Specialities, Inc.).

is that the dermal-epidermal separation in cryosurgical bullae formation occurs above the PAS-positive basement membrane, while in bullous scarring diseases the separation is below this membrane.

Dr. Daniels also has shown that enzymes, represented in this study by diphosphopyridine nucleotide diaphorase (DPNH diaphorase) as a mitochondrial enzyme and lactic acid dehydrogenase as a cytoplasmic enzyme, after a lag period of several hours are completely inacti-

Figure 72–3 Epidermal-dermal separation six hours after freezing, showing intact PAS-positive membrane. *Luxol-fast blue.* (Courtesy of Dr. Farrington Daniels, Jr.)

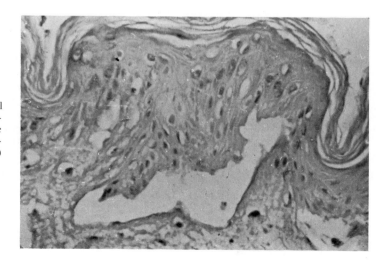

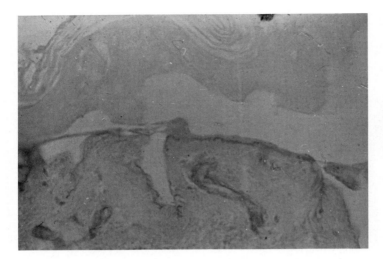

Figure 72–4 Twenty-four hours after freezing. *Alcidin blue PAS.* (Courtesy of Dr. Farrington Daniels, Jr.)

vated. The loss begins in the basal layer and progresses up through the prickle cell layer. The role of lysosomal enzymes is not clear. However, Dr. Daniels and Dr. Johnson have evidence that these compo-

nents are differently affected by hyperthermal and hypothermal insult. With a cryosurgical "blister" at the dermal-epidermal junction, epithelial repair is rapid. Tongues of new epidermis grow in from the sides, rapidly spreading over the surface.

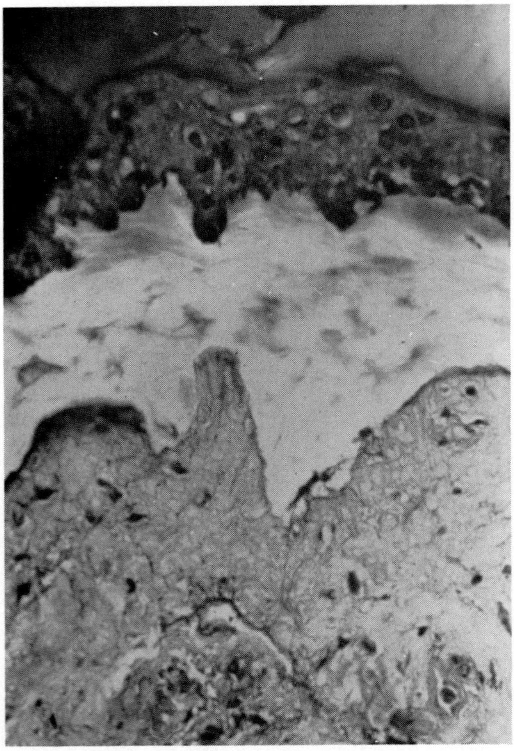

Clinical experience in treating thousands of superficial keratoses and areas of lentigo seems to confirm these histologic findings.

However, with cryosurgery of deep skin lesions, the variation in response of different tissue components must account for the variation in scar formation. The relative resistance of fibrocytes, collagen, bone, and cartilage is a positive factor. The sensitivity of nerve tissue is useful in treating painful lesions, such as metastatic carcinoma of the skin overlying or adjacent to this tissue.

The relative sensitivity of the melanocytes versus the keratinocytes in the skin is used commercially in "cryobranding" of cattle, but in dermatologic research treatment of pigmented nevi and melanomas is still in the experimental stage.

MEASUREMENT OF DEPTH OF FREEZING

Depth of freezing can be estimated clinically by observation, palpation, and ballottement of the frozen mass (ice ball). With experience these estimates are usually adequate for treating superficial

Figure 72–5 Flat, pigmented nevus 24 hours after freezing. Note retained oxytalan fibers in dermis. (Courtesy of Dr. Farrington Daniels, Jr.) (See also Color Plate XI-E.)

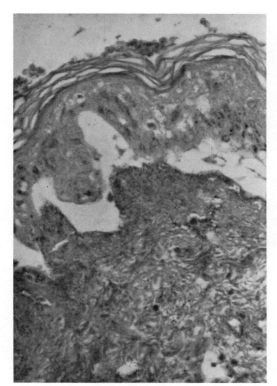

Figure 72–6 Twenty-four hours after freezing. *Reinhardt.* (Courtesy of Dr. Farrington Daniels, Jr.) (See also Color Plate XI-F.)

benign or premalignant lesions. In treating malignancies, more accurate methods of determining the depth of tissue destruction are necessary. Since tumor cells are not all irreversibly damaged at 0° C. or even −1° C., it is desirable to determine

directly or indirectly the isothermic penetration of subzero cold into the tissue. Although −20° C. is frequently advocated as representing a lethal temperature, even its advocates realize that this is an arbitrary figure and that the critical lethal temperature varies with the type of cell being frozen, the rate of freezing and thawing, and whether there is only one freeze-thaw cycle or repeated cycles.

The movement of temperature in depth in treating lesions is most accurately determined by thermocouples (or thermistors) emplaced in the skin at various known depths and positions.

Dr. Holger Brodthagen (1961) of Denmark designed acrylic jigs for positioning thermocouple-tipped needles at set depths in the skin for his experiments using carbon dioxide as a cryogen.

For our studies I designed a circular autoclavable nylon jig with central opening (Torre, 1968). Thermocouple-tipped hypodermic needles inserted into tracks in the jig automatically center the thermocouples at a 1, 2, 3, 5, 7, or 10 mm. depth, depending on the track chosen (Fig. 72–9). Using a Linde (Union Carbide) tissue temperature indicator, up to four depths can be monitored visually by switching from one channel to another. Using polygraphs, such as the Gilson Model II, up to six depths can be simultaneously monitored with continuous recording. Accurate depth positioning of thermocouples is valuable in research and in relating clinical criteria to movements of tempera-

Figure 72–7 Red cell thrombus 24 hours after freezing. *KPM.* (Courtesy of Dr. Farrington Daniels, Jr.) (See also Color Plate XII-A.)

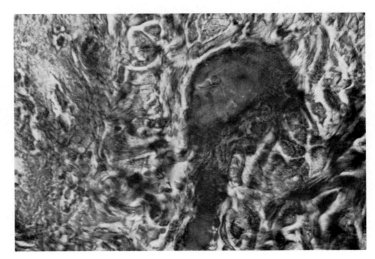

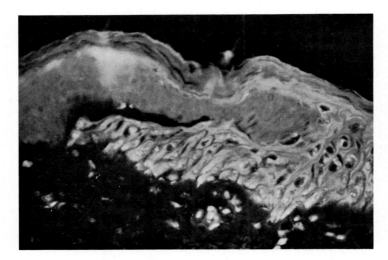

Figure 72–8 Regrowth of epithelium at margin of cryoinjury at 48 hours. *Acridine orange.* (Courtesy of Dr. Farrington Daniels, Jr.) (See also Color Plate XII-B.)

ture in depth but is of limited value in the practical clinical treatment of skin malignancies. When margins and depth of a tumor are definite, a thermocouple-tipped needle can be emplaced under the tumor by palpation without using a jig. This is particularly true in nodular epitheliomas occurring over bony areas such as the forehead. In such cases if the tumor were freely movable, the needle would be inserted under the tumor, but superficial to the periosteum, and the freezing continued until the desired temperature at that depth was attained.

When thermocouples are not used, accurate clinical criteria must be determined. In instances in which the cryo-

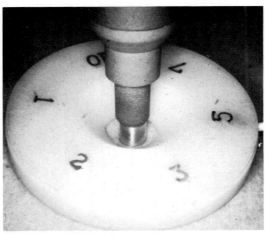

Figure 72–9 Measuring depth of cold penetration. Nylon jig positioning thermocouple-tipped hypodermic needle at predetermined depth beneath lesion being treated.

probe can be maintained at a constant temperature and similar interface contact with a homogenous tissue can be duplicated (Fig. 72–10), the depth of freezing is time-related. Thus we can determine from previous monitoring that an "x-" diameter cryoprobe at $-196°$ C. should yield a $-20°$ C. temperature under its

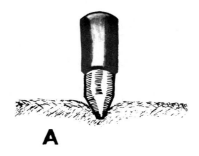

A

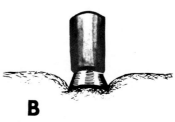

B

Figure 72–10 Effect of pressure. *A,* With a probe of this shape, not only is the tissue compressed and the contact between the probe and skin improved but also a "wall" effect comes into play, increasing the contact area between probe and skin (interface.) *B,* With a probe of this shape, "wall" effect does not play a role.

midpoint, at "y" depth, in "z" minutes. This method is used by some head and neck surgeons for treating intraoral malignancies by contact freezing, as well as for treating tumors by inserting a cryoprobe into the mass of the lesion. The method is of limited value in treating skin cancers, because with a large proportion of lesions the interface contact and pressure cannot be kept consistent owing to surface irregularity.

For contact surface freezing of skin tumors with flat cryoprobes, we have found a way of determining depth of freeze which is not critically dependent on exact duplication of interface contact of pressure. From experiments with agar gel as well as skin lesion monitoring, we have found that for every size cryoprobe the depth of freezing has a mathematical relationship to the lateral spread of freezing, and this lateral spread can be easily seen and measured (Fig. 72–11). Therefore, for each size probe we can determine that the freezing front will be at a central depth of "y" when the frozen surface reaches a certain "x"-diameter. With thermocouple-monitored experiments, it is also possible to approximate the location of the −20° C. front in relation to the

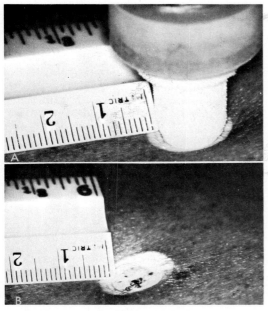

Figure 72–11 Measuring lateral spread of freezing. While cryoprobe is in place *(A)*, and after cryoprobe is removed *(B)*.

freezing (0° C.) front for each cryoprobe. This constant relationship is dependent on the cryoprobe being maintained at −196° C. The ratio varies with the rate of cooling. The faster the rate of cooling, the closer the −20° C. front approximates the 0° C. front.

When using the spray technique, the cooling rate varies tremendously, freezing time is unpredictable, and lateral spread of freezing cannot be accurately determined. Consequently, other criteria must be used to predetermine depth of destruction. Thermocouple monitoring is the most accurate, but a fairly reliable clinical criterion is "thaw time." This is closely related to depth of freeze, although there is variation with different types of lesions and different areas of the body.

It is important that the lesion be allowed to thaw at room temperature without using means of slowing down (such as obstruction circulation) or speeding up (such as palpating the lesion with warm fingers) the process. Thaw time is more valuable in treating epitheliomas, for which repeated freeze-thaw cycles are used routinely. The second freeze can be adjusted by information gained from the thaw time clocked following the first freeze, and a third freeze-thaw cycle can be used if the first two thaw times are considered inadequate (Torre, 1970).

TREATMENT OF PREMALIGNANCIES

Prophylactic treatment of skin malignancies includes treatment of premalignant lesions. Cryosurgery is ideally suited to the treatment of many of these lesions, including actinic keratoses, Bowen's disease, lentigines, leukoplakia, keratoacanthomas, and cutaneous horns (Torre, 1973). Actinic keratoses are the most common and can be treated by application of carbon dioxide sticks or liquid nitrogen on a cotton swab. In my own practice thousands of lesions have been treated with liquid nitrogen using the spray method without local analgesics. The nitrogen was sprayed on the lesion for a few seconds until the frozen area extended throughout the involved area plus a peripheral zone of

2 to 3 mm. In larger lesions the spray was moved over the area in the same manner as a paint spray gun. A thaw time of 15 to 60 seconds (depending on the adjudged thickness of the lesion being treated) was considered satisfactory. Suspicious areas were biopsied (shave biopsy technique) while the lesions were frozen. Trichloroacetic acid was applied to the biopsy site for hemostasis.

Areas of lentigo were treated similarly, with a thaw time of 15 to 30 seconds. Leukoplakia was treated more vigorously, with a thaw time of 60 to 120 seconds and repeated freeze-thaw cycles in many cases. When the lip was extensively involved, the entire vermilion border was frozen, starting at one oral commissure and slowly advancing along the lip to the other commissure.

Cutaneous horns, verrucous keratomas, and suspected keratoacanthomas were first infiltrated at the base with 2 percent aqueous lidocaine, the central portion was removed for biopsy, and the raw surface was painted with a 100 percent trichloroacetic acid. The nitrogen spray was then directed into the central cavity until the entire lesion and a 2 to 3-mm. margin of normal tissue was frozen. For cutaneous horns and keratomas, a thaw time of 30 to 45 seconds was considered sufficient. For keratoacanthomas, a thaw time of 1′ 30 to 3′ was sought and frequently a second freeze-thaw cycle instituted. Lesions of Bowen's disease was handled like multicentric superficial epitheliomas.

The precancerous condition known as the melanotic freckle of Hutchinson should be an ideal target, on theoretic grounds, for cryosurgery, since the cells involved (melanocytes) are more sensitive to freezing than are keratinocytes. In this condition pathologic cells are found not only in the surface epidermis but also along the hair follicles, so that electrosurgery, if used, has to be carried out deeply and vigorously (with resultant scarring), or soft x-ray treatment can be administered by the Miescher technique (given in the dosage range of approximately 10,000 R. with resultant scarring and other postirradiation sequelae). In a commercial application of cryosurgery known as "cryobranding," animal skin has been subjected to liquid nitrogen or solid carbon dioxide–cooled applicators, and the pigment cells of the hair follicle are destroyed without destroying the hair-forming cells (thus the hair in a treated area grows back white instead of resuming its previous color). This method causes minimal damage to the hide (skin), as compared with high-temperature branding. However, no study on the treatment of melanotic freckles has yet been published, and such treatment must be considered as strictly experimental. In my own practice, only those lesions without nodules are treated (nodular lesions being excised and examined for evidence of melanoma). Since about 3 mm. is the average depth of the hair follicle, in treatment I try for freezing beyond this depth.

With experience it should be possible to obtain a cure rate of close to 100 percent with keratoses and lentigines. However, as the best cosmetic end result is desirable, when first starting to use cryosurgery it is better to undertreat than overtreat in managing nonmalignant lesions. It is a simple matter to retreat in three to four weeks if the lesion is not completely gone. The cure rate for leukoplakia, Bowen's disease, and keratoacanthomas is encouraging, but too few cases have been treated for too short a time for reliable statistics. The relatively excellent cosmetic result obtained in treating superficial premalignant lesions with cryosurgery may be due at least in part to the fact that the blister formed after this procedure usually causes epidermal-dermal separation above the PAS-positive basement membrane, while in scarring diseases the separation is below the membrane. This finding has been consistent in our experimental studies at cornell.

TREATMENT OF MALIGNANCIES

More than 2000 lesions in over 700 patients have been treated by cryosurgery since early 1965. Many different experimental techniques with various types of apparatus were used. When cryoprobes were applied, in all cases a tip temperature of $-190°$ C. to $-196°$ C. was maintained. The great majority of lesions were treated with liquid nitrogen spray utilizing successive prototypes of my "cryoderm system" Early cases were treated with a single freeze-thaw cycle. Most early cases were treated so that the epithelioma and a small rim of normal tissue were frozen. Depth of freezing was usually determined clinically by palpation but in a few was monitored by thermocouple-tipped hypodermic needles attached to a Linde depth temperature indicator apparatus. In some a special jig was used to position the needle tip at a known depth. It is only within the past seven years that a standardized system of treatment has evolved. This standard treatment utilizes only the cryoderm system apparatus. Cryoprobes are used on flat or slightly elevated, roughly circulated lesions 1½ cm.

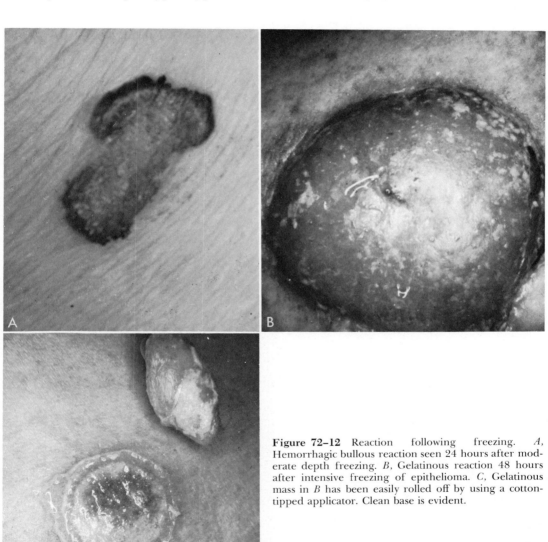

Figure 72–12 Reaction following freezing. *A,* Hemorrhagic bullous reaction seen 24 hours after moderate depth freezing. *B,* Gelatinous reaction 48 hours after intensive freezing of epithelioma. *C,* Gelatinous mass in *B* has been easily rolled off by using a cotton-tipped applicator. Clean base is evident.

or less in diameter. Following infiltration of the area with a 2 percent lidocaine solution, a shave biopsy of the lesion is taken, 100 percent trichloroacetic acid is applied for hemostasis, and a flat-faced cryoprobe is applied firmly. A cryoprobe the size of the lesion or slightly larger is selected. Freezing is continued until the easily visible surface ice front extends peripherally to double the diameter of the probe. If a 1-cm. probe is used, the diameter of the frozen surface area would be 2 cm. If a 0.5 cm. probe is used, the surface area would be 1 cm. The lesion is then allowed to thaw, and the freeze-thaw cycle is repeated. For large, irregular, ulcerated, or fungating lesions, a spray technique is used. For large and irregular lesions, a biopsy is taken from one margin and hemostasis obtained with 100 percent trichloroacetic acid. The lesion is then sprayed until the entire surface of the tumor and a peripheral normal skin zone of 3 to 5 mm. are frozen. In large lesions the spray is moved back and forth over the surface. The thaw time is then clocked. The lesion is then refrozen and the thaw time again measured. Thaw

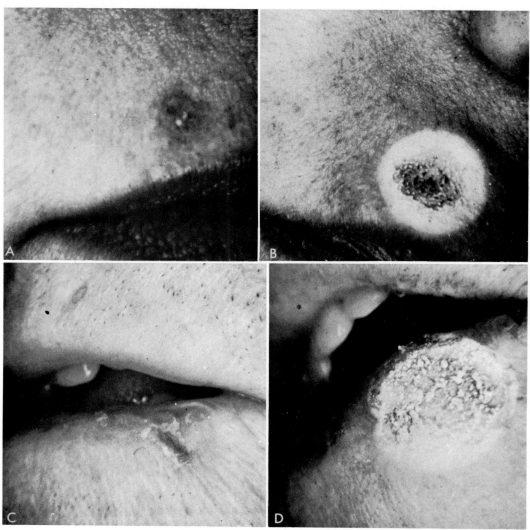

Figure 72–13   Treatment. *A*, Basal cell epithelioma of upper lip. *B*, Area frozen with spray. *C*, Basal cell epithelioma of lower lip. *D*, Area frozen with spray.

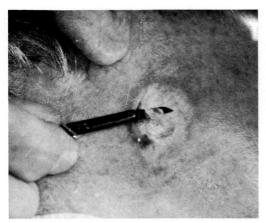

Figure 72–14 Shave biopsy of a lesion while frozen (use of local anesthetic unnecessary).

times varying from one to three minutes each cycle seem desirable (depending on the adjudged depth of the lesion). If the thaw times are less then desired, a third freeze-thaw cycle is used. Only in patients with multiple large, superficial, multicentric epitheliomas is a single freeze-thaw cycle used, and this only if the thaw time is satisfactory.

In fungating or ulcerated lesions, the mushy gelatinous tissue is removed by a curet for biopsy and hemostasis obtained by application of 100 percent trichloroacetic acid. Occasionally it is necessary to electrocoagulate a bleeder. The lesion is then sprayed as in the previous paragraph (see Figs. 72–12 to 72–15).

RESULTS

Statistical cure rate is difficult to establish in our series of over 2000 epitheliomas in the past ten years owing to the great variation in technique in the early years and the fact that we were attempting to find the minimal amount of cryosurgery which would give a reasonable cure rate. By reasonable cure rate, we mean one comparable to that obtained by alternate methods of treatment, such as curettage and electrodesiccation, ionizing irradiation, and scalpel surgery. We set a 95 percent cure rate as a target and have now followed enough patients for five years to confirm that, with patients treated by the standardized techniques, this cure rate is reasonable.

The cure rate varied according to location of the tumor. Our overall cure rate for lesions followed over five years was between 95 and 97 percent. Recurrence was very high for scalp lesions, being 43 percent (three out of seven). Eyelid lesions also had

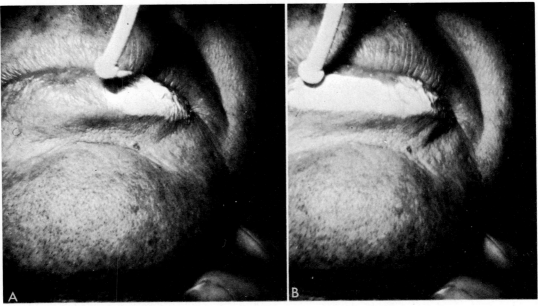

Figure 72–15 Spray technique for lip. *A*, Spraying is started at one margin of lip. *B*, Spray tip is gradually advanced along lip until entire lip is covered.

a recurrence rate of over 10 percent, but this figure compares favorably with the results obtained by scalpel surgery. Domonkos (1965), however, reported a recurrence rate of less than 3 percent with 242 epitheliomas of the eyelid treated by Phillips contact tube roentgen irradiation. Graham (1975), who has treated a large series of patients (653 malignant tumors) with cryosurgery, had no recurrence in ten eyelid tumors and ten scalp tumors, although her overall recurrence rate was higher than 5 percent.

Zacarian (1973 and 1975) has reported in detail on a large number of malignancies treated by cryosurgery. He treated 2193 malignant tumors occurring in 1323 pa-tients. The tumors consisted of 1981 basal cell epitheliomas, 115 epidermoid carcinomas, 67 basosquamous carcinomas, 27 Bowen's lesions, and 3 cases of Kaposi's sarcoma. Twenty percent of his tumors were on the nose, 8 percent on the ears, and 5 percent on the eyelids. His recurrence rate was 2 percent for individual lesions, 3.8 percent for patients. This is not a five-year follow-up rate, but Dr. Zacarian states that 75 percent of the patients have been followed for between three and ten years. Most of his recurrences involved cases early in the series treated by a liquid nitrogen–chilled copper disk technique now discontinued in favor of a liquid nitrogen spray method.

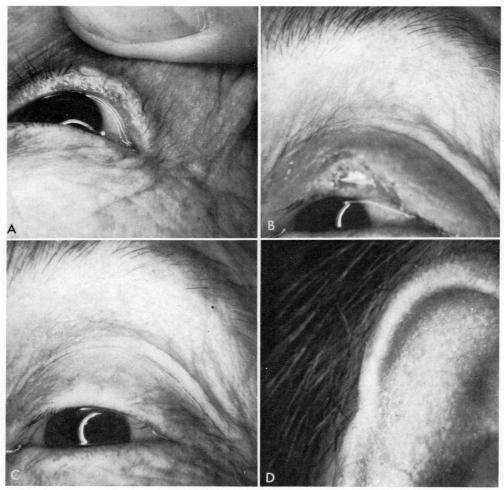

Figure 72–16　Results. *A*, Basal cell epithelioma of eyelid margin. Note that eyelashes in tumor region are missing, indicating tumor extension deeper than hair bulb. *B*, Central portion of tumor removed by curet for biopsy before freezing. Note exposure of tarsal plate. *C*, End result after cryosurgery. *D*, End result of treatment of basal cell epithelioma infiltrating to cartilage of ear.

topical 5-fluorouracil. South. Med. J., 60:185, 1967.

Klein, E., Milgrom, H., Helm, F., Ambrus, J., Traenkle, H. L., and Stoll, H. L.: Tumors of the skin. I. Effects of local use of cytostatic agents. Skin, 1:81, 1962.

Klein, E., Stoll, H. L., Milgrom, H., Case, R. W., Traenkle, H. L., Graham, S., Laor, Y., and Helm, F.: Tumors of the skin. IV. Double blind study of effects of local administration of anti-tumor agents in basal cell carcinoma. J. Invest. Dermatol., 44:351, 1965a.

Klein, E., Stoll, H. L., Milgrom, H., Traenkle, H. L., Case, R. W., Laor, Y., Helm, F., and Nadel, R. S.: Tumors of the skin. V. Local administration of anti-tumor agents to multiple superficial basal cell carcinoma. J. Invest. Dermatol., 45:489, 1965b.

Klein, E., Stoll, H. L., Milgrom, H., Traenkle, H. L., Graham, S., and Helm, F.: Tumors of the skin. VI. Study on effects of local administration of 5-fluorouracil in basal cell carcinomas. J. Invest. Dermatol., 47:22, 1966.

Waldorf, D. S.: Mycosis fungoides-response topical nitrogen mustard. Arch. Dermatol., 97:608, 1968.

74

Systemic Chemotherapy and Tissue Culture*

Jane C. Wright, M.D.

The types of skin cancer which, when treated by the systemic administration of the cancer chemotherapeutic agents available today, respond with some measure of success are mycosis fungoides, Hodgkin's disease, lymphosarcoma, leukemia cutis, squamous cell carcinoma, and the malignant melanoma. Important regressions can be as volatile as any cure in these diseases. The degree of successful therapy varies with the tumor type involved, with the selection of the drug, and with the sensitivity of the tumor to the drug employed.

MYCOSIS FUNGOIDES

Mycosis fungoides, first described as a disease entity in 1806 by Alibert, poses several well-established disease stages wherein the recommended treatment is different. Excellent studies on the clinicopathologic nature and natural history of the disease have been reported by Sequeira (1914), Pusey (1924), Allen (1954), Gall (1955), Belisario (1959a), Bluefarb (1959), Andrews and Domonkos

(1963), Block et al. (1963), and Epstein (1970).

Mycosis fungoides develops gradually. In the premycotic stage, it is characterized by various types of cutaneous eruptions that are extremely difficult to differentiate from several other skin diseases, either on clinical or histologic grounds. Later, irregular thickening and infiltration of the skin develop. In the last stage, there is the formation of nodular growths that frequently ulcerate and form mushroom-like tumors in the skin. The disease may begin with skin tumors. Severe pruritus almost universally accompanies the disease.

In the early stage when the diagnosis is suspected but not established, the treatment is generally conservative in nature. Therapy at this time usually consists of the use of ultraviolet light, emollients, and topical corticosteroids (Haynes and Van Scott, 1968).

---

*This chapter is dedicated to the Cancer Service League, Inc. and to the Ancient Egyptian Arabic Order Nobles Mystic Shrine of North and South America and its Jurisdictions, Inc.

1594

Treatment

Ultraviolet Rays. While ultraviolet rays are either natural or artificial, the latter are currently preferred. It is especially valuable in the early stage of mycosis fungoides, and following the use of ultraviolet light approximately 60 to 70 percent of patients will become pruritus-free and will show resolution of their skin lesions. As presently used, ultraviolet light is beneficial as an antipruritic and also serves to clear the cutaneous lesions (Bluefarb and Ihrke, 1952).

Ionizing Irradiation. Radiation therapy with ionizing rays in one form or another is employed in all three stages of mycosis fungoides for as long as it provides remissions. These remissions may last for weeks to months and occasionally for a year or more. Among the first to report remissions with the use of irradiation were Scholtz (1902), Jamieson (1903), and Allen (1904a). The types of irradiation employed in the plaque and infiltrative states are grenz, teleroentgen, contact, and superficial (with and without an aluminum filter) (Petratos, 1968). Mycosis fungoides lesions found in such difficult locations as the mouth and external auditory canal are best treated with radium (Wise, 1938). When the lymph nodes are involved, then high voltage therapy is necessary (Craver, 1934).

Electron Beam. Electron beam therapy is recommended for those patients with mycosis fungoides whose disease has become resistant to the conventional forms of teleroentgen therapy. This form of therapy provides total body surface irradiation. Adjunct treatment is individualized to the patient. The important series reported by Fromer and colleagues (1961) comprised a nine-year follow-up on 200 cases, and the majority of patients responded dramatically to electron beam therapy. Reported remissions lasted from three to four months; at that time repeat therapy was administered. As adjunct therapy, the corticosteroids, antimalarials, and cytotoxic agents were administered to some patients. Fromer and his colleagues believed that patients in the advanced stages of the disease would be salvaged for many months beyond the usual course, and that patients treated in the early stages of the disease had a better prognosis than those treated in the later stages. The survival rate of patients from the time of institution of electron beam therapy in this series of 200 cases was as follows: 80 patients living from one to four years; 24 patients living from five to nine years.

Garb (1948) reported upon a patient with mycosis fungoides in whom a long remission occurred following therapy with antimonials.

Alkylating Agents

NITROGEN MUSTARD (MUSTARGEN, HN2). With the advent of the clinical use of nitrogen mustard in 1946 by Gilman and Philips, the compound was administered systemically in cases of mycosis fungoides with fair to good success (Karnofsky et al., 1947; Henstell and Tober, 1947; Henstell and Newman, 1947; Osborne et al., 1947; Block and Murphy, 1948; Goldberg and Mason, 1949; Evans et al., 1950). The usual dosage was 0.4 mg. per kg., given intravenously in two or four divided doses over two to four days. In 1956, Sipos and Jakso first described the use of topical nitrogen mustard in three patients with mycosis fungoides and reported fairly good results. In a later work on the painting treatment with nitrogen mustard, they concluded that the erythema in phase I, the infiltrations in phase II, and the ulcerated lesions in phase III disappeared following either a single or double treatment in every case. However, the large, nonulcerated tumors in phase III did not respond to treatment. In 1959, Haserick and colleagues demonstrated the rapid clearing of the plaque lesions associated with relief of the pruritus in one patient following the use of topical nitrogen mustard given to 12 patients with mycosis fungoides; the remissions lasted from one to 18 months, and no systemic toxicity occurred. In a later review of over 50 patients from the Cleveland Clinic in 1968, the value of painting with nitrogen mustard in producing cutaneous remissions was confirmed. Sipos (1965), Waldorf et al. (1967), and Van Scott and Winters (1970) all noted that topical mustard therapy can result in hypersensitivity, as manifested by contact dermatitis, urticaria, and fever following serial paintings with the drug.

When it is administered intravenously, the usual daily dose of nitrogen mustard is 0.1 mg. per kg. of body weight for four days. This course may be repeated at intervals of from four to six weeks. The toxic effects of nitrogen mustard when given systemically are nausea, vomiting, bone marrow depression, and localized phlebitis. The use of anti-emetic drugs has been found helpful in reducing the severity of the nausea and vomiting. The further addition of barbiturates improves the overall effect.

In its topical administration, generally 10 mg of a fresh mixture of nitrogen mustard dissolved in 20 to 50 ml. of water and applied daily for from four to seven days, then once per week, is usually adequate. Because nitrogen mustard deteriorates rapidly after being dissolved, it is important to apply it immediately after its preparation. In its application, the skin of the affected areas are thoroughly cleansed of their natural oils. With the use of rubber gloves, small gauze sponges held by a hemostat are used in the topical painting. The lesions are kept moist by the solution for five or more minutes and then air-dried. Three to six hours later the patient is given a soap and water bath.

Triethylenemelamine (TEM), azetepa (thiadiazole phosphoramide), and cyclophosphamide (endoxan, Cytoxan) are three other alkylating agents in the same class as nitrogen mustard which have clearly demonstrated their activity against mycosis fungoides when given orally.

TRIETHYLENEMELAMINE (TEM). In a series of patients with various incurable neoplasms treated with triethylenemelamine, one patient was in the advanced stages of mycosis fungoides. Following the administration of TEM, the ulcerated lesions dried and the tumors regressed temporarily (Wright et al., 1950). The major side effect of TEM is bone marrow depression, which was not manifest in this case.

AZETEPA (THIADIAZOLE PHOSPHORAMIDE). Azetepa, an oral form of thio-TEPA, was first shown to have antitumor effects by Sloboda and Vogel (1962).

Bateman in 1964 demonstrated its effectiveness in the treatment of advanced cancer. Wright and colleagues (1964) demonstrated the beneficial effects of azetepa in two of four patients with mycosis fungoides. Remissions lasted from three weeks to seven months. The average oral daily dose of azetepa is from 30 to 70 mg. The major side effect is bone marrow depression; occasionally nausea and vomiting may occur.

CYCLOPHOSPHAMIDE (ENDOXAN, CYTOXAN). Cyclophosphamide was synthesized by Arnold and Bourseaux (1958) with the hope of developing a compound which theoretically would have a greater selective affinity for neoplastic cells. Some neoplastic cells, as well as some rapidly growing normal cells, contain increased amounts of the enzymes phosphatase and phosphamidase, which are active in the breakdown of cyclophosphamide. Initial trials in Germany by Gross and Lambers (1958) indicated that cyclophosphamide produced remissions in lymphosarcoma, Hodgkin's disease, and the chronic leukemias. Later reports by Abele and Dobson (1960) and Van Scott et al. (1962) showed the drug to be of importance in the production of remissions in patients with mycosis fungoides.

Cyclophosphamide can be administered either intravenously or orally in doses of 50 mg. every other day, or 50 to 100 mg. per day. Daily dosages are adjusted to the status of bone marrow function. The major side effects of Cytoxan are bone marrow depression, alopecia, and hemorrhagic cystitis. If hemorrhagic cystitis occurs, it is wise to discontinue therapy at once (Talley, 1970). Pulmonary fibrosis has also been reported as a complication (Andre et al., 1967).

The alkylating agents have been called radiomimetics since they act upon tissue in a fashion similar to radiotherapy.

Hormones. The clinical effectiveness of cortisone and ACTH in the treatment of mycosis fungoides was demonstrated by Hench and associates in 1949. Subsequent studies by Thorn et al. (1950) and others at the First Clinical ACTH Conference demonstrated the effectiveness of hormones in the control of mesenchymal disorders, as well as some of their other effects on the body tissues. In the early 1950's, the literature contained many series of various skin conditions which were treated systemically by either ACTH or cortisone, and they generally included patients with mycosis fungoides (Tulipan, 1950; Taylor et al., 1950; Sulzberger et al., 1951; Costello, 1951; Newcomer et al., 1952; Hopkins et al., 1952; Steiner and Frank, 1952; Lowenfish, 1957). In 1957 Tolman reported on a patient with mycosis fungoides whose skin remained clear of lesions following steroid therapy. Haynes and Van Scott (1968) advocated large doses of systemic steroids over short periods in order to effect a reduction in the disease.

When ACTH is administered intramuscularly, the daily dosage is from 60 to 200 mg.; the intravenous dosage ranges from 25 to 50 mg. daily. Cortisone is administered orally in divided doses of from 100 to 300 mg. daily. The daily oral dosage of prednisone ranges from 15 to 60 mg. The undesirable side effects which may occur with the use of these hormones consist of sodium retention, alkalosis, hypokalemia, weight loss, edema, diabetes, high blood pressure, hirsutism, acne, and psychic changes.

The topical steroid creams and ointments are chiefly used in the early stages of mycosis fungoides; occasionally they afford the patient comfort in the later stages, particularly in the event of pruritus. Topical steroid creams are especially effective when they are covered with plastic occlusive dressings (Farber et al., 1966 and 1968). Local steroid injections are partially absorbed and may produce some of the steroid side effects; their use is generally reserved for a later stage of the disease.

Antimetabolites

FOLIC ACID ANTAGONISTS. As a folic acid antagonist, methotrexate is one of a group of antimetabolites of clinical value and, as such, is a substance which competes with the action of a normally occurring essential metabolite in the body and usually has a chemical structure similar to that metabolite. Methotrexate has been

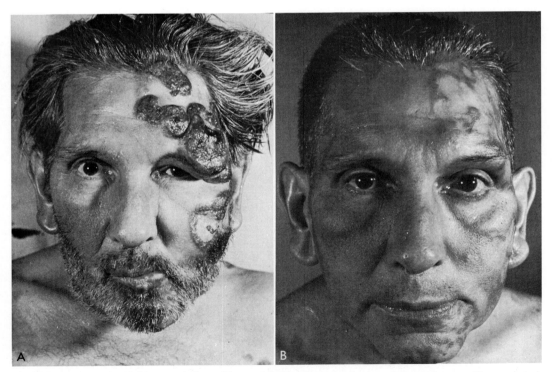

Figure 74–1 *A*, Patient with mycosis fungoides on 6/2/60 prior to institution of chemotherapy. Note tumors in skin. *B*, Same patient in remission on 7/7/60. Observe regression of tumors, which occurred following five weeks on cancer chemotherapy with oral methotrexate. Remission lasted eight months.

demonstrated to produce significant and important remissions in patients with mycosis fungoides (Wright et al., 1960, 1963, and 1964; Haynes and Van Scott, 1968; Van Scott and Haynes, 1968).

The author and associates presented a series of 20 patients who had moderate to far advanced mycosis fungoides and who were treated with methotrexate. Three patients received insufficient therapy, and one patient developed septicemia and multiple skin abscesses. Accordingly, of 16 patients in the series who could be evaluated, nine showed definite subjective and objective improvement, and seven were unimproved. Remissions ranged from 1½ to 24½ months. Figures 74–1 to 74–3 show the remissions obtained in four patients.* Haynes and Van Scott (1968) presented 30 patients treated with methotrexate at the Dermatology Branch of the National Cancer Institute. Remissions occurred in six of the 30 patients which lasted from 5+ to 20+ months.

---

*All the photographs of patients in this chapter were taken by Mr. Kim Massey.

The intermittent administration of methotrexate via either oral or intravenous routes, twice to three times per week, is 2.5 to 10 mg. Massive doses of 50 mg. may sometimes be administered once per week. New dosage schedules wherein the drug is given on four to five consecutive days with subsequent rest periods being studied. In a personal communication, Haynes (1971) wrote:

It is of interest that patients who have high mitotic indices in their mycosis fungoides infiltrates, do poorly on weekly Methotrexate and better on a more frequent dosage regimen, whereas those with a low mitotic index do well on a weekly dose. Although there are several alternate explanations for this observation, I feel that the clinical failure of the high count group on weekly doses is "schedule resistance"; i.e., the increase in cell numbers during the intervals between administration of the drug more than compensates for the cell-kill obtained from the pulse of Methotrexate.

The side effects of methotrexate administration are bone marrow depression, mucous membrane ulcerations, nausea,

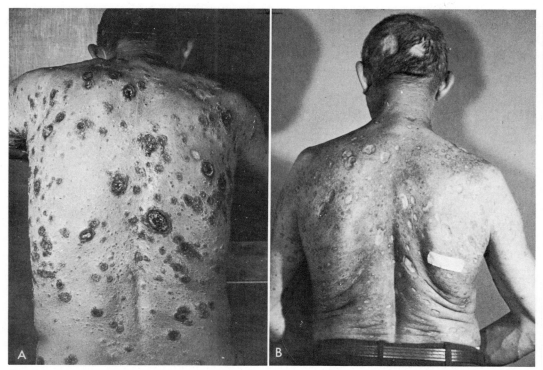

Figure 74–2   *A*, Patient with mycosis fungoides on 4/7/60 prior to institution of chemotherapy. Note ulcerated tumors on skin. *B*, Same patient in remission on 5/26/60. Observe regression of tumors, which occurred following seven weeks of cancer chemotherapy with methotrexate.

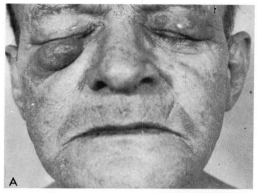

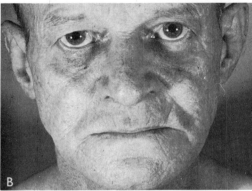

Figure 74–3 *A*, Patient with d'emblee form of mycosis fungoides prior to treatment with methotrexate on 1/15/62. Note tumors in skin around eyes. *B*, Same patient after six months of treatment with methotrexate. Note the regression of tumor masses.

vomiting, diarrhea, bleeding from all mucosal surfaces, liver damage (especially fibrosis), pulmonary fibrosis, and varying degrees of epilation. Our experience has shown that, with the oral dosages recommended for adults, the only side effects are a slight drop in the total white blood count and minimal mucosal ulceration; over a long period of time, slight epilation may occur (if the dosage is titrated to the individual's tolerance).

PYRIMIDINE ANTAGONIST. The pyrimidine antagonist, 6-azauridine (AzUR), developed by Welch and associates (1960), is a compound which functions through the inhibition of pyrimidine nucleotide synthesis. Preliminary clinical studies indicated that AzUR induced remissions in patients with both acute leukemia and chronic granulocytic leukemia without concomitant toxicity to normal cellular elements in the bone marrow (Handschumacher, et al., 1962). Further investigations by Calabresi and associates (1964) indicated that AzUR induced remissions in patients with mycosis fungoides. The optimum dosage of the oral form of AzUR is 135 mg. per kg. body weight per day. The side effects of the drug consist of minimal leukopenia, anemia, stomatitis, and crystalluria.

Antitumor Antibiotics

ACTINOMYCIN D (DACTINOMYCIN, COSMEGEN). Actinomycin D is the best known of the antibiotic class of antineoplastic compounds. Farber and coworkers (1956) introduced actinomycin D into clinical use in this country, noting its beneficial effects in Wilms' tumor, Hodgkin's disease, and rhabdomyosarcoma of childhood. Wright and associates (1964) reported a series of seven cases of mycosis fungoides treated with the drug in which one patient had a remission lasting $1\frac{3}{4}$ months. Therapy was discontinued because the patient refused further treatment due to the nausea, vomiting, and diarrhea caused by the drug. Actinomycin D may be given intravenously daily for from five to ten days, to a total of 75 μg. per kg. body weight, or for twenty days, to a total of 100 μg. per kg. body weight. The local toxic effects are due to the vesicant action of the drug. Systemic effects include glossitis, cheilosis, vaginitis, proctitis, bone marrow depression, and alopecia.

STREPTONIGRIN. Streptonigrin, another antitumor antibiotic, was isolated from broth filtrates of *Streptomyces* flocculus by Rao and Cullen (1959–1960). Wilson and associates in 1961 demonstrated the temporary antitumor effects in a variety of solid tumors with the use of this drug. In 1964, Harris and workers reported on seven patients with mycosis fungoides treated with streptonigrin, and remissions were produced in five (Fig. 74–4). The usual oral dosage of the drug is 0.2 to 0.4 mg. daily until the occurrence of toxicity. An adequate course of therapy consists of at least a total oral dosage of approximately 5.0 mg. The major toxic effect of streptonigrin is bone marrow depression, which may be quite virulent.

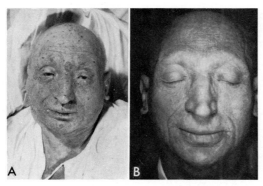

Figure 74–4 *A,* Patient with advanced mycosis fungoides prior to chemotherapy with streptonigrin. *B,* Same patient 36 weeks after institution of streptonigrin. Note marked clearing of skin and face.

Vinca Alkaloid. Vinblastine (Velban) is a *Vinca* alkaloid isolated from the periwinkle plant, which was noted to have antitumor activity by Cutts et al. (1960). Armstrong and associates (1962) reported upon the initial effectiveness of this drug in several tumor types. In 1962, Wright and colleagues noted remissions produced by Velban in six of 13 patients with mycosis fungoides. The remissions lasted from one week to over 11 months. The average adult can tolerate from 2.5 to 10 mg. of Velban given either orally or intravenously once weekly. Therapy is titrated according to the individual hematopoietic picture. The chief toxic reaction to Velban is hematologic; gastrointestinal and neurologic toxicities are less common and usually not as severe. Epilation is occasionally seen as a toxic reaction.

Other Therapy. As in cancer chemotherapy for tumors other than those of the skin, multiple drug therapy is now being used. One report by Haynes and Van Scott (1968) showed a poor result with the use of a combination of nitrogen mustard, vincristine, methylhydrazine, and prednisone in several patients with mycosis fungoides. Of course, numerous drug combinations await further clinical investigation in order to establish the efficacy of this mode of therapy as compared to single drug therapy.

HODGKIN'S DISEASE AND LYMPHOSARCOMA OF THE SKIN

In patients with Hodgkin's disease and lymphosarcoma, the cutaneous manifestations are infrequent in occurrence. According to Bluefarb (1959), the cutaneous lesions of Hodgkin's disease occurred in 13 to 53 percent of patients. In a study of 196 cases of lymphosarcoma, Sugarbaker and Craver (1940) described skin involvement in 5.5 percent. Unlike mycosis fungoides, which usually involves only the skin and mucous membranes, Hodgkin's disease and lymphosarcoma have usually become generalized in the body before skin involvement occurs. Hodgkin's disease of the skin usually originates in the lymph nodes with extension in-continuity or elsewhere in the skin. The specific lesions may be circumscribed infiltrations or papules, usually occurring in crops and accompanied by itching. The nonspecific eruptions may be erythematous, urticarial, vesicular, or bullous, accompanied by pruritus. Lymphosarcoma of the skin may be primary, but more usually it is a metastatic manifestation occurring in papules or subcutaneous nodules of varying sizes. Pruritus may or may not accompany the lesions. However, in Hodgkin's disease the most common skin affliction is a generalized pruritus.

Treatment in both diseases is aimed at the basic disease process, and radiation therapy and systemic cancer chemotherapy either singly or in combination are usually employed (Bluefarb, 1959; Lewis and Wheeler, 1967; Aisenberg, 1970; Van Scott and Haynes, 1971).

Treatment

Radiation Therapy. In the consideration of the treatment regimen for Hodgkin's disease and lymphosarcoma, radiation therapy must be mentioned because of its importance.

In the 1960's, as the newer methods and equipment of radiation therapy were evolved, there was a significant improvement in the survival rate in patients with

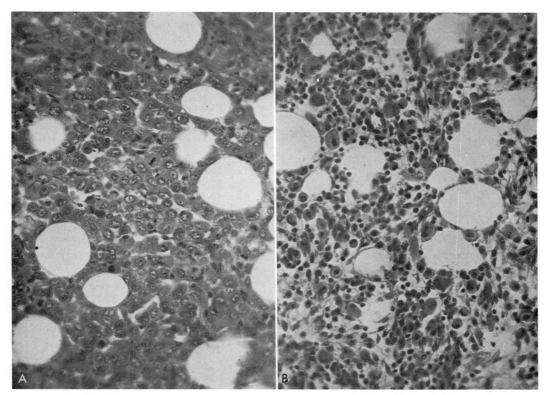

Figure 74–7 *A,* Photomicrograph of malignant melanoma in a patient prior to chemotherapy. *B,* Photomicrograph of a repeat biopsy from the same patient following therapy with treithylenethiophosphoramide. Note the ballooning of the cells and the pyknotic nuclei.

phenylalanine mustard (melphalan, Alkeran), another one of the polyfunctional alkylating agents, in the treatment of metastatic melanoma of the skin.

The most effective chemotherapeutic drug, when administered systemically, for the malignant melanoma is imidazole carboxamide, which is both a DNA inhibitor and an alkylating agent. Experience from a variety of cooperative groups, as reported to the National Cancer Institute, with the use of this agent in patients with malignant melanoma showed an overall response rate of 19.5 percent (81 out of 419 patients). The median remission duration of those responding was 16+ weeks at the last report. Cornell and Pasmantier (1971) had one patient with malignant melanoma who had multiple small pulmonary nodules in both lung fields. These apparent tumors disappeared after one year of therapy. The patient has had no evidence of disease in the past two years.

The side effects of imidazole carboxa-mide are hematologic and gastrointestinal.

Imidazole carboxamide is generally administered in courses at monthly intervals, and the dosage schedule is usually 4.5 mg. per kg. body weight, intravenously and daily for 10 days. In Cornell's case described above, the patient received 4.5 mg. per kg. body weight intravenously, once per week, for one year.

Chemotherapy as administered by the perfusion technique will be discussed in detail in the following chapter under Methods of Treatment.

TISSUE CULTURE STUDIES OF SKIN TUMORS

The growth of human tumors in vitro dates back to 1911 when Carrel and Burrows reported on the growth of "human sarcomata and carcinomata." Since that time a number of investigators have grown human tumors for a variety of purposes. Notable among the works which provided guidelines and which allowed for correlations or served as reference sources are the investigations of Murray and Stout (1954), Cobb (1955), Cobb et al. (1955), Orr and McSwain (1955), Hu et al. (1957), Lasfarques and Ozzello (1958), Cobb and Wright (1959), Cobb and Walker (1960), Papanicolaou and Maddi (1961), Dobrynin (1963), and Di Paolo (1964).

The first five-year study of human tumors in tissue culture, conducted by Cobb et al. (1961), was concerned with the growth characteristics and cellular morphology of a variety of human tumors, as well as the determination of an optimal culture medium for the majority of these tumors. A small number of normal tissues were also studied. Some of the distinguishing features of the various tumor types were recorded. Lymphoma cultures were characterized by the presence of a large number of immature lymphocytic forms. Sarcoma cultures, although identified with some difficulty, exhibited cells with rounder nuclei as compared with other fibroblastic cells and showed marked fibrinolysis and a swirling growth pattern. Melanoma cultures generally exhibited radial outgrowths. The melanocyte was observed in various stages of differentiation, ranging from the undifferentiated unipolar or bipolar form in cultures of amelanotic melanomas to the differentiated dendritic form in cultures of more heavily pigmented melanomas (Cobb and Walker, 1960). Carcinomas in culture were distinguished by the following criteria: cells with polygonal to round shape, round vesicular nuclei, prominent large nucleoli, marked basophilic cytoplasm, and a variation in nuclear and total cell diameter within groups of cells.

A variety of media were used in an attempt to improve the rate and extent of growth. These included Eagle's basal medium, NCTC 109, and medium 199 supplemented with varying proportions (10, 20, and 40 percent) of human, horse, and calf sera. A comparative study evaluating the effects of heterologous (horse), homologous (pooled human), and autologous sera, each combined with Eagle's basal medium, was reported by Cobb and Walker (1961). Of 21 normal and malignant culture series, 19 exhibited better outgrowths in Eagle's medium with autologous serum.

Results of the in vitro growth were recorded. A total of 549 tissue, pleural, and peritoneal effusion specimens from 366 patients were prepared in vitro, and 364 specimens, or 66.4 percent, grew in culture. The percent growth of the major groups studied was lymphomas, 84 percent; sarcomas, 70.3 percent; melanomas, 72.1 percent; skin carcinomas, 43.7 percent; breast carcinomas, 54.6 percent; respiratory system, 73.3 percent; alimentary system, 61.2 percent; primary site undetermined, 70.5 percent; male and female urogenital system, 54.1 percent; malignant tumors of the nervous system, 78.5 percent; benign tumors, 72.7 percent; and normal tissues, 69.5 percent.

Materials of Tissue Cultures

In the second five-year study, the specimens cultured included fresh biopsies of primary or metastatic solid tumor masses and pleural and peritoneal effusions from patients with far advanced neoplastic disease (Walker et al., 1965). A total of 607 tumor specimens were isolated from 580 patients. The solid tumor specimens were collected aseptically in 1-oz. jars containing 5 cml.^{3} of medium 199 (without bicarbonate) plus 150 μg. per ml. of neomycin. The fluid specimens were centrifuged and the sedimented cells redistributed in medium 199 plus 40 percent of the supernatant fluid.

Results

A total of 81 (70.3 percent) malignant melanoma specimens were grown in tissue culture, and 57 demonstrated positive growth. The growth rate is represented as 15.3 percent exhibiting fast growth, 47.5 percent moderate growth, and 37.2 percent slow growth.

Several patterns of growth were ob-

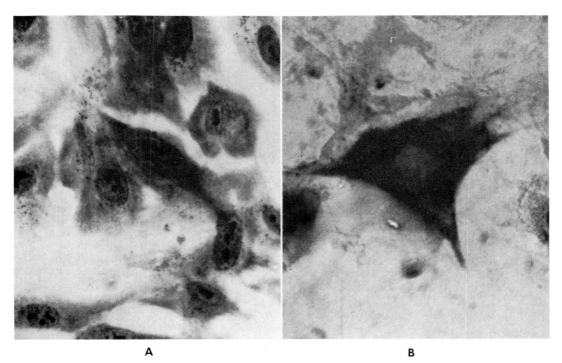

Figure 74–8 *A*, Tissue culture of mycosis fungoides cells showing intact polygonal and multipolar cells. *B*, Tissue culture of same cells treated with 0.05 mg. per ml. of methotrexate. Note heavily granular cell and surrounding degenerating cells and cellular debris.

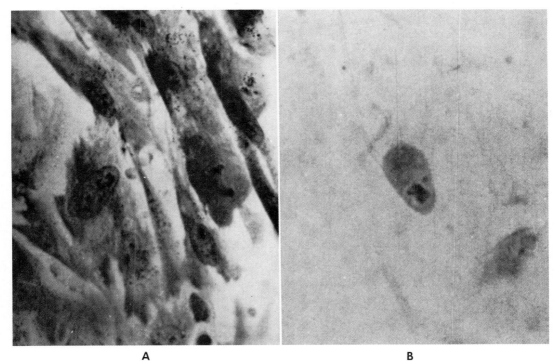

Figure 74–9 *A*, Tissue culture of mycosis fungoides showing numerous cells with one cell in anaphase. *B*, Tissue culture of same cells treated with 0.1 µg. per ml. of streptonigrin showing few remnants of degenerating cells.

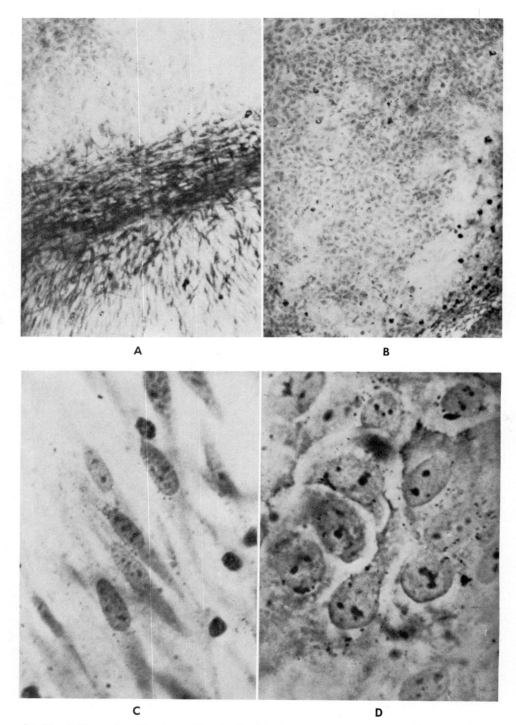

Figure 74–10   *A*, Eleven day old culture of basal cell epithelioma showing a varied growth pattern. Top, epithelial sheet; middle, "fibroblastic cells oriented circumferentially around the epithelial sheet"; bottom, fibroblastic cells oriented radially. ×90. *B*, Another view of same epithelial sheet. *C*, Higher magnification of same fibroblastic cells. ×900. *D*, Higher magnification of same epithelial cells. ×900.

served, but they were not specific for given tumor groups: (1) the simple spreading out of the explant and a drifting out of cells; (2) the random migration of single cells, observed to some degree in all cultures and the dominant pattern of growth in a majority of tumor and tissue specimens in culture; (3) the migration of cells in confluent sheets with or without a fringe of spindle cells, generally observed in carcinoma and other tissue specimens of epithelial origin (this was never observed in the lymphomas, except in one case of mycosis fungoides, and it was believed to be an outgrowth of skin); and (4) the organotypic migration, in which the cells appeared to be structurally oriented in a three-dimensional matrix.

The cell types observed, like the growth patterns, were not specific for a given tumor type. In general, the cells were round, polygonal, bipolar, and multipolar spindle-shaped; one or all of these cell types were found in a single culture. Whether they represent one or multiple origins in a given culture is not known.

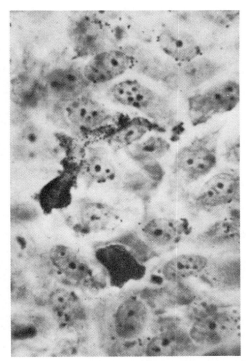

Figure 74–12   Two cells in basal cell carcinoma containing fine metachromatic granules. ×*900.*

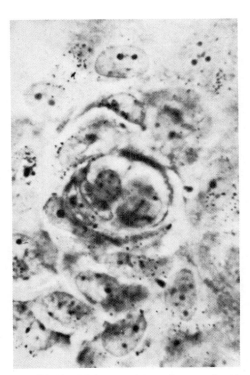

Figure 74–11   High power view of a nest of epithelial cells in culture of basal cell carcinoma. ×*900.*

In our laboratory, several cells having some of the characteristics observed in tissue sections were seen, notably the signet-ring cells of adenocarcinoma, the immature lymphoid and reticulum cells of the polymorphic infiltrate in mycosis fungoides, and the melanin-containing or -producing cells in the melanotic and in the amelanotic melanoma, respectively. (See Figures 74–8 to 74–27).

Ten of 11 basal cell tumors were grown in culture (Walker et al., 1964). Different morphologic types of cellular outgrowths were found to occur from basal cell epithelioma explants. Of particular interest were the outgrowths of sheets of epithelial cells which occurred in three of the 11 culture series. In two series it seemed likely that the epithelial cells represented in vitro proliferations of the epithelial component of the basal cell epithelioma. It is thought, although unproven, that the sheets of epithelial cells arise from the tumor tissue. Both Söltz-Szötz (1963) and Dobrynin (1963) have described similar findings in their studies of the tissue cul-

Text continued on page 1614

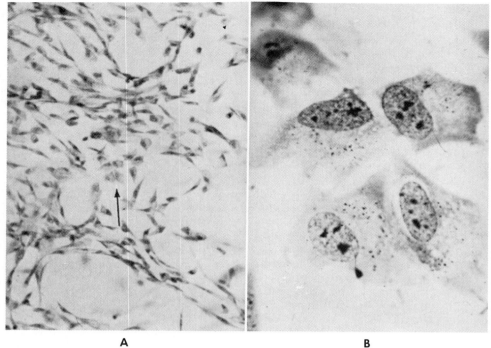

A   B

Figure 74–13   *A*, Tissue culture of basal cell carcinoma showing highly unorganized growth pattern with marked pleomorphism. ×900. *B*, Higher power. Note the increased nuclear to cytoplasmic ratio and prominent irregular nucleoli of these bizarre epithelial-like cells. ×900.

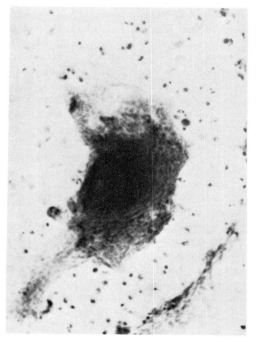

Figure 74–14   Culture of basal cell carcinoma showing the explant as a dark central area with surrounding sheet of outgrowing epithelial cells. ×90.

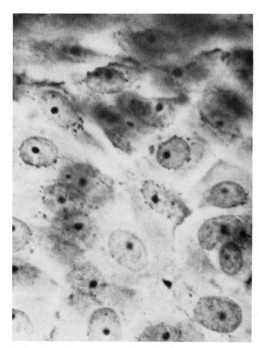

Figure 74–15   Culture of basal cell carcinoma showing high power view of epithelial cells with constant nuclear size and single round nucleoli. ×900.

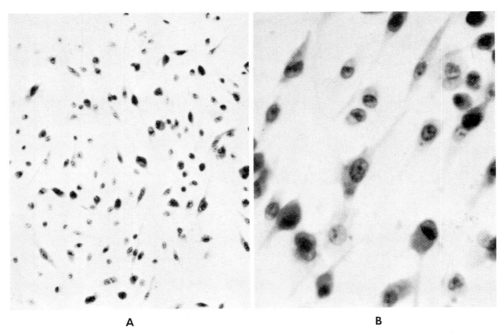

A   **B**

Figure 74–16 *A*, Melanoma cells and macrophages in culture of a primary lesion which arose de novo. ×*300.* *B*, Higher magnification of same. ×*470.* (*From* Cobb, J. P., and Walker, D. G.: Studies on human melanoma cells in tissue culture. I. Growth characteristics and cytology. Cancer Res., 20:858, 1960.)

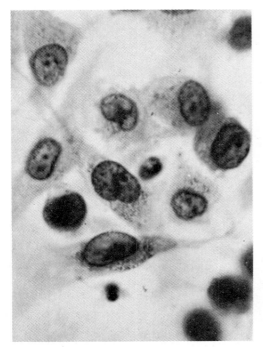

Figure 74–17 Several large, relatively undifferentiated melanocytes in tissue culture of primary malignant melanoma. ×*1100.* (*From* Cobb, J. P., and Walker, D. G.: Studies on human melanoma cells in tissue culture. I. Growth characteristics and cytology. Cancer Res., 20:858, 1960.)

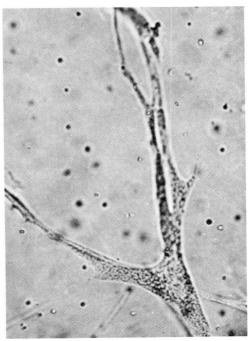

Figure 74–18 Living dendritic melanocyte in culture of pigmented recurrent melanoma unstained. ×*845.* (*From* Cobb, J. P., and Walker, D. G.: Studies on human melanoma cells in tissue culture. I. Growth characteristics and cytology. Cancer Res., 20:858, 1960.)

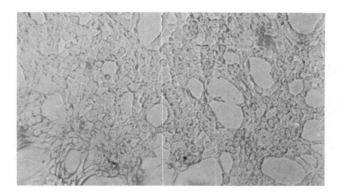

Figure 74–19 Living undifferentiated melanocytes in culture of nonpigmented recurrent melanoma unstained. ×*110.* (*From* Cobb, J. P., and Walker, D. G.: Studies on human melanoma cells in tissue culture. I. Growth characteristics and cytology. Cancer Res., 20:858, 1960.)

Figure 74–20 Highly branched melanocyte in culture of pigmented metastatic skin nodule. ×*470.* (*From* Cobb, J. P., and Walker, D. G.: Studies on human melanoma cells in tissue culture. I. Growth characteristics and cytology. Cancer Res., 20:858, 1960.)

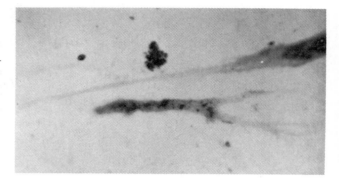

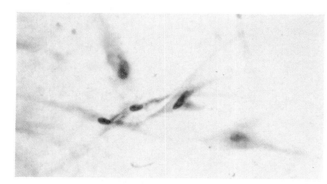

Figure 74–21 Dendritic melanocyte in culture of another pigmented metastatic skin lesion. ×*300.* (*From* Cobb, J. P., and Walker, D. G.: Studies on human melanoma cells in tissue culture. I. Growth characteristics and cytology. Cancer Res., 20: 858, 1960.)

Figure 74–22 Living, highly branched, dendritic melanocyte in culture of gray metastatic subcutaneous mass. *Phase contrast,* ×*430.* (*From* Cobb, J. P., and Walker, D. G.: Studies on human melanoma cells in tissue culture. I. Growth characteristics and cytology. Cancer Res., 20:858, 1960.)

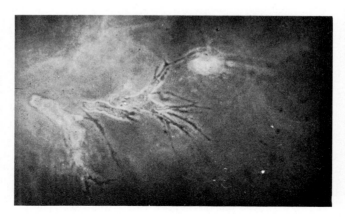

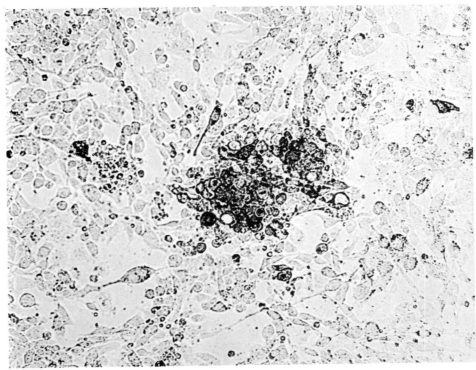

Figure 74–23 Living cells of trypsinized melanoma specimen growing directly on glass. ×75. (*From* Cobb, J. P., and Walker, D. G.: Studies on human melanoma cells in tissue culture. I. Growth characteristics and cytology. Cancer Res., 20:858, 1960.)

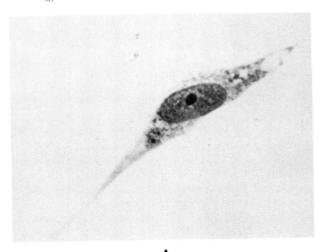

A

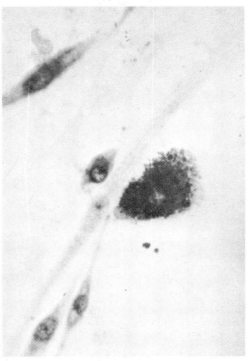

B

Figure 74–24 *A,* Fibroblast with coarse melanin granules in cytoplasm in culture from lymph node with metastatic melanoma. *B,* Macrophage with coarse to fine melanin granules in cytoplasm in tissue culture of same specimen as in *A.* (*From* Cobb, J. P., and Walker, D. G.: Studies on human melanoma cells in tissue culture. I. Growth characteristics and cytology. Cancer Res., 20:858, 1960.)

ture of the basal cell and other epithelial tumors of human origin.

In Vitro Testing of Human Neoplasms

The wide variation noted in the responsiveness of human tumors of the same histopathologic type emphasizes the need for a method of selecting the most effective therapeutic agent for each given patient with neoplastic disease. Discrepancies have been noted in the comparative study of clinical data with experimental systems employing animal tumors, transplantable human tumors in heterologous hosts (hamster, rat, mouse, and chick egg), and both animal and human malignant cell lines.

A number of investigators have studied the individual patients' tumor tissue or the neoplastic cells or both, using a variety of laboratory test systems, in an attempt to determine human tumor sensitivity to cancer chemotherapeutic agents. Tumor

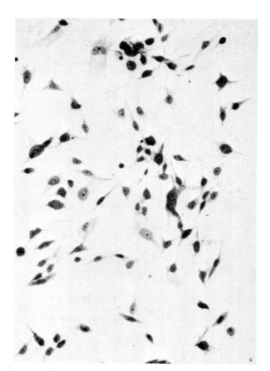

Figure 74–25 Melanoma cells in culture of an ascitic effusion. ×330. (*From* Cobb, J. P., and Walker, D. G.: Studies on human melanoma cells in tissue culture. I. Growth characteristics and cytology. Cancer Res., 20:858, 1960.)

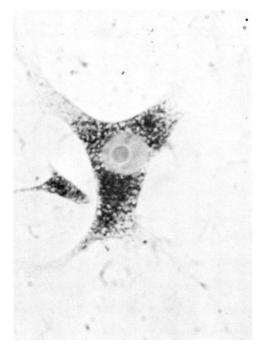

Figure 74–26 Large, stellate, DOPA-positive melanocyte stained for DOPA-oxidase. Enzyme sites appear black. ×1290. (*From* Cobb, J. P., and Walker, D. G.: Studies on human melanoma cells in tissue culture. I. Growth characteristics and cytology. Cancer Res., 20:858, 1960.)

specimens or cells are prepared for testing in the following ways: primary short-term explant cultures of solid tumors (Antikajian et al., 1951; Cobb, 1955; Hirschberg et al., 1956; Gellhorn et al., 1957; Cobb and Walker, 1958 and 1961; McDonald and Cole, 1960; McDonald and Baxter, 1961; Walker and Wright, 1961, 1962a, and 1962b); Golomb et al., 1962; Liss, 1963; McDonald et al., 1963; Hurley and Yount, 1964; Jackson, 1964); short-term cultures of cell suspensions from minced or trypsinized portions of the primary tumor (Di Paolo and Dowd, 1960 and 1961; Ambrose et al., 1962; Krahe, 1962); modified organ cultures (McDonald et al., 1963); short-term cultures of malignant effusions (Cobb and Walker, 1958 and 1961; Di Paolo, 1964; Hurley and Yount, 1964); short-term buffy coat cultures (Richmond et al., 1961; Cohen et al., 1963); cultures of purified suspension of lymphocytes (Holland and Ebaugh, 1962; Schrek, 1960 and 1964); short-term bone marrow aspirates (Hiraki et al.,

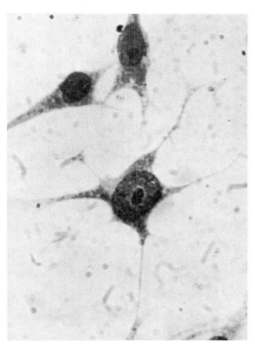

Figure 74–27 Large, stellate melanocyte. ×*1290*. (*From* Cobb, J. P., and Walker, D. G.: Studies on human melanoma cells in tissue culture. I. Growth characteristics and cytology. Cancer Res., 20:858, 1960.)

logic evidence of cytotoxicity. Some of the investigators who have undertaken these studies are Black and Speer (1953 and 1954), Laszlo et al. (1958), Di Paolo and Dowd (1961), Wolberg and Curreri (1961), Birnie and Heidelberger (1962 and 1963), Holland and Ebaugh (1962), Wolberg and Brown (1962), Bertino (1963), and Di Paolo (1964).

The morphologic evaluation of the response to cancer chemotherapeutic agents is generally used when cell cultures comprise a heterogeneous population. Quantitative measurements of responsiveness in such systems are difficult. Semiquantitative determinations (cell counts and mitotic indexes) have been obtained when sufficiently large numbers of cells are available. In our study, the gradation of cytotoxity was based on the criteria presented in Table 74–1.

The cytologic criteria used in evaluating drug action in fresh or cultured specimens of bone marrow and peripheral blood are defined within the limits of these particular cell systems. Thus, as evidence of cytotoxicity, Hirake and workers (1961b) used the inhibition of platelet formation, inhibition of erythropoiesis, inhibition of myelocyte growth, altered growth patterns, and the appearance of crystals in various myeloid cells.

The degree of correlation between laboratory and clinical results is also dependent on the interpretation of the clinical responses. As a result of this caution and conservatism in grading the clinical results, we have perhaps tended to underrate the degree of the therapeutic responses.

In our earlier studies (Cobb, 1955; Cobb and Walker, 1958 and 1961; Cobb et al., 1955 and 1961), the in vitro drug dosages were based on effective threshold concentrations which had been determined in cultures of HeLa cells. Details of our initial clinical and tissue culture results have been previously published (Golomb et al., 1962; Wright et al., 1962). Since 1960 our evaluations have been based on the results observed with drug concentrations equal to the cytotoxic end point (CE) (Toplin, 1959), a value determined in HeLa and other human malignant cell lines. The effects of graded

1961a); freshly dispersed cells from bone marrow aspirates (Kusumoto, 1959); freshly dispersed cells from peripheral blood samples (Laszlo et al., 1958; Bertino, 1963); and tissue slices of freshly excised solid tumors (Wolberg and Curreri, 1961; Wolberg and Brown, 1962; Birnie and Heidelberger, 1962 and 1963).

The in vitro dosage schedules (i.e., drug concentration and exposure time) are usually based on the following data: (1) cytotoxic levels determined in tissue culture (LD_{50}, ID_{50}) or cytotoxic end point (CE); (2) animal primary screening data; and (3) clinical dosage levels (the daily dose by systemic routes, the dose administered by perfusion or infusion, and the full therapeutic dose and selected subfractions).

Three parameters are generally used in evaluating the in vitro sensitivity of tumor cells to the various antitumor compounds: (1) biochemical measurements of metabolic activity; (2) inhibition of established cell growth in tissue culture; and, (3) morpho-

TABLE 74–1   CYTOTOXIC CRITERIA

Mild Sensitivity (S+) Grade 1°	Marked Sensitivity (S++++) Grade 2°
Nuclear changes:	
Nuclear membrane folding Nuclear lobulation Reduced punctate nucleoli	Membrane thickening Large intranuclear vacuoles Chromatin clumping Pyknotic nuclei Anucleate forms
Cytoplasmic changes: Cytoplasmic vacuolation Coarse granulation Retraction of cytoplasmic processes	Cytoplasmic blebbing Loss of cytoplasmic material
Mitotic changes:	
Lowered mitotic index Aberrant anaphases (unequal divisions, lagging chromosomes)	Aberrant metaphases (fractured chromosomes, condensed chromosomes in bizarre orientation) Metaphase arrest
Overall cellular damage:	
Some retraction and increased cell density	Cell ghosting (moribund, pale-staining cellular remnants) Cytolysis

*Rating ascribed for correlation with patient responses.

dosages were also studied and separate correlations were determined at three in vitro drug concentrations: the lethal end point (LE), cytotoxic end point (CE), and subtoxic dose (ST) for human malignant cell lines. The correlation results obtained with each chemotherapeutic agent are presented in Table 74–2. In Table 74–3, the results according to the major tumor types studied are listed.

A total number of 109 patients were studied for their in vivo, in vitro responses to chemotherapy. Of these, 33 patients were excluded from the final evaluation because of inadequate therapy, unexpected early demise, or other unavoidable events which precluded an evaluation of the clincal responses. The data in Table 74–2 show that a higher percentage correlation is achieved when the in vitro responses to the lowest dosage (column ST) are used for the evaluation. The degree of this correlation is 70.7 percent when grade I responses (slight decrease in the patient's tumor and mild sensitivity in tissue culture) are considered as "no response" (grade 0). Using cytotoxic criteria as an indication of in vitro drug effectiveness, Hurley and Yount (1964) obtained a 58 percent correlation between the clinical responses and laboratory findings.

Many difficulties were encountered in the use of several of these sensitivity test systems. Some of these studies have been abandoned because of the inability to obtain a suitable number of viable cells from preparations of cell suspensions or satisfactory growth of explants. These conditions are sometimes further complicated by the lack of reliable indicators of drug activity. With the advent of more refined in vitro techniques which can be applied directly to the patient's own tumor tissue, additional information may be obtained which may permit a more critical evaluation of the laboratory findings. Thus far, efforts to develop a reliable in vitro drug sensitivity test system capable of predicting the clinical response in an individual patient with cancer have been partially successful in a few but by no means solve all of the different aspects of this problem.

TABLE 74–2 CORRELATION RESULTS ACCORDING TO TYPE OF DRUG*

Drug	Tissue Culture Doses		
	LE†	CE†	ST†
Antimetabolites:			
Methotrexate	5/6‡	8/8	4/4
5-Fluorouracil	4/7	5/8	6/7
Hydroxyurea (Hydrea)	1/1	1/1	1/1
Alkylating agents:			
Thio-TEPA (TSPA)	0/6	4/7	6/6
Chlorambucil (CB-1348)	2/4	1/4	1/2
L-Phenylalanine mustard (CB-3025)	0/0	1/1	1/1
AB-132 (Turloc) (dimethylurethimine)	0/1	1/2	1/2
Antibiotics:			
Actinomycin D	1/2	1/3	0/2
Mithramycin (PA-144)	1/6	2/7	6/6
Mitomycin C	1/3	2/3	2/2
Streptonigrin	1/10	5/11	6/6
Botanicals:			
Vinblastine (Velban)	7/18	7/20	7/19
Totals:	23/64	38/75	41/58
Percent positive correlation	35.9%	50.6%	70.7%

*Grade 0 and 1 responses considered 0 (no response).
†LE, lethal end point; CE, cytotoxic end point; ST, subtoxic dosage level.
‡Ratio of the number of positive correlations versus the total number of specimens tested at that dosage level.

CONCLUSION

The slow but steady progress in the control of certain neoplasms in humans by chemical means has been encouraging. Chemical compounds capable of producing worthwhile therapeutic responses in some types of cancers are now available.

With the optimal clinical application of

TABLE 74–3 CORRELATION RESULTS ACCORDING TO TUMOR TYPE*

Tumor Type	Tissue Culture Doses		
	LE†	CE†	ST†
Carcinomas	7/20‡	12/22	15/18
Melanomas	4/17	10/19	11/16
Lymphomas and sarcomas	10/22	14/28	11/19
Miscellaneous	2/5	2/6	4/5

*Grade 0 and 1 responses considered 0 (no response).
†LE, lethal end point; CE, cytotoxic end point; ST, subtoxic dosage level.
‡Ratio of the number of positive correlations versus the total number of specimens tested at that dosage level.

currently available compounds, laboratory techniques, and clinical knowledge, physicians can now achieve better therapeutic results in patients with certain forms of skin cancer than was ever possible at any time in the past.

REFERENCES

Abele, D. C., and Dobson, R. L.: The treatment of mycosis fungoides with a new agent, cyclophosphamide (Cytoxan). Arch. Dermatol., 82:725, 1960.
Aisenberg, A. C.: Hodgkin's disease. *In* Maddin, S. (Ed.): Current Dermatologic Management. St. Louis, Mo., The C. V. Mosby Company, 1970, pp. 132, 133.
Alibert, J. L. M.: Description des maladies de la peau observées à l'Hopital St. Louis et exposition des meilleures méthodes suivies pour leur traitement. Paris, Barroid l'Aine et Fils, 1806, p. 157.
Allen, A. C.: The Skin: A Clinicopathologic Treatise. St. Louis, Mo., The C. V. Mosby Company, 1954.
Allen, C. W., discussion *in* Sherwell: A Case of Mycosis Fungoides. J. Cutan. Dis., 22:281, 1904a.
Allen, C. W.: Radiotherapy and Phototherapy. New York, Lea Brothers & Company, 1904b, pp. 257–264.
Ambrose, E. J., Andrews, R. D., Easty, D. M., Field, E. O., and Wylie, J. A. H.: Drug assays on cultures of human tumour biopsies. Lancet, 1:24, 1962.
Andre, R., Rochant, H., Dreyfus, B., Duhamel, G., and Fechere, J. C. L.: Fibrose interstitielle diffusé du poumon au cours d'une maladie de Hodgkin traitée par des doses élevées d'endoxan. Bull. Mem. Soc. Med. Hop. Paris, 118:1133, 1967.
Andrews, G. C., and Domonkos, A. U.: Diseases of the Skin. Ed. 5. Philadelphia, W. B. Saunders Company, 1963, pp. 591–681.
Antikajian, G., Wright, L. T., Plummer, J. I., and Weintraub, S.: The effect of triethylene melamine, aureomycin, and some 4-amino derivatives of folic acid on tissues in vitro. J. Natl. Cancer Inst., 12:269, 1951.
Armstrong, J. G., Dyke, R. W., Fouts, P. J., and Gahimer, J. E.: Hodgkin's disease and carcinoma of the breast and other tumors treated with vinblastine sulfate. Cancer Chemother. Rep., 18:49, 1962.
Arnold, H., and Bourseaux, F.: Syntheses und Abbau cytostatisch wirksamer cyclischer N-phosphamidester des bis (B-chloroethylamines). Agew. Chem. [Engl.], 70:539, 1958.
Aso, X., Asano, M., Hirose, K., and Takayasu, H.: Evaluation of Bleomycin treatment. Progress in antimicrobial and anticancer chemotherapy. Tokyo, University of Tokyo Press, 1969, pp. 9–17.
Bateman, J. C.: Chemotherapy of solid tumors with triethylene thiophosphoramide. New Engl. J. Med., 252:879, 1955.

Bateman, J. C.: Clinical studies with azetpa in the treatment of advanced cancer. Acta Unio Internationalis Contra Cancrum, 20:345, 1964.

Belisario, J. C.: Sarcoma: Lesions of reticuloendothelial origin, follicular lymphoblastoma and mycosis fungoides. *In* Cancer of the Skin. London, Butterworth & Company Ltd., 1959a, pp. 236–243.

Belisario, J. C.: Leukaemia cutus. *In* Cancer of the Skin. London, Butterworth & Company Ltd., 1959b, pp. 250–257.

Bernard, J.: Acute leukemia treatment. ASC-NCI Conference on acute leukemia and Burkitt's tumor. Cancer Res., 27:2565, 1967.

Bertino, J. R.: The mechanism of action of the folate antagonists in man. Cancer Res., 23:1286, 1963.

Birnie, G. D., and Heidelberger, C.: Biochemical experiments towards the prediction of clinical responses to fluorinated pyrimidines. Proc. Am. Acad. Cancer Res., 3:304, 1962.

Birnie, G. D., and Heidelberger, C.: In vitro synthesis of acid soluble thymidine compounds by human neoplastic tissue. Cancer Res., 23:420, 1963.

Black, M. M., and Speer, F. D.: Effects of cancer chemotherapeutic agents on dehydrogenase activity of human cancer tissue in vitro. Am. J. Clin. Pathol., 23:218, 1953.

Black, M. M., and Speer, F. D.: Further observations on effects of cancer chemotherapeutic agents on in vitro dehydrogenase activity of cancer tissue. J. Natl. Cancer Inst., 14:1147, 1954.

Block, M., and Murphy, J. C.: Effect of nitrogen mustard in mycosis fungoides. Arch. Pathol., 46:519, 1948.

Block, J. B., Edgcomb, J., Eisen, A., and Van Scott, J.: Mycosis fungoides; natural history and aspects of its relationship to other malignant lymphomas. Am. J. Med., 34:228, 1963.

Bluefarb, S. M.: Cutaneous Manifestations of Malignant Lymphomas. Springfield, Ill., Charles C Thomas, Publisher, 1959.

Bluefarb, S. M., and Caro, W. A.: Lymphoma cutis. *In* Maddin, S. (Ed.): Current Dermatologic Management. St. Louis, Mo., The C. V. Mosby Company, 1970, pp. 219, 220.

Bluefarb, S. M., and Ihrke, R.: Psoriasis and mycosis fungoides. Quart. Bull. Northwest. Univ. Med. School, 26:93, 1952.

Boggs, D. P., Wintrobe, M. M., and Cartwright, G. E.: The acute leukemias; analysis of 322 cases and review of literature. Medicine, 41:163, 1962.

Burchenal, J. H.: Treatment of the leukemias. Semin. Hematol., 3:122, 1966.

Burchenal, J. H.: Long-term survival in Burkitt's tumor and in acute leukemia. ACS-NCI Conference on acute leukemia and Burkitt's tumor. Cancer Res., 27:2616, 1967.

Burchenal, J. H., Murphy, M. L., Ellison, R. R., Sykes, M. P., Tan, T. C., Leone, L. A., Karnofsky, D. A., Craver, L. F., Dargeon, H. W., and Rhoads, C. O.: Clinical evaluation of a new antimetabolite, 6-mercaptopurine in the treatment of leukemia and allied disease. Blood, 8:965, 1953.

Calabresi, P., Turner, R., and Lefkowitz, E.: Beneficial effects of azauridine in psoriasis and mycosis fungoides. Proc. Am. Acad. Cancer Res., 5:10, 1964.

Carrel, A., and Burrows, M.: Cultivation in vitro of malignant tumors. J. Exp. Med., 13:571, 1911.

Clinical Screening Cooperative Group of the European Organization for Research on the Treatment of Cancer: Study of the clinical efficiency of Bleomycin on human cancer. Br. Med. J., 2:643, 1970.

Cobb, J. P.: Tissue culture observations of the effects of chemotherapeutic agents on human tumors. Trans. N.Y. Acad Sci., 17:237, 1955.

Cobb, J. P., and Walker, D. G.: Effect of actinomycin D on tissue cultures of normal and neoplastic cells. J. Natl. Cancer Inst., 21:263, 1958.

Cobb, J. P., and Walker, D. G.: Studies on human melanoma cells in tissue culture. I. Growth characteristics and cytology. Cancer Res., 20:858, 1960.

Cobb, J. P., and Walker, D. G.: Effect of heterologous, homologous, and autologous serums on human normal and malignant cells in vitro. J. Natl. Cancer Inst., 27:1, 1961.

Cobb, J. P., and Wright, J. C.: Studies on a craniopharyngioma in tissue culture. I. Growth characteristics and alterations produced following exposure to two radiomimetic agents. J. Neuropathol. Exp. Neurol., 18:563, 1959.

Cobb, J. P., Kiefer, J. H., and Wood, F. H.: Human bladder neoplastic cells in tissue culture. J. Urol., 73:1039, 1955.

Cobb, J. P., Walker, D. G., and Wright, J. C.: Comparative chemotherapy studies on primary short-term cultures of human normal, benign and malignant tumor tissues—A five-year study. Cancer Res., 21:583, 1961.

Cohen, M., Shaw, M. W., and Craig, A. P.: The effects of streptonigrin on cultured human leukocytes. Proc. Natl. Acad. Sci., 150:16, 1963.

Cohen, S. S.: Introduction to the biochemistry of D-arabinosyl nucleosides. *In* Davidson, J. N., and Cohn, W. E. (Eds.): Progress in Nucleic Acid Research and Molecular Biology. New York, Academic Press, 1966, pp. 1–68.

Cornell, G. N., and Pasmantier, M.: Personal communication, 1971.

Costello, M. J.: Cortisone in the treatment of cutaneous diseases. New York J. Med., 51:2017, 1951.

Craver, L. F.: The treatment of the more important lymphadenopathies, with special reference to irradiation. Med. Clin. North Am., 18:703, 1934.

Cutts, J. H., Beer, C. T., and Nobel, R. L.: Properties of vinca leukoblastine, an alkaloid in Vinca rosea Linn, with reference to its antitumor action. Cancer Res., 20:1023, 1960.

Diamond, H. D.: The natural history and management of lymphosarcoma. Med. Clin. North Am., 40:721, 1956.

Diamond, L. K., and Luhby, A. L.: Pattern of "spontaneous" remission in leukemia of childhood observed in 26 of 300 cases. Am. J. Med., 10:238, 1951.

Di Paolo, J. A.: The use of human tumor effusions in primary culture for testing chemotherapeutic compounds (a preliminary report). Cancer, 17:391, 1964.

Di Paolo, J. A., and Dowd, J. E.: In vitro sensitivity of human tumors toward potential chemotherapeutic compounds. Proc. Am. Acad. Cancer Res., 31:107, 1960.

Di Paolo, J. A., and Dowd, J. E.: Evaluation of

inhibition of human tumor tissue by cancer chemotherapeutic drugs with an in vitro test. J. Natl. Cancer Inst., 27:807, 1961.

Dobrynin, Y. U.: Establishment and characteristics of cell strains from some epithelial tumors of human origin. J. Natl. Cancer Inst., 31:1173, 1963.

Dolowy, W. C., Henson, P., Cornet, J. A., and Sellin, H.: Toxic and antineoplastic effects of L-asparaginase. Study of mice with lymphoma and normal monkeys and report on a child with leukemia. Cancer, 19:1813, 1966.

Eichenlaub, F. J., and Olivo, M. A.: Nitrogen mustard therapy of lymphosarcoma. Report of a case. Med. Ann. D.C., 17:391, 1948.

Ellison, R. R., Holland, J. F., Silver, T., Bernard, J., and Boiron, M.: Cytosine arabinoside—A new agent for induction of remission in acute leukemia. (9th Internatl. Cancer Congress). Tokyo Abs., S1181:645, 1966.

Epstein, E. (Ed.): Skin Surgery. Ed. 3. Springfield, Ill., Charles C Thomas, Publisher, 1970.

Evans, A. E., Farber, S., Brunet, S., and Mariano, P. J.: Vincristine in the treatment of acute leukemia in children. Cancer, 16:1302, 1963.

Evans, T. S., Cipriano, A. P., and Hirsch, E. O.: Mycosis fungoides with "tumor d'emblee"; report of a case treated with nitrogen mustard. Ann. Intern. Med., 33:1294, 1950.

Farber, S.: The effect of therapy on the life history and biologic behavior of leukemia. Tenth R. Kretschmer Memorial Lecture. Proc. Inst. Med. Chicago, 18:311, 1951.

Farber, S., Diamond, L. K., Mercer, R. D., Sylvester, R. F., and Wolff, J. A.: Temporary remission in acute leukemia in children produced by folic acid antagonist, 4-aminopterylglutamic acid (aminopterin). New Engl. J. Med., 238:787, 1948.

Farber, S., Schwachman, H., Toch, R., Downing, V., Kennedy, B. H., and Hyde, J.: The effect of ACTH in acute leukemia in childhood. Proc. 1st Clin. ACTH Conf., 1:328, 1949.

Farber, S., Downing, V., Schwachman, H., Toch, R., Appleton, R., King, J. P., Heald, F., and Feriozi, D.: The action of ACTH and cortisone in acute leukemia. Proc. Clin. ACTH Conf., 2:251, 1950.

Farber, S., Appleton, R., Downing, V., Heald, F., King, J., and Toch, R.: Clinical studies on triethylene phosphoramides and diethylene phosphoramide compounds with nitrogen mustard–like activity. Cancer, 6:135, 1953.

Farber, S., Maddock, D., and Swaffield, M.: Studies on the carcinolytic and other biological activity of actinomycin D. Proc. Am. Acad. Cancer Res. 2:104, 1956.

Farber, E. M., Zackheim, H. S., McClintoak, R. P., and Cox, A. J., Jr.: Therapy of mycosis fungoides with topically applied fluocinolone acetonide under occlusive dressing. Cancer, 19:237, 1966.

Farber, E. M., Zackheim, H. S., McClintoak, R. P., and Cox, A. J., Jr.: Treatment of mycosis fungoides with various strengths of fluocinolone acetonide cream. Arch. Dermatol., 97:165, 1968.

Fernbach, D. J., Sutow, W. W., Thurman, W. G., and Vietti, T. J.: Preliminary report. Clinical trials with cyclophosphamide in children with acute leukemia. Cancer Chemother. Rep., 8:102, 1960.

Frei, E., and Freireich, E. J.: Chemotherapy of acute leukemia. *In* Advances in Chemotherapy. New York, Academic Press. 1965, pp. 283–284.

Fromer, J. L., Johnston, D. O., Salzman, F. A., Trump, J. G., and Wright, K. A.: Management of lymphoma cutis with low megavolt electron beam therapy; nine year follow-up in 200 cases. South. Med. J., 54:769, 1961.

Gall, E. A: Enigmas in lymphoma, reticulum-cell sarcoma and mycosis fungoides. Minn. Med., 38:674, 1955.

Galton, D. A. G.: Myleran in chronic myeloid leukemia. Br. Med. J., 1:208, 1953.

Garb, J.: Mycosis fungoides (granuloma fungoides), tumor stage, responding rapidly to antimony preparations; preliminary report. J. Invest. Dermatol., 10:43, 1948.

Gellhorn, A., Murray, M. R., Hirschberg, E., and Eising, R. F.: In vitro and in vivo effects of chemical agents on human and mouse glioblastoma multiforme. London, Proc. 2nd Int. Congress Neuropathol., 1957, pp. 265–271.

Gilman, A., and Philips, F. S.: The biological and therapeutic applications of the B-chlorethylamines and sulfides. Science, 103:409, 1946.

Goldberg, L. C., and Mason, L.: Treatment of cutaneous blastomas and other diseases with nitrogen mustard. Arch. Dermatol. Syph., 60:181, 1949.

Golomb, F. M., Cobb, J. P., Walker, D. G., and Wright, J. C.: In vitro selection of chemotherapeutic agents for perfusion therapy of human cancer. Surgery, 51:639, 1962.

Gross, R., and Lambers, K.: Erste Erfabrungen in der Behandlung maligner Tumoren mit einem aeven N-Lost-Phosphamidester. Dtsch. Med. Wochenschr., 83:458, 1958.

Gumport, S. L., Wright, J. C., and Golomb, F. M.: The treatment of advanced malignant melanoma with triethylene thiophosphoramide (Thio-TEPA or TSPA). Ann. Surg., 147:232, 1958.

Haddow, A., and Timmis, G. M.: Bijunctional sulphonic acid esters with radiomimetic activity. Acta Un. Int. Cancr., 7:469, 1951.

Handschumacher, R. E., Calabresi, P., Welch, A. D., Bono, V., Fallon, H., and Frei, E.: Summary of current information on 6-azauridine. Cancer Chemother. Rep., 21:1, 1962.

Harris, M. N., Medrek, T. J., Golomb, F. M., Gumport, S. L., Postel, A. H., and Wright, J. C.: Chemotherapy with streptonigrin in advanced cancer. Cancer, 18:49, 1965.

Haserick, J. R., Richardson, J. H., and Grant, D. J.: Remission of lesions in mycosis fungoides following topical application of nitrogen mustard. Cleveland Clin. Quart., 26:146, 1959.

Haynes, H. A.: Personal communication, 1971.

Haynes, H. A., and Van Scott, E. J.: Therapy of mycosis fungoides. Progr. Dermatol., 3:1, 1968.

Hency, P. S., Kendall, E. C., Slocumb, C. H., and Polley, J. F.: The effect of a hormone of the adrenal cortex (17-hydroxy-11-dihydrocortisone: compound E) and of the pituitary adrenocorticotropic hormone on rheumatoid arthritis. Proc. Mayo Clin., 24:181, 1949.

Henstell, H. H., and Newman, B. A.: The influence of nitrogen mustard on mycosis fungoides. Blood, 2:564, 1947.

Henstell, H. H., and Tober, J. N.: Treatment of mycosis fungoides with nitrogen mustard. J. Invest. Dermatol., 8:183, 1947.

Higuchi, K.: Chemotherapy of skin cancer with Bleomycin. Progress in antimicrobial and anticancer chemotherapy. Proc. 6th Int. Congress Chemother. Tokyo, University of Tokyo Press, 1969, pp. 33–34.

Hiraki, E., Ofuji, M., Kadonami, H., Ota, Z., Sanada, H., Kitajima, S., Nabeshima, S., Sato, T., Sezaki, S., Arimori, S., and Matsumori, H.: Study on bone marrow (IX). Study on the treatment of leukemia by tissue culture and the formation of new crystals in the myelocytes. J. Jap. Soc. Intern. Med., 50:100, 1961a.

Hiraki, K., Ofuji, S., Suminami (Kadonami), H., Ota, Z., Sanada, H., Kitazawa, Y., Nabeshima, M., Sato, S., Sezaki, T., Arimori, S., and Matsumori, H.: Tissue culture evaluation of the screening of anti-leukemia agents. The appearance of crystals in various myeloid cells (Japi). J. Jap. Soc. Intern. Med., 50:992, 1961b.

Hirschberg, E., Gelhorn, A., Reiner, L., Eising, R. F., and Murray, M. R.: In vivo and in vitro effects of quinacrine and related acridines on human and mouse brain tumors. Proc. Am. Acad. Cancer Res., 2:117, 1956.

Holland, F. C., and Ebaugh, F. G., Jr.: The effects of various antimetabolites on DNA synthesis in normal and leukemic human leukocytes in tissue culture and correlation with effective in vivo therapeutic concentrations. Clin. Res. N.Y., 10:201, 1962.

Holland, J. F., and Regelson, W.: Studies of phenylalanine nitrogen mustard (CB3025) in metastatic malignant melanoma of man. Ann. N.Y. Acad. Sci., 68:1122, 1958.

Hopkins, J. G., Kesten, B. M., Nelson, C. T., Hambrick, G. W., Jr., Jennings, R. G., Jr., and Machacek, G. F.: Pituitary adrenocorticotropic hormone (ACTH) and cortisone in diseases of the skin. II. Allergic and other dermatoses; report of 67 cases. Arch. Dermatol., 65:401, 1952.

Hu, F., Staricco, R. J., Pinkus, H., and Fosnaugh, R. P.: Human melanocytes in tissue culture. J. Invest. Dermatol., 28:15, 1957.

Hurley, J. D., and Yount, L.: Personal communication, 1964.

Ichikawa, R.: Bleomycin, a new antitumor antibiotic—as a specific against the squamous cell carcinoma. J. Jap. Med. Assoc., 61:487, 1969.

Ichikawa, T.: The clinical effect of Bleomycin against squamous cell carcinoma and further developments. Proc. 6th Int. Congress Chemother. Tokyo, University of Tokyo Press, 1969, pp. 1–3.

Ishizuka, J., Takayama, H., Takeuchi, T., and Umezawa, H.: Activity and toxicity of Bleomycin. J. Antibiot. (A) (Tokyo), 20:15, 1967.

Jackson, L. G.: Personal communication, 1964.

Jamieson, W. A.: Mycosis fungoides and its treatment by the x-rays. Br. J. Dermatol., 15:1, 1903.

Jelliffe, A. M., and Thomson, A. D.: Prognosis in Hodgkin's disease. Br. J. Cancer, 9:21, 1955.

Kaplan, H.: Report, Radiological Society of North America. Newer Techniques in Radiation Therapy in Hodgkin's disease. Chicago, Ill., Dec., 1969.

Karnofsky, D. A., Craver, L. F., Rhoads, C. P., and Abels, J. C.: An evaluation of methyl-bis (B-chloroethyl) amine hydrochloride and tris (B-chloroethyl) amine hydrochloride (nitrogen mustard) in the treatment of lymphomas, leukemia and allied diseases. In Mouton, F. R. (Ed.): Approaches to Tumor Chemotherapy. American Association for the Advancement of Science. 1947, pp. 37–55. Washington, D.C.

Karnofsky, D. A., Burchenal, J. H., Armistead, G. C., Jr., Southam, C. M., Bernstein, J. L., Craver, L. F., and Rhoads, C. P.: Triethylene melamine in the treatment of neoplastic disease. Arch. Intern. Med., 87:477, 1951.

Karon, M. R., Freireich, E. J., and Frei, E., III: A preliminary report on vincristine sulfate—A new active agent for the treatment of acute leukemia. Pediatrics, 30:791, 1962.

Kidd, J.: Regression of transplanted lymphomas induced *in vivo* by means of normal guinea pig serum. I. Course of transplanted cancers of various kinds in mice and rats given guinea pig serum, horse serum or rat serum. J. Exp. Med., 98:565, 1953.

Krahe, M.: Studies of the selective effect of cytostatic agents on explanted cells from female genital carcinomas. Geburtshilfe Frauenheilkd., 22:1139, 1962.

Kusumoto, H.: In vitro studies on the influences of antitumor substances upon morphologic changes of leukocytes in the bone marrow. 3. Phase contact microscopic observation of morphologic changes provoked by some of the anti-tumor substances in the purified bone marrow leukocytes. J. Osaka City Med. Center, 8:1253, 1959.

Lasfarques, E. Y., and Ozzello, L.: Cultivation of human breast carcinoma. J. Natl. Cancer Inst., 21:1131, 1958.

Laszlo, J., Stengle, J., Wight, K., and Burk, D.: Effects of chemotherapeutic agents on metabolism of human acute leukemia cells in vitro. Proc. Soc. Exp. Biol. Med., 97:127, 1958.

Lewis, G. M., and Wheeler, C. E., Jr. (Eds.): Practical Dermatology. Ed. 3. Philadelphia, W. B. Saunders Company, 1967, pp 576–581, 596–598.

Liss, L.: A test to determine susceptibility of neoplasms to anti-neoplastic drugs. Abs. 14th Annual Meeting, Tissue Culture Ass., May, 1963.

Livingston, R. B., and Carter, S. K. (Eds.): Single Agents in Cancer Chemotherapy. New York, Plenum Press, 1970, pp. 326–331.

Lowenfish, F. P.: Intramuscular administration of prednisolone in dermatoses. Comparison with oral and topical therapy. Int. Rec. Med., 170:636, 1957.

McDonald, G. O., and Baxter, M. A.: Response of human benign and malignant cells in culture to anti-tumor agents. Proc. Am. Acad. Cancer Res., 3:49, 1961.

McDonald, G. O., and Cole, W. H.: The use of human tumors in primary culture for testing anti-cancer compounds. Surg. Forum, 10:67, 1960.

McDonald, G. O., Stroud, A. N., Brues, A. M., and Cole, W. H.: In vivo and in vitro assay for drug effect on cancer cells. Ann. Surg., 157:787, 1963.

Murray, M. R., and Stout, A. P.: The classification and diagnosis of human tumors by tissue culture methods. Tex. Rep. Biol. Med., 12:898, 1954.

Newcomer, V. D., Sternberg, T. H., and Linden, I. H.: An evaluation of ACTH and cortisone in dermatologic patients. Am. Pract. Dig. Treat., 3:912, 1952.

Oettgen, H. F., Old, L. J., Boyse, E. A., Campbell, H. A., Philips, F. S., Clarkson, B. D., Tallal, L., Leeper, R. D., Schwarta, M. D., and Kim, J. H.: Inhibition of leukemia in man by L-asparaginase. Cancer Res., 27:2619, 1967.

Orr, M. F., and McSwain, B.: Tissue culture of human breast carcinoma. Am. J. Pathol., 31:125, 1955.

Osborne, E., Jordan, J. W., Hoak, F. C., and Pschierer, F. J.: Nitrogen mustard therapy in cutaneous blastomatous diseases. J.A.M.A., 135:1123, 1947.

Papanicolaou, G. N., and Maddi, F. U.: Diagnostic value of cells of endometrial and ovarian origin in human tissue culture. Acta Cytol., 5:1, 1961.

Pearson, O. H., Eliel, L. P., and Talbot, T. R.: The use of ACTH and cortisone in neoplastic disease. N.Y. Acad. Med. Bull., 26:235, 1950.

Peters, M. V.: Study of survivals in Hodgkin's disease treated radiologically. Am. J. Roentgen., 63:299, 1950.

Peters, M. V.: Prophylactic treatment of adjacent areas in Hodgkin's disease. Cancer Res., 26:1232, 1966.

Petratos, M. A.: Current practice of teleroentgen therapy. Cutis, 4:716, 1968.

Piffard, D.: A case of mycosis fungoides; presented by Dr. Sherwell. J. Cutan. Dis., 22:279, 1904.

Pinkel, D. P., Simone, J. V., Hustu, H. O., and Phomes, J.: Total therapy of childhood acute lymphatic leukemia. Proc. Am. Pediatr. Soc., 19:90, 1971.

Pusey, W.: The Principles and Practice of Dermatology. Ed. 4. New York, Appleton, 1924.

Rao, K. V., and Cullen, W. P.: Streptonigrin, an antitumor substance; I. Isolation and characterization. Antibiot. Ann., 7:950, 1959–1960.

Richmond, H. G., Ohnuki, Y., Awa, A., and Pomerat, C. M.: Multiple myeloma in an in vitro study. Br. J. Cancer, 15:692, 1961.

Scholtz, W.: Ueber den Einfluss der Röntgenstrahlen auf die Haut in gesundem und Krankem Zustande. III. Klinischer Thell, Arch. Dermatol. Syph. (Berl.), 59:421, 1902.

Schrek, R. A.: Method for screening chemotherapeutic agents against normal and leukemic cells of man. Proc. Am. Acad. Cancer Res., 3:148, 1960.

Schrek, R. A.: In vitro measurement of cytotoxicity of reagents to normal and leukemic lymphocytes. Proc. Am. Acad. Cancer Res., 5:57, 1964.

Sequeira, J. H.: Discussion on mycosis fungoides. Proc. R. Soc. Med. (Derm.), 7:190, 1914.

Shay, H., and Sun, D. C. H.: Clinical studies of triethylene thiophosphoramide in the treatment of inoperable cancer. Cancer, 8:498, 1955.

Shay, H., Zarafonetis, C., Smith, N., Woldow, I., and Sun, D. C. H.: Treatment of leukemia with triethylene thiophosphoramide (Thio-TEPA); preliminary results in experimental and clinical leukemia. Arch. Intern. Med., 92:628, 1953.

Sipos, K.: Painting treatment of nitrogen mustard in mycosis fungoides. Dermatologia (Mex.), 130:3, 1965.

Sipos, K., and Jasko, G.: A mustárnitrogen helyi

alkalmazása héhány börbelegségben. Börgyögy. Vener. Szle., 32:198, 1956.

Sloboda, A. E., and Vogel, A. W.: Comparison of two anti-neoplastic compounds with Thiotepa; laboratory evaluation. Cancer Chemother. Rep., 24:7, 1962.

Söltz-Szötz, J.: Soziales verhalten von zellen maligne entarteter tumoren der menschlichen haut in der gewebkultur. Arch. Klin. Exp. Dermatol., 216:36, 1963.

Steiner, K., and Frank, L.: Clinical experiences with cortisone and corticotropin (ACTH) in some cutaneous diseases. Arch. Dermatol., 65:524, 1952.

Sugarbaker, E. D., and Craver, L. F.: Lymphosarcoma, a study of 196 cases with biopsy. J.A.M.A., 115:17, 112, 1940.

Sulzberger, M. B., Sauer, G. C., Herrmann, F., Baer, R. L., and Milberg, J. L.: Effects of ACTH and cortisone on certain diseases and physiologic functions of the skin. I. Effects of ACTH. J. Invest. Dermatol., 16:323, 1951.

Sykes, M. P., Philips, F. S., and Karnofsky, D. A.: Comparative therapeutic activity of the nitrogen mustards and allied compounds. Med. Clin. North Am., 40:837, 1956.

Talley, R. W.: Systemic chemotherapy of human malignant neoplasms. In Cole, W. H. (Ed.): Chemotherapy of Cancer. Philadelphia, Lea & Febiger, 1970.

Tan, C. T., and Aduna, N. S.: Preliminary clinical experience with leucocristine in children. Proc. Am. Assoc. Cancer Res., 3:367, 1962.

Tan, C. T., Phoa, J., Lyman, J., Murphy, M. L., Dargeon, H. W., and Burchenal, J. H.: Hematological remissions in acute leukemia with cyclophosphamide. Blood, 18:808, 1961.

Tan, C., Tasaka, H., and Di Marco, A.: Clinical studies of daunomycin. Proc. Am. Assoc. Cancer Res., 6:64, 1964.

Taylor, S. G., Ayer, J. P., and Morris, R. S.: Cortical steroids in treatment of cancer. J.A.M.A., 144:1058, 1950.

Thorn, G. W., Forsham, P. H., Frawley, T. F., Hill, S. R., Roche, M., Staehelm, D., and Wilson, D. L.: Medical progress; the clinical usefulness of ACTH and cortisone. New Engl. J. Med., 242:783, 824, 865, 1950.

Tolman, M. M.: Mycosis fungoides; remission following steroid therapy. Arch. Dermatol., 75:146, 1957.

Toplin, I. A.: Tissue culture cytotoxicity test for large scale cancer chemotherapy screening. Cancer Res., 19:959, 1959.

Tulipan, L.: Failure of ACTH (adrenocorticotropic hormone) in the treatment of a case of mycosis fungoides. J. Invest. Dermatol., 15:349, 1950.

Ultman, J. E.: Personal communication, 1957.

Umezawa, H: Bleomycin and other antitumor antibiotics of high molecular weight. Progress in Antimicrobial and Anticancer Chemotherapy. Washington, D. C., Proc. 4th Int. Congress Chemother., 5:1079, 1965.

Van Scott, E. J., and Haynes, H. A.: Therapy of mycosis fungoides, lymphoma. 6th National Cancer Conference Proc. Philadelphia, J. B. Lippincott Company, 1968, pp. 553–557.

Van Scott, E. J., and Haynes, H. A.: Cutaneous

lymphomas. *In* Fitzpatrick, T. B., Arndt, K. A., Clark, W. H., Jr., Eisen, A. Z., Van Scott, E. J., and Vaughan, J. H. (Eds.): Dermatology in General Medicine. New York, McGraw-Hill, 1971, pp. 556–573.

Van Scott, E. J., and Winters, P. L.: Responses of mycosis fungoides to intensive external treatment with nitrogen mustard. Arch. Dermatol., 102:507, 1970.

Van Scott, E. J., Auerbach, R., and Clendenning, W. E.: Treatment of mycosis fungoides with cyclophosphamide. Arch. Dermatol., 85:499, 1962.

Waldorf, D. S., Haynes, H. A., and Van Scott, E. J.: Cutaneous hypersensitivity and desensitization to mechlorethamine in patients with mycosis fungoides, lymphoma. Ann. Intern. Med., 67:282, 1967.

Walker, D. G., Goldstein, N., Kopf, A. W., and Wright, J. C.: Epithelial outgrowths from tissue cultures of basal cell epitheliomas. J. Invest. Dermatol., 42:435, 1964.

Walker, D. G., and Wright, J. C.: The effect of vincaleukoblastine on primary cultures of human neoplasms: a preliminary report. Cancer Chemother. Rep., 10:139, 1961.

Walker, D. G., and Wright, J. C.: Intracellular changes in cells from human neoplasms following exposure to several antibiotics. 13th Annual Meeting of Tissue Culture Assoc., May, 1962a.

Walker, D. G., and Wright, J. C.: Cytological alterations in primary explant cultures of human neoplasms exposed to vincaleukoblastine. Cancer Res., 22:1267, 1962b.

Walker, D. G., Lyons, M. M., and Wright, J. C.: Observations on primary short-term cultures of human tumors. A second 5-year study. Europ. J. Cancer, 1:265, 1965.

Welch, A. D., Handschumacher, R. E., Finch, S. C., Jaffee, J. J., Cardosa, S. S., and Calabresi, P.: A synopsis of recent investigations of 6-azauridine (NSC-32074). Cancer Chemother. Rep., 9:39, 1960.

Wilson, W. L., Labra, C., and Barrist, E.: Preliminary observations on use of streptonigrin as an antitumor agent in human beings. Antibiot. Chemother. (N.Y.), 11:147, 1961.

Wise, F.: Diseases of the hematopoietic system. *In* McKee, G. M.: X-rays and Radium in the Treatment of Diseases of the Skin. Ed. 3. Philadelphia, Lea & Febiger, 1938, pp. 567–583.

Wolberg, W. H., and Brown, R. R.: Autoradiographic studies of in vitro incorporation of uridine and thymidine by human tumor tissue. Cancer Res., 22:1113, 1962.

Wolberg, W. H., and Curreri, A. P.: A method for the determination of human tumor sensitivity to cancer chemotherapeutic agents — A preliminary report. Cancer Chemother. Rep., 12:25, 1961.

Wright, J. C., and Walker, D.: Tissue culture as a test model for sensitivity of chemotherapeutic agents on tumors. Proc. Internatl. Symposium in Münster/Westfalen, 1972. Stuttgart, Georg Thieme Verlag, 1974, pp. 17–28.

Wright, J. C., Gumport, S. L., and Golomb, F. M.: Remissions produced with the use of methotrexate in patients with mycosis fungoides. Cancer Chemother. Rep., 9:11, 1960.

Wright, J. C., Cobb, J. P., Gumport, S. L., Safadi, D., Walker, D. G., and Golomb, F. M.: Further investigation of the relation between the clinical and tissue culture response to chemotherapeutic agents on human cancer. Cancer, 15:284, 1962.

Wright, J. C., Golomb, F., and Gumport, S. L.: Observations on the use of cancer chemotherapeutic agents in patients with mycosis fungoides. Proc. Am. Acad. Cancer Res., 4:73, 1963.

Wright, J. C., Lyons, M. M., Walker, D. G., Golomb, F. M., Gumport, S. L., and Medrek, T. J.: Observations on the use of cancer chemotherapeutic agents in patients with mycosis fungoides. Cancer, 17: 1045, 1964.

Wright, L. T., Wright, J. C., Prigot, A., and Weintraub, S.: Remissions caused by triethylene melamine in certain neoplastic diseases. J. Natl. Med. Assoc., 42:343, 1950.

Yu, K. P., Howard, J. P., and Clarkson, B. D.: Comparative studies of cytosine arabinoside (CA) and 5-fluoro-2'-deoxyuridine (FUDR) in leukemia in man. Proc. Am. Assoc. Cancer Res., 7:78, 1966.

Zubrod, C. G.: Treatment of the acute leukemias. Cancer Res., 27:2557, 1967.

75

Perfusion

Frederick M. Golomb, M.D.

Techniques of regionally administered chemotherapy are of some usefulness in the study and treatment of skin cancers. Since these lesions are visible and accessible, their response to therapy can be readily observed. Melanoma and sarcoma of the extremities and squamous cell carcinoma of the head and neck, in particular, have been of interest to surgeons who use techniques of regional chemotherapy. Some therapeutic usefulness now exists for several other skin cancers as well.

DEFINITIONS

Perfusions

Regional perfusions are techniques designed to isolate, either partially or completely, a tumor-bearing area by mechanically limiting its arterial inflow and venous outflow. Because the amount of drug reaching the nonperfused parts of the body can be controlled, high concentrations of anticancer agents may be delivered to the cancer area. In practice, an extracorporeal circuit is required. Short-acting drugs, generally alkylating agents, are used since they can be washed out of the perfused area at the completion

of the procedure. The duration of a regional perfusion is usually a few hours or less.

Infusions

Intra-arterial infusion chemotherapy is the technique of administering drugs into the arterial supply of a tumor-bearing area. This approach is based on the rationale that a high concentration of drug can be delivered to the cancer cells in the infused area, where a significant amount of the agent will be removed by the first circulation through the capillary bed. Thus the concentration outside the tumor area is kept to levels low enough to prevent severe systemic toxicity. This procedure is usually done by pumping an antimetabolite solution steadily or intermittently into the artery. The technique also takes into account the fact that each cell in a cancer mass is not necessarily in the drug-sensitive phase of its mitotic cycle at the same time as its neighbor. The infusion, therefore, proceeds for a period of several days or weeks to expose each cell to the chemotherapeutic agent as it enters its vulnerable stage. When it is feasible to administer a specific antidote to

1623

neutralize the drug leaving the infused area, higher doses of an antimetabolite may be safely used.

HISTORY

Bierman et al. (1949) described a method of catheterizing visceral arteries with a radiopaque cardiac catheter introduced into the femoral or brachial arteries for intra-arterial cancer chemotherapy. Klopp et al. (1950) described the treatment of head and neck cancer with fractionated intra-arterial nitrogen mustard instilled via a catheter placed in the external carotid artery. In the same article, he suggested the use of the heart-lung machine for isolated chemotherapy, but it was not until 1957 that Creech and coworkers (Ryan et al., 1957) described the first isolated perfusions. The concept of continuous antimetabolite infusion chemotherapy with systemic metabolite injections was advanced by Sullivan et al. (1959). In the ensuing years, many new contributions and refinements have been added; however, the basic concepts are unchanged.

BIOLOGIC FACTORS IN PERFUSION THERAPY

Rationale of Regional Therapy

An ideal treatment would fix a high concentration of drug in the tumor only and prevent systemic toxicity and minimize local nontumor tissue toxicity. Isolated perfusion achieves the objective of minimal systemic toxicity, but occasionally it is at the expense of local tissue damage. Continuous intra-arterial infusion with chemical neutralization prevents both forms of toxicity but may not achieve its objective owing to incomplete distribution of the drug to the tumor. Both techniques may spare the immune centers, such as the spleen, regional lymph nodes, and reticuloendothelial system, from the harmful effects of the drugs.

Optimum Therapy Design and Kinetics

Tumor cell generating or doubling time varies greatly from neoplasm to neoplasm. With a long doubling time, the effectiveness of a brief therapeutic program may be inadequate. The most vulnerable phase for these cells is while they are dividing; therefore, intermittent, prolonged, or combined therapy is logical. The doubling time for rapid growing tumors, such as teratocarcinoma or Ewing's sarcoma, is 11 to17 days, while that for squamous cell and basosquamous cell carcinoma of the skin is 130 to 143 days. Early treatment is desirable whenever possible, since the doubling time is geometrically adverse once tumors are visible. A tumor with a doubling time of 30 days will take more than 1000 days to achieve a volume of 20 ml., but only 90 days later it will be 160 ml. in size.

Other biologic factors, such as tumor-specific sensitivity to various chemotherapeutic agents, are of great importance. Efforts have been made to improve the selection of drugs for perfusion, such as the tissue culture sensitivity test which was described in 1962 (Golomb et al., 1962a), but as yet no such in vitro tests are of practical value. Drug selection is now based, for the most part, on empirical criteria gathered from clinical experience.

The vascular supply of tumors, as studied by Fontaine et al. (1954) and Lindgren (1945), is richest at the periphery among the viable cells, while the vessels in the necrotic center are often sparse or absent. This vascular complex may be affected by factors which limit the effectiveness of the drugs perfused through them. These include infection, effects of inflammation, collaterals, arteriovenous shunts, radiation changes, prior surgery, and scarring.

TECHNIQUES

Isolated perfusion, originated by Ryan and Creech et al. (1957), requires an extracorporeal circuit which contains an oxygenator and heat exchanger (Fig. 75–1). Creech advanced the hypothesis

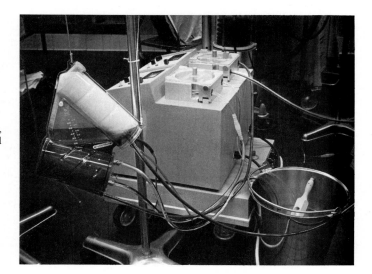

Figure 75–1 Pump, oxygenator, and heat exchanger used for isolated perfusions.

that the action of many of the drugs used was potentiated by high oxygen tension, which was reinforced by the laboratory studies of Krementz. There is some evidence that lowered pH levels and vascular spasm are aggravated in a high oxygen perfusion (Golomb et al., 1961). However, local tissue tolerance is better with an oxygenated circuit, and it is recommended for all extremity perfusions. Hyperthermia

Figure 75–2 *A,* Intra-arterial infusion: skin areas reached by infusion. *B,* Intra-arterial infusion: arteries which may be cannulated for infusion.

Abbreviations: I.C., internal carotid; E.C., external carotid; C.C., common carotid; V.A., vertebral; T.C., transverse cervical; Ax.A., axillary; I.M., internal mammary; Br.A., bronchial; I.A., intercostal; B.A., brachial; H.A., hepatic; C.Ax., celiac axis; R.A., renal; I.I.A., internal iliac; S.G., superior gluteal; E.I., external iliac.

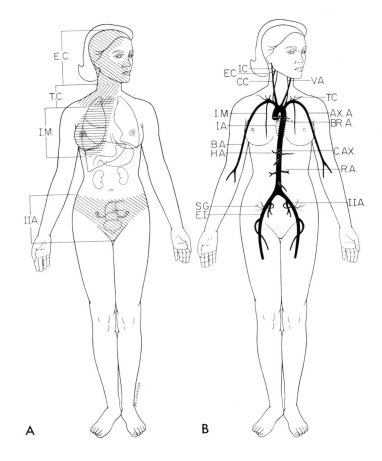

perfusions were first advocated by Shingleton et al. (1960) and Woodall et al. (1959). Since Cavaliere et al. (1967) reported on the efficacy of hyperthermia alone without chemotherapy, the addition of a heat exchanger to the circuit is generally routine. Stehlin has reported significant improvement in results of perfusion with hyperthermia as compared to prior experience with normothermic perfusions (Stehlin et al., 1975). We employ a heat exchanger which raises the circulating blood temperature to 43° C. and have increased the duration of the perfusion to 1½ or 2 hours (Fig. 75–1).

Intra-arterial infusion requires the placement of a catheter into the artery and the use of a pump to overcome the resistance of arterial blood pressure (Fig. 75–2). While essentially a simple procedure, its proper application requires close

attention to details to achieve the desired results and to prevent complications. These include such factors as localization of the infusate by dye studies, selection and care of catheters, pumps, and drugs, and prevention of catheter dislodgement and infection as the site of exit from the skin. For a detailed presentation of these techniques the reader is referred to the papers of Creech et al. (1958), Benson et al. (1963), Bierman et al. (1951), Sullivan and McPeak (1962), Sullivan et al. (1959), Woodhall et al. (1959), Shingleton et al. (1960), Clarkson and Lawrence (1961), Lawrence (1963a), and Golomb et al. (1962b).

The sites which are suitable for infusion and perfusion are illustrated in Figures 75–2 and 75–3. Isolation is more complete in locations where tourniquets may be applied. Infusions are more effective when arteries are used which supply a small area, such as the branches of the external carotid.

Drugs and Dosage

Infusions. The dose of methotrexate most commonly used is that advocated by Sullivan et al. (1959). A dose of 50.0 mg. of methotrexate is infused evenly over a 24-hour period, while 6.0 mg. of the citrovorum factor (leucovorin) is given intramuscularly every four to six hours. Other metabolite and antidote combinations have not been used as widely.

Other agents are administered in doses based on systemic intravenous or oral experience. The exceptions are 5-fluorouracil, which can be given in larger doses by continuous infusion than by intermittent intravenous injections, and 5-FUDR, which must be given in far smaller doses by continuous infusion than by intermittent intravenous injection.

Perfusions. The dosage of nitrogen mustard (Mustargen) and other short-acting agents is limited by local toxicity more often than by systemic effect. For example, the dosage recommended for the femoral artery is 0.4 to 0.8 mg. per kg. body weight. For longer acting drugs, such as actinomycin D (dactinomycin), the

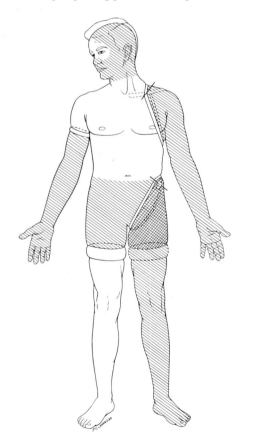

Figure 75–3 Isolated perfusion sites. The shaded areas indicate regions treated by perfusion. The location of the tourniquets restricts the distribution of the drugs during the perfusion.

dose is 25 μg. per kg. body weight, and that of phenylalanine mustard (melphalan) is 1.0 to 2.0 mg. per kg. These doses are appropriately adjusted for other locations by taking into consideration the extent of the drug leak and the size of the area perfused. Thus the doses of nitrogen mustard for the external carotid artery should not exceed 7.0 to 10.0 mg.

INDICATIONS FOR PERFUSION

Most patients selected for this form of treatment have extensive, recurrent, malignant tumors considered to be incurable by any modality. The objective is palliation of pain and regression of tumor growth. Lesions which are localized to anatomic regions supplied by single arterial and venous channels are suitable (Figs. 75–2 and 75–3). In general, patients with distant metastases are not so treated unless the local lesion presents sufficient symptoms to justify the procedure. In certain patients with primary malignant melanoma who would be treated by discontinuous excision and regional lymph node dissection, perfusion may be employed as an adjuvant.

COMPLICATIONS

In addition to complications expected from surgery, others resulting from the chemotherapeutic agents, indwelling catheters, tourniquets, and other equipment must be anticipated. Superimposed on these is the clinical status of patients who are often debilitated, poorly nourished, and in pain. Anticipation of complications will often serve to minimize untoward events.

Isolated perfusion often leads to local edema and inflammation. If severe, corticosteroids may be necessary. Hemorrhage from arteriotomy can occur from technical error, incompletely neutralized systemic heparinization, or wound breakdown; however, this is not a common problem. Hypotension may result from the redistribution of body fluids after tourniquet release and may require vigorous fluid

and electrolyte replacement. Arteritis, especially in smaller vessels, and phlebitis may be expected with any of the alkylating agents, actinomycin D, mithramycin, or hyperthermia. Pulmonary embolization is always a threat associated with phlebitis. Other local effects, which can be moderate to severe, include inflammatory changes in skin and muscle and neurologic deficits. Systemic toxicity is a risk associated with incomplete isolation or flush of the perfused part. Some agents, particularly the antineoplastic antibiotics, may be reabsorbed slowly from a perfused area even after an adequate flush. This may result in subsequent bone marrow depression, gastrointestinal tract ulcerations, and alopecia.

Infusions, while more simple to perform, are associated with a high incidence of problems. Sepsis is perhaps the cause of most of the severe complications and can result in bacteremia, late hemorrhage, and arteritis. The catheter may dislodge or crack, causing leakage of the infusate into tissues along its course. Hemorrhage is surprisingly uncommon even when catheters are dislodged accidentally. Indeed, they may be removed from patients after a few weeks with little danger of subsequent bleeding. Air embolization can be prevented by knowing it can happen and by being alert to this possibility. Reservoir bottles in tandem or plastic bag infusors can minimize this danger. Clogged catheters may be forcibly opened by aspirating or, if necessary, by injecting fluid into them as long as the emboli dislodged into the cannulated vessels do not infarct uncollateralized end vessels, such as those of the extremities or brain. This practice is to be avoided whenever possible by using a heparinized infusate and continuous infusion. Systemic toxicity is usually manifested by signs of bone marrow depression, and the drugs should be discontinued immediately on detection of leukopenia below 3500 and thrombocytopenia below 80,000.

REASONS FOR TREATMENT FAILURE

All too often the objectives of tumor regression and prolongation of life are not achieved. While the cause may be an inadequate amount of or ineffective drugs, other factors may play a role. The most common cause is the advanced stage of disease and the patient's inability to mobilize those host resistant factors necessary to contain his cancer. Prior surgery or irradiation might occlude or distort the circulation in a tumor and deflect the drug from the neoplasm. Advanced age, unusual drug sensitivity, technical failures, and improper dosage schedules all could contribute to failure. The technical problems are paradoxically more serious in the seemingly less technical infusion than in perfusion.

RESULTS

Perfusion for skin cancer has found its greatest usefulness in the treatment of melanoma of the extremities and squamous cell carcinoma of the head and neck area. While it has been employed in the treatment of other neoplasms which involve the skin, such as Kaposi's sarcoma, lymphosarcoma, reticulum cell sarcoma, basal cell epithelioma, carcinoma of the breast, and other sarcomas, experience with these cancers is more limited. Perfusion, however, has its place along with the other therapeutic modalities available to us in certain specific instances.

Melanoma

In 1957 Oscar Creech, Edward Krementz, and Robert Ryan treated the first patient, a 76 year old farmer, by isolated perfusion. At the time of treatment he had multiple satellites over his leg. Eleven years later he was well and free of disease. Since then many centers throughout the world have employed this treatment on hundreds of patients. While technique and patient sampling vary somewhat, the clinical results are quite similar.

Patient Selection. The patients fall into two major categories: (1) those with primary melanoma grossly limited to an isolated anatomic area, and (2) those with recurrent disease.

Patients in the latter category have a poor prognosis, and treatment would otherwise consist of amputation or systemic chemotherapy. Stehlin (1968) states that his indications for radical amputation have been significantly reduced since employing perfusion.

Advances in systemic chemotherapy have been somewhat disappointing. A collective review by Lawrence and Carter (1970) revealed that, while a variety of drugs and drug combinations can produce up to a 32 percent response rate, these remissions are almost invariably short lived and are of a minor degree. The most impressive responses reported were with the combination of BCNU [1,3-bis(2-chloroethyl)-1-nitrosourea], vincristine, and DTIC, 32 percent; Cytoxan, 32 percent; hydroxyurea, 24 percent; DTIC, 24 percent; BCNU, 19 percent; procarbazine, 19 percent; and vincristine, 12 percent. Moon (1970) reported objective regression in nine of 20 patients (45 percent) treated with the combination of BCNU and vincristine. Immunotherapy with intralesional BCG, C-Parvum, or transfer factor is of value in treating melanoma recurrence limited to the skin. The systemic application of these agents by vaccination is of promise.

Complete remissions have been reported by intra-arterial infusion chemotherapy, but Krementz and Creech (1968) have seen only eight short-lived responses in 21 patients treated by a combination of methotrexate, thio-TEPA, and melphalan. Bierman (1969) reported on responses following single injections of 10.0 to 20.0 mg. of nitrogen mustard into the femoral artery of the affected extremity but intimated that regional perfusion is more likely to achieve total tumor sterilization. Others, such as Freckman (1970), are more enthusiastic about continuous intra-arterial infusion chemotherapy. However, in the patient with recurrent melanoma limited to an isolated area, such as the extremity, pelvis, shoulder girdle, or the head and neck area, isolated perfusion appears to be the treatment of choice at the present time.

Perfusion As an Adjuvant to the Primary Surgical Treatment of Melanoma. More than 17 years have elapsed since the first regional perfusions were carried out. Most current reports of this technique consider perfusion of recurrent melanoma to be an established part of our armamentarium. Since it can arrest disease once it becomes widespread in an extremity, Creech (1962) stated, "in view of the remarkable results observed in some cases of advanced regional melanoma, chemotherapy by perfusion should become an integral part of the surgical treatment of patients with this disease." Evidence has since accrued which seems to support this thesis. Stehlin and Clark (1965) reported the results in a study at the M. D. Anderson Hospital and Baylor University where perfusion was used as an adjuvant to the surgical treatment of melanoma. They compared the results in 112 patients conventionally treated with those in 215 perfused. While the overall survival totals are similar — 49 percent in the surgical group compared to 55 percent in the perfused group — 15 percent more cases in the perfused group were in stages III and IV. The results are expectedly similar in stage I when the disease is limited to the primary lesion. However, in stage III, when spread has occurred to adjacent skin, lymphatics, or regional nodes, a marked improvement in the perfused group (46 percent) was seen as compared to the surgical group (16 percent).

At New York University we have treated 62 patients with primary melanoma by surgery plus perfusion. These operations were performed by the techniques illustrated in Figures 75–5 and 75–6, with the exception of one patient whose lesion developed in the parotid area. In this case perfusion plus radical neck dissection in continuity with the primary lesion appeared to control the local disease, but the patient died of lung metastases three years later. The 61 extremity lesions included seven of the upper extremity and 54 of the lower. Forty-four patients (72 percent) are free of disease; eight (13 percent) are living with disease; and nine (15 percent) have died of recurrent melanoma with distant metastases within two years of treatment. Of 35 patients treated more than five years ago, 23 (66 percent) are living. Nineteen patients were in stage III (with regional lymph node metastases) at the time of their operations five or more years ago. Eight (42 percent) of these stage III patients are living. Ten patients

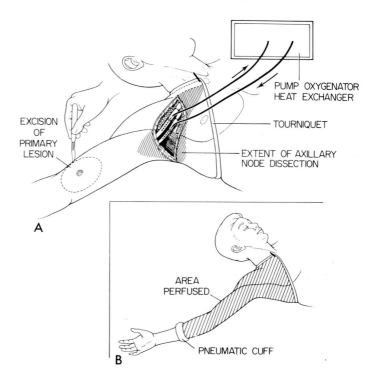

Figure 75–4 Technique for simultaneous perfusion of upper extremity, radical axillary dissection, and excision of primary lesion for melanoma *(A)*. During one anesthesia a radical axillary dissection is performed, after which the axillary artery and vein are cannulated and a tourniquet is secured about the shoulder and lower arm. The limb is then perfused between the tourniquets. During the perfusion, which prevents blood-borne dissemination of tumor cells, the primary lesion is excised and the site skin grafted. The perfused zone *(B)* is then flushed of residual drug before the tourniquets and catheters are removed.

EXCISION OF PRIMARY LESION

PUMP OXYGENATOR HEAT EXCHANGER

TOURNIQUET

EXTENT OF AXILLARY NODE DISSECTION

A

AREA PERFUSED

PNEUMATIC CUFF

B

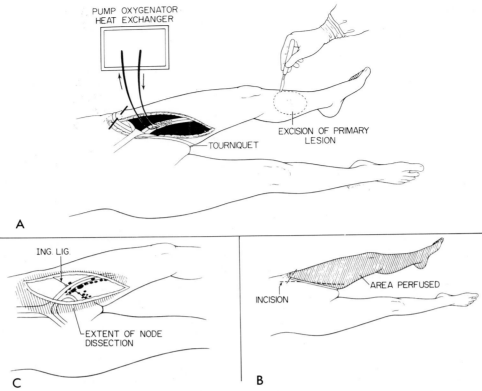

Figure 75–5   Technique for simultaneous perfusion of lower extremity, radical groin dissection, and excision of primary melanoma lesion *(A)*. All stages are performed at one operation. At the completion of the radical ilio-inguinal groin dissection *(C)*, the external iliac vessels are cannulated and a tourniquet is placed across the inguinal area and secured with a Steinmann pin in the iliac crest. While the extremity is being perfused, the primary lesion is excised and the resultant defect skin grafted. The chemotherapeutic agent is then flushed from the leg before removal of the tourniquet. Any tumor cells in transit between the primary lesion and the groin are subjected to hyperthermia and to a large concentration of drug during this procedure *(B)*.

received actinomycin D as the chemotherapeutic agent; of these, two recurred. Five were given Thio-TEPA alone and four TSPA and melphalan combined. The rest received melphalan alone.

Krementz and Creech (1968) reported the five-year survival rate in patients treated at Tulane University by combined perfusion and surgery. Of 118 patients followed for more than five years, there were 60 (50.8 percent) survivors. Stehlin (1975) reported a five-year survival rate in 48 percent of a similar group of patients. These results are better than the 20 percent reported for similar cases treated by surgery alone (McNeer and Canton, 1969).

The eventual role of perfusion in the management of the primary operable case of malignant melanoma cannot be determined until controlled and randomized studies have been completed with a statistically significant number of cases followed for a sufficient period of time. Such studies are now being conducted in this country by the Central Oncology Group, a cooperative venture of several university and hospital centers.

Perfusion For Recurrent Melanoma. Sixty-six patients with recurrent melanoma limited to an extremity were perfused. Forty-four, or 67 percent, had complete disappearance of detectable tumor. The disease eventually recurred in over two-thirds of these patients, but 13 (30 percent) are still free of tumor six to 176 months later. Seventeen percent are alive five to 14 years since their recurrent disease was perfused. Eleven of those whose disease recurred were perfused a second or third time.

To achieve uniformity in their results, Creech and his coworkers employed melphalan as the chief chemotherapeutic agent in their perfusions. Stehlin and Clark (1965), Rochlin and Smart (1965), and others have also used this agent almost exclusively, and the results have been rather consistent among these workers. We have employed a variety of drugs in our perfusions. Some interesting results were obtained in melanoma patients treated with actinomycin D. Thirty-six of our patients with extensive recurrent melanoma were perfused with this agent, and nine (25 percent) are still free of disease. Another five are living with disease at least nine months following treatment. In some the remissions appear to have been induced by a different mechanism than that in those perfused with melphalan and the other agents. In these patients treated with actinomycin D, an initial objective tumor response was followed a few weeks later by regrowth of the lesions. Actinomycin D was then given intravenously at weekly intervals over a period of months, and it caused eventual complete regression which persists after the termination of therapy. The first such patient is an example:

Mrs. R. A. at age 52 had a melanoma of the left leg excised in November, 1959. It recurred four months later. A radical groin dissection, three local excisions with skin grafts, and an isolated perfusion with melphalan and thio-TEPA were done over the next five months. The dosage of melphalan was 62.5 mg. (0.9 mg. per kg.) and of thio-TEPA 62.0 mg. (0.9 mg. per kg.) delivered in five aliquots at 5- to 10-minute intervals during a 60-minute isolated perfusion of the left lower extremity on August 26, 1960.

All skin nodules softened or disappeared at the time of discharge from the hospital five days later. No toxicity developed. On September 27, 1960, the lesions recurred. A 60-minute isolated perfusion with 12.0 mg. (0.2 mg. per kg.) of mithramycin (PA–144) of the leg distal to the mid-thigh was performed. All lesions were excised, and skin was grafted to the leg during the perfusion.

On November 17, 1960, recurrent lesions were noted in the leg. At the time of the final perfusion, five skin lesions were present on the lower leg and ankle which varied in size from 1.0 × 4.0 mm. to 8.0 × 15.0 mm.

On December 19, 1960, an isolated perfusion of the left lower extremity was performed through the external iliac artery and vein. Actinomycin D, 6.0 mg. (0.1 mg. per kg.) in six aliquots at five-minute intervals was administered. After 60 minutes the extremity was flushed with 500 ml. of dextran and 400 ml. of 5 percent dextrose in saline. Inflammatory changes distal to the tourniquet were first detected 24 hours postoperatively. These progressed to induration and cellulitis by the third postoperative day and bullae and edema by the next. Regression in these changes began on the ninth postoperative day and subsided on the twelfth postoperative day; however, muscular weakness necessitated the use of crutches for two months.

Systemic toxicity was manifested by nausea and vomiting for the first three postoperative days; it then subsided only to recur on the eleventh postoperative day. The vomitus became "coffee ground" in appearance three days later. Diarrhea occurred on the thirteenth postoperative day. Pharyngitis, stomatitis, and glossitis began on the fifth postoperative day and did not improve until the twelfth. The white blood count reached its nadir of 1900 on the eleventh postoperative day and the platelets on the eighth postoperative day at 80,000. When the hemoglobin, preoperatively 11.5 g., fell to 8.8 g. on the fourth postoperative day, transfusions totaling 2000 ml. of whole blood were given. Alopecia developed and persisted for two months.

On January 18, 1961, or one month after the perfusion, new skin lesions developed on the leg. Biopsy confirmed these to be melanoma. Systemic actinomycin D was instituted intravenously on February 21, 1961, and was continued weekly in doses of 400 μg. through July 11, 1961; then 800 μg. were administered weekly through May 16, 1962, when the use of the drug was discontinued due to severe nausea and vomiting. A total of 39.75 mg. was administered during 432 days. On March 28, 1961, the lesions, which had continued to grow and increase in number, appeared (Fig. 75–4A). These began to soften, pale, and gradually disappear until on June 27, 1961, all were gone (Fig. 75–4B). No further therapy was given after May 16, 1962.

An area of induration in the incision in the lower left quadrant, present since the last perfusion, was biopsied on April 3, 1963, and revealed melanoma. However, no new lesions have occurred, and the patient was healthy and free of disease on March 31, 1971, or ten years and three months after the initial perfusion with actinomycin D. Six additional patients experienced a similar sequence of events.

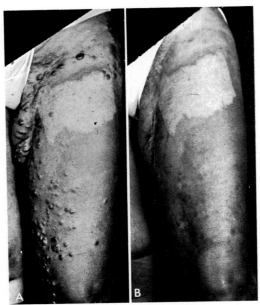

Figure 75–6 *A,* Leg of 52 year old woman with extensive recurrent melanoma. *B,* Same patient seven months after perfusion with actinomycin D. Patient is free of disease 14 years and three months later.

The consensus of experience with perfusion for melanoma of the extremities appears to indicate that marked regression or gross destruction of lesions lasting upwards of six months will occur in one-third of all cases. An additional 20 to 40 percent may be expected to have regression lasting a shorter period of time. Only 25 percent will not be expected to respond at all.

Perfusion of advanced melanoma of the extremity has resulted in five-year survivals of almost 30 percent. Krementz and Ryan (1971) reported ten patients out of 34 surviving for five or more years, and we have six of 21. This compares with 10 to 16 percent for those whose recurrent lesions were treated by surgery alone. Stehlin and Clark (1965) have observed that perfusion reduced materially the incidence of recurrence within the extremity in advanced cases from 64 percent in those treated by conventional means to 13 percent in those perfused. In patients who are not cured, perfusion has delayed the appearance of local recurrence in the treated extremity until systemic disease becomes overwhelming. Thus its trial as

an adjuvant to the conventional surgical approach seems justified.

Squamous Cell Carcinoma

Head and Neck. The external carotid artery supplies most of the skin above the cricoid cartilage except that of the orbit, the frontal scalp, and the posterior neck (Fig. 75–2). It supplies, in addition, most of the dura, the skull bones, external and middle ear, the oral cavity, and maxillary sinus, as well as partially supplying the frontal, ethmoid, and sphenoidal sinuses and nasal cavity. Perfusions using rapidly fixed agents, such as nitrogen mustard, have been satisfactorily employed for cancers in these locations. More often, however, intra-arterial infusions of the external carotid artery cannulated either directly or retrograde via the superficial temporal artery have been employed. Details of these techniques have been reported by Ramsden and Duff (1963) and by Golomb (1964).

Results measured by objective tumor regression have been reported in more than 60 percent of 959 cases reviewed (Table 75–1). In 104 (10.1 percent) cases complete gross disappearance of tumor occurred. While complete regression occurred in one-tenth of all cases, this was short lived, lasting less than three months in nearly all those patients not receiving further therapy.

Methotrexate by intra-arterial infusion plus intramuscular citrovorum factor for neutralization of systemic drug leakage was the most commonly used therapy. Two hundred and sixty cases of squamous cell carcinoma treated with this combination were evaluated to determine the occurrence of objective tumor regression. In 175 cases (67 percent) regression occurred, and in 43 cases (16.5 percent), this was complete (Golomb, 1962b).

Other Locations. There is limited objective data on skin cancers elsewhere in the body. Large squamous cell carcinomas arising in sinus tracts and burn scars have been treated by fractionated HN2, continuous methotrexate infusion, and isolated perfusion, usually with thio-TEPA or

TABLE 75–1 SUMMARY OF OBJECTIVE TUMOR RESPONSE TO INFUSION AND PERFUSION THERAPY OF HEAD AND NECK CANCER*

Procedure	Total Cases Suitable For Study	Number With Objective Response	% With Objective Response	Number With Complete Regression	% With Complete Regression
Methotrexate infusion and citrovorum factor systemically for squamous cell carcinoma	498	328	65	47	9
All other infusions	292	165	57	35	12
All infusions	790	493	62	82	10
All perfusions	169	95	56	22	13
All cases	959	588	60.6	104	10.1

*From Golomb (1964).

NH2. Good objective regression has been reported in isolated cases by Lawrence (1963b) and others. Four of our patients, two with cancer of the vulva, one with cancer of the buttock, and one with cancer of the leg responded dramatically to isolated perfusion with NH2. However, the results were transient, and recurrences were noted in all after less than three months.

Adenocarcinoma

While considerable experience and success have been obtained with regional chemotherapy of adenocarcinoma in visceral organs, such as the liver, only a small number of skin lesions have been so treated. These include breast cancer and adenocarcinoma of the head and neck area, where a limited response to isolated perfusion and intra-arterial infusion has been noted by Ariel (1957), Creech et al. (1958), and Krementz et al. (1962). Isolated perfusion for perineal recurrence of rectal cancer has been ineffective in achieving objective tumor regression; however, pain relief usually will occur and justify this form of therapy. Intra-arterial infusion has been of objective and subjective value for these cases.

The internal iliac arteries supplying the pelvic viscera and skin may be catheterized by percutaneous selective angiography or by direct surgical cannulation. The surgical method we have found most practical has been to expose the superior gluteal arteries via incisions over the lateral buttocks. Catheters are then advanced retrograde into the internal iliac arteries. This spares the patient an abdominal operation and prevents the drug from reaching the buttocks where it would ordinarily be of no therapeutic value.

Sarcoma

Sarcomatous lesions which affect the skin do lend themselves to treatment by perfusion. Our experience with Kaposi's sarcoma (Fig. 75–7), liposarcoma, leiomyosarcoma, rhabdomyosarcoma, and reticulum cell sarcoma (Fig. 75–8) indicates that an objective regression may be anticipated in two-thirds of the patients perfused. This response rate may be increased with the addition of pre- or postperfusion irradiation and hyperthermia, as reported by Stehlin (1969). The agents most frequently employed in perfusion for sarcoma are melphalan and actinomycin D combined. Intra-arterial infusion with nitrogen mustard has been effective in one-third of the patients reported by Ariel (1957) and Byron et al. (1961). Persistence of residual tumor is the rule with both these methods of treatment, and unless further extirpation or irradiation can be administered, recurrence is to be expected.

Lymphosarcoma is usually treated with a combination of systemic chemotherapy and radiation. However, 80 to 90 percent of patients presenting local recurrences after such forms of therapy will respond to regional chemotherapy. Again, re-

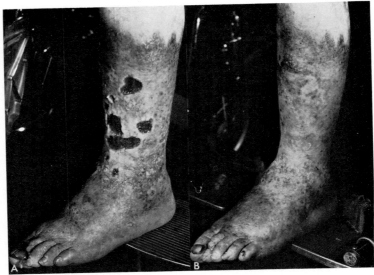

Figure 75–7 *A*, Leg and foot of a 71 year old man with recurrent Kaposi's sarcoma after maximum irradiation therapy. *B*, Same patient 21 weeks after perfusion with 48 mg. of nitrogen mustard.

growth within a few weeks or months is the rule.

Kaposi's sarcoma is usually sensitive to nitrogen mustard and may be considered suitable for therapy by regional tech-

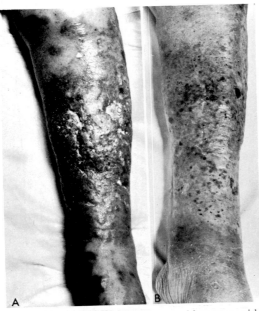

Figure 75–8 *A*, Leg of a 71 year old woman with cutaneous manifestations of reticulum cell sarcoma. Severe bone marrow depression precluded further systemic chemotherapy. *B*, Same patient three weeks after perfusion with 18.0 mg. of nitrogen mustard. Local response was associated with no further bone marrow depression.

niques in certain instances. Cook (1961) reported from Africa the complete disappearance of disease in nine of 60 patients treated with intra-arterial nitrogen mustard. These regressions lasted an average of 23 months. Twenty-seven of 60 patients had objective evidence of regression persisting an average of seven months. The response to isolated perfusion, as reported by Monaco and Austen (1959), Lawrence (1963b), and Golomb et al. (1962b), in patients who have received prior irradiation indicates that regressions may be achieved which last up to a year in patients whose limbs have been adequately irradiated.

DISCUSSION

Cancer therapists have long accepted the concept that, in order to cure patients, radical approaches are justified. For cancers with a high recurrence rate, the addition of another method of treatment might produce better results than one method alone. Thus combination therapy, using surgery plus radiation or surgery plus chemotherapy, has been widely advocated. Regional chemotherapy added to surgery or radiation in selected cases is also to be considered. For melanoma of the extremities, the combined use of isolated perfusion and surgery is being studied and appears to improve the survival rates in certain cases. Occasionally, for example, preoperative infusion or perfusion therapy can convert an unresectable oral cavity lesion into a resectable one. Or, in the case of sarcomas of the extremities, the results of combined therapy employing hyperthermic perfusion, local excision, and irradiation suggest that amputations may be less frequently indicated.

What constitutes desirable palliation in each case must be determined before attempting a regional chemotherapeutic procedure. Is diminution of the size of the lesion for a few weeks or months a sufficient reward for a major operative procedure? Does transient reduction in local cancer-caused pain justify the substitution of pain and discomfort from the procedures employed to achieve this end? Will the patient leave the hospital in more comfort and with a better emotional outlook than before treatment? These are some of the questions to ask before advocating therapy or deciding on the type of regional techniques to employ.

Should palliative radiation therapy be used before, after, or instead of regional therapy? After radiation the blood vessels supplying certain cancers may be narrowed or closed, thus reducing the efficiency of subsequent regional chemotherapy. Lesions such as recurrent pelvic or facial cancer are particularly susceptible to this. In these cases the author prefers to employ a regional perfusion technique first and then radiation, since local chemotherapy is more likely to be of value prior to radiation than following it. The staging of procedures has proved useful in many cases in which the combination of modalities can offer more than either one alone.

Reducing the total mass of a tumor by partial resection, or destruction by electrodesiccation or cryosurgery can improve the results of subsequent regional therapy.

CONCLUSIONS

Perfusion, or regional chemotherapy, has a place in the treatment of skin cancers. Its use must be advocated, however, with restraint and with the knowledge that serious complications may be encountered. Perfusion is to be advocated with the knowledge that, in the majority of patients, its palliative effects are short lived, and, when used as an adjuvant to curative modalities of treatment, its supplemental value is for the most part unproved. Nevertheless, with increasing experience it is becoming apparent that regional techniques of chemotherapy have a definite usefulness in the treatment of certain types of skin cancer.

REFERENCES

Ariel, I. M.: Treatment of inoperable cancer by intra-arterial administration of mechlorethamine. Arch. Surg., 74:516, 1957.

Benson, J. W., Kiehn, C. L., and Holden, W. D.: Cancer chemotherapy by arterial infusion. Arch. Surg., 87:125, 1963.

Bierman, H. R.: Selective Arterial Catheterization: Diagnostic, Therapeutic and Investigative. Springfield, Ill., Charles C Thomas, Publisher, 1969.

Bierman, H. R., Miller, E. R., Byron, R. L., Dod, K., Black, D., and Kelley, K.: Intra-arterial catheterization in man. Bull. Univ. Calif. Med. Center, 1:84, 1949.

Bierman, H. R., Byron, R. L., Jr., and Kelly, K. H.: Therapy of inoperable visceral and regional metastases by intra-arterial catheterization in man. Cancer Res., 11:236, 1951.

Byron, R. L., Jr., Perez, F. M., Yonemoto, R. H., Bierman, H. R., Gildenhorn, H. L., and Kelly, K. H.: Left brachial arterial catheterization for chemotherapy in advanced intra-abdominal malignant neoplasms. Surg. Gynecol. Obstet., 112:689, 1961.

Cavaliere, R., Ciocatto, E. C., Giovanella, B. C., Heidelberger, C., Johnson, R. O., Margottini, M., Mondovi, B., Moricca, G., and Rossi-Fanelli, A.: Selective heat sensitivity of cancer cells. Cancer, 20:1351, 1967.

Clarkson, B., and Lawrence, W., Jr.: Perfusion and infusion techniques in cancer chemotherapy. Med. Clin. North Am., 45:689, 1961.

Cook, J.: The treatment of Kaposi's sarcoma with nitrogen mustard. E. Afr. Med. J., 38:510, 1961.

Creech, O. J., Jr.: Regional chemotherapy. Surg. Gynecol. Obstet., 114:504, 1962.

Creech, O. J., Jr., Krementz, E. T., Ryan, R. F., and Winblad, J. N.: Regional perfusion utilizing an extracorporeal circuit. Ann. Surg., 148:616, 1958.

Creech, O. J., Jr., Krementz, E. T., Ryan, R. F., Reemtsma, K., and Winblad, J. N.: Experiences with isolation-perfusion technics in the treatment of cancer. Ann. Surg., 149:627, 1959a.

Creech, O. J., Jr., Krementz, E. T., Ryan, R. F., Reemtsma, K., and Elliot, J. L.: Perfusion treatment of patients with cancer. J.A.M.A., 171:2069, 1959b.

Fontaine, R., Walter, P., Kim, M., and Kieny, R.: De l'utilité de l'artériographie pour le diagnostic des tumeurs des membres d'origine osseuse et extra-osseus. J. Radiol. Electrol., 35:165, 1964.

Freckman, H. A.: Results of regional intra-arterial cancer chemotherapy in 1,150 patients. *In* Tenth International Cancer Congress Abstracts. Houston, Medical Arts Publishing Company, 1970, p. 454.

Golomb, F. M.: Perfusion and infusion chemotherapy for cancer of head and neck tumors. Proc. Natl. Cancer Conf., 5:561, 1964.

Golomb, F. M., Hall, A. B., Cox, K. R., Schetlin, C. F., Gumport, S. L., and Wright, J. C.: A simplified technic for regional perfusion. Report of its use in a series of twenty-three cases of malignancies of the head and neck. Am. J. Surg., 102:839, 1961.

Golomb, F. M., Cobb, J. P., Walker, D. G., and Wright, J. C.: In vitro selection of chemotherapeutic agents for perfusion therapy of human cancer. Surgery, 51:639, 1962a.

Golomb, F. M., Postel, A. H., Hall, A. B., Gumport, S. L., Cox, K. R., and Wright, J. C.: Chemotherapy of human cancer by regional perfusion. Report of 52 perfusions. Cancer, 15:828, 1962b.

Klopp, C. P., Alford, T. C., Bateman, J., Berry, G. M., and Winship, T.: Fractionated intra-arterial cancer chemotherapy with methyl bisamine hydrochloride: A preliminary report. Ann. Surg., 132:811, 1950.

Krementz, E. T.: Regional perfusion for tumors other than melanoma. Proc. Natl. Cancer Conf., 5:533, 1964.

Krementz, E. T., and Creech, O. J., Jr.: Advances in the treatment of malignant melanoma. Proc. Natl. Cancer Conf., 6:529, 1968.

Krementz, E. T., and Ryan, F. R.: Chemotherapy of melanoma of the limb by regional perfusion. Presented at an exhibit of the same name at the Southeast Surgical Congress, Miami, April 18–21, 1971.

Krementz, E. T., Creech, O. J., Jr., Ryan, F. R., and Reemstma, K.: An appraisal of cancer chemotherapy by regional perfusion. Ann. Surg., 156:417, 1962.

Lawrence, W., Jr.: Current status of regional chemotherapy. Part I. Technics. N.Y. J. Med., 63:2359, 1963a.

Lawrence, W., Jr.: Current status of regional chemotherapy. Part II. Results. N.Y. J. Med., 63:2518, 1963b.

Lindgren, A. G. H.: The vascular supply of tumors with special reference to the capillary angioarchitecture. Acta Pathol. Microbiol. Scand., 22:493, 1945.

Livingston, R. B., and Carter, S. R.: Single Agents in Cancer Chemotherapy. New York, IFI/Plenum, 1970.

Mcneer, G., and Canton, J.: Local failure in the treatment of melanoma. Am. J. Roentgenol., 99:791, 1969.

Monaco, A. P., and Austen, W. G.: Treatment of Kaposi's sarcoma at lower extremity by extracorporeal perfusion with chemotherapeutic agents. New Engl. J. Med., 261:1045, 1959.

Moon, J. H.: Combination chemotherapy in malignant melanoma. Cancer, 26:468, 1970.

Ramsden, C. H., and Duff, J. K.: Continuous arterial infusion of head and neck tumors. Cancer, 16:133, 1963.

Rochlin, D. B., and Smart, C. R.: Treatment of malignant melanoma by regional perfusion. Cancer, 18:1544, 1965.

Ryan, R. F., Krementz, E. T., Creech, O., Jr., Winblad, J. P., Chamblee, W., and Cheek, H.: Selected perfusion of isolated viscera with chemotherapeutic agents using an extracorporeal circuit. Surg. Forum, 8:158, 1957.

Shingleton, W. W., Parker, R. T., and Mahaley, S.: Abdominal perfusion for cancer chemotherapy. Ann. Surg., 152:583, 1960.

Stehlin, J. S., Jr.: Malignant melanoma: An appraisal. Surgery, 64:1149, 1968.

Stehlin, J. S., Jr.: Hyperthermic perfusion with chemotherapy for cancer of the extremities. Surg. Gynecol. Obstet., 129:305, 1969.

Stehlin, J. S., Jr., and Clark, R. L.: Melanoma of the extremities: Experiences with conventional treatment and perfusion in 339 cases. Am. J. Surg., 110:366, 1965.

Stehlin, J. S., Giovanella, B. C., Ipolyi, P. D., Muenz, L. R., and Anderson, R. F.: Results of hyperthermic perfusion for melanoma of the extremities. Surg. Gynec. Obstet., 140:339, 1975.

Sullivan, R. D., and McPeak, C. J.: A favorable response in tongue cancer to arterial infusion chemotherapy. J.A.M.A., 179:293, 1962.

Sullivan, R. D., Miller, E., and Sikes, M. P.: Antimetabolite-metabolite combination cancer chemotherapy. Effects of intra-arterial methotrexate-intramuscular citrovorum factor therapy in human cancer. Cancer, 12:1248, 1959.

Woodhall, B., Hall, K., Mahaley, S. J. R., and Jackson, J.: Chemotherapy of brain cancer: Experimental and clinical studies in localized hyperthermic cerebral perfusions. Ann. Surg., 150:60, 1959.

76

Laser Cancer Surgery

Leon Goldman, M.D.

One of the important fields of current laser surgical research is cancer. The laser is a form of intense light, the most powerful light in the world. The name laser is an acronym for *l*ight *a*mplification of *s*timulated *e*mission of *r*adiation. Its basic properties briefly are (1) coherency, (2) monochromatism, (3) high energy and power densities, and (4) selective color absorption of some laser systems, therefore, of selective value in pigmented tissues.

The laser emission may be continuous (CW) or pulsed, with pulses lasting milliseconds, nanoseconds, or even picoseconds. The following types of lasers have been used in dermatology:

Laser	Spectral Region	Wavelength (nm.)
Ruby	Red	694.3
Neodymium	Infrared	1060.0
Neodymium–YAG	Infrared	1060.0
Argon	Blue-green	499.5–514.5
Krypton	Visible	476.2–647.1
CO_2	Far infrared	10,600.0
Helium-neon	Red	632.8
Ultraviolet	Ultraviolet	265.0–360.0

To transmit these beams from various laser systems so that accessible cancers of the skin may be treated, the following types of optical systems may be used:

1. Lenses
2. Prisms
3. Mirrors
4. Curved, tapered quartz rods
5. Fiber optics—quartz and special crystalline fiber optics
6. Gas lenses

Actually, laser cancer research starts with cytologic studies. With the laser attached to a microscope, ruby or argon, it is possible to use microirradiation of single cells and tissues. Beam diameters can vary from less than 1 to 50 microns. Studies have been done on selective effects of the laser on chromosomes, mitochondria, and lysosomes. With such instrumentation, it is possible to do microsurgery on selected areas of chromosomes. Such studies have been done by Berns et al. (1969) on the large chromosomes of the salamander. In addition, tissue cultures of amelanotic and melanotic melanomas have also been exposed to the laser to study the protective effect of pigment, the development of pigment following laser irradiation, and the absorption of the laser through pigment granules and pigment masses in the cells of tissue cultures.

Moreover, with the laser attached to a

microscope it is possible to do microemission laser spectroscopy in situ on actual tumors in man and animals. This technique uses only a small area, 50 microns or less, of the sample without complete destruction of the whole tumor. This technique serves to identify cations in tissue. Of special value in the field of cancer would be such chemicals as lead, calcium, phosphorus, nickel, arsenic, and beryllium. With this technique it is possible to analyze living tumors without the destruction of the entire sample as is often necessary in spectroscopy. This form of spectroscopy can be used also in deparaffinized microscopic sections. Then staining can be done, both routine and special.

The interest of the dermatologist, however, is in the use of the laser as a surgical instrument for treatment of cancer. Is the laser necessary? The credo which is used in all studies of the applications of the laser is the oft repeated, "If you don't need the laser, don't use it." With the help of the engineer and the physicist, the surgeon has now added the laser to his scalpel, the high frequency electrosurgical unit, the liquid nitrogen cryosurgical unit, the liquid nitorgen cryosurgical probe, and, recently, the plasma scalpel. Perhaps not so much for dermatologic surgery but for visceral surgery, there are many problems involving hemorrhage. These include especially hemorrhage of the liver, the lungs, and the heart. Even in the field of dermatology there is often need for arrest of hemorrhage, as in the treatment of vascular lesions such as cavernous angiomas, port-wine spots, areas of telangiectasia, and angiosarcomas.

The special quality of the laser that makes it of use in surgery is the fact that it is a precise light beam, a collimated light beam. This makes it possible to have a knife edge, as it were, thinner than any razor blade. As a matter of fact, it is possible to have the beam of such magnitude that it is not even visible. Because of the high output of lasers, a very high degree of thermal coagulation necrosis can be induced; consequently, relatively bloodless surgery can be accomplished. Moreover, because of the color absorption of some lasers, it is possible to have selective color

absorption in areas which are pigmented. Therefore, selective surgery can be done. No other physical modality in dermatologic surgery has this property of selective color absorption. If the lesion is not pigmented, melanin or hemoglobin skin pigments may be added, such as vital dyes, ferrofluids, carbon, and so forth.

Another feature of laser surgery of interest to the dermatologist is the relatively good cosmetic result of laser surgery, as mentioned above. With certain lasers the duration of the impact of the laser is in terms of milliseconds; therefore, the pain is only minimal. Other lasers of the pulsed type include impacts of nanoseconds and even picoseconds. The lasers of interest to the surgeon are those of the continuous wave (CW) type.

The responsibility for introducing a new modality of treatment into medicine is well realized. This means a thorough investigation of its early and delayed effects on living tissue and of the safety programs necessary for protection of the patient as well as the operator. Finally, there is the need to develop a flexible, easy, usable apparatus at a low cost.

To provide for dermatologic surgery, the laser beam must be transmitted so that the dermatologist can use it. This involves the transmission techniques previously listed: lenses, mirrors, prisms, curved glass quartz rods, and fiber optics. There is not an excessive loss of output with these various systems of transmission except for the fiber optics. Now there are new developments in fiber optics, especially in crystalline fiber optics, which may make for transmission of relatively high outputs, especially of the CW systems and the Nd–YAG lasers. With fiber optics, a safe, flexible operating probe can be used so that precision surgery is possible.

The pulsed lasers destroy cancer tissue after impact by a tissue reaction which is essentially a thermal coagulation necrosis plus elastic recoil and pressure waves. With high output systems there are also electrical field changes as yet not understood. In pigmented tissues especially, free radical formation may be produced by these impacts. The impact is visible in the form of a plume cloud of particles of high velocity. In animals these plume fragments may contain living cells and may develop new foci of the tumor about the target area. As yet, this has not been found in any of our experiments with the pulsed laser treatment of malignancy in man. The pulsed lasers destroy tumor masses in situ with relatively little bleeding. This laser would be used in the same manner that the dermatologist would use the high frequency electrosurgical unit for local or metastatic masses in which excisional procedures are not required or are impractical.

The CW lasers are used for excisions. The ones most commonly used today are the argon laser, the carbon dioxide laser, and the Nd–YAG lasers. In laser surgical research today, the high output carbon dioxide laser, 100 to 300 watts, has been used because of its relatively high efficiency, its compactness as a portable type of unit, and its relatively cheaper cost. Special expensive infrared optics are needed to transmit the beam. Our experiences have been chiefly with the American Optical carbon dioxide laser with its flexible manipulator arm and its endoscope. We have also used the argon laser with the manipulator arm composed of multiple mirrors. Current research is now being done with fiber optic systems capable of transmission of high output argon laser beams. Recently we have used the special crystalline fiber optics of Nath and Schindler with high output Nd–YAG lasers on various types of skin cancer.

After the laser instrument has been analyzed and studied and is ready for experimental use, the next important step is the development of a laser safety program, safe for the physicist who develops it and safe for the patient and the operator. Because of the intensity of the laser light, the absorption of the incident beam on the cornea, and its focusing by the lens, severe burns of the retina can be produced. This reaction is used as a basis for the marvelous developments of laser ophthalmologic surgery. To avoid retinal damage, the eyes must be protected. This is done first through area control, namely, the construction of special facilities where safety is the consideration in construction. The laser system is to be enclosed, if possible. The control area may have laser safety windows through which transmission of the laser beam is reduced. Another consideration is the avoidance of specular surfaces to prevent development of highly reflectant beams. Finally, there is the necessity of training personnel in laser safety and appointing or employing a laser safety officer.

Specific protective glasses are used for necessary eye protection. There is no single laser protective glass. Different glasses must be used for the ruby, the argon, and the neodymium lasers. For the carbon dioxide laser, ordinary glasses or plastic glasses may be used. For the high output carbon dioxide lasers on white surfaces, such as bones, ruby protective glasses may be used to reduce the intensity of the visible light. For Nd–YAG laser surgery, the Schott KG protective glass is preferred to the Schott BG-18. The glasses should be marked and fit well. It is emphasized that the protective glasses reduce visual acuity, and for the argon laser, for example, the glasses will erase the beam entirely. The hazard in the use of invisible beams is the reflection from instruments, such as the hemostat or forceps. Guide beams, such as red lights or helium-neon or krypton lasers, are often used with infrared, invisible laser systems. It has been shown that, with planned laser safety programs, the laser is safe.

The other consideration in the safety program is protection of the skin of the patient as well as that of the operator. Because of the reflection of the beam, the area about the skin should be protected with materials such as sterile cardboard, which reflects the beam, barrier creams of titanium dioxide or zinc oxide, and cloths. Because so little is known about chronic exposure, the hands of the operator should also be protected with gloves. In our experience, the black leather glove is more highly protective against the laser systems than are other types of gloves. In the operating room rubber gloves are sufficiently protective. For operating room techniques, instrument heads must be sterilizable. When local anesthesia is used, the anesthesia is ranged about the local lesion to avoid changing the optical properties of the target area for maximum laser absorption. For general anesthesia,

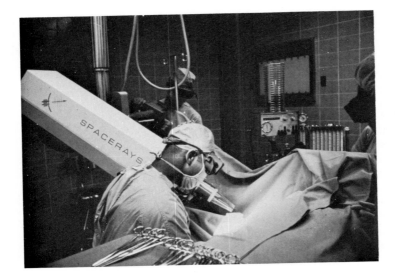

Figure 76–1 The pulsed ruby laser in the operating room. Protective glasses worn by operator and nurse.

halothane is preferred. For brief operations in children, ketamine has been used. Standardization of permitted exposures has recently been developed by the American National Standards Institute Z-136 committee with the following provisions: for pulsed laser systems, 0.4 to 1.4 micrometer region (visible and near-infrared visible), the maximum intensity incident on the skin should not exceed 0.10 joule per cm.^{2} per pulse for exposure times greater than 0.1 millisecond and should not exceed 0.01 joule per cm.^{2} for a pulse of shorter duration. With continuous wave laser systems for exposure times greater than one second, the power density shall not be in excess of 0.1 watt per cm.^{2}; with an exposure time of one second or less, the power output shall not exceed 1.0 watt per cm^2. With laser systems in the 1.4 to 1000 micrometer spectral region (infrared), the exposure levels permitted are the same as in the other. It is admitted that, because of the lack of experience with the ultraviolet lasers (0.2 to 0.4 micrometer), there is actually little information available. It is hoped that the Committee will have more information available when high output ultraviolet lasers are used extensively in biologic and medical experimentation. Farrington Daniels and John Knox have indicated the

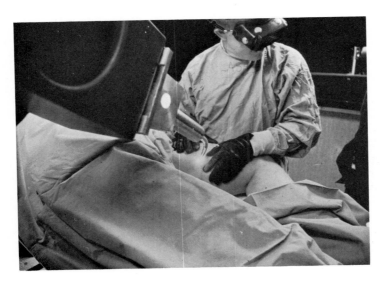

Figure 76–2 Ruby laser impact of metastatic melanoma of the thigh through curved, tapered quartz rod. Note draping of the patient and protective gloves and glasses of the operator.

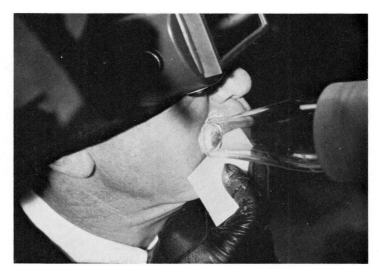

Figure 76–3 Safety technique for laser treatment of carcinoma of the face. Note eye protection of patient, cardboard template to protect lips by reflecting laser beam, plume trap over head of pulsed laser to prevent dispersion of fragments from tumor on laser impact, and protective gloves worn by operator to prevent chronic exposure of fingers to laser radiation.

need for data on permissible levels of ultraviolet exposures to the skin with new laser systems.

Air pollution, which is another feature of laser safety, is not a significant factor in dermatologic surgery. Whether the viable tumor fragments in pulsed laser system operations are harmful to the operator is not known. In our experience with plume traps on the head of the laser instrument and with vacuum installation, plume fragments are removed as air pollutants. Since such plume fragments do not arise with the CW lasers used at the present time, there is no concern about such hazards with these CW laser systems.

After adequate understanding and development of a laser safety program have evolved and with the availability of reliable, flexible, safe instrumentation, one can proceed with laser investigative surgery. This is done first in animals and then in man. In our experience, the skin of the miniature pig is a practical test model for laser skin surgery, as the pig skin is a good model, even for excisional surgery, knot tying, wound closure, and so forth, when expensive monkeys cannot be used. Extensive dermatologic investigative laser surgery in animals has been done for wound healing experiments and for the treatment of tumors such as the melanoma, types of angiosarcoma, and those induced by the polyomavirus. Controls have included scalpel surgery, high frequency electrosurgery, cryosurgery, and plasma scalpel surgery.

Twelve years ago, the initial experiments were started with the treatment of cancer of the skin in man. Cancer of the skin is of importance for investigative laser surgery because of the accessibility of the tumor. Unlike that in the use of x-ray, the target area must be available and accessible to the laser. The tumors treated have been the following:

1. Melanomas, primary and metastatic types
2. Angiosarcomas
3. Paget's disease
4. Bowen's disease
5. Squamous cell carcinomas
6. Varied metastatic malignancies
7. Malignant lymphomas, including mycosis fungoides

Sixteen patients with melanomas have been treated; four of these were primary melanomas. The follow-up period has been more than seven years. The black color of the melanoma means increased laser absorption with the ruby, the neodymium, the argon, and the Nd–YAG lasers and subsequent thermal coagulation destruction of the tumor mass. However, the serious prognosis of the cutaneous metastases of melanoma has not been changed at all with the laser treatment of multiple metastases. There has been no evidence in any of our experiments that the laser has served to spread the individually treated lesion. Only four cases of primary melanoma were treated, because the conventional treatments are preferred since laser therapy is a form of investigative surgery.

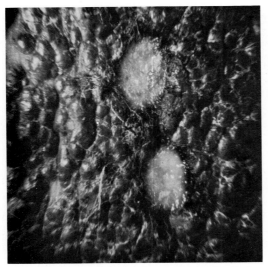

Figure 76–4 Metastatic melanoma of thigh five days after laser treatment. Biopsy negative in clear zone.
(See also Color Plate XII–C.)

Follow-up studies were available in only two patients, one elderly, cachectic, and in his 90's with multiple basal carcinomas as well as an extensive facial superficial melanoma, and the other elderly with primary melanoma of the neck. He had refused all surgery or radiation. Follow-up of one year in the first patient, with autopsy following renal infection, showed no evidence of melanoma. Four-year follow-up in the second patient has shown no recurrence or any evident metastatic lesions.

Three patients with angiosarcoma were treated. When the lesion was small and the laser output was high, the laser was effective locally. For large lesions the laser was not practical. One angiosarcoma of the finger was excised with the American Optical carbon dioxide laser. Also, in Kaposi's hemorrhagic sarcoma, the ruby laser was effective for small lesions.

Eighty basal cell epitheliomas were treated. There was an initial recurrence rate of 12 percent. With the new high output laser systems, this figure was reduced to 5 percent in a small series. The cosmetic results were good. Nonpigmented basal cell malignancies responded better to laser impacts if vital dyes were used to increase the absorption. These vital dyes

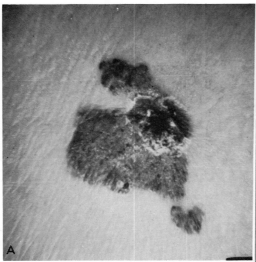

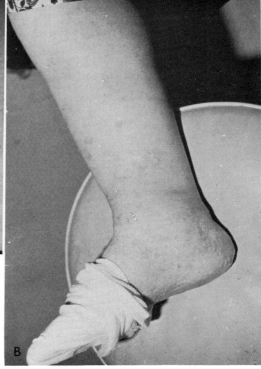

Figure 76–5 Melanoma of the lower leg with skin metastases in an elderly woman with congestive heart failure *(A)* before laser treatment and *(B)* one year after laser treatment. Later metastatic lesions developed elsewhere on leg.
(See also Color Plate XII-D.)

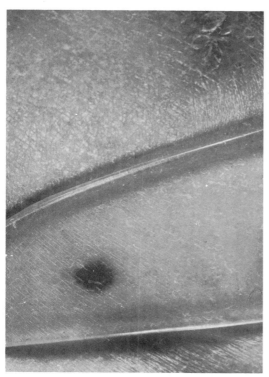

Figure 76–6 Hemorrhagic sarcoma of leg in elderly woman. Three years after the laser treatment, biopsy was negative; fresh lesion shown under the diascope. This also was treated by the laser with clearing.

may be injected or tattooed into the basal cell epithelioma. Recent experiments have also been done with ferrofluids to try to determine whether they can provide increased color absorption for nonpigmented basal cell epitheliomas.

Ferrofluids also have the advantage of providing a system which can be moved by magnetic fields into the lesion. Here laser and even microwaves may be used to induce local thermal coagulation necrosis. Radioactive Fe may also be used for localized radiation.

The most suitable type of patient for whom laser treatment may be used at present is a patient with multiple basal cell epitheliomas. In two patients with recurrent basal cell epitheliomas of the face, even on the ala nasi, the laser was effective. Mohs' controlled chemosurgery has been used to study the initial effects of the laser treatment. This was used to determine the initial extent of the laser necrosis on the tumor cords. The difficulty of doing properly controlled studies with the laser as an adjuvant is obvious.

Small lesions of squamous cell epithelioma responded to laser treatment. Metastatic malignancies were treated in two patients with effective destruction of small lesions and incomplete destruction of large types of lesions. These included metastases from the breast and carcinoma of the cervix. The laser was ineffective in the treatment of large plaques of mycosis fungoides and in the treatment of leukemia.

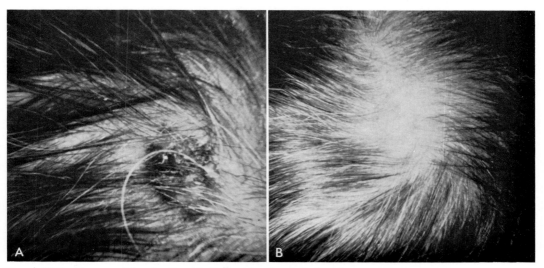

Figure 76–7 Pigmented basal cell epithelioma of scalp *(A)* before laser treatment and *(B)* four years after laser treatment.
(See also Color Plate XII-E.)

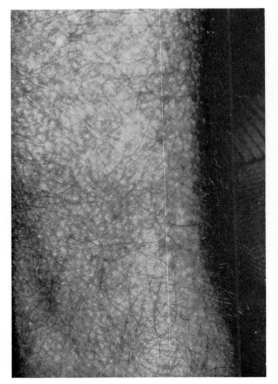

Figure 76–8 Basal cell epithelioma of the forearm eight years after laser treatment. Area clear, biopsy negative.

For actinic keratoses, the laser treatment was effective provided the lesions were small. Painting with dye increased the absorption of the laser. Leukoplakia of the lip and cheek areas painted with toluidine blue or Evans' blue was treated effectively with the pulsed ruby laser.

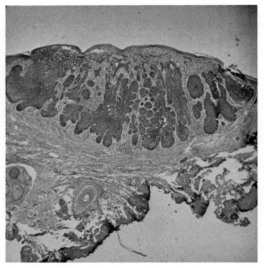

Figure 76–9 Bloodless excision of basal cell epithelioma by CO_2 laser. There is only a narrow band of thermal coagulation necrosis deep in the tissue. (See also Color Plate XII-F.)

The carbon dioxide laser was used also for excision of basal cell epitheliomas. The lesions showed good healing in the two patients in whom this technique was tried. In addition, carcinoma of the vulva has been treated by Schellas in our laser laboratory. More experiments are underway now. Current research is directed toward the development of laser operating microscopes for the detection and treatment of preinvasive carcinoma, especially in the cervix and buccal mucosa, as well as in the skin.

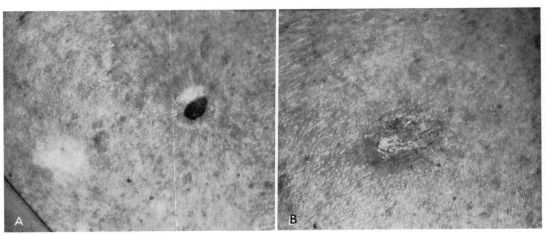

Figure 76–10 Nd–YAG surgery of recurrent basal cell carcinoma of the back with 20 to 25 watts *(A)*. *(B)* Two months later, biopsy negative.

mation of infected host cells that possibly later are eliminated.

More directly, Goldner et al. (1964) could interrupt tumorigenesis by SV40 in hamsters by intraperitoneal injection of syngeneic, morphologically intact, non-virus producing, SV40 transformed cells that had been rendered nonviable by x-irradiation. Similar findings also were reported by Girardi et al., (1965) using viable human cells transformed by SV40 in vitro rather than x-irradiated hamster cells. Essential for successful suppression of tumor induction was the fact that the cells used for immunization were morphologically intact. Cells disrupted by freezing and thawing were inactive.

The immune mechanism responsible for graft rejection is intimately associated with lymphoid cells (Gibson and Medawar, 1943; Mitchison and Dube, 1955) and is related to delayed hypersensitivity. Most likely, this mechanism is also involved in control of neoplastic growth. Circulating antibodies undoubtedly also play a role in graft rejection; cytotoxic antibodies have been demonstrated in vitro (Gorer, 1943; Gorer and O'Gorman, 1956). At present, it is felt that different classes of immunoglobulins may act differently on tumor cells, and some immunoglobulins may in one way or another interfere with the cell-mediated immunity. The latter is probably the basis for the immunologic enhancement phenomenon. This phenomenon refers to a seemingly paradoxical situation. Homografts of tumor cells are successfully established and grow faster and in increased numbers where the recipients previously have been immunized with the same tumor used for grafting (Kaliss, 1958 and 1962). Enhancement can be seen after both active immunization and passive transfer of isoantiserum to the graft recipient. When it is induced by active immunization, factors that are of importance seem to be the use of repeated injections and of relatively large doses of antigen. The physical state of the antigen used may also influence the result. Repeated freezing and thawing of a tumor cell antigen preparation was found to increase the degree of enhancement (Kaliss, 1962).

A major point in immunologic enhancement is undoubtedly direct exposure of the grafted cells to antibody. Treatment of tumor cells in vitro with enhancing isoantiserum prior to transplantation will result in enhanced growth (Kaliss, 1962). The antibodies involved are probably of the 7S immunoglobulin class (Möller, 1966; Takasugi and Hildemann, 1969). Immunization procedures that will favor 7S antibody formation are therefore likely to induce enhancement.

The human tumors that have been most often reported as having specific—usually common—antigens are Burkitt's lymphoma, nasopharyngeal carcinoma, cancer of the colon, hepatocarcinoma, osteogenic sarcoma, malignant melanoma, and neuroblastoma. Burkitt's lymphoma and nasopharyngeal carcinoma have a definite association with Epstein-Barr virus, but no causal relationship has been established. These rumors often respond dramatically to chemotherapy.

The methods used to demonstrate tumor antigens are complex and subject to interpretation, but they have provided an insight into possible future studies (Hellström et al., 1968a and 1968b). The variable clinical course of malignant melanoma and the frequency of dormancy and notable spontaneous regressions suggest that there may be a melanoma-specific antigen. Patients with metastatic melanoma and no evident primary tumor, or with a specific history of a lesion that "fell off" or disappeared, form about 2 to 5 percent of all new patients. One might guess that at least an equal number of persons may have primary melanomas that spontaneously regress without metastasizing.

A word of caution about cancer antigens such as the colon carcinoembryonic antigen (CEA) concerns their practical value. The studies by Gold (1967) are important, but one must remember that specific antibodies to the antigen may not be detected once the tumor enlarges or metastasizes. Morton (1969) also showed that the incidence and titer of antibodies to a melanoma antigen was higher in patients with localized disease than in those with widespread metastases.

IMMUNOTHERAPY OF MALIGNANCIES

In general, immunotherapy has been divided into passive, active, and adoptive immunity. This division is an artificial one, and usually it is more accurate to state that the reaction is predominantly "passive" or "active"; most therapeutic attempts include elements of both kinds of reaction.

Injections of sera and gamma globulins from patients with cancer or from normal persons have been unavailing, although several isolated regressions of melanoma and leukemia after multiple transfusions with blood from "cured" patients have been reported. An example from a host of negative studies was an attempt to treat patients with Burkitt's lymphoma by injecting them with 5 ml. of plasma (per kg. body weight) from patients with the same disorder during periods of remission (Fass et al., 1970a). In our opinion the host defenses against malignancies are primarily cellular; therefore, humoral agents are unlikely to be useful therapeutic agents. Even the danger of the enhancement of tumor growth is probably remote because of the ineffectiveness of such sera.

Active immunity requires that the host's defense mechanisms are capable of being stimulated. Specific anticancer stimulation would be the ultimate goal. The fact that a tumor has developed is evidence that either the host was not stimulated to respond or he was incapable of responding. One can also envision local factors that may determine whether or not carcinoma in situ survives and grows. These important but ill-defined factors, such as cell-cell recognition and inhibition, have been studied primarily in cell cultures.

Nonspecific adjuvant stimulants are illustrated by the use of BCG vaccines with and without adjuvants (Mathé, 1969); the effectiveness of the hoped for boost of existing resistance to tumor growth is limited by the severity of the local reactions.

More specific methods include the injection of cancer cell homogenates, irradiated autogenous tumor cells, and irradiated cultured cells derived from the same kind of malignancy. Some investigators have conjugated proteins to cancerous cells in the hope that these cell complexes would induce a therapeutic hypersensitivity reaction.

Specific cancer viruses have not been associated with human malignancies, but virus-specific immune reactions have provided excellent preventive and therapeutic reactions in experimental animals.

An interesting example of the clinical study of active cancer immunity is the attempt of Mathé (1969) to treat patients with leukemia. He reduced the amount of leukemia cells by chemotherapy and then instituted active immunotherapy by applying BCG vaccine to large areas of scarified skin every few days. In a second series of similar patients, intradermal and subcutaneous injections of frozen allogeneic leukemia cells were used. Eilber and Morton (1969) injected BCG vaccine directly into metastatic melanoma nodules. In those patients who were immunologically competent, the injected nodules regressed and even distant nodules regressed in a few instances. Other investigators have not been able to duplicate these results.

Specific active immunity has been tried by many investigators for many years without valid evidence of practical clinical accomplishment. In most instances the patient's tumor cells were either irradiated or frozen, then reinjected. Many of these studies suffered from the handicap of being done in patients with large amounts of residual tumor. Under such circumstances it is difficult to see how even minor observable effects on the tumors could be detected. Nadler and Moore (1969) used allogeneic cultured cancer cells of the same kind as those of the patient. One out of nearly a hundred patients in the study had a complete remission of his lung metastases from osteogenic sarcoma and others had significant regressions.

In a study combining some of the elements of active, passive, and adoptive immunity, Nadler and Moore (1969) cross-injected tumor tissue in paired patients with the same diagnosis and blood types. Subsequently reciprocal infusions of 2 to 5 g. of peripheral leukocytes were performed daily for 10 to 15 days. About 15 percent of the patients so treated and surviving one month (Moore and Gerner, 1971) had objective regressions, and five of 130 patients had complete regressions of metastases. The interesting results on patients with malignant melanoma are described in the next section.

An unusual kind of adoptive immunity with cultured human lymphocytes has been reported by Moore and Gerner (1970). Permanent lymphocyte cell lines were established from peripheral blood samples. The cultured immature lymphocytes were grown in 200-liter vessels and, when possible, exposed to a brei of irradiated tumor cells of the patient to be treated. Several patients were infused with over 300 g. of lymphocytes, and two patients were reported to have had significant regressions. This technique will require much more study of the isoantigen compatibilities of the cultured cells, survival studies, and evidence of localization of the lymphocytes in the tumors. In the future, effective methods of providing specific stimulation to lymphocytes will be required. These studies have a firm base of experimental support, including work on lymphocyte–tumor cell interactions in vitro and preliminary animal experiments by Alexander et al. (1966).

MALIGNANT MELANOMA

There has been much clinical evidence suggesting the important role of "immunity" or host resistence in the pathogenesis of malignant melanoma. As mentioned previously, there are objective observations of spontaneous regressions of primary lesions with and without metastases. Further, in rare instances established metastases have regressed; more commonly, metastatic lesions have remained dormant for from three to 20 years. Patients with melanomas of the foot or leg who have had a radical groin dissection may develop a bizarre pattern of metastases called satellitosis. In this condition there seems to be a complete loss of regional defensive measures, and literally thousands of metastases may develop in the leg below the level where the lymphatics were severed. The rest of the body often remains free of disease, or the usual pattern of relatively few metastases may be present. This iatrogenic demonstration of the potential numbers of metastases from a melanoma shows the effect of the altered tissue environment on growth of the tumor cells.

Regressions of melanomas have been reported after administration of rabies vaccine by Pack (1950); after administration of smallpox vaccine by Burdick and Hawk (1964), Milton and Brown (1966), and Hunter-Craig et al. (1970); and after BCG vaccine inoculations by Morton et al. (1970).

These reports were accompanied by independent findings of melanoma-associated antigens by Lewis et al. (1969), Morton (1970), and Romsdahl and Cox (1970). Hellström et al. (1968b) claimed that melanoma antigens could be detected by the inhibition of melanoma cells growing in cultures.

Passive immunologic therapy with serum and whole blood from patients cured of melanoma was reported to give sporadic regressions by Summer and Foraker (1960) and Teimourion and McCune (1963). In our opinion this kind of therapy is unlikely to be effective. The role of cellular immunity in the care of malignant melanoma has been emphasized by many investigators, including Golomb et al. (1967), Nadler and Moore (1968), Jehn et al. (1970), Fass et al. (1970b), as well as those mentioned previously.

Active immunologic therapy with irradiated autochthonous melanoma cells, inducing cytotoxic antibodies but having no observable effect on established metastases, was found by Ikonopisov et al. (1970). Human allogeneic melanoma cell lines reported by Nadler and Moore (1966) were irradiated and inoculated at intervals in 25 patients with metastases that no longer responded to chemotherapy. The few objective regressions were incidental to this evaluation of the safety of the method; no enhancement of tumor growth was observed. Probably all of these investigators realized the need for a prospective study in which active immunity would be initiated in patients from whom all gross tumor was excised but who had a high risk of recurrence.

Attempts to stimulate recognition by the host lymphocytes of the "nonself" or antigenic foreigners of the melanoma by the injections of irradiated tumor cells are worthwhile efforts, but there is an equal need for information as to how the efficiency of the technique can be increased. Further, reports of melanoma antigenicity would indicate that the patient's lymphocytes are coded to recognize and destroy the melanoma cells (Morton, 1969) but are unable to cope with large numbers of tumor cells. The problem may be that the patient's lymphocytes are "smothered" or neutralized by an excess of tumor antigen or inhibited by humoral "blocking" or "enhancing" antibodies.

One method of immunization may involve both active and adoptive immunity—the so-called "double-cross immunotherapy". Cross-immunization of pairs of patients with melanoma presupposed that there is a common tumor antigen and that the introduction of foreign lymphocytes from a melanoma patient might be able to stimulate the recipient's lymphocytes or, less likely, directly attack the recipient's tumor cells. Moore and his colleagues (Nadler and Moore, 1969; Moore and Gerner, 1971) paired volunteer melanoma patients with advanced disease according to blood type. Each patient was injected with 1 to 5 g. of cells from his partner; after five days reciprocal daily infusions of leukocytes were done. About 5 to 15 g. of leukocytes were recovered each day by leukapheresis and infused intravenously into the partner. The cell infusions were continued daily for 10 to 15 days. Eighteen of 86 patients with widespread melanoma had regressions of 50 percent or more of the measurable lesions, and two patients had complete regressions. The authors concluded that these remarkable regressions in patients with advanced disease provided evidence for a therapeutic trial in high risk patients with primary melanoma. The limitations of these studies were the relatively small number of lymphocytes that could be given, allogeneic reactions, and the difficulty in pairing. As a result of these limitations, it was concluded that some other form of adoptive immunity might be useful and feasible.

Moore and Gerner (1970) have reported initial studies in which several hundreds of grams of autochthonous and allogeneic cultured lymphocytes were infused into patients with metastatic melanoma. Several striking regressions were reported despite the disparity of the amount of tumor cells in the patients to the amount of lymphocytes infused. Valid evaluation of this technique would require a prospective controlled study in patients with occult disease.

Despite the excitement generated by these reports of immunologic defenses against malignant melanoma, none of them are ready for use in clinical practice. Wide surgical excision of the primary lesion still provides the best chance of cure; radical removal of metastases may be effective in some situations but ineffective in others (Moore and Gerner, 1971). X-ray therapy provides palliation by controlling the growth of large metastases in a few patients. The best chemotherapeutic agent is imidazole carboxamide, but it is clinically effective in only one out of seven patients, and it has immunosuppressive activity.

At present, immunotherapeutic procedures should be studied only in patients who have failed to respond to standard therapy.

EPIDERMAL NEOPLASMS

Immunotherapy of epithelial tumors of the skin had its origin in the studies of topical chemotherapy by several dermatologists. Madison and Haserick (1962) applied alkylating agents to the cutaneous lesions of mycosis fungoides. Klein et al. (1962) treated cutaneous metastasis and keratoacanthoma by the local administration of an antimetabolite, 5-fluorouracil (5-FU). They noted a more intense inflammatory response at the sites of primary and secondary tumors than on the normal skin and deduced that a selective antitumor reaction might be occurring. These intense reactions eradicated coexisting premalignant keratoses and superficial basal cell and squamous cell carcinomas. Similarly, Dillaha et al. (1963) noted that topical administration of 5-FU produced selective inflammation of keratoses and skin cancers after analogous effects had been observed in a patient treated with intravenous injections of 5-FU. Klein et al. (1965) and Dillaha et al. provided definite evidence for resolution of cutaneous cancers and premalignant lesions of the skin by topical application of 5-FU. In Europe an alkylating agent, Trenimon, has been injected directly into various cancers and metastases. Spiessl (1960), Peschke (1962), and Belisario (1965) applied this drug topically to skin cancers and observed regressions. In the course of parallel studies with this drug, Helm et al. (1965) observed that delayed hypersensitivity reactions were more intense at tumor sites than in the normal skin.

Skin tumors, because they provide considerable flexibility for the study of tumor biology, were investigated as to immunologic factors affecting premalignant and malignant epidermal neoplasms. Immediate hypersensitivity reactions were difficult to induce with most antigens under controlled conditions and did not appear to have selective effects on cutaneous neoplasms. But as noted previously, several chemotherapeutic agents (Klein, 1968a and 1968b) produced delayed cutaneous hypersensitivity reactions on the skin of patients with epitheliomas. Of these drugs, 2,3,5-tris-ethylene-imino-1,4-benzo-quinone (Trenimon, or TEIB) was investigated further; it produced a more intense challenge reaction at sites involved by cutaneous neoplasms than in the normal skin (Helm et al., 1965; Helm and Klein, 1965). The inflammatory reaction was a typical challenge response of the delayed hypersensitivity type. When the concentration of the challenging dose was reduced sufficiently, the reaction was almost entirely confined to the sites of neoplastic involvement with minimal or no reaction in the adjacent skin (Klein, 1968a and 1968c). The intense reaction resolved superficial basal cell carcinomas, squamous cell carcinomas in situ, premalignant keratoses, and leukoplakia (Helm et al., 1965). The hypersensitivity could be transferred by peripheral leukocytes from sensitized to nonsensitized patients; following transfer of immunity, the response of patients to challenge with the same drug resulted in tumor resolution.

Since TEIB was an alkylating agent with chemotherapeutic activity, dinitro-chlorobenzene (DNCB) was investigated as a "pure" sensitizer in order to determine whether the therapeutic hypersensitivity reactions required cytostatic activity or whether they could be induced by chemicals which did not have antimitotic activities. It was found that cytostatic activity was not necessary. Subsequent studies included patients with advanced disseminated malignant diseases and patients with intractable multiple epitheliomas. Patients with multiple superficial basal cell carcinoma syndromes, xeroderma pigmentosum, arsenical dermatoses and associated epidermal neoplasms, radiation dermatitis with malignant degeneration, widespread multiple solar keratoses, intraepithelial squamous cell carcinomas, and oral leukoplakia were treated successfully with topical immunotherapy.

BASAL CELL CARCINOMAS

The essential features of cell-mediated immunotherapy of epidermal neoplasms are demonstrated by the reactions of basal cell carcinomas. Hypersensitivity is induced by topical application of a cream containing 0.01 to 0.05 percent DNCB or TEIB. This preparation is applied daily under an occlusive dressing to an area of approximately 1 cm. until hypersensitivity becomes apparent. Hypersensitivity to topical application of these concentrations of DNCB or TEIB usually becomes apparent after two to three weeks of daily administration. It may, however, appear within one week or require up to 10 weeks.

After hypersensitivity is induced, the lowest concentration of the sensitizing agent which results in a response to challenge is determined. For this purpose a range of concentrations of the sensitizing agent is applied by a modified occlusive patch test technique to the normal skin. Since the effects on the tumor are markedly more intense than on the normal skin, a concentration of the sensitizing agent which barely produces a challenge response in the normal skin will produce an intense reaction in the tumor. It is

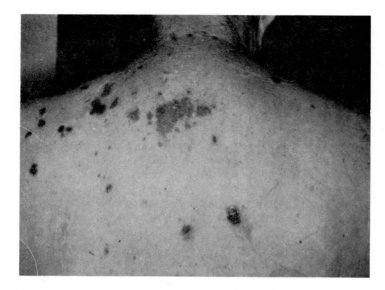

Figure 77–1 Patient with multiple basal cell nevoid syndrome and a 30-year history of large numbers of basal cell carcinomas involving both sun-exposed and unexposed areas of the skin. Upper back of patient is shown here prior to immunotherapy.

therefore not necessary to produce a challenge reaction in the normal skin in order to induce adequate effects on epidermal tumors. Effective concentrations of DNCB or TEIB for the challenge reaction usually range from 1 part per 100,000 to 1 part per 10 million. The reaction to the patch test is observed at 24-hour intervals for up to five days. As soon as the onset of a challenge response to a given concentration of the sensitizing agent is observed, the patch test is discontinued at that concentration, but others are continued at progressively lower concentrations until the minimal effective level is established. A preparation containing the minimal effective concentration of the sensitizing agent is then applied topically to the areas involved with neoplastic lesions (Fig. 77–1). The sensitizing agent is applied to the entire area. Usually the inflammatory reaction to the challenging application becomes apparent within 24 to 72 hours. Erythema, edema, and vesiculation develop, followed by erosion, exudation, necrosis (Fig. 77–2), and subsequent re-epithelialization (Fig. 77–3). This sequence of events may take from 10 days

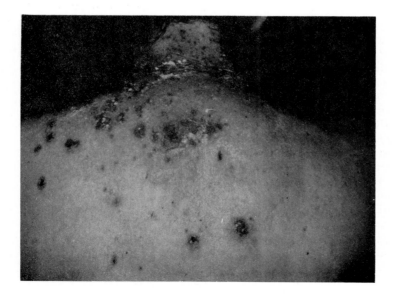

Figure 77–2 Two weeks after initiating immunotherapy by daily local application of a cream containing dinitrochlorobenzene (DNCB) at a concentration of 1:100,000. Clinically evident lesions have undergone immune challenge reactions. Additional lesions, particularly on the sun-exposed area of the neck, have become apparent as a result of their reactivity. Some lesions, notably the large lesion in the scar located in the interscapular area, already show re-epithelialization. Note that the normal tissues, including scar tissue free of tumor, do not show a reaction.

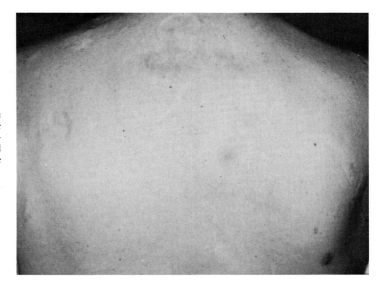

Figure 77–3 Patient shown 1½ years following a six-week course of immunotherapy. Patient has remained free of recurrence and clinically detectable lesions in the area treated.

to several weeks. At higher concentrations (i.e., above the minimal effective concentration of the sensitizer), the onset and severity of the reactions is accelerated.

There was no recurrence of the specific lesions which were resolved by topical therapy during an observation period of more than five years (Klein, 1969). Many patients with damaged skin subsequently developed new lesions at sites which had not previously been involved and were successfully treated by subsequent challenges with DNCB or TEIB. A note of caution is necessary since, for subsequent therapeutic courses, the sensitizing agent should be titrated again. A lower concentration (10^{-8} DNCB in the case of the patient shown in Figures 77–1 to 77–3) than in the first course (10^{-5}) may be required. Although the lower concentration may produce considerably milder reactions on the normal skin, resolution of the neoplastic lesions and subsequent recovery is often more rapid. Topical therapy in patients with multiple superficial basal cell carcinomas is very successful, and more than 98 percent of the lesions can be eradicated by immunologic challenge treatment.

It is noteworthy that many more punctate reactive sites may develop than those that have the discrete appearance of basal carcinomas. These areas include precancerous and minute lesions which cannot be clinically detected prior to the onset of the hypersensitivity reaction. Biopsies of these reactive lesions, not previously suspected as neoplastic, will reveal them to be basal cell carcinomas. Thus the hypersensitivity reaction not only unmasks clinically undetectable lesions but also eradicates them. The differential effect of the immune reaction on abnormal cells is further demonstrated by the observation that normal re-epithelialization proceeds while cancer cells are being destroyed and an exudate containing the debris of necrotic tumor cells is forming.

Systemic toxicity, other severe side effects, and generalized allergic reactions have not occurred in more than 100 patients treated with topical immunotherapy (Klein, 1969) over the past decade. The discomfort resulting from the cutaneous reaction is adequately controlled by mild analgesics and topical or brief courses of systemic corticosteroids. Steroid administration does not interfere with the resolution of the neoplasms once a challenge response is initiated, although the inflammatory component of the reaction is suppressed.

Therapeutic challenge reactions in malignant and premalignant lesions may be induced by topical administration of concentrations of 1 part per 100,000,000 or less of DNCB or TEIB, but usually concentrations of 1:1,000,000 to 1:100,000 are employed.

SQUAMOUS CELL CARCINOMAS

Topical immunotherapy for intraepidermal squamous cell carcinomas produces effects similar to those observed in basal cell carcinomas. Suitable lesions for topical immunotherapy are those seen in patients with intractable multiple squamous cell carcinomas associated with arsenical dermatitis, late radiation dermatitis, and severe actinic degeneration and xeroderma pigmentosum. Squamous cell carcinoma in situ responded more intensely than did premalignant keratoses to topical challenge with TEIB or DNCB. In general, however, the reaction to challenge of squamous cell carcinomas is similar to that of actinic keratoses, and early, undetectable lesions of squamous cell carcinoma become apparent. More than 90 percent of squamous cell carcinomas in situ have been found to undergo regressions following immunologic challenge. As might be expected, deeper invasive lesions are less amenable to therapy. Deeper lesions which do not regress completely become smaller and may then respond to a second course of immunotherapy or topical chemotherapy.

For example, residual lesions of squamous cell carcinoma in patients with xeroderma pigmentosum can be treated by a second course of immunotherapy to which topical 5-fluorouracil (5-FU) is added. The reaction of neoplasms to the combination of topical chemotherapy and immunotherapy is considerably more intense than with either agent given alone. Recurrent squamous carcinomas following surgery or x-irradiation are difficult to treat with topical immunotherapy, and even two to five successive courses of immune challenge may be less than 60 percent effective.

PREMALIGNANT EPIDERMAL LESIONS

At least 75 percent of the premalignant keratoses in patients with arsenical dermatoses can be successfully treated with topical immunotherapy. In an adequately responsive patient, a concentration of 0.0005 percent TEIB will produce selective erythema at the sites of arsenical keratoses without adverse effects on the adjacent normal skin. Higher concentrations of TEIB (up to 0.01 percent) will improve the results. At a concentration of 0.1 percent or more, however, the uninvolved skin becomes inflamed without appreciable increase in the therapeutic results.

The effects of topical immunotherapy with TEIB or DNCB in solar keratoses are essentially similar to those described for superficial basal cell carcinomas and squamous cell carcinomas. At an appropriate concentration of the sensitizing agent, the challenge reaction is usually limited to the lesions, and at higher concentrations, the intensity of the reaction is still more marked at sites of actinic keratoses than in the adjacent normal skin. The intensity of the reaction in developing keratoses is less marked than in clinically obvious lesions and may be limited to a punctate area of erythema lasting 24 to 72 hours. Complete resolution of more than 95 percent of the actinic lesions can be expected.

LEUKOPLAKIA

Leukoplakia of the external aspects of the lips and of the vulva responds adequately to local chemotherapy; intraoral leukoplakia unsuitable for topical chemotherapy is amenable to immunotherapy in some patients. The lowest concentration of TEIB at which a response to challenge is elicited on the skin is applied under an occlusive dressing (Oradhesive, Squibb) to the areas of leukoplakia. The reaction within 24 to 48 hours varies in intensity but is usually mild. The regional lymph glands may become swollen and tender. Partial to complete remission of leukoplakia may be induced, but recurrences in seven of 14 patients were observed within four to six weeks following discontinuation of immunotherapeutic challenge. Recurring lesions may be retreated by intermittent challenge at intervals of four to six weeks and have been controlled for periods of up to five years. Immunotherapy of leukoplakia should not be considered a routine therapeutic modality at present.

PREVENTIVE TOPICAL IMMUNOTHERAPY

Intermittent topical therapy with TEIB and DNCB is of value as preventive therapy in patients with extensive, frequent, de novo formation of multiple superficial basal cell carcinomas, squamous cell carcinomas in situ, or premalignant keratoses. Immune challenge reactions can be induced in skin areas of various extent (e.g., face to entire body surface) for many years at intervals ranging from two months to two years. Resolution of premalignant lesions reduces the expected incidence of new tumors in patients with xeroderma pigmentosum and multiple basal cell carcinoma syndromes.

INVESTIGATIVE ASPECTS OF TOPICAL IMMUNOTHERAPY

Studies were carried out to determine whether the effects of the hypersensitivity reaction on skin tumors were due to cell-mediated immunity or to humoral antibodies (Klein, 1968c and 1969). Peripheral white blood cells were collected by leukaphoresis from patients who had been sensitized to TEIB and DNCB. Concentrated WBC preparations (10^6 to 10^8 WBC per ml.) were injected into the subcutaneous tissue of 12 patients who were not sensitive to these agents. Within eight to 24 hours after administration of the cells, systemic transfer of hypersensitivity was demonstrated by challenge reactions to the respective sensitizing agents in eight of 12 subjects. This remarkable response to challenge by TEIB or DNCB following cell-mediated transfer of immunity produced selective resolution of cutaneous neoplasms. The sequence of inflammatory changes following challenge was similar to the reactions in patients prepared by topical sensitization.

As might be expected, the challenge reaction was more marked and more rapid in onset at sites where the white cells had been injected. It was evident, however, that the recipients' own cells acquired reactivity to the sensitizing drug following the administration of white cells from sensitized donors. The therapeutic effect was limited to superficial lesions.

In a related study, intravenous administration of the sensitizer (0.4 mg. TEIB) did not result in cutaneous or systemic hypersensitivity reactions in patients sensitized by topical application of the drug. Since it is known that agents which produce specific cell-mediated hypersensitivity reactions are also capable of producing humoral antibodies which may block the cell-mediated response, an attempt was made to utilize WBC-mediated transfer of immunity in order to avoid the initial formation of humoral antibodies. In patients with mycosis fungoides to whom immunity had been transferred, a temporary reduction in the degree of infiltration at areas involved by plaques and nodules was observed following intravenous administration of TEIB.

Plaques of mycosis fungoides were injected with immune lymphocytes, and topical challenging doses of the sensitizer were applied. Complete regression of some lesions for periods of six to eight months were confirmed by clinical and microscopic examinations. In the same patients, topical application of challenging doses to lesions that had not been injected with lymphocytes provided a variable response. Complete resolution of some lesions lasted for from three to nine months. These observations are in agreement with the work of Ratner et al. (1968) and Van Scott and Winters (1970), who reported regression of mycosis fungoides lesions following induction of hypersensitivity to nitrogen mustard or DNCB and subsequent challenge with these agents.

The effect of combinations of two sensitizing agents was studied in patients with multiple superficial epitheliomatosis (xeroderma pigmentosum, arsenical dermatitis, multiple basal cell carcinoma syndromes, and actinic keratoses). Simultaneous sensitization with TEIB and DNCB did produce additive therapeutic effects. The intensity of the reaction of neoplastic lesions to the combination of two or more sensitizers was markedly increased at concentrations at which the agents separately produced no apparent reaction (Klein, 1968c and 1969). The reaction of the adjacent normal skin, however, was not increased by the combination topical immune therapy.

COMBINATION OF TOPICAL CHEMOTHERAPY AND IMMUNOTHERAPY

The systemic administration of most cytotoxic agents produces some degree of immunosuppression. However, local administration of cytotoxic agents did not suppress the response to challenge with DNCB in experimental animals (Klein et al., unpublished data). Topical 5-FU actually enhanced the reaction following challenge with DNCB or TEIB in patients with xeroderma pigmentosum and multiple basal cell syndromes. These patients continued to develop new lesions when treated with topical chemotherapy or immunotherapy alone, and better control was effected with courses of concurrent local chemotherapy and immunotherapy. A selectivity of response for neoplastic lesions was retained; therefore, this method can be used in areas with atrophic scars and sites of skin grafting.

BIOLOGIC SIGNIFICANCE OF TOPICAL IMMUNOTHERAPY

These experimental and clinical studies indicate that immune reactions of the delayed hypersensitivity type will selectively eradicate superficial cutaneous premalignant and malignant lesions.

The reduced incidence of new lesions in patients who had persistently developed new skin tumors in the past suggests that immunotherapy provides a mechanism for surveillance and recognition of abnormal cells and clumps of cells which are too small to become apparent by their reaction to a hypersensitivity-inducing agent. If these lesions had remained viable, they would have developed into clinically significant neoplasms.

The resolution of premalignant keratoses in patients with arsenical dermatitis, xeroderma pigmentosum, or x-ray or solar-induced actinic keratoses also indicates the selective nature and the potentially prophylactic value of immunotherapy, since the involution of premalignant lesions prevents their transformation into squamous cell carcinomas.

The removal of neoplastic cells by immune challenge reactions appears to be related to either qualitative or quantitative differences between the antigenic composition of normal cells and the composition of their premalignant and malignant counterparts. These differences may be present in neoplastic cells before their premalignant or malignant state can be recognized by morphologic criteria. A less selective mechanism, namely, preferential binding of the sensitizing agents to abnormal but not necessarily malignant cells, may also produce the desirable attraction of lymphocytes to the sera.

The studies of the transfer of immunity by peripheral leukocytes suggest that the reaction is associated with cell-mediated immunity. The mechanisms by which lymphocytes recognize and selectively destroy altered epidermal cells are not understood. One possibility is that the sensitizing agent interacts with both normal and neoplastic epidermal cells and elicits an immune response on the part of the host cells. The more intense reaction at the sites involved by premalignant and malignant lesions may indicate that proportionately larger amounts of the sensitizing agent have access to, or into, the neoplastic cells.

Another possibility is the formation of different antigen complexes in normal and neoplastic cells under the influence of the same sensitizing agent. The sensitizing agent may act as a hapten by combining with or otherwise altering different components of normal and malignant cells. In their natural states these do not differ sufficiently from each other to provide a basis for immunologic incompatibility. Following interaction with an appropriate hapten, the antigenicity of the neoplastic cells may be sufficient to stimulate an effective immune response. Recruitment of lymphocytes and macrophages occurs, and larger numbers of mononuclear cells, which may be sensitized to tumor antigens, concentrate in the tumor site.

Cell-mediated immune reactions are usually more specifically directed toward the carrier protein than toward the haptene, while humoral antibodies are more responsive to the haptene. The observation that reactions following sensitization with potential haptene drugs are associated with cell-mediated immune mechanisms is consistent with a lymphocyte-cell interaction in which the haptene is firmly bound to the abnormal cell.

The effects of combining two or more sensitizing agents indicate at least an additive, if not a synergistic, effect on the immunologic reaction. This might be interpreted as representing a reaction to several haptenes that bind to the same protein complex. The enhancement of the selective destructive effects of topical cytostatic agents following induction of hypersensitivity also suggests a selective immune response on the tumors. Even if the increased effects of cytostatic agents are merely the result of altered absorption of the cytostatic agent due to increased permeability, they suggest that the delayed hypersensitivity reaction at the sites involved by neoplasia produces additive effects.

From a clinical standpoint the effects of topical challenge are largely limited to superficial lesions. In the vascular environment of the epidermis, the cellular immune reaction may predominate, since it depends on actively migrating cells rather than on passive diffusion of immunoglobulins. In lesions which have penetrated into the dermis, both the humoral antibodies and the cellular elements would have access to the sensitized cells. Noncytotoxic humoral antibodies could more readily combine with the sensitized cells and thus block or reduce the intensity of the lymphocyte-cell reaction. If the antigenic stimulation for a cell-mediated immune reaction is relatively weak, the humoral antibody effects may predominate. These considerations may explain the reduced effect of the intravenous administration of TEIB following the induction of topical hypersensitivity.

The therapeutic effects following induction of specific cell-mediated hypersensitivity by the chemical agents that have been studied differ in epidermal neoplasms and in neoplasms arising from other tissues. This suggests that these agents behave differently towards cells of different origin. This might have been expected in view of the high degree of specificity of cell-mediated immunity and specificity of hypersensitivity-inducing agents for particular target cells. At least some agents which induce cutaneous delayed hypersensitivity reactions have some selectivity for cutaneous neoplasms. Further studies are needed to find agents which may produce hypersensitivity in other neoplasms and which can be utilized for therapeutic purposes.

The utilization of delayed hypersensitivity evoked by a simple chemical in the management of neoplastic lesions provides a new approach to the management of disease. This approach exploits the therapeutic potential of delayed hypersensitivity reactions. Until recently these reactions have been considered primarily causes of disease or obstacles to therapy.

REFERENCES

Alexander, P., and Hamilton-Fairley, G.: Cellular resistance to tumors. Br. Med. Bull., 23:86, 1967.

Alexander, P., Delorme, E. J., and Hall, J. G.: The effect of lymphoid cells from the lymph of specifically immunized sheep on the growth of primary sarcomata in rats. Lancet, 1:1186, 1966.

Belisario, J. C.: An appraisal of therapeutic methods for skin carcinomas by scalpel or electrosurgery, ionizing radiation, electrochemosurgery and local chemotherapy. Acta Derm. Venereol. (Stockh.), Suppl. 56, 1964.

Belisario, J. C.: Carcinoma of the skin: Etiology and therapy with special emphasis on topical preparations. Dermatol. Digest, March, 1965.

Burdick, K. H., and Hawk, W. A.: Vitiligo in a case of vaccinia virus–treated melanoma. Cancer, 17:708, 1964.

Cooper, H. L.: Lymphocyte stimulation in malignant melanoma. New Engl. J. Med., 283:369, 1970.

Defendi, V., and Roosa, R. A.: Effect of thymectomy on induction of tumors and on the transplantability of polyoma-induced tumors. Cancer Res., 25:300, 1965.

Delorme, E. J., and Alexander, P.: Treatment of primary fibrosarcoma in the rat with immune lymphocytes. Lancet, 2:117, 1964.

Dillaha, C. J., Jansen, G. T., Honeycutt, W. M., and Bradford, A. C.: Selective cytotoxic effect of topical 5-fluorouracil. Arch. Dermatol., 88:247, 1963.

Dillaha, C. J., Jansen, G. T., Honeycutt, W. M., and Holt, G. A.: Further studies with topical 5-fluorouracil. Arch. Dermatol., 92:410, 1965.

Eddy, B. E., Grubbs, G. E., and Young, R. D.: Tumor immunity in hamsters infected with adenovirus type 12 or simian virus 40. Proc. Soc. Exp. Biol. Med., 117:575, 1964.

Eilber, F. R., and Morton, D. L.: Cutaneous anergy and prognosis following cancer surgery. Surg. Forum, 10:116, 1969.

Fass, L., Herberman, R. B., Ziegler, J., and Morrow, R. H., Jr.: Evaluation of the effect of remission plasma on untreated patients with Burkitt's lymphoma. J. Natl. Cancer Inst., 44:145, 1970a.

Fass, L., Herberman, R. B., Ziegler, J. L., and Kiryabwire, J. W. M.: Cutaneous hypersensitivity reactions to autologous extracts of malignant melanoma cells. Lancet, 1:116, 1970b.

Foley, E. J.: Attempts to induce immunity against mammary adenocarcinoma in inbred mice. Cancer Res., 13:578, 1953.

Gibson, T., and Medawar, P. B.: Fate of skin homografts in man. J. Anat., 77:299, 1943.

Girardi, A. J., Jensen, F. C., and Koprowski, H.: SV$_{40}$-induced transformation of human diploid cells: Crisis and recovery. J. Cell. Comp. Physiol., 65:69, 1965.

Gold, P.: Circulating antibodies against carcinoembryonic antigens of the human digestive system. Cancer, 20:1663, 1967.

Goldner, H. A., Girardi, A. J., Larson, V. M., and Hilleman, M. R.: Interruption of SV-40 virus tumorigenesis using irradiated homologous tumor antigen. Proc. Soc. Exp. Biol. Med., 117:851, 1964.

Golomb, F. M., Solowey, A. C., Postel, A., Gumport, S. L., and Wright, J. C.: Induced remission of malignant melanoma with actinomycin D. Immunologic implications. Cancer, 20:656, 1967.

Gorer, P. A.: Experimental studies on leukemia and allied conditions. Guy's Hosp. Gaz., 57:166, 1943.

Gorer, P. A., and O'Gorman, P.: Cytotoxic activity of isoantibodies in mice. Transplant. Bull., 3:142, 1956.

Habel, K.: Resistance of polyoma virus immune animals to transplanted polyoma tumors. Proc. Soc. Exp. Biol. Med., 106:722, 1961.

Hellström, I., Hellström, K. E., Pierce, G. E., and Bill, A. H.: Demonstration of cell-bound and humoral immunity against neuroblastoma cells. Proc. Natl. Acad. Sci. USA, 60:1231, 1968a.

Hellström, I., Hellström, K. E., Pierce, G. E., and Yang, J. P. S.: Cellular and humoral immunity to different types of human neoplasms. Nature (Lond.), 220:1352, 1968b.

Helm, F., and Klein, E.: Effects of allergic contact dermatitis on basal cell epitheliomas. Arch. Dermatol., 91:142, 1965.

Helm, F., Klein, E., Traenkle, H. L., and Rivera, E. P.: Studies on the local administration of 2,3,5-triethylene-iminio-1, 4-benzoquinone (Trenimon) to epitheliomas. J. Invest. Dermatol., 45:152, 1965.

Hirszfeld, L., Halber, W., and Laskowski, J.: Über die serologische spezifität der krebszellen. Klin. Wochenschr., 8:1563, 1929.

Holland, J. F.: Epidemic acute leukemia. New Engl. J. Med., 283:1165, 1970.

Hunter-Craig, I., Newton, K. A., Westbury, G., and Lacey, B. W.: Use of vaccinia virus in the treatment of metastatic malignant melanoma. Br. Med. J., 2:512, 1970.

Ikonopisov, R. L., Lewis, M. G., Hunter-Craig, I. D., Bodenham, D. C., Phillips, T. M., Cooling, C. I., Proctor, J., Hamilton Fairley, G., and Alexander, P.: Auto-immunization with irradiated tumour cells in human malignant melanoma. Br. Med. J., 2:752, 1970.

Jehn, U. W., Nathanson, L., Schwartz, R. S., and Skinner, M.: In vitro lymphocyte stimulation by a soluble antigen from malignant melanoma. New Engl. J. Med., 283:329, 1970.

Kaliss, N.: Immunological enhancement of tumor homografts in mice: A review. Cancer Res., 18:992, 1958.

Kaliss, N.: The elements of immunologic enhancement: A consideration of mechanisms. Ann. N.Y. Acad. Sci., 101:64, 1962.

Klein, E.: Local cytostatic chemotherapy and immunotherapy. Geriatrics, 23:154, 1968a.

Klein, E.: Tumors of the skin. IX. Local cytostatic therapy of cutaneous and mucosal premalignant and malignant lesions. N.Y. J. Med., 68:886, 1968b.

Klein, E.: Tumors of the skin. X. Immunotherapy of cutaneous and mucosal neoplasms. N.Y. J. Med., 68:900, 1968c.

Klein, E.: Hypersensitivity reactions at tumor sites. Cancer Res., 29:2351, 1969.

Klein, E., Milgrom, H., Helm, F., Ambrus, J., Traenkel, H. L., and Stoll, H. S.: Tumors of the skin: Effects of local use of cytostatic agents. Skin, 3:81, 1962.

Klein, E., Stoll, H. L., Jr., Milgrom, H., Case, R. W., Traenkle, H. L., Graham, S., Laor, Y., and Helm, F.: Tumors of the skin. IV. Double-blind study on effects of local administration of anti-tumor agents in basal cell carcinoma. J. Invest. Dermatol., 44:351, 1965.

Law, L. W.: Studies of experimental transmission of leukemogenic virus infection in mice. J. Natl. Cancer Inst., 34:543, 1965.

Lewis, M. G.: Possible immunological factors in human malignant melanoma in Uganda. Lancet, 2:921, 1967.

Lewis, M. G., Ikonopisov, R. L., Nairn, R. C., Phillips, T. M., Hamilton Fairley, G., Bodenham, D. C., and Alexander, P.: Tumour-specific antibodies in human malignant melanoma and their relationship to the extent of the disease. Br. Med. J., 3:547, 1969.

Madison, J. F., and Haserick, J. R.: Topically applied mechlorethamine on twelve dermatoses. Arch. Dermatol., 86:663, 1962.

Mathé, G.: Approaches to the immunological treatment of cancer in man. Br. Med. J., 4:7, 1969.

Miller, J. F.: Analysis of the thymus influence in leukaemogenesis. Nature (Lond.), 191:248, 1961.

Miller, J. F.: Effect of neonatal thymectomy on the immunological responsiveness of the mouse. Proc. R. Soc. Lond. (Biol.), 156:415, 1962.

Miller, J. F., Doak, S. M., and Cross, A. M.: Role of the thymus in recovery of the immune mechanism in the irradiated adult mouse. Proc. Soc. Exp. Biol. Med., 112:785, 1963.

Milton, G. W., and Brown, M. M. L.: The limited role of attenuated smallpox virus in the management of advanced malignant melanoma. Aust. N. Z. J. Surg., 35:286, 1966.

Mitchison, N. A., and Dube, O. L.: Studies on immunological response to foreign tumor transplants in mouse; relation between hemagglutinating antibody and graft resistance in normal mouse and mice pretreated with tissue preparations. J. Exp. Med., 102:179, 1955.

Möller, G.: Biologic properties of 19S and 7S mouse isoantibodies directed against isoantigens of the H-2 system. J. Immunol., 96:430, 1966.

Moore, G. E., and Gerner, R. E.: Cancer immunity-hypothesis and clinical trial of lymphocytotherapy for malignant diseases. Ann. Surg., 172:733, 1970.

Moore, G. E., and Gerner, R. E.: Malignant melanoma. Surg. Gynecol. Obstet., 132:427, 1971.

Morton, D. L.: Acquired immunological tolerance and carcinogenesis by the mammary tumor virus. I. Influence of neonatal infection with the mammary tumor virus on the growth of spontaneous mammary adenocarcinomas. J. Natl. Cancer Inst., 42:311, 1969.

Morton, D. L.: Cancer immunology and the surgeon. Surgery, 67:396, 1970.

Morton, D. L., Malmgren, R. A., Holmes, E. C., and Ketcham, A. S.: Demonstration of antibodies against human malignant melanoma by immunofluorescence. Surgery, 64:233, 1968.

Morton, D. L., Eilber, F. R., Malmgren, R. A., and Wood, W. C.: Immunological factors which influence response to immunotherapy in malignant melanoma. Surgery, 68:158, 1970.

Muna, N. M., Marcus, S., and Smart, C.: Detection of immunofluorescence of antibodies specific for human malignant melanoma cells. Cancer, 23:88, 1969.

Nadler, S. H., and Moore, G. E.: Clinical immunologic study of malignant disease: Response to tumor transplants and transfer of leukocytes. Ann. Surg., 164:482, 1966.

Nadler, S. H., and Moore, G. E.: Immunotherapy of malignant melanoma. Geriatrics, 23:150, 1968.

Nadler, S. H., and Moore, G. E.: Immunotherapy of malignant disease. Arch. Surg., 99:376, 1969.

Nurse, D. S.: Effect of antimetabolites on epidermal structures. Arch. Dermatol., 87:258, 1963.

Oleinick, A.: Altered immunity and cancer risk: A review of the problem and analysis of the cancer mortality experience of leprosy patients. J. Natl. Cancer Inst., 443:775, 1969.

Omura, E. F., and Torre, D.: Inflammation of actinic keratoses due to systemic fluorouracil therapy. J.A.M.A., 208:150, 1969.

Pack, G. T.: Note on experimental use of rabies vaccine for melanomatosis. Arch. Dermatol. Syph., 62:694, 1950.

Park, S. K., Brody, J. I., Wallace, H. A., and Blakemore, W. S.: Immunosuppressive effect of surgery. Lancet, 1:53, 1971.

Peschke, M.: Mykosis fungoides. Dermatol. Wochenschr., 145:19, 1962.

Pfehn, R. T., and Main, J. M.: Immunity to methylcholanthrene-induced sarcomas. J. Natl. Cancer Inst., 18:769, 1957.

Piessens, W. F.: Evidence for human cancer immunity: A review. Cancer, 26:1212, 1970.

Ratner, A. C., Waldorf, D. S., and Van Scott, E. J.: Alterations of lesions of mycosis fungoides lymphoma by direct imposition of delayed hypersensitivity reactions. Cancer, 21:83, 1968.

Romsdahl, M. M., and Cox, I. S.: Human malignant melanoma antibodies demonstrated by immunofluorescence. Arch. Surg., 100:491, 1970.

Sjogren, H. O., Hellström, I., and Klein, G.: Transplantation of polyoma virus–induced tumors in mice. Cancer Res., 21:329, 1961.

Snyderman, R. K., and Starzynski, T. E.: The clinical application of 5-flourouracil in the treatment of skin lesions. Plast. Reconstr. Surg., 41:549, 1968.

Spiessl, B.: Moeglichkeiten und bisherige ergebnisse bei der anwendung des trenimon bei malignen tumoren in kiefer-und gesichtsbereich. Symposien Aktueller Therapeutischer Probleme. Stuttgart, Enke, 1960.

Summer, W. C., and Foraker, A. C.: Spontaneous regression of human melanoma, clinical and experimental studies. Cancer, 12:79, 1960.

Takasugi, M., and Hildemann, W. H.: Regulation of immunity toward allogeneic tumors in mice. J. Natl. Cancer Inst., 43:843, 1969.

Teimourion, B., and McCune, W. S.: Surgical management of malignant melanoma. Am. Surg., 29:515, 1963.

Van Scott, E. J., and Winters, P. L.: Responses of mycosis fungoides to intensive external treatment with nitrogen mustard. Arch Dermatol., 102:507, 1970.

Index

Page numbers in italics indicate illustrations